Performing the Small Animal Physical Examination

To my mother Jill, father Richard, and brother Brent –
for teaching me how to dream

To Mountainside Veterinary Hospital –
for seeing value in my dream

To my veterinary mentor, Dr. Abraham Bezuidenhout –
for helping my dream take flight

To my veterinary colleagues, Drs. Brian Collins, Zenny Ng, and Troy Holder –
for dreaming beside me

To my veterinary patients –
for inspiring my dream into reality

To my beautiful "fur babies" Bailey and Nina –
for being dreams come true

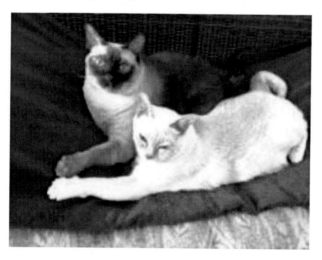

And to Lowell E. Fox and Marshall Strife of Arrowhead Arthur Murray –
for teaching me new ways to dream, on and off the dance floor.

Performing the Small Animal Physical Examination

Ryane E. Englar, DVM, DABVP (Canine and Feline Practice)
Assistant Professor, Small Animal Primary Care,
Midwestern University College of Veterinary Medicine,
Glendale, AZ, USA

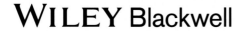

Registered Office
John Wiley & Sons, Inc., 111 River Street, Hoboken, NJ 07030, USA

Editorial Office
John Wiley & Sons, Inc., 111 River Street, Hoboken, NJ 07030, USA

For details of our global editorial offices, customer services, and more information about Wiley products visit us at www.wiley.com.

Wiley also publishes its books in a variety of electronic formats and by print-on-demand. Some content that appears in standard print versions of this book may not be available in other formats.

Library of Congress Cataloging-in-Publication Data

Names: Englar, Ryane E., author.
Title: Performing the small animal physical examination / Ryane E. Englar.
Description: Hoboken, NJ : Wiley, 2017. | Includes bibliographical references and index. |
Identifiers: LCCN 2017025865 (print) | LCCN 2017027039 (ebook) | ISBN 9781119295327 (pdf) | ISBN 9781119295310 (epub) | ISBN 9781119295303 (cloth)
Subjects: | MESH: Physical Examination—veterinary | Veterinary Medicine—methods | Cats | Dogs
Classification: LCC SF772.5 (ebook) | LCC SF772.5 .E54 2017 (print) | NLM SF 772.5 | DDC 636.089/6075—dc23
LC record available at https://lccn.loc.gov/2017025865

Cover image: Courtesy of Ryane E. Englar
Cover design by Wiley

Set in 10/12pt Warnock Pro by Aptara Inc., New Delhi, India

10 9 8 7 6 5 4 3 2 1

Contents

About the Author

Ryane E. Englar, DVM, DABVP (Canine and Feline Practice), is a 2008 graduate of Cornell University College of Veterinary Medicine. Following graduation, she spent 5 years as an associate veterinarian in small animal practice, split between her home state of Maryland and upstate New York. She then became a Clinical Instructor of Community Practice Service at Cornell's Companion Animal Hospital and a Consultant for the Louis J. Camuti Hotline in association with Cornell's Feline Health Center. She joined the Midwestern University College of Veterinary Medicine in February 2014 as an Assistant Professor of Small Animal Primary Care, and was on faculty when Midwestern opened its doors to its inaugural class, the Class of 2018. Her special interests are feline medicine, clinical communication, relationship-centered care, and the human–animal bond.

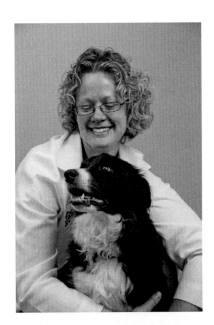
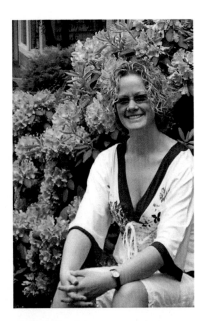
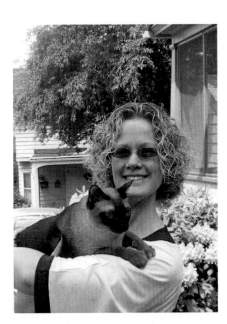

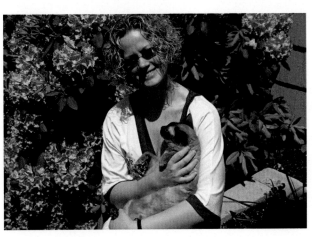
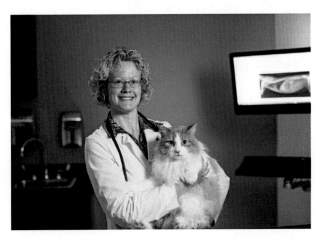

Preface

Veterinary medicine is an ever-growing field of knowledge. Much like its human counterpart, the profession of veterinary medicine has expanded into a great many specialty areas of interest that have collectively magnified the standard of care that today's veterinary patient is able both to expect and to receive. Veterinary clients are often astounded when I recommend referral of their companion animal to any number of board-certified specialists. It may come as a surprise to our clients that we are so well represented as a profession to be able to offer such specialties as anesthesiology, cardiology, critical care, dentistry, dermatology, internal medicine, soft tissue and orthopedic surgery, neurology, nutrition, and oncology, to name just a few. To the veterinary student, these areas of expertise are often captivating and represent opportunities that did not exist within the profession 50 years ago: open doors through which we can practice a standard of medicine that is increasingly progressive and state of the art.

With all the bells and whistles available to the veterinary student in the modern teaching hospital, it is easy to forget that at the heart of every successful veterinary encounter is a basic, comprehensive physical examination. No matter how many diagnostic tests and procedures are developed to provide answers to our patients and clients alike, there is still no substitute for a thorough examination. The physical examination links the generalist to the specialist because all veterinary practitioners must master this set of skills that collectively paints a picture of our patient and its needs.

As a veterinary student, I found this content area to be immensely lacking.

This is my attempt, as faculty, to correct that deficit by providing a comprehensive resource that takes any member of the veterinary team through the canine and feline physical examination.

Acknowledgements

I am a firm believer that the only way any of us succeed in the profession of veterinary medicine is by having the support of colleagues to give us a leg up on the gargantuan climb up the ladder of lifelong learning. Some colleagues are there to weather the storms of vet school; others offer us refuge that first day, week, month, or year out in the trenches. We all have that one colleague we called to celebrate the "firsts" – our first patient, our first surgery, our first case that beat the odds. But how many of us are blessed enough to have that one colleague to call when work just isn't going right?

Rachel Beard, DVM, was my "on call" colleague for all the rough spells that first year out in practice. We had shifts that overlapped at a 24-7 practice: I practiced as a generalist by day; she practiced as a criticalist at night. No matter how many emergencies Rachel had lined up to see her, she was never too busy for me: to review a case, to critique a radiograph, but most importantly, to serve as that warm, friendly, peaceful face we all need to see at the end of the day to know we're on the right path. It also didn't hurt that she brought Kali, her German Shepherd, to work with her every night. When I close my eyes, I still remember that dynamic duo coming down the corridor to greet me. It's been years since then, but you never forget those who climb the mountain beside you.

Rachel, this book is for you. Thank you for teaching by example the importance of paying it forward.

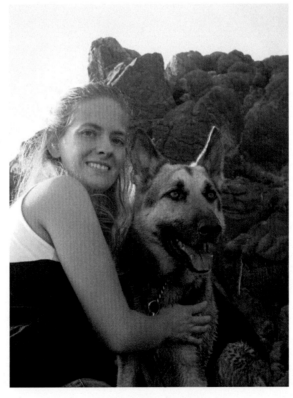

Rachel Beard, DVM
January 17, 1980 – August 24, 2011

Part One

Performing the Feline Physical Examination

1

Setting the Stage: Feline-Friendly Practice

1.1 Challenges Faced in Feline Practice

Every 5 years, the American Veterinary Medical Association conducts a national survey to track trends in pet ownership. In 2012, the number of owned cats exceeded the number of owned dogs in the United States by over four million [1]. Yet despite their growing popularity and the increased perception that cats are members of the family, cats remain underserved when it comes to veterinary care [1–4].

By their own admission, cat-owners are less likely than dog-owners to pursue annual wellness examinations. According to the Bayer Veterinary Care Usage Study, a four-phase analysis of companion animal practice, only 37% of cat-owners over a 12-month period visited a veterinary clinic for routine examination [2]. Indoor-only [2, 5] and aged populations [6] were at increased risk of escaping veterinary medical attention. The former were perceived as being less likely to succumb to illness [2], and the overall value of the veterinary wellness visit was lost on cat-owners, 83% of whom believed their cat to be in "excellent health" [2]. Were it not for vaccinations, many cat-owners would not pursue routine veterinary care at all [6].

The Bayer Veterinary Care Usage Study concluded that cat-owners' reluctance to seek veterinary medical care is multifactorial [2]. One major driving force is lack of owner education [2, 6]. Many cats are unplanned acquisitions: "I didn't necessarily find the cat, the cat found me" [2]. As a result, cat-owners may receive limited, if any, initial guidance as to when to pursue veterinary care [2]. By contrast, dog-owners tend to plan the introduction of a new pet into the household and are more likely to seek out instructions on proper care from breeders and shelters.

Many cat-owners are unaware that routine wellness care is essential [7]. Further compounding the issue is that cats effectively mask subtle signs of illness. Cat-owners often find it difficult to determine when their cat is sick [3, 8]. When cat-owners do recognize illness, over one-third of them look to the Internet for veterinary medical advice rather than pursue veterinary medical attention [5, 6].

Of those cat-owners who do perceive value in preventive medicine, the toll that veterinary visits take on the cat and cat-owner alike represents a significant barrier to follow-up care [2]. Cat-owners view the veterinary visit as an ordeal, the stress of which begins well before the client and cat ever set foot in the clinic [2, 6].

Owners must first capture the cat, which is easier said than done. The cat may hightail it at the sight of a cat carrier or aggressively resist being confined to it. As a result, cat-owners look forward to this aspect of the veterinary visit the least [6], yet of those surveyed, only 18% had been instructed by the veterinary team on how to decrease transportation-associated stress [2].

Once confined to the cat carrier, the cat may vocalize for the duration of the journey to and from the clinic. Upon arrival to the clinic, cats become visibly stressed in the waiting room, especially when their space is encroached upon by other patients. When they finally reach the examination room, their tolerance may be sufficiently limited [6].

To summarize their veterinary experience, the Bayer Veterinary Care Usage Study asked 1938 cat-owners to create a collage representing their veterinary experience. The majority of cat-owners used pictures from horror films [2]. Fifty-eight percent of cat-owners described their cats as hating veterinary visits [9].

This perception of the veterinary experience adversely impacts the profession's ability to attract and retain cat-owners and to provide consistent, high-quality medical care. The veterinary visit is undoubtedly a source of feline stress, the net result of which may be provoked aggression. When cats are fractious, the veterinary team is unable to examine them thoroughly. Feline stress may artificially create abnormal physical examination findings such as tachycardia and tachypnea. The intensity of the stress response may also induce abnormalities in routine screening and other diagnostic tests. Stress hyperglycemia is common, and can be challenging to differentiate from diabetes mellitus without additional testing. If stress is not recognized as the culprit for these abnormalities, the veterinary team may use the test results to support a diagnosis that is inaccurate. This places the patient at increased risk of being

Performing the Small Animal Physical Examination, First Edition. Ryane E. Englar.
© 2017 John Wiley & Sons, Inc. Published 2017 by John Wiley & Sons, Inc.

subjected to irrelevant or inappropriate treatment plans [10, 11].

Of equal concern is that cats' behavior in the home appears to be altered for some period of time after the veterinary visit. Cats may become standoffish after visiting the clinic, and this may last for several days [6]. In addition, the residual effect of the veterinary visit may transiently impact inter-cat dynamics in multi-cat households. The hospital-goer is not always welcomed back into the fold with open arms, and inter-cat aggression may ensue.

As a result of the many challenges that cat-owners face when committing to a veterinary visit, most prefer to avoid the clinic altogether [6]. This, combined with feline resistance, represents two significant obstacles to cats receiving veterinary care.

1.2 The Emergence of Feline-Friendly Practice

As a result of feline and owner resistance, cats are a largely untapped resource for the veterinary profession: between 2001 and 2011, annual feline visits decreased by 14% [2]. Hence cats represent a rich opportunity area to increase veterinary revenue. Practice management tools may help to capture this underrepresented population through the use of social media and by relying upon business metrics more effectively to identify patients with lapsed appointments [9]. However, without addressing cat-specific issues surrounding the veterinary visit, marketing campaigns focused strictly on data may not be as effective.

The concept of feline-friendly practice emerged from the realization that the burden is on the veterinary profession to adapt to cats, not the other way around. Cats are not small dogs. Cats have different behavioral, physiological, medical, and psychological needs. Furthermore, owners hold different expectations when it comes to their care [6]. The American Association of Feline Practitioners developed the Cat Friendly Practice program to cater to this distinct population of companion animals [12]. Although practitioners are not required to participate, those who do are provided with the tools necessary to adopt a feline-centered practice philosophy [12]. It is hoped that participating institutions will elevate their approach to feline care in order to attract, medically manage, and retain cat-owning clientele.

1.3 Key Principles of Feline-Friendly Practice

Feline-friendly practice philosophy centers on an understanding of normal cat behavior and communication. Cats are often misunderstood, especially when it comes to our perception of how cats respond to conflict [13, 14]. Cats are by nature solitary: prior to domestication, they lived and hunted alone [13, 14]. Hence they avoid altercations with other cats rather than engage in conflict whenever possible [13–15]. This explains why the provision of escape routes and hideaways is so important when dealing with inter-cat aggression in the home [16]. Cats need to feel that they can get away. They need both to be able to hide a visual source that is distressing to them and to be themselves hidden from view (Figure 1.1). Cat trees with hideaways that have a separate entrance and exit are preferred so that cats do not become trapped by an aggressor.

Cat trees and shelves are also used to create a buffer between cats in shared living quarters. This vertical space serves a dual function: an elevated escape route or a way to increase distance between cats [16]. Cats are able to seat themselves where they feel comfortable based upon their preexisting social hierarchy (Figure 1.2).

One can take these same principles and adapt them to feline-friendly practice by creating a clinic setting in which cats are minimally exposed to other cats and other species [17]. The ideal feline-friendly practice has a designated cat-only waiting room (Figure 1.3).

Preferably, shelving is provided to keep carriers off of the ground to build a sense of security through the simulation of vertical space [18].

When at all possible, the practice should structure its appointment schedule to minimize wait times. When unforeseen circumstances extend the wait, feline patients should be directed into cat-only examination rooms as soon as possible.

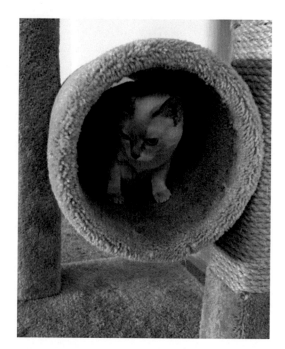

Figure 1.1 Cat tree demonstrating a hideaway with a separate entrance and exit.

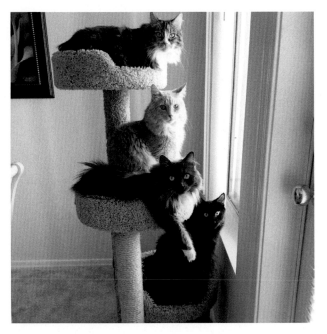

Figure 1.2 Cat tree demonstrating how vertical space allows cats to share living space. Source: Courtesy of Bianca J. Hartrum.

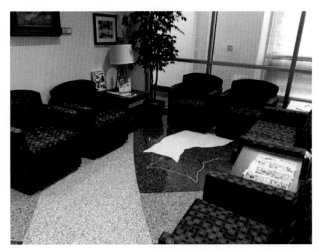

Figure 1.3 Separate waiting area designated for cats.

If the examination rooms have windows facing the interior of the corridor, blinds may be installed to reduce visual stimuli (Figure 1.4).

The exterior to cat-designated examination rooms may be fitted out with a sliding card to denote when the rooms are occupied. This prevents unknowing staff from entering an occupied room with closed blinds and inadvertently allowing a cat to escape into the hospital corridor (Figure 1.5).

When feline patients are required to be admitted into the hospital, a cat-designated ward should be available to decrease inter-species exposure [18]. Cages may be stacked, taking a "kitty condo" approach. However, cages should not face each other (Figure 1.6). When they do, cats see other cats, and this may be a significant source of stress.

Once confined to a cage, the cat may be offered a hideaway, provided that the cat is stable enough not to require constant supervision that would be hindered by blocking the support staff's full view of the patient (Figure 1.7) [18]. As an alternative to physical hideaways placed within the cage itself, a towel hung over the cage door serves the same purpose (Figure 1.8). The towel will also minimize light reflection that is caused by cages

Figure 1.4 Blinds installed in cat-designated examination rooms may be either (a) open to allow bold cats to appreciate their surroundings or (b) closed to reduce visual stimuli in fearful or timid patients.

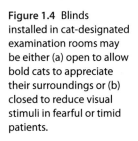

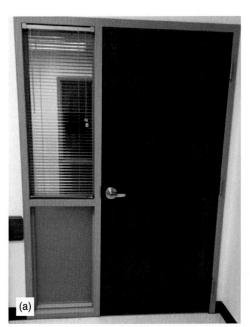

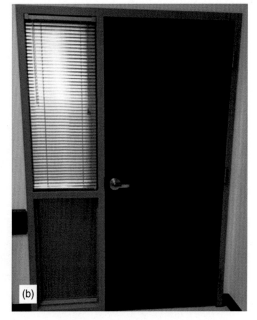

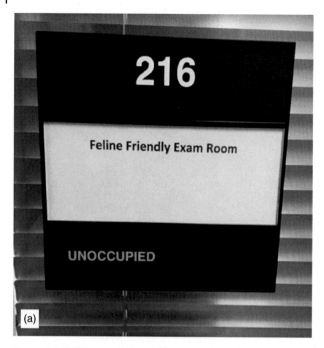
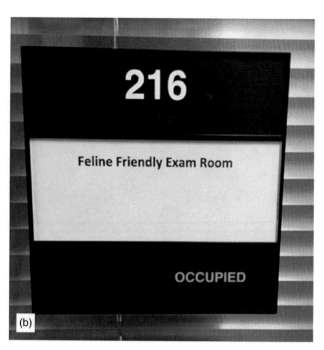

Figure 1.5 (a) Unoccupied and (b) occupied cat-designated examination room.

constructed of stainless steel [17]. Laminate materials are preferred because they do not cause light to bounce off of the sides of the cage and create glare.

The lighting of hospital wards should also be considered when planning for patient comfort. Light should be sufficient for patient monitoring but not so austere as to compound the reflection of light within stainless-steel cages.

The quality and type of light may be important in veterinary medicine; lighting has been studied in both the human classroom and critical care settings. The use of cool-white fluorescent lighting has been linked to irritability, fatigue, and difficulty focusing in people.

By contrast, full-spectrum lighting, as from natural daylight, reduces the body's response to cortisol. A patient exposed to full-spectrum lighting adapts better to stress [19].

When intensive and critical care units in human medicine do not have full-spectrum lighting and are instead fitted out with fluorescent overhead lighting, with continuous light exposure, the body's circadian rhythm is disrupted. This may contribute to prolonged hospital stays [19, 20]. One solution to this problem is to reduce lighting in intensive and critical care units. Clinicians were initially concerned that this would compromise

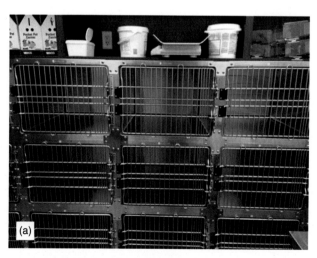
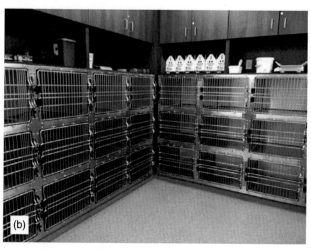

Figure 1.6 Stacked cages (a) alongside one wall of the feline ward and (b) on neighboring walls that make up a corner, allowing cats to see one another.

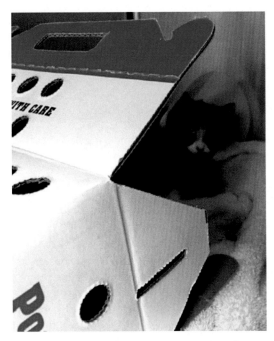

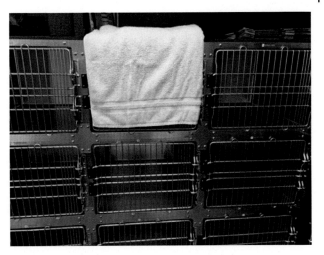

Figure 1.8 A towel hung over the cage door provides an alternative means of reducing visual stimuli.

Figure 1.7 Disposable pet carrier used as a hideaway for a patient convalescing from an ovariohysterectomy. The patient is able to decrease visual stimuli and may feel more secure by being out of view.

patient care. However, studies have demonstrated that reducing the intensity of light decreases anxiety in people [19].

The color of light may also influence patient outcomes owing to color's ability to alter emotional states [20]. The Society of Critical Care Medicine promotes the use of blues, greens, and violets in intensive and critical care unit lighting to inspire a sense of calm [19, 21].

Although more research is needed to evaluate the relevance to veterinary medicine, studies have confirmed

that intense or continuous light is a source of anxiety for animals [22–24]. The tapetum lucidum in companion animals intensifies their perception of light and they may be averse to lighting that is comfortable to humans [25, 26]. As a result, many feline-friendly practices have adopted from human medicine the practice of dimming lights, with or without colored lighting, for patient comfort (Figure 1.9).

Another visual stimulus that may be aversive to cats is the white coat. "White coat syndrome" is not unique to companion animals: it is well documented in human medicine that stress in the clinic setting activates the sympathetic nervous system in some but not all patients, and this results in hypertension. Although transient, it still may damage target organs [27–30]. White coat syndrome has been reported in dogs in addition to cats [31, 32]. More concerning is that in cats with preexisting

Figure 1.9 Feline and canine intensive care unit with (a) overhead fluorescent lighting and (b) dimmed and green overhead fluorescent lighting.

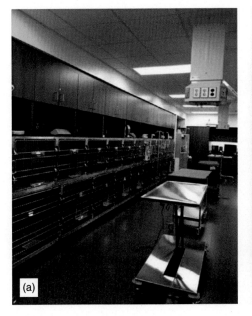

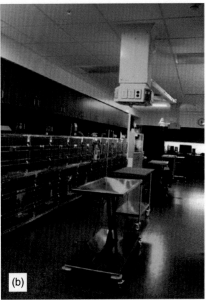

(a)

(b)

target organ disease, such as renal insufficiency, the magnitude of white coat-induced hypertension is greater and prolonged [32]. Feline-friendly practice may better serve its patients by altering the definition of what is considered to be professional attire and leaving the white coat out of the examination room [33, 34].

1.4 The Role of Sound

Noise stress has been documented in laboratory rodents: when ambient noise approaches 85 decibels, rodents exhibit behavioral and physiological signs of stress [35]. Although the same research is lacking in companion animal medicine, it is logical to consider using softer voices and a relaxed tone to convey a sense of calm. Maintaining ambient noise below 60 decibels is preferred [33].

Similarly, consideration should be applied to the type of sounds that are directed at cats. Although shushing is done with good intentions, to quiet a patient, the sound of shushing is remarkably similar to hissing [17]. Shushing at a cat may therefore be viewed as a threat no different than a direct stare.

Background music also impacts patient stress, although it has been studied more extensively in dogs than cats. In both shelter and kennel environments, hard rock and heavy metal music induces stress whereas classical music induces calm, provided that the noise level is appropriate as outlined above [36, 37].

A current concern in human medicine should be addressed as it relates to veterinary medicine, namely the use of music in operating rooms. High-capacity airflow systems and positive-pressure ventilation cause operating rooms to be noisy even when not in use [38]. Music has an additive effect and may contribute as much as 87 decibels [39]. There is potential risk that anesthetized patients may become hearing impaired if they are exposed to sound of that magnitude. The cochlea is typically protected by the stapedius muscle, which contracts in response to loud sounds. However, anesthetic drugs damp this protective reflex [38]. Hearing acuity may be diminished, and the fight or flight response may be activated if exposure to high-intensity sounds is prolonged. Therefore, veterinary professionals need to manage sound volume whether or not the patient is conscious to minimize the stress response and hearing loss.

1.5 The Role of Tactile Stimulation

Metal surfaces on examination room tables may be cold and slippery. Consider the use of non-slip mats or soft foam covering that can be easily laundered so that patients feel secure in their footing (Figure 1.10) [33].

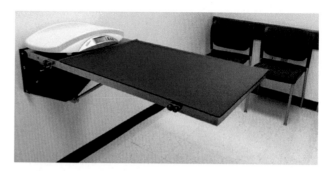

Figure 1.10 Non-slip mat on table in feline-dedicated examination room.

Tactile stimulation also refers to our use of touch to handle and comfort feline patients. Cats typically only exhibit allorubbing and allogrooming toward those within their social group. When cats exhibit these behaviors toward members of the same species, they typically limit themselves to the head and neck. Likewise, cats prefer the same locations when they accept physical touch from humans [13, 40]. Cats may react adversely to being stroked down the back or abdomen [41]. Cats may respond with skin crawling, which is attributed to increased arousal, or they may extend their claws in self-defense [41, 42].

1.6 The Role of Scent

Scent in cats can be conveyed through a number of mechanisms. Cats have sebaceous glands around their lips and chin. Through head-bunting, cats are able to deposit their scent on both inanimate objects and other animals. When cats scratch, they deposit scent via the sebaceous glands between their digits. Cats also scent-mark through feces and urine. Urine marking is a common and natural form of communication between cats. However, it can be exaggerated in situations involving inter-cat conflict [40, 43].

Compared with humans, who have 2–4 cm^2 of olfactory epithelium, cats are estimated to have 20 cm^2. Cats rely heavily on olfaction to communicate. Unlike visual cues, which are fleeting, olfactory messages persist in the environment. Veterinary professionals often forget that these olfactory cues can overwhelm feline patients because the scents are much less intense to the human nose [17, 40, 44]. Scents that humans do not detect may easily assault feline patients. Cats that are placed in an unclean examination room may be distracted by odors that the veterinary team is not aware of. These odors may communicate uncertainty that then in turn heightens the cat's anticipatory stress regarding the veterinary visit.

Examination rooms should be cleaned thoroughly before use. However, care should be taken to avoid cleaning agents and disinfectants that contain citrus, aloe, pine, or eucalyptus [13]. Many cats find these scents to be unpleasant. Remember that these scents may also be present in room air fresheners.

Avoid the use of rubbing alcohol when possible because this scent is equally aversive [33]. Past negative experiences with this scent are etched into the patient's memory [45–47]. Olfaction is processed by the brain in such a way that it has widespread effects and may also influence emotion [47]. As a result, patients have the potential for powerful negative association with this scent [33].

Avoid exposing feline patients to canine scent. Having feline-dedicated examination rooms will help (Figure 1.11). However, care must be taken to wipe down any and all exposed surfaces between patients: not just the floor, but also walls and cabinets [33].

In addition to thorough cleaning protocols and the airing out of rooms between patients, feline-friendly practices often make use of synthetic feline facial pheromone. Cats produce five functional pheromones in their facial secretions: F1–F5 [48]. Cats preferentially deposit the F3 fraction on familiar objects, so it is thought that the F3 fraction induces a sense of security. The F3 fraction also promotes the cat exploring its environment, and reduces urine marking [48].

The F3 fraction has been commercially produced for use in veterinary medicine (Feliway; Ceva Santé Animale) to curb undesired behaviors. It was initially marketed as an intervention for inappropriate urination because cats rarely urine mark sites that have already been marked with facial pheromone [49]. Indeed, its use does appear to reduce urine marking successfully [50–53]. Its proposed use has since expanded to include generalized stress reduction at the veterinary clinic, reduced anxiety during technical procedures, increased grooming

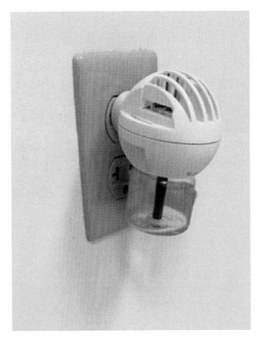

Figure 1.12 Synthetic feline facial pheromone diffuser.

behavior, enhanced appetite, and medical management of cystitis [13, 50, 54–56].

This product is sold over-the-counter as a plug-in diffuser that is marketed as covering an area of approximately 700 square feet: just the right size for an examination room (Figure 1.12). Diffusers should be continuously plugged in, and must be refilled once per month. The product is also sold as a spray that can be spritzed onto hands, clothing, and towels that are stocked in the examination room to "mark" veterinary professionals as "familiar" to the cat and less threatening. Studies have demonstrated that the spray is successful at reducing stress levels in cats when used on the examination room table within a consultation room [48]. The spray may also be used by owners on and inside cat carriers to facilitate transport to and from the veterinary clinic.

1.7 The Role of Advance Preparation

The first veterinary visit sets the tone for both the current and subsequent visits. Plan ahead for what you may encounter and anticipate your patient's needs. Easily laundered toys and highly palatable treats are effective distractors to have on hand when preparing for the arrival of kittens, and soft surfaces are important to consider when examining seniors that may have underlying osteoarthritis [13].

Stock the examination room in advance of the appointment, and have equipment and other essentials ready

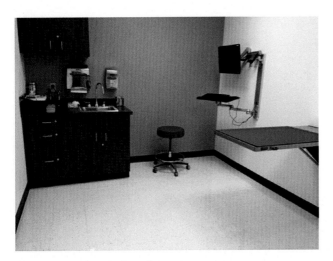

Figure 1.11 Feline-dedicated examination room.

and available for use to minimize unnecessary noise and a flurry of activity. Cats do not appreciate sudden movements, and can pick up on anxiety within the veterinary team. A slow, calm, and methodical approach sets the tone for a visit that is both respectful to the patient and efficient [13].

It is often said that to succeed in feline medicine, you must "go slow to go fast" [13]. What this refers to is the importance of adapting to the patient's pace. Cats should not be rushed through an examination. They need time to acclimate to feel that they are in control and secure in their current state [40]. This reduces stress, lessens aggressive tendencies, and decreases the likelihood of stress-induced hyperglycemia, which may complicate diagnostic test results [57].

In the author's experience, cats are subject to "kitty minutes": they have only so much tolerance. Forcing a feline patient through aspects of a physical examination is counterproductive. One quickly runs out of "kitty minutes." When this occurs, the patient becomes a safety hazard to the veterinary team. More concerning is the negative and long-lasting effect that the experience will have on the patient and its memory. The patient now has a very sour view of the veterinary experience, and this perception will color subsequent encounters [16]. The patient is likely to anticipate similar adverse outcomes even if the subsequent experience is intended by the veterinary team to be very different [16].

It is said that patience is a virtue, and this is especially true in feline medicine. It is critical that the veterinary team takes its time, even if this means that the appointment has to be staged in order to complete all aspects of the comprehensive examination [58].

1.8 Examination Room Etiquette: Accessing the Cat

Historically, the veterinary profession has prioritized efficiency. Past handling of companion animals did not always take the welfare of the patient into consideration [59]. Unfortunately, what was safe and efficient for veterinary professionals was not always psychologically safe and desirable to veterinary patients. Cats in particular were handled with "brudacaine" before it was understood that by removing a cat's perception of having control over the situation, feline anxiety and aggression were intensified. So-called "problem cats" were bound to become worse problems during subsequent visits owing to the vicious cycle of fear and the power of memory.

In the past, feline patients that were reluctant to leave the safety of their transport carrier were "dumped" onto the examination room table. Cardboard carriers that could not be easily disassembled facilitated this process because, short of tipping them upside down, there was little chance of extracting a resistant patient (Figure 1.13).

Tipping carriers or shaking them in any way to force the cat out into full range of view is no longer advised [17]. Doing so eliminates the cat's choice to come out on its own. Lack of control creates stress for the patient, which is now more likely to become defensively aggressive [40]. Instead of "dumping" cats from carriers onto examination room tables, the cat should be given the option to come out on its own once the client has settled into an examination room. This provides the cat with control over the situation: it decides whether or not to extract itself from the carrier and to explore the new environment. Most importantly, the cat has time to decide: the

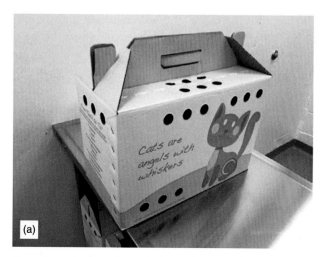
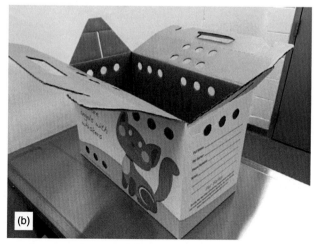

Figure 1.13 Cardboard carrier (a) sealed at the top for transport purposes and (b) opened at the top in the examination room to allow for visualization of the patient. Note that there is no easy way to extract the patient other than reaching down into the carrier, which could be perceived as threatening, or tipping the carrier to "dump" the cat out onto the examination room table.

carrier can be opened while the veterinary team converses with the client and takes a comprehensive history. Providing treats near the carrier's exit may coax an otherwise shy or unsure patient out into the open [13, 17, 40, 60]. While the cat is deciding its approach, the veterinary team may discretely observe the patient during history taking, noting the patient's body posture and respiration to add to the overall picture of its emotional state.

Initially, the cat may be tucked into the back of the carrier (Figure 1.14a). As the cat acclimates to the environment, its interest may be piqued in terms of what is going on outside the carrier and it may be tempted to investigate (Figure 1.14b). The cat may or may not leave the safety of the carrier at this point, but it is at least nearer to the exit. If given sufficient time, the cat may take the next step and peek out of the carrier with its head, still taking care to keep the rest of its body hidden. If the cat feels secure enough, it may begin the process of exiting the carrier entirely of its own accord (Figure 1.14c).

If the patient is reluctant to exit the carrier, it helps to have a plastic carrier that can be easily disassembled. The top half of the carrier can be removed quietly and without jostling the patient so that the patient is not required to leave the safety of the carrier to be examined (Figure 1.15). Observation of the patient's body posture will be instrumental in knowing how best to approach safely and proceed with the examination.

If the patient is exceptionally fearful or agitated, the mindful practitioner may slide a towel between the two halves of the carrier as the top half is removed. In so

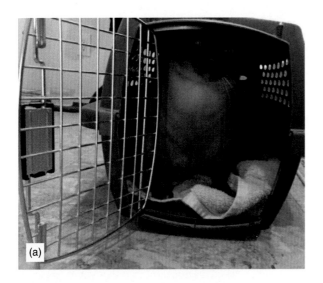

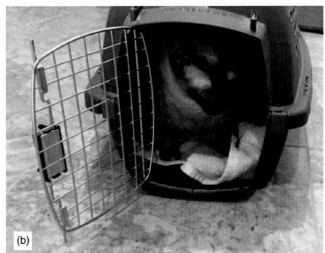

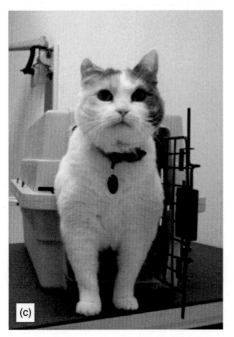

Figure 1.14 (a) This feline patient is reluctant to leave its carrier. (b) The patient has yet to leave the carrier, but is starting to migrate toward the carrier's opening. Its interest has been piqued, and it is beginning to look around to see what is outside the carrier. (c) This feline patient has partially exited the carrier. It is not all of the way out, so any sudden gesture or noise may cause it to retreat, but it is feeling confident enough to explore.

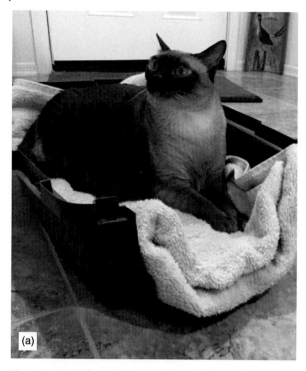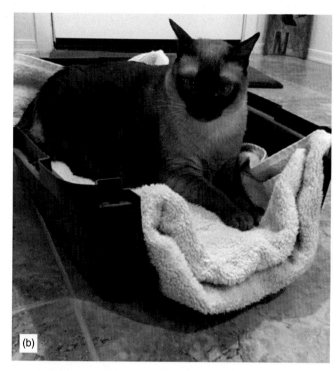

(a) (b)

Figure 1.15 (a) The patient is initially startled upon having the top half of the carrier removed. (b) The patient's ears denote irritation. This tells the veterinary professional to approach slowly, methodically, and cautiously.

doing, the patient is covered with a towel and may benefit from the illusion of feeling "hidden" [40].

Cats may remain under cover for the duration of the examination. Others may elect to emerge from hiding once the carrier is disassembled. Some but not all cats prefer to be handled on the examination room table (Figure 1.16a), some may prefer to tuck themselves up onto the feline-friendly scale (Figure 1.16b), others may migrate to examination room chairs (Figure 1.16c), and some prefer to be handled on the floor or on a lap (Figure 1.16d).

The most important aspect of the veterinary visit is that the cat is allowed to choose [40].

1.9 Recognizing Body Language

Cats communicate with each other and with other species through their eyes, ears, mouth, tail, and coat [44]. Because they prefer to avoid physical conflict when possible [13], cats have become adept at reading each other's visual cues [44].

Assuming that ambient lighting is adequate and is not a contributing factor, pupil size and shape accurately reflect the cat's underlying emotional state. A fearful cat exhibits mydriasis due to activation of the body's sympathetic "fight or flight" response (Figure 1.17a). Not only are the pupils dilated, they are rounded, sometimes so much so that it becomes very difficult to see each

iris. Contrast that with the pupils of a non-adrenalized feline patient: they tend to be more elliptical or slit-like (Figure 1.17b). When cats are at ease, they sometimes exhibit what is referred to as a "slow blink": in this case, the pupils are normal in size and shape, and the eyelids are halfway closed as if to convey security and a sense of restfulness (Figure 1.17c).

Feline ears are dynamic and can convey a series of visual cues over a very short amount of time [44]. Alert cats typically have symmetrical ear carriage, with both ears erect and directed toward a shared stimulus (Figure 1.18a). Cats that are uncertain or are exhibiting heightened awareness of their surroundings tend to have asymmetric ears, meaning that one or both ears are swiveled with the inner pinnae directed sideways (Figure 1.18b). Symmetrically flatted ears, pinned down against the top of the head, denote defensiveness: the patient is on guard and may feel forced to strike out aggressively as a means of self-defense (Figure 1.18c). Cats that are defensively aggressive may also hiss or spit at the perceived threat (Figure 1.19).

The tail is another great source of visual communication for cats. Its position in space and whether or not it is piloerect may be used to gauge a patient's emotional state. Relaxed, calm, and confident cats tend to keep their tails out and behind them (Figure 1.20a). By contrast, fearful cats tuck their tails underneath of their bodies (Figure 1.20b). As cats adapt a more offensive posture, they hold their tails perpendicular to the

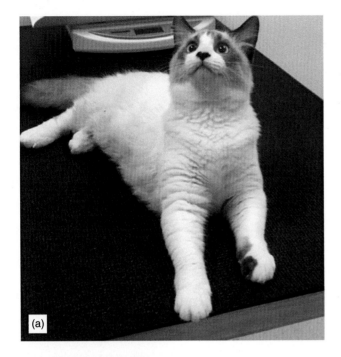

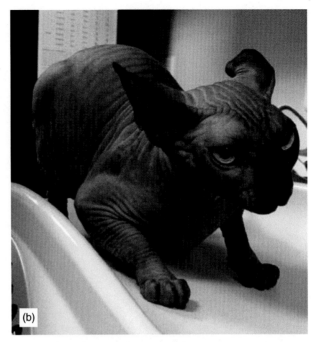

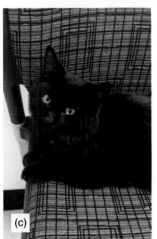

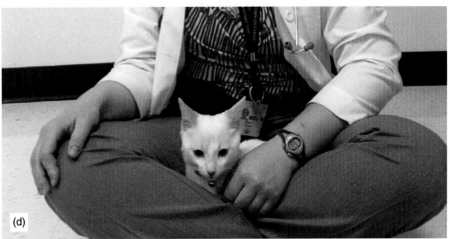

Figure 1.16 (a) The patient appears to be comfortable sprawled out onto the examination room table. Source: Courtesy of Lydia T. McDaniel. (b) The patient has elected to tuck itself up into a ball on the examination room scale. As in Figure 1.15b, its ears denote irritation. This tells the veterinary professional to approach slowly, methodically, and cautiously. Source: Courtesy of Brittany Hyde. (c) The patient has chosen to be examined on the examination room chair. Source: Courtesy of Amanda Coleman. (d) The patient's preference is to be examined on the floor in the clinician's lap.

ground (Figure 1.20c). Cats with bristled tails are hyper-aroused and are poised to attack (Figure 1.20d) [44].

Body posture, combined with pupil size and shape, ears, and tail carriage, collectively paints a picture of how each individual cat is perceiving the environment and helps observers to determine how that cat is likely to react [61]. The adept veterinary professional can identify the gamut of signals from curiosity and tolerance (Figure 1.21a) to warning signs of impending intolerance (Figure 1.21b). Potential complicating factors are that human observers are not always as quick to identify behavioral

cues [44] and that play behavior can bear a striking resemblance to aggression (Figure 1.21c).

Cats rarely expose their ventrum. When they do, it may be in the context of a fight, in which case it may be intended to reflect deferential behavior. Alternatively, cats may be doing so to adapt a defensive posture, in which case they concurrently raise their paws up over the abdomen, with claws unsheathed, as a warning that they are poised to attack if forced to [44].

Context is exceptionally important when interpreting the feline belly-up display. Cats that are immensely

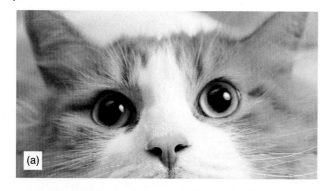

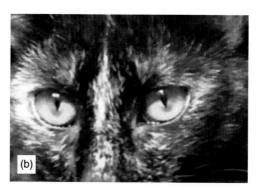

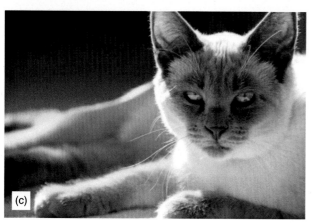

Figure 1.17 (a) The patient is startled, as is evident by its appreciably dilated pupils. Source: Courtesy of the Media Resources Department at Midwestern University. (b) The patient has normal size and shape and is less likely to be under the influence of "fight or flight." Source: Courtesy of Leigh Ann Howard. (c) The patient appears to be relaxed and is exhibiting a "slow blink." This is a patient that is exceptionally tolerant and malleable. Source: Courtesy of Amanda Rappaport.

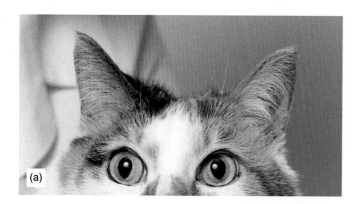

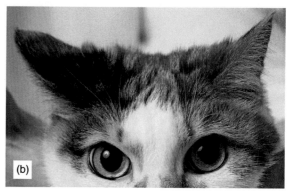

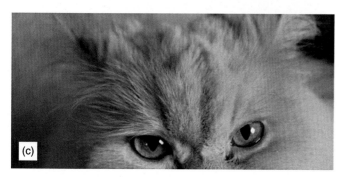

Figure 1.18 (a) The patient is alert and focused. Source: Courtesy of the Media Resources Department at Midwestern University. (b) The patient's swiveled ears are conveying uncertainty about the current situation. Source: Courtesy of the Media Resources Department at Midwestern University. (c) The patient's ears are pinned back. This is a "red flag" to practitioners that the patient is feeling threatened. Source: Courtesy of Marissa Haglund, Midwestern University CVM 2019.

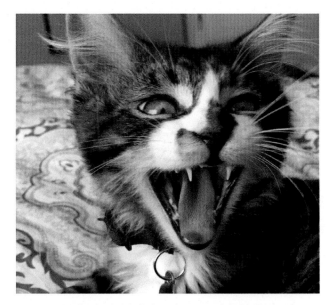

Figure 1.19 The patient is feeling threatened and is hissing as a means of communicating its desire to be left alone. Source: Courtesy of Hilary Lazarus.

relaxed may also demonstrate this behavior, especially when they are in their home environment surrounded by the familiar presence of comforting housemates (Figure 1.22).

Veterinary professionals should make an effort to read the visual cues that the patient is communicating from the moment they enter the examination room. This will facilitate the interaction by allowing the clinician to anticipate how best to approach a given patient. In the presence of a patient that is demonstrating fear, for instance, a savvy feline-friendly practitioner would make a conscientious effort to avoid direct stares [33]. This may be interpreted by the patient as a threat. Instead, the best approach would be to avert one's gaze and to allow the patient to acclimate to the clinician's presence. Furthermore, it may be wise to consider performing the physical examination in reverse, from tail to head, instead of from head to tail, so as to minimize eye contact in a fearful patient.

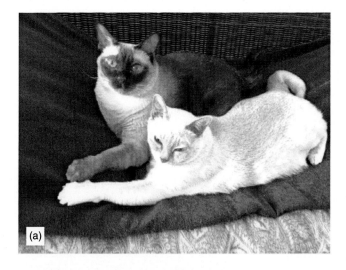

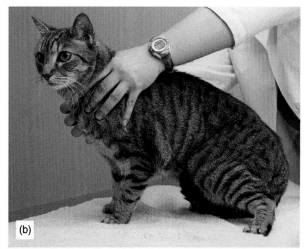

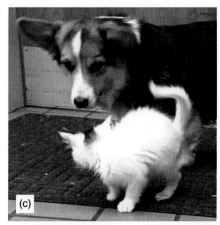

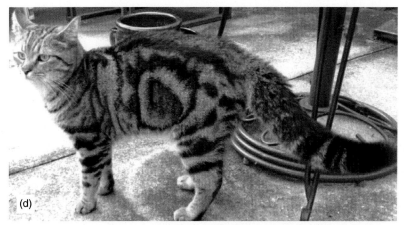

Figure 1.20 (a) Note the tail position in these two relaxed cats. (b) This patient's uncertainty is conveyed by its tail being tucked up underneath of its abdomen. Source: Courtesy of the Media Resources Department at Midwestern University. (c) Note this patient's offensive posture and the corresponding tail position perpendicular to the ground. Source: Courtesy of Cora R. Zenko. (d) This patient is exhibiting piloerection. Its awareness of its surroundings is heightened and the puffed tail conveys "stay away or I may be forced to attack." Source: Courtesy of Karen Burks, DVM.

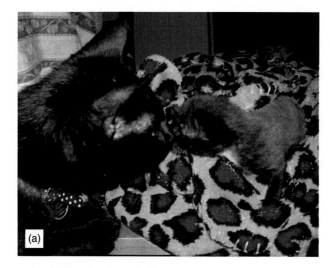

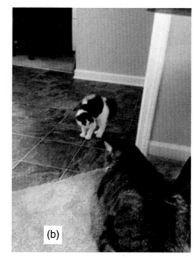

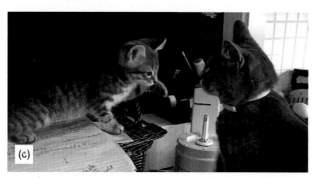

Figure 1.21 (a) The adult black cat depicted is investigating the situation with curiosity and without defensive or offensive facial expressions. Source: Courtesy of Alexandra Aczona-Velasquez. (b) The cat in the background has an arched back, demonstrating fear. Source: Courtesy of Kat Mackin. (c) This kitten is practicing striking behavior with a paw and the adult cat at which the behavior is directed is tolerating it. Source: Courtesy of Cora R. Zenko.

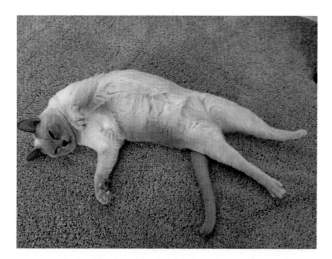

Figure 1.22 This cat is exhibiting belly-up behavior; however, its claws remain retracted and its feet are not tautly held over the abdomen. This cat is not on the attack. This cat is resting and feels safe and secure enough to do so.

1.10 Feline-Friendly Handling

It is tempting to anticipate that a patient will become aggressive and to respond accordingly, without patience and with excessive force [59]. It is equally tempting to label these patients as "difficult" or, simply put, "bad cats." However, it is important to understand that in a clinical setting, the primary reason underlying a patient's aggressive tendencies is fear [13]. Recognizing early signs of fear by assessing body posture and promoting feline-friendly handling may help to prevent the escalation of such fear into full-out aggression that worsens with each subsequent visit [13].

Veterinary practice lacks uniform guidelines as to what constitutes proper handling and restraint in a clinical setting [62]. Feline-friendly practice advocates that the veterinary team take a "less is more" approach with patients. Handling that uses the least amount of restraint necessary to achieve to desired outcome is preferred.

Accordingly, feline-friendly practice has moved away from the tendency to "scruff" all cats as a default means of restraint [13]. Scruffing refers to the clasping of skin at the nape of a cat's neck to exert a variable amount of pressure, thus inducing immobility [13]. One advantage of scruffing is that it provides control of the head and neck. When used properly, it can be a safe means of restraint for the veterinary team.

Cats use scruffing with conspecifics in natural settings under very limited circumstances: mating, dominating during a fight, and transporting young [63]. When the

veterinary team uses scruffing, the cat perceives it as an attempt by the practitioner to dominate it [40], and as a loss of control [40]. Although the action may result in the desired effect of immobility, it neither calms nor comforts the cat [13]. Cats may either freeze into submission or ramp up the attack. Naturally, there are circumstances when scruffing may be the only alternative to ensure staff safety; however, it should not be the default method by which cats are restrained. When it is used, scruffing should be done properly (1.23**a–d**). Adult cats should never be suspended freely in the air, lifted by the nape of

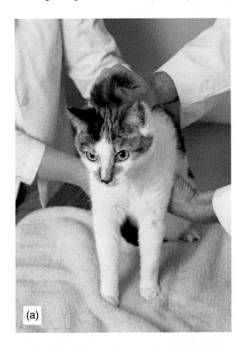
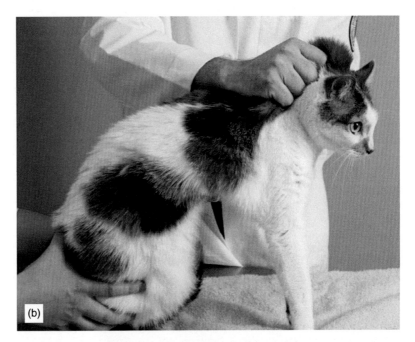
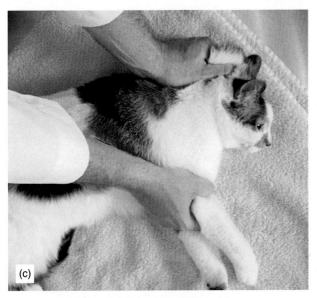
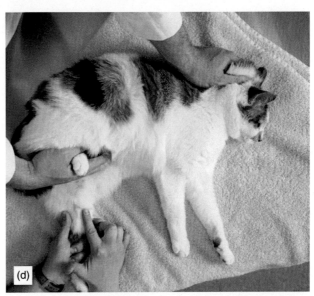

Figure 1.23 (a) Scruffing a cat properly. Note how the restrainer is supporting the chest and underbelly. (b) Side view of scruffing a cat properly. The cat is not suspended freely in the air. All four feet are planted on the ground so that the patient feels secure and grounded. (c) The properly scruffed cat can also be placed with ease into lateral recumbency. Note how the restrainer is resting his palm against the patient's neck for support. (d) Once in lateral recumbency, the properly scruffed cat can be securely positioned for venipuncture. Note how the restrainer is holding off the left hindlimb with his right hand. Source (a)–(d): Courtesy of the Media Resources Department at Midwestern University.

the neck. When scruffing is used, care should be taken not to stretch or extend the cat's body beyond what is comfortable and natural for the patient. Pulling on the feet should be minimized.

That being said, rather than default to scruffing, the veterinary team should adopt the "less is more" approach and experiment with alternative strategies. Maintaining the patient in a natural position is preferred, and hands are used as a means of gentle tactile communication rather than as gripping utensils to force the patient into submission (Figure 1.24a–c).

Another means of feline-friendly restraint that is gaining in popularity is the "kitty burrito" technique [60]. This method manages "challenging" cats by swaddling them with a towel, blanket, or comparable wrap. This provides several advantages:

- The wrapped cat is less able to thrash about or "alligator roll."
- The wrapped cat is less able to use its claws in self-defense.
- The wrapped cat can be hidden except for the part of the body that is actively being examined. The hidden cat may feel more secure and less likely to strike out.

To employ the "kitty burrito" technique, the veterinary technician starts the process by "cloaking" the cat with a towel when it is sternal. Next, the towel is wrapped under and around the patient in a swaddling effort to envelop all four feet (Figure 1.25a–e). The patient is unable to "alligator roll" when restrained using this technique. As a result, this technique allows the restrainer to feel in control of the cat without using extreme force. Because the cat is securely and safely restrained, the veterinarian is now able to proceed with the examination by taking a peek at the patient in "parts." The veterinary technician exposes only the part of the patient that they need at any given time so that the patient feels more secure and less exposed.

This technique can also be used to expedite procedures such as venipuncture. Only the limb from which blood will be sampled needs to be exposed and the rest of the cat can "hide." For example, exposure of the forelimb enables the veterinary technician to hold off at the proper location to facilitate venipuncture from the cephalic vein (Figure 1.26a). Similarly, exposure of the hind limb enables the veterinary technician to hold off at the proper location to facilitate venipuncture from the medial saphenous vein (Figure 1.26b).

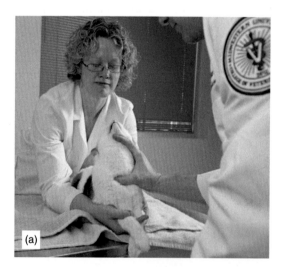

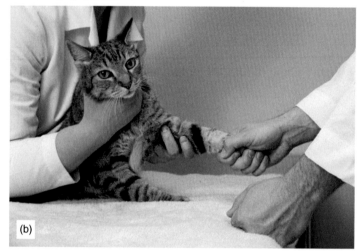

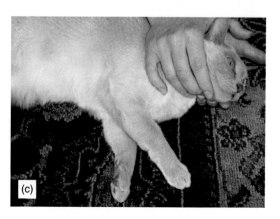

Figure 1.24 (a) Preparing a feline patient for jugular venipuncture without scruffing. Source: Courtesy of the Media Resources Department at Midwestern University. (b) Preparing a feline patient for cephalic venipuncture without scruffing. Source: Courtesy of the Media Resources Department at Midwestern University. (c) Alternative method of restraining a feline patient in lateral recumbency without scruffing. Note that the restrainer's grip around the neck is firm but not overly forceful. The patient can breathe normally without any airway constriction.

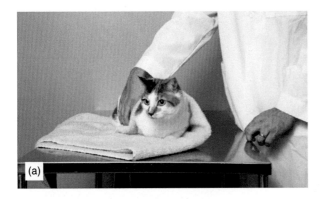

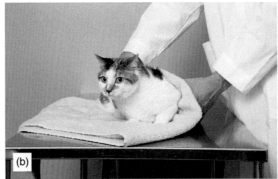

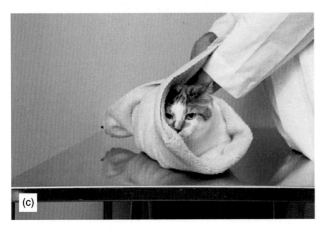

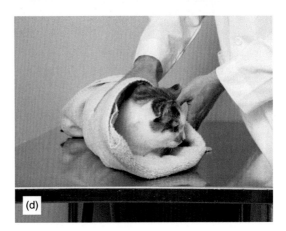

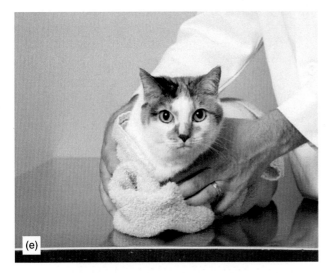

Figure 1.25 (a) Step 1 of the "kitty burrito" technique: position the cat on the towel. (b) Step 2: curl the towel around one side of the increasingly suspicious cat. (c) Step 3: swaddle the cat by curling the other side of the towel around the cat. (d) Now the cat is fully encased in the "kitty burrito." However, the restrainer's grip on the "kitty burrito" is weak and needs to be more secure or else the cat could escape. (e) The restrainer's grip has been tightened so that the cat is more snuggly encased in the "kitty burrito." This will make it more difficult for the cat to escape. Source (a)–(e): Courtesy of the Media Resources Department at Midwestern University.

Some veterinary teams find that the use of acupressure calms the feline patient. The restrainer's hand gently caps the cat's head with the restrainer's three middle fingers falling along the dorsum of the skull. These three fingers can be used to stroke the head gently, slowly, and methodically while the restrainer's first and fifth digits provide a means by which to control the cat's head [60].

There is ongoing controversy regarding a newer restraint technique, pinch-induced behavioral inhibition [33, 64], otherwise known as "clipnosis." This is a form of scruffing in which clips rather than hands are used to apply firm pressure along the dorsal midline to dampen the cat's response to external stimuli. Cats retain some mobility, although they appear to be less resistant to diagnostic procedures such as venipuncture [64]. Several studies have reported success in using this method of restraint [65, 66], and cats in which this technique was tested did not display changes in heart rate, respiratory rate, or blood pressure that might suggest that clipnosis was painful [64]. However,

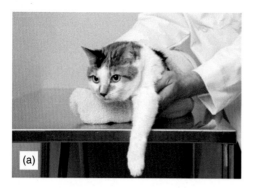
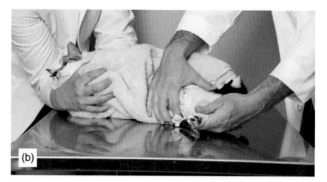

Figure 1.26 (a) The left forelimb has been uncovered in preparation for venipuncture. (b) The right hindlimb has been uncovered in preparation for venipuncture. Source (a), (b): Courtesy of the Media Resources Department at Midwestern University.

some clinicians, including the present author, have reservations about inhibiting normal behaviors to curb behavior that is clinic induced [13].

1.11 Other Feline Handling Tools

There is a precarious balance between feline-friendly practice and the need to protect the veterinary team. Animal-related injuries such as bite wounds are commonplace in the veterinary profession [67–69] and measures must be taken to maximize safety while addressing patient welfare. There are times when the use of a cat muzzle is indicated. Cat muzzles serve two functions: to prevent biting and to reduce visual stimuli because they cover the eyes. When feline patients are fearful, a soft muzzle is the best approach to block the cat's ability to see what is causing distress (Figure 1.27). Although the soft muzzle covers both the mouth and eyes, the material is such that if a cat is motivated enough to bite, it can bite through the fabric [33].

For cats that are known to be on the offensive and are poised to attack, stiffer muzzles are preferred (Figure 1.28). It is much less likely that a cat will be able to bite through this, thus more effectively protecting staff.

As an alternative approach to muzzling and in the event that a site distal to the cat's face and head needs to be examined, an Elizabethan collar may be placed on the feline patient to prevent it from reaching the clinician with its mouth (Figure 1.29). In this case, the Elizabethan collar must be longer than anticipated to make sure that it exceeds well beyond the muzzle.

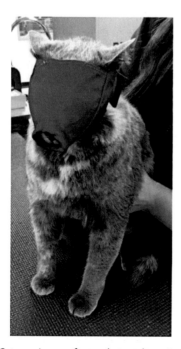

Figure 1.27 Cat wearing a soft muzzle to reduce visual stimulation.

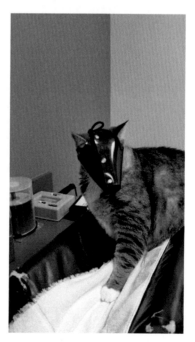

Figure 1.28 Cat wearing a leather muzzle to reduce the risk of the restrainer sustaining a bite wound injury. Source: Courtesy of Kat Mackin.

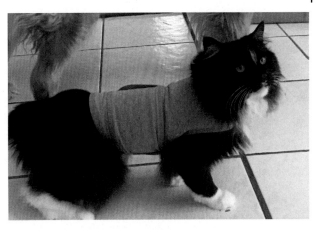

Figure 1.30 Cat wearing a body wrap to reduce anxiety. Source: Courtesy of Christiana Otterson, Kaylee Otterson, and Sarah McN. Sykes, Midwestern University CVM 2019.

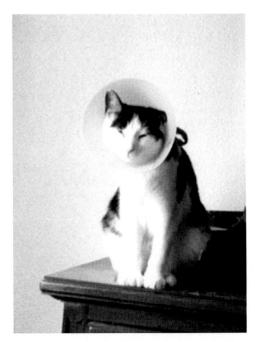

Figure 1.29 Cat wearing an Elizabethan collar as a means of distancing the patient's mouth from the clinician's hand, without requiring the use of a muzzle. Source: Courtesy of Kat Mackin.

A fearful patient may also benefit from wearing a body wrap such as a Thundershirt that applies pressure to the torso non-invasively to simulate swaddling. These are marketed for both cats and dogs (Figure 1.30). It is believed that anxiety is diminished when evenly applied pressure is provided over the body's core [70–72].

Finally, there are times when chemical restraint is appropriate both to ensure the safety of the veterinary team and to minimize the stress on the patient.

Anxiolytic drugs can facilitate feline-friendly handling and diminish negative associations between the cat and the veterinary team. Intramuscular injections that are reversible are preferred because they are fast-acting, easy to administer in a fractious patient, and their duration can be terminated when the physical examination or the diagnostic procedure is completed. Sedation protocols should be tailored to the individual based upon age, health status, underlying disease processes, and the duration for which sedation is required. All of these can be difficult to predict in a patient that has never before been examined and is intolerant of handling. However, it is the responsibility of the attending clinician to weigh risks versus benefits. These should be effectively communicated to clients in order to assist them with decision-making, a significant component of relationship-centered care [33].

References

1 American Veterinary Medical Association Center for Information Management (2012) *U.S. Pet Ownership and Demographics Sourcebook*, Center for Information Management, Schaumburg, IL.

2 Volk, J.O., Thomas, J.G., Colleran, E.J., and Siren C.W. (2014) Executive summary of phase 3 of the Bayer Veterinary Care Usage Study. *Journal of the American Veterinary Medical Association*, **244** (7), 799–802.

3 Nolen, R.S. (2011) Feline-friendly handling guidelines aim for perfect veterinary visits. Veterinary team, pet owner have a hand in limiting stress in cat patients. *Journal of the American Veterinary Medical Association*, **239** (1), 26–27.

4 Vogt, A.H., Rodan, I., Brown, M. *et al.* (2010) AAFP–AAHA feline life stage guidelines. *Journal of the American Animal Hospitals Association*, **46** (1), 70–85.

5 Burns, K. (2011) 6 factors in declining veterinary visits. *Journal of the American Veterinary Medical Association*, **238** (5), 538–540.

6 Volk, J.O., Felsted, K.E., Thomas, J.G., and Siren, C.W. (2011) Executive summary of the Bayer Veterinary Care Usage Study. *Journal of the American Veterinary Medical Association*, **238** (10), 1275–1282.

7 Vogt, A.H., Rodan, I., Brown, M. *et al.* (2010) AAFP–AAHA feline life stage guidelines. *Journal of Feline Medicine and Surgery*, **12** (1), 43–54.

8 Lue, T.W., Pantenburg, D.P., and Crawford, P.M. (2008) Impact of the owner–pet and client–veterinarian bond on the care that pets receive. *Journal of the American Veterinary Medical Association*, **232** (4), 531–540.

9 Volk, J.O., Felsted, K.E., Thomas, J.G., and Siren, C.W. (2011) Executive summary of phase 2 of the Bayer

Veterinary Care Usage Study. *Journal of the American Veterinary Medical Association*, **239** (10), 1311–1316.

10 Greco, D.S. (1991) The effect of stress on the evaluation of feline patients, in *Consultations in Feline Internal Medicine* (ed. J.R. August), Saunders, Philadelphia, pp. 13–17.

11 Carlstead, K., Brown, J.L., and Strawn, W. (1993) Behavioral and physiological correlates of stress in laboratory cats. *Applied Animal Behaviour Science*, **38**, 143–158.

12 American Association of Feline Practitioners (2013) *Ten Solutions to Increase Cat Visits*, http://www.catvets.com/public/PDFs/Education/Solutions/solutionsbrochure.pdf (accessed 23 December 2016).

13 Rodan, I., Sundahl, E., Carney, H. *et al.* (2011) AAFP and ISFM feline-friendly handling guidelines. *Journal of Feline Medicine and Surgery*, **13** (5), 364–375.

14 Rodan, I., Sundahl, E., Carney, H. *et al.* (2011) Feline focus: AAFP and ISFM feline-friendly handling guidelines. *Compendium: Continuing Education for the Practicing Veterinarian*, **33** (12), E3.

15 Bowen, J. and Heath, S. (2005) An overview of feline social behaviour and communication, in *Behaviour Problems in Small Animals: Practice Advice for the Veterinary Team*, Saunders, Philadelphia, pp. 29–36.

16 Levine, E.D. (2008) Feline fear and anxiety. *Veterinary Clinics of North America: Small Animal Practice*, **38** (5), 1065–1079, vii.

17 Scherk, M. (2013) The cat-friendly practice, in *BSAVA Manual of Feline Practice: A Foundation Manual* (eds. A. Harvey and S. Tasker), British Small Animal Veterinary Association, Gloucester.

18 Brunt, J. (2012) The cat-friendly practice, in *The Cat* (ed. S. Little), Saunders Elsevier, St. Louis, pp. 20–25.

19 Rubert, R., Long, L.D., and Hutchinson, M.L. (2007) Creating a healing environment in the ICU, in *Critical Care Nursing: Synergy for Optimal Outcomes* (eds. R. Kaplow and S.R. Hardin), Jones and Bartlett, Sudbury, MA, pp. 27–39.

20 Starkweather, A., Witek-Janusek, L., and Mathews, H.L. (2005) Applying the psychoneuroimmunology framework to nursing research. *Journal of Neuroscience Nursing*, **37** (1), 56–62.

21 Fontaine, D.K., Briggs, L.P., and Pope-Smith, B. (2001) Designing humanistic critical care environments. *Critical Care Nursing Quarterly*, **24** (3), 21–34.

22 Morgan, K.N. and Tromborg, C.T. (2007) Sources of stress in captivity. *Applied Animal Behaviour Science*, **102** (3–4), 262–302.

23 Veranic, P. and Jezernik, K. (2001) Succession of events in desquamation of superficial urothelial cells as a response to stress induced by prolonged constant illumination. *Tissue and Cell*, **33** (3), 280–285.

24 Pollard, J.C. and Littlejohn, R.P. (1994) Behavioral effects of light conditions on red deer in a holding pen. *Applied Animal Behaviour Science*, **41** (1–2), 127–134.

25 Gunter, R. (1951) The absolute threshold for vision in the cat. *Journal of Physiology*, **114** (1–2), 8–15.

26 Miller, P.E. and Murphy, C.J. (1995) Vision in dogs. *Journal of the American Veterinary Medical Association*, **207** (12), 1623–1634.

27 Verdecchia, P., Schillaci, G., Borgioni, C. *et al.* (1995) White coat hypertension and white coat effect – similarities and differences. *American Journal of Hypertension*, **8** (8), 790–798.

28 Ogedegbe, G. (2008) White-coat effect: unraveling its mechanisms. *American Journal of Hypertension*, **21** (2), 135.

29 Cardillo, C., Defelice, F., Campia, U., and Folli, G. (1993) Psychophysiological reactivity and cardiac end-organ changes in white coat hypertension. *Hypertension*, **21** (6), 836–844.

30 Palmer, B.F. (2001) Impaired renal autoregulation: implications for the genesis of hypertension and hypertension-induced renal injury. *American Journal of Medical Science*, **321** (6), 388–400.

31 Marino, C.L., Cober, R.E., Iazbik, M.C., and Couto, C.G. (2011) White-coat effect on systemic blood pressure in retired racing greyhounds. *Journal of Veterinary Internal Medicine*, **25** (4), 861–865.

32 Belew, A.M., Barlett, T., and Brown, S.A. (1999) Evaluation of the white-coat effect in cats. *Journal of Veterinary Internal Medicine*, **13** (2), 134–142.

33 Herron, M.E. and Shreyer, T. (2014) The pet-friendly veterinary practice: a guide for practitioners. *Veterinary Clinics of North America: Small Animal Practice*, **44** (3), 451–481.

34 Crowell-Davis, S.L. (2007) White coat syndrome: prevention and treatment. *Compendium: Continuing Education for the Practicing Veterinarian*, **29** (3), 163–165.

35 Anthony, A., Ackerman, E., and Lloyd, J.A. (1959) Noise stress in laboratory rodents. 1. Behavioral and endocrine response of mice, rats, and guinea pigs. *Journal of the Acoustic Society of America*, **31** (11), 1430–1437.

36 Wells, D.L., Graham, L., and Hepper, P.G. (2002) The influence of auditory stimulation on the behaviour of dogs housed in a rescue shelter. *Animal Welfare*, **11** (4), 385–393.

37 Kogan, L.R., Schoenfeld-Tacher, R., and Simon, A.A. (2012) Behavioral effects of auditory stimulation on kenneled dogs. *Journal of Veterinary Behavior*, **7** (5), 268–275.

38 Katz, J.D. (2014) Noise in the operating room. *Anesthesiology*, **121** (4), 894–898.

39 Gloag, D. (1980) Noise and health: public and private responsibility. *British Medical Journal*, **281** (6252), 1404–1406.

40 Rodan, I. (2010) Understanding feline behavior and application for appropriate handling and management. *Topics in Companion Animal Medicine*, **25** (4), 178–188.

41 Heath, S. (2009) Aggression in cats, in *BSAVA Manual of Canine and Feline Behavioural Medicine*, 2nd edn. (eds. D. Horwitz and D.S. Mills), British Small Animal Veterinary Association, Gloucester, p. 233.

42 Soennichsen, S. and Chamove, A.S. (2002) Responses of cats to petting by humans. *Anthrozoos*, **15** (3), 258–265.

43 Pageat, P. and Gaultier, E. (2003) Current research in canine and feline pheromones. *Veterinary Clinics of North America: Small Animal Practice*, 33 (2), 187–211.

44 Overall, K.L. (1997) *Clinical Behavioral Medicine for Small Animals*, Mosby, St. Louis.

45 Mazur, J.E. (2006) *Basic principles of classical conditioning, in Learning and Behavior*, 6th edn., Prentice Hall, Upper Saddle River, NJ, pp. 76–81.

46 Yin, S. (2009) Classical conditioning (aka associative learning), in *Low Stress Handling, Restraint, and Behavior Modification of Dogs and Cats*, Cattle Dog Publishing, Davis, CA, pp. 83–84.

47 Bear, M.F., Connors, B.W., and Paradiso, M.A. (2007) The chemical senses, in *Neuroscience: Exploring the Brain*, 3rd edn., Lippincott Williams & Wilkins, Baltimore, pp. 271–272.

48 Pereira, J.S., Fragoso, S., Beck, A. *et al.* (2016) Improving the feline veterinary consultation: the usefulness of Feliway spray in reducing cats' stress. *Journal of Feline Medicine and Surgery*, 18 (12), 959–964.

49 Herron, M.E. (2010) Advances in understanding and treatment of feline inappropriate elimination. *Topics in Companion Animal Medicine*, 25 (4), 195–202.

50 Griffith, C.A., Steigerwald, E.S., and Buffington, C.A. (2000) Effects of a synthetic facial pheromone on behavior of cats. *Journal of the American Veterinary Medical Association*, 217 (8), 1154–1156.

51 Hunthausen, W. (2000) Evaluating a feline facial pheromone analogue to control urine spraying. *Veterinary Medicine*, 95 (2), 151–155.

52 Frank, D.F., Erb, H.N., and Houpt, K.A. (1999) Urine spraying in cats: presence of concurrent disease and effects of a pheromone treatment. *Applied Animal Behaviour Science*, 61 (3), 263–272.

53 Mills, D.S. and Mills, C.B. (2001) Evaluation of a novel method for delivering a synthetic analogue of feline facial pheromone to control urine spraying by cats. *Veterinary Record*, 149 (7), 197–199.

54 Gunn-Moore, D.A. and Cameron, M.E. (2004) A pilot study using synthetic feline facial pheromone for the management of feline idiopathic cystitis. *Journal of Feline Medicine and Surgery*, 6 (3), 133–138.

55 Frank, D., Beauchamp, G., and Palestrini, C. (2010) Systematic review of the use of pheromones for treatment of undesirable behavior in cats and dogs. *Journal of the American Veterinary Medical Association*, 236 (12), 1308–1316.

56 Kronen, P.W., Ludders, J.W., Erb, H.N., *et al.* (2006) A synthetic fraction of feline facial pheromones calms but does not reduce struggling in cats before venous catheterization. *Veterinary Anaesthesia and Analgesia*, 33 (4), 258–265.

57 Rand, J.S., Kinnaird, E., Baglioni, A., *et al.* (2002) Acute stress hyperglycemia in cats is associated with struggling and increased concentrations of lactate and norepinephrine. *Journal of Veterinary Internal Medicine*, 16 (2), 123–132.

58 International Cat Care and American Association of Feline Practitioners (2012). *A Guide to Creating a Cat Friendly Practice*. American Association of Feline Practitioners, Hillsborough, NJ.

59 Moffat, K. (2008) Addressing canine and feline aggression in the veterinary clinic. *Veterinary Clinics of North America: Small Animal Practice*, 38 (5), 983–1003, vi.

60 Rodan, I. (2012) Understanding the cat and feline-friendly handling, in *The Cat* (ed. S. Little), Saunders Elsevier, St. Louis, pp. 2–19.

61 Leyhausen, P. (1979) *Cat Behavior: the Predatory and Social Behavior of Domestic and Wild Cats*, Garland STPM Press, New York.

62 Patronek, G.J. and Lacroix, C.A. (2001) Developing an ethic for the handling, restraint, and discipline of companion animals in veterinary practice. *Journal of the American Veterinary Medical Association*, 218 (4), 514–517.

63 Allbrook, A. (2013) Handling the 'challenging' cat. *Veterinary Nursing Journal*, 28 (9), 299–301.

64 Pozza, M.E., Stella, J.L., Chappuis-Gagnon, A.C., *et al.* Pinch-induced behavioral inhibition ('clipnosis') in domestic cats. *Journal of Feline Medicine and Surgery*, 10 (1), 82–87.

65 Tarttelin, M.F. (1991) Restraint induced by skin clips. *International Journal of Neuroscience*, 57, 288.

66 Tarttelin, M.F. (1993) Restraint induced by non-noxious skin clips: modifications of this technique results in a greater success rate in the adult cat. *International Journal of Neuroscience*, 71, 131.

67 Drobatz, K.J. and Smith, G. (2003) Evaluation of risk factors for bite wounds inflicted on caregivers by dogs and cats in a veterinary teaching hospital. *Journal of the American Veterinary Medical Association*, 223 (3), 312–316.

68 August, J.R. (1988) Dog and cat bites. *Journal of the American Veterinary Medical Association*, 193 (11), 1394–1398.

69 Jeyaretnam, J., Jones, H., and Phillips, M. (2000) Disease and injury among veterinarians. *Australian Veterinary Journal*, 78 (9), 625–629.

70 Grandin, T. (1992) Calming effects of deep touch pressure in patients with autistic disorder, college students, and animals. *Journal of Child and Adolescent Psychopharmacology*, 2 (1), 63–72.

71 Grandin T. (1989) Voluntary acceptance of restraint by sheep. *Applied Animal Behaviour Science*, 23 (3), 257–261.

72 Cottam, N., Dodman, N.H., and Ha, J.C. (2013) The effectiveness of the Anxiety Wrap in the treatment of canine thunderstorm phobia: an open-label trial. *Journal of Veterinary Behavior*, 8 (3), 54–61.

2

Assessing the Big Picture: the Body, the Coat, and the Skin of the Cat

2.1 Forms of Identification

Over two million owned cats go missing annually in the United States [1], and it is estimated that twice that number enter shelters each year [2]. Of those cats that enter shelters, less than 2% are recognized as being owned and returned home, due in large part to lack of owner identification [3]. Lord *et al.* [4] found that nationwide, 86% of cats lack visual forms of identification at the time they are reported missing, and only 7% have an implanted microchip. Regionally, owners may demonstrate even less compliance with veterinary recommendations to provide pets with identification. In Ohio, only 3% of surveyed cat-owners had microchips implanted in their cats [5]. A popularly voiced reason against microchipping was that indoor-only cats did not require identification because they did not get lost [3], and microchips were therefore viewed as an unnecessary expense [3]. However, the presence of a microchip immensely increases the chance for a missing cat to be reunited with its owner: owner recovery of cats from a shelter increased from 2 to 39% due to microchips alone [6].

Microchips are electronic forms of patient identification that are approximately the size of a grain of rice and are typically implanted between the shoulder blades. Once implanted, they are not visible to the naked eye. In a lean cat one can often feel the microchip, but in an average-sized to overweight cat it is typically impossible.

For microchips to be an effective form of patient identification, their data must be detected by a scanner that then displays the unique identifying number of each chip. The unique identifier of each chip can then be registered to the pet-owner, whose contact information can be accessed from a database. One complicating factor is that the United States lacks standardization among microchip frequencies. This means that unless a scanner is said to be "universal," it may be incapable of displaying an identifying number that is outside its frequency range [7].

An additional complication is that the burden is on the owner to both register the microchip and maintain updated contact information. Lord *et al.* [6] found that only 58.1% of microchipped lost dogs and cats that ended up at shelters had been registered. When owner

registrations were found, there were additional obstacles that delayed, if not prevented, the missing patient from being reunited with its owner. Owner telephone numbers were often incorrect or disconnected; or the chip was registered to a past owner who no longer claimed responsibility for the patient [6].

The veterinary team should take a leadership role in considering patient identification as a form of preventive medicine. First-time patients and clients that are new to the practice present the ideal opportunity to discuss patient identification and to relay practice recommendations. Even better, scanning for microchips can be integrated into the physical examination to ensure that they are still functional, and allows the veterinary team to remind owners to update contact information [7].

Scanning should also be performed following implantation to be certain that the process was successful. Rarely, the microchip can back out of the injection site before the skin seals.

Another form of permanent patient identification is an ear tattoo, although this is more typically performed in laboratory cats rather than client-owned cats (Figure 2.1).

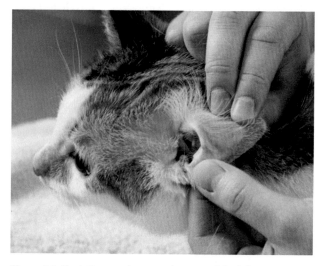

Figure 2.1 Ear tattoo on the ventral aspect of the left pinna. Source: Courtesy of the Media Resources Department at Midwestern University.

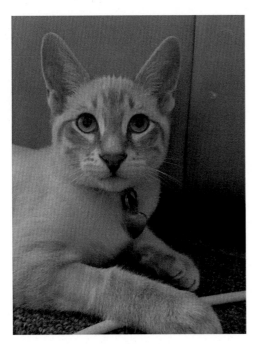

Figure 2.2 Cat donning collar. Source: Courtesy of Jessica Herrod.

Permanent forms of patient identification are preferred because they cannot be removed, intentionally or unintentionally. They also cannot be altered [7]. Less permanent, but visible forms of patient identification include collars (Figure 2.2). Three main types of collars are used in cats: plastic buckle, breakaway, and elastic stretch safety.

Lord *et al.* [3] found that approximately three-fourths of cats will tolerate a collar, and that safety risks are minimal: only 3.3% of cats got their collars caught. Like microchips, collars are infrequently used in cats because of the perception that indoor-only cats do not get lost, and the misperception that cats would tolerate them poorly. However, in a study that examined cat and cat-owner compliance over a 6-month period, 56.3% of owners noted that their cats tolerated the collars better than expected [3]. Collar-wearing compliance also increased by 70% when practices provided free collars with identification tags during wellness visits [7].

2.2 Body Condition Scoring

It is the responsibility of the veterinary team to make nutritional recommendations to cat-owners with the aim of providing whole-body wellness through maintenance of an ideal body weight. Increased body weight adversely impacts the musculoskeletal, urinary, gastrointestinal, and endocrine systems by predisposing cats to lameness, lower urinary tract disease, hepatic lipidosis, and diabetes mellitus [8, 9]. Weight gain is increasing in

frequency in the companion animal population, as is the trend toward sedentary, indoor-only lifestyles [10–13]. As a result, over one-third of pet cats are said to be overweight (>10% above ideal body weight) or obese (>20% above ideal body weight) [8, 10, 12, 13].

On the other hand, being underweight is also risky to health and may hasten death [14]. Age-related loss of lean body mass results in whole-body weakness, increasing the risk of falls and fractures, and may also damp the body's immune response [15]. When weight loss is disease-related, as in the case of cardiac and renal cachexia, it compounds owners' perceptions of quality of life and may contribute to premature decision-making regarding euthanasia [15, 16].

As an objective, repeatable measurement, body weight is an important vital sign that should be documented at every visit [8]. This allows for the discovery of trends that prompt the veterinary team to intervene when a patient's plane of nutrition is inappropriately matched to that particular individual's needs. However, it does not take into account anticipated differences in body weight based upon breed: an adult cat's ideal body weight may range from 2 to 7 kg [12].

In human medicine, the body mass index as a measurement of weight relative to height is used to extrapolate body composition in order to fine-tune nutritional recommendations to the individual. The equivalent measurement has been attempted in feline medicine using ribcage circumference and limb length. However, the accuracy of the feline system is questionable owing to the challenges associated with obtaining measurements from an awake, active cat [8].

A more commonly used and validated method in veterinary medicine is the Purina nine-point system of body condition scoring [17]. This system is useful for approximating the percentage of body fat in cats, and can be used to calculate energy requirements for cats based on their respective body condition score (BCS) [8]. BCS is measured along a sliding scale, in which the extremes of one and nine reflect emaciation and morbid obesity, respectively. As demonstrated in Figure 2.3, BCS is determined by assessing visible and/or palpable landmarks. When evaluating the BCS, it is important to take into account both lateral and aerial views.

In breeds with thick, plush coats that dwarf otherwise typically visible characteristics, palpation becomes even more important (Figure 2.4). Skeletal landmarks that are emphasized include the ribcage, lumbar vertebrae, waist line, and wings of the ilia. Palpating for soft tissues such as an abdominal fat pad and fat coverage over the ribs is equally important [18].

Unlike body weight, BCS is a subjective measurement and may vary between observers who are evaluating the same patient [18]. However, it provides a starting point to initiate a conversation about the patient's current plane of nutrition.

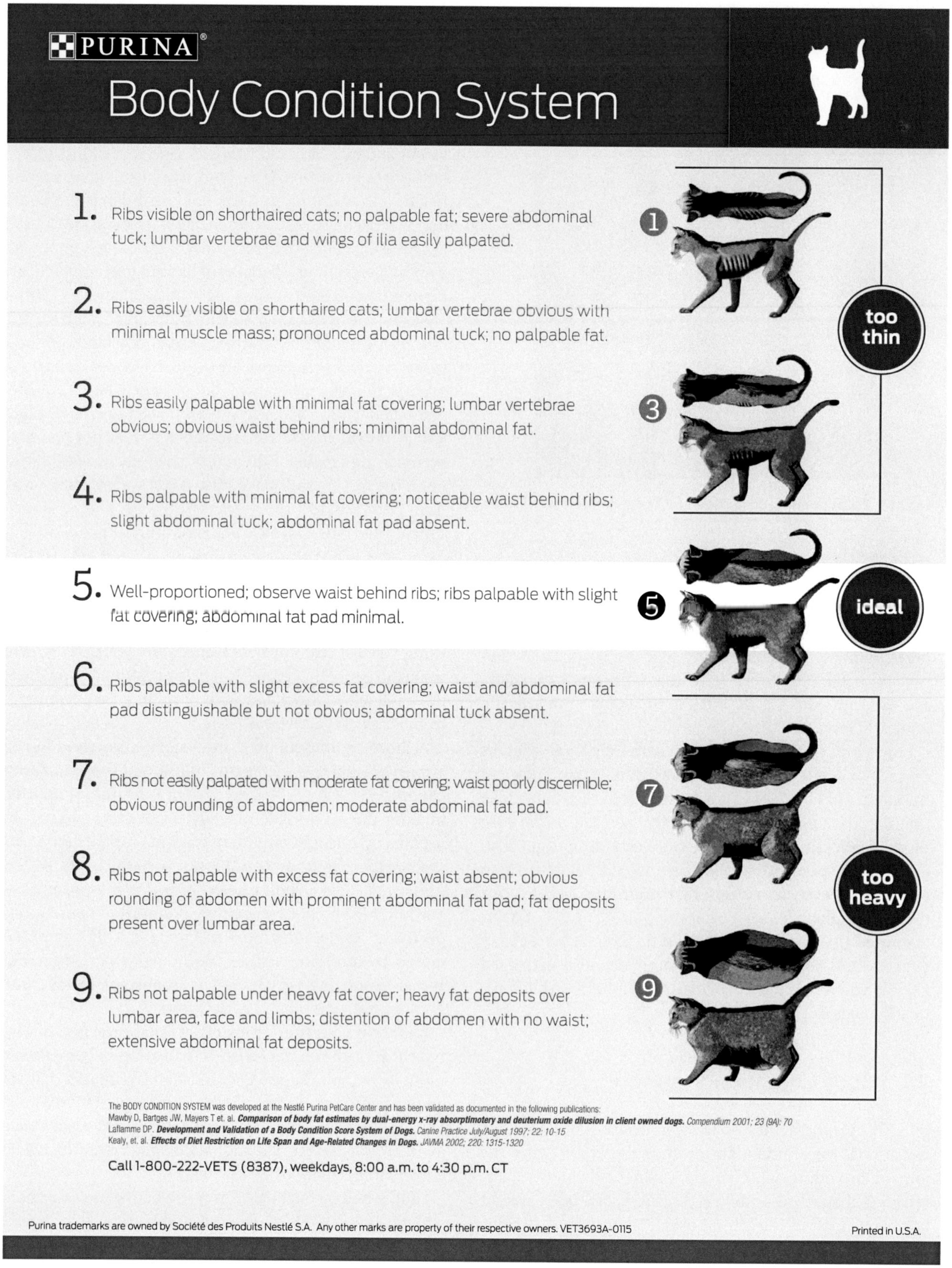
PURINA®
Body Condition System
1. Ribs visible on shorthaired cats; no palpable fat; severe abdominal tuck; lumbar vertebrae and wings of ilia easily palpated.
2. Ribs easily visible on shorthaired cats; lumbar vertebrae obvious with minimal muscle mass; pronounced abdominal tuck; no palpable fat.
3. Ribs easily palpable with minimal fat covering; lumbar vertebrae obvious; obvious waist behind ribs; minimal abdominal fat.
4. Ribs palpable with minimal fat covering; noticeable waist behind ribs; slight abdominal tuck; abdominal fat pad absent.
5. Well-proportioned; observe waist behind ribs; ribs palpable with slight fat covering; abdominal fat pad minimal.
6. Ribs palpable with slight excess fat covering; waist and abdominal fat pad distinguishable but not obvious; abdominal tuck absent.
7. Ribs not easily palpated with moderate fat covering; waist poorly discernible; obvious rounding of abdomen; moderate abdominal fat pad.
8. Ribs not palpable with excess fat covering; waist absent; obvious rounding of abdomen with prominent abdominal fat pad; fat deposits present over lumbar area.
9. Ribs not palpable under heavy fat cover; heavy fat deposits over lumbar area, face and limbs; distention of abdomen with no waist; extensive abdominal fat deposits.
1
3
5
7
9
too thin
ideal
too heavy
The BODY CONDITION SYSTEM was developed at the Nestlé Purina PetCare Center and has been validated as documented in the following publications:
Mawby D, Bartges JW, Mayers T et. al. Comparison of body fat estimates by dual-energy x-ray absorptimotery and deuterium oxide dilusion in client owned dogs. Compendium 2001; 23 (9A): 70
Laflamme DP. Development and Validation of a Body Condition Score System of Dogs. Canine Practice July/August 1997; 22: 10-15
Kealy, et. al. Effects of Diet Restriction on Life Span and Age-Related Changes in Dogs. JAVMA 2002; 220: 1315-1320
Call 1-800-222-VETS (8387), weekdays, 8:00 a.m. to 4:30 p.m. CT
Purina trademarks are owned by Société des Produits Nestlé S.A. Any other marks are property of their respective owners. VET3693A-0115
Printed in U.S.A.

Figure 2.3 Assessing feline BCS using the Purina 9-point system. Source: Courtesy of Nestlé Purina PetCare.

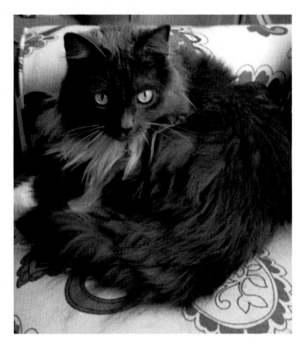

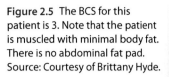

Figure 2.5 The BCS for this patient is 3. Note that the patient is muscled with minimal body fat. There is no abdominal fat pad. Source: Courtesy of Brittany Hyde.

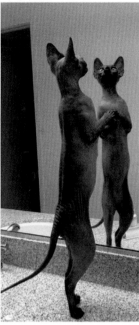

Figure 2.4 Note the challenges that a medium-haired coat presents when body condition scoring using visible landmarks alone. This patient may be overscored unless palpation is used, given that visual landmarks are difficult to appreciate under this plush coat. Source: Courtesy of Bianca J. Hartrum.

According to the Purina nine-point system for assessing BCS for cats, cats are underweight if they score a BCS of 1, 2, or 3:

- A cat that is classified as having a BCS of 1 is considered to be emaciated. If short-haired, these cats have ribs that are easy to appreciate visually without palpation. There is no palpable fat and whole-body muscle mass is scant to non-existent. The waist line is exaggerated.
- A cat that is classified as having a BCS of 2 is considered to be moderately underweight. The abdominal tuck is pronounced but not to the extent of a cat with a BCS of 1. Whole-body muscle mass is poor, and there is still no palpable fat.

- A cat that is classified as having a BCS of 3 is considered to be mildly underweight (Figure 2.5). The ribs are not visible; however, they are easily palpable. There is minimal body fat. The abdominal fat pad is absent. The waistline is obvious.

The author considers cats with a BCS of 4 to be a "lean normal."

According to the Purina nine-point system for assessing BCS for cats, cats are considered ideal if they score a BCS of 5 (Figure 2.6). These patients are well proportioned and they have a visible waist and palpable ribs with slight fat coverage. If there is an abdominal fat pad, it is minimal. The author considers cats with a BCS of 6 to be slightly overweight.

According to the Purina nine-point system, cats are overweight if they score a BCS of 7, 8, or 9:

- A cat that is classified as having a BCS of 7 is considered to be mildly overweight (Figure 2.7). It is possible, but

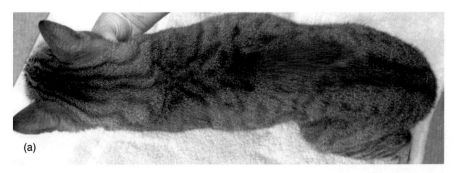

(a)

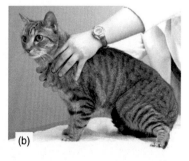

(b)

Figure 2.6 The BCS for this patient is 5. (a) In this aerial view, the patient's tuck at the waist is apparent. (b) In this lateral view, the patient's tuck at the waist is less easy to appreciate. This is why taking a two-view approach in addition to palpation is preferred.
Source (a), (b): Courtesy of the Media Resources Department at Midwestern University.

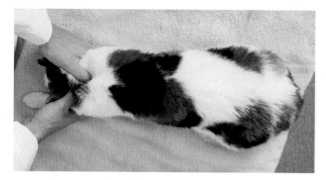

Figure 2.7 The BCS for this patient is 7. In this aerial view, the patient's tuck at the waist is difficult to appreciate. Source: Courtesy of the Media Resources Department at Midwestern University.

challenging, to feel the ribcage, and the waistline is difficult to appreciate. There is a decent abdominal fat pad with rounding of the abdomen (Figure 2.8).

- A cat that is classified as having a BCS of 8 is considered to be moderately overweight (Figure 2.9). It is not possible to feel the ribcage due to fat coverage, and there is no waistline. Not only is there a prominent abdominal fat pad, there are also fatty deposits palpable in the lumbar region bilaterally.
- A cat that is classified as having a BCS of 9 is considered to be morbidly obese. Fat deposits are extensive: in addition to a prominent fat pad and lumbar "love handles," fat is present over the face and limbs.

BCS is a tool that tends to be underutilized by the veterinary team [18], yet it should be measured at each visit. It is important to keep in mind that just as is the case with human beings, not all cats are "built" the same in terms of size and shape. Some cats will score a BCS of

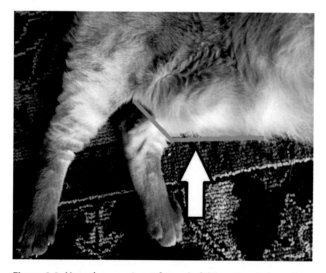

Figure 2.8 Note the prominent fat pad of this patient in lateral recumbency. This patient has a BCS of 7.

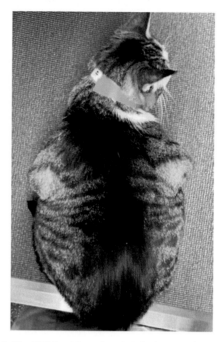

Figure 2.9 The BCS for this patient is 8. In this aerial view, there is a much rounder appearance to the whole cat, it is not just that the waistline has disappeared. The cat has taken on a more ovoid silhouette than is normal.

7 for their entire life: they always have been, and always will be, simply put, "big cats." Other cats will score a BCS of 3 for their entire life: they always have been, and always will be, simply put, "skinny." Noting trends over time is a good way to be proactive. Changes in body size or shape may occur prior to the development of overt clinical signs that owners may recognize. The "big cat" that was always a BCS of 7 and is now a 5 on physical exam, without any identifiable changes in diet or feeding routine at home, should be flagged as needing a more extensive work-up.

It is the responsibility of the veterinary team to engage the client in a discussion about the risks of being under- or overweight. Many owners do not recognize weight as an issue for their pet such that the burden is on the veterinary team to address the topic of weight management [19]. Cat-owners especially have difficulty recognizing and accepting that weight is a health concern for their pet [20]. The BCS is an excellent opportunity to elicit the client's perspective and to include them in the process of identifying weight as a primary problem.

To incorporate the BCS successfully into the veterinary approach to preventive medicine, clients need to become familiar with the scoring system and educated on how to make use of it. Studies in canine medicine have compared BCS as determined by dog-owners with BCS as determined by the veterinary professional and have found that 27% of owners underscore by two marks. In other words, a dog that is scored a BCS of 7 by a veterinarian is scored a BCS of 5 by an owner [21]. This may not seem like a significant discrepancy; however, it reflects failure on the part of the owner to recognize an excess of 20–30% body weight [21]. Comparison studies involving the cat-owner and the veterinary team are lacking; however, underscoring on the part of the cat-owner is likely. Taking the time to review the approach to BCS and to train the owner to be an accurate assessor may facilitate discussions on weight management at future visits and may help to acquire owner buy-in.

2.3 Assessing Hydration

In addition to BCS, the hydration status of a patient is one of many indicators of whole-body wellness.

In order to estimate a patient's hydration status, the veterinary team needs to start with a thorough patient history. Insight into the patient's presenting complaint may help the practitioner to anticipate fluid losses that may induce dehydration. For instance, if a patient presents for protracted vomiting and diarrhea, they are unlikely to be well hydrated. In addition to the digestive tract, patients may experience loss of water through alternative routes such as increased urinary output. A polyuric cat, for example, with a diagnosis of chronic renal failure is likely to experience an appreciable deficit in whole-body water balance. Similarly, burn patients may undergo extreme losses of water, and other traumatic injuries may lead to extensive blood loss, a large proportion of which includes water. A thorough history provides insight not only into the route of water loss, but also the duration: peracute versus acute versus chronic. The timeline may help to determine if the patient's hydration status is as expected [22].

The history serves to augment physical examination findings to paint a consistent picture of the patient's hydration status. To characterize hydration status for each patient, the veterinary professional should examine skin turgor, mucous membrane moistness, eye position within the orbits, heart rate, peripheral pulse quality, capillary refill time, and whether or not there is jugular distension [22].

Cardiovascular findings are described in Chapter 5; this section emphasizes skin turgor.

Skin turgor is an assessment of the skin's elasticity. It can be performed in human medicine on the skin of the forearm. The veterinary practitioner does not tend to make use of limbs for this measurement, but rather relies upon grasping a generous fold of skin at the nape of the neck or between the shoulder blades. This skin fold is classically lifted up, pinched between the examiner's thumb and index fingers or twisted to one side by the examiner's flick of the wrist. Some refer to this process as intentionally "tenting the skin" (Figure 2.10). The skin fold is then released and the experienced practitioner observes that one of two outcomes is possible:

1) In a euhydrated patient, there is appreciable skin elasticity. The fold of skin returns to its normal position almost instantaneously. In other words, there is not a persistent "skin tent."
2) As the patient dehydrates, there is a progressive loss of skin elasticity, which leads to slow-to-bounce-back skin – the skin is said to be "sluggish" and it does not seem motivated to return to its normal position. As dehydration progresses, the skin fold eventually does not return at all, it remains "tented."

Keep in mind that assessing hydration status is not an exact science – it is somewhat subjective. The skin tent

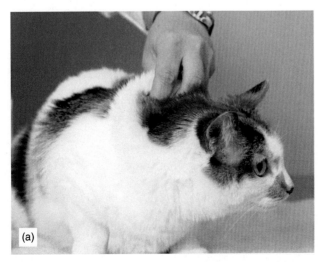 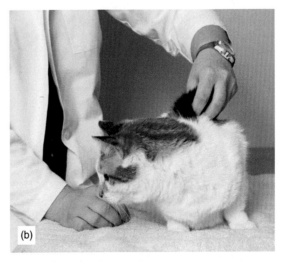

Figure 2.10 Assessing the patient's hydration status by tenting the skin (a) over the nape of the neck and (b) between the shoulder blades. Source (a), (b): Courtesy of the Media Resources Department at Midwestern University.

test can also be deceiving: the presence of a skin tent is suggestive of but not pathognomonic for dehydration. The following are situations in which the outcome of the skin tent test may be supportive of dehydration when in fact the patient is anything but at a loss for fluids:

- Geriatric patients often have decreased elasticity regardless of hydration status.
- Patients who have experienced excessive weight loss may have extensive skin folds. These may create the illusion of skin tenting in the absence of dehydration.
- Obese patients may be dehydrated in the absence of skin tenting.

As a result of these discrepancies, it is important to compare physical examination findings with the results of baseline diagnostic tests. In particular, the complete blood count, serum chemistry panel, and urinalysis are important clinical reasoning tools that clinicians should use to ask themselves whether or not their assessment of hydration makes sense in light of the data [22].

In cases of dehydration, the following clinicopathologic data are typically seen:

- CBC: hemoconcentration with increased total solids.
- Serum Chemistry Panel: azotemia.
- Urinalysis: increased urine specific gravity.

In cases of dehydration, the azotemia is said to be pre-renal. However, it is important to remember that elevations in BUN and creatinine can also be of renal or post-renal origin, and that azotemia alone does not have to indicate dehydration.

When the history, physical examination findings, and clinicopathologic data collectively suggest dehydration, the veterinarian should estimate the percentage of dehydration that is detected. The smallest percentage at which dehydration is clinically detectable is 5%.

- A patient is said to be 5% dehydrated when the skin tents slightly, meaning that the skin fold returns to its original position but less rapidly than expected. There will also be a subtle tackiness to the mucous membranes. The veterinarian's finger does not "stick" to the gums, but the gums are not as moist as they ought to be [22].
- A patient is said to be 6–8% dehydrated when there is moderate skin tenting. The skin fold does ultimately return to its proper anatomic location but it is sluggish to do so. The mucous membranes are dry [22].
- A patient is said to be 10–12% dehydrated when there is severe skin tenting and the skin fold remains tented. It never returns to its anatomic location. The veterinarian's fingers stick to the mucous membranes because they are so tacky. The eyes take on a sunken appearance as in the case of enophthalmos. As a result, the nictitating membranes appear to be prominent [22].

- A dehydration state of 15% is incompatible with life if protracted [22].

It is important to remember that dehydration is a continuum and these percentages are, simply put, guidelines to help the clinician to prognosticate and to provide appropriate patient care. Understanding the severity of dehydration will help establish fluid therapy guidelines for the patient, including the route and rate of administration. Fluid therapy is patient driven and ever-changing in response to the patient's needs. Frequent reevaluation of hydration status is necessary to tailor the treatment plan to the individual.

2.4 Inspecting the Coat: First Impressions

If this is the patient's first visit to the practice, it behooves the clinician to take a moment to recognize distinguishing features that may be unique to the patient's breed. These breed-specific identifiers are important to note in any medical record and may assist with patient identification. Cat-owners frequently self-identify the patient's breed – they may or may not be accurate in their assessment. Adopted gray cats are frequently identified as Russian Blue cats on account of coat color whether or not they share additional traits that match the breed standard. Likewise, "big cats" are often referred to as Maine Coons based on their size alone rather than any confirmed pedigree.

One of the most important characteristics to recognize and record is coat length and whether or not the patient belongs to a "furless" breed. The Sphynx is perhaps the best known breed of cat that is said to be "furless" and indeed, at a cursory glance, from a distance, it appears to be just that (Figure 2.11a). However, touching the skin reveals fine hairs that yield a texture of chamois. These hairs are the result of underlying hair follicle dysplasia: the Sphynx cat has the same number of hair follicles as a furred cat, but the hair shafts are abnormal [23].

The skin of a Sphynx cat is the color that the coat would have been. As a result, there is great variety in skin color and mottling (Figure 2.11b and c). Because they lack a coat, Sphynx cats require more maintenance than one might assume. There is no coat to absorb the oils that are produced by the skin. These oils accumulate on the skin, between skin folds, and under nails. Sphynx cats also accumulate excess debris in their ears because they have less ear hair, if any at all, to filter out particulate matter. The breed as a whole therefore requires routine bathing and ear cleaning. These responsibilities are important to convey to cat-owners if they are unfamiliar with the breed so that these cats are maintained in a way that is most conducive to their health [24, 25].

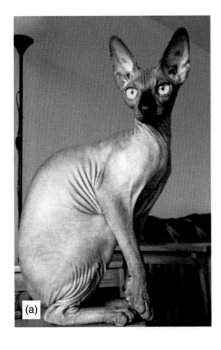

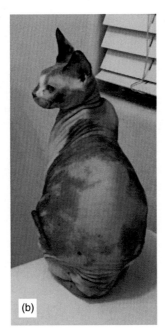

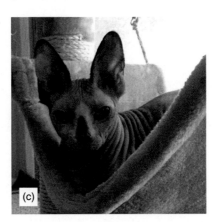

Figure 2.11 (a) The Sphynx cat as an example of a furless breed. (b) The skin of a Sphynx cat varies in color: its color is what the coat color would have been. (c) A second example of how the skin of a Sphynx cat can vary based upon the color that the coat would have been. Source (a)–(c): Courtesy of Brittany Hyde.

Sphynx cats are not the only "furless" breed, but they are the most popular of this variety in the United States. There is also the Levkoy cat and the Donskoy from Russia and the Bambino cat, a cross between a Sphynx and a Munchkin cat.

If the patient has a coat, it should be described in terms of texture, especially if it is unique. The majority of cats will have straight coats. However, the Cornish and Devon Rex breeds have coats that are not naturally straight. Their coats are rexed (curled) [24–26].

Also if the patient has a coat, it should be described in terms of coat length. The majority of cats in the United States are Domestic Short-Haired (DSH) cats. DSH cats are not an official or recognized breed, but rather a hodgepodge of cats of mixed ancestry sharing one common trait: a short coat (Figure 2.12). Some might refer to them as the "mutts" of the cat world. These cats are not to be confused with the British Shorthair or the American Shorthair, which are in fact recognized by cat breed registries [24, 25].

Domestic Medium-Haired (DMH) and Domestic Long-Haired (DLH) cats are also groupings of cats based upon coat length (Figure 2.13). As above, these are not to be confused with purebreds such as Himalayans and Persians, which are known for their plush, long-haired coats. Note that it can be difficult at times to differentiate between DMH and DLH cats, as they sometimes take on an in-between appearance (Figure 2.14).

Coat length may seem obvious as a visible characteristic and may therefore be easy to overlook, but it is important to recognize, record, and review with the client because the coat at its current length may require routine upkeep to maintain it in good health [24, 25].

Owners may look to veterinarians for information as to proper care and coat maintenance, and some owners may elect to alter the coat length accordingly to prevent matting and other complications associated with coats of certain lengths. For instance, the "lion cut" is becoming an increasingly popular method by which to manage cats with long coats, especially if the cats are prone to excessive shedding, matting, and/or heat stress in regions of the

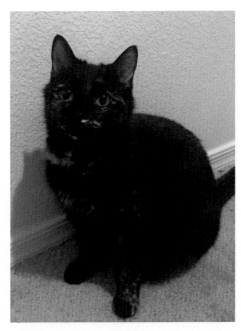

Figure 2.12 The domestic short-haired cat as example of a cat with a short coat length. Source: Courtesy of Amanda D. Schellinger.

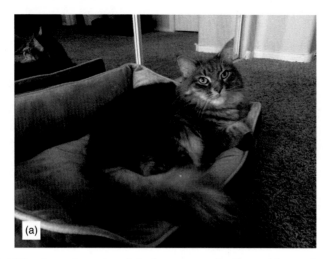
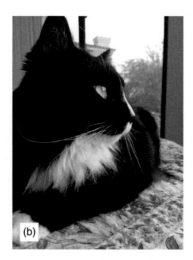

Figure 2.13 (a) The domestic medium-haired cat as example of a cat with a medium coat length. Source: Courtesy of Garrett Rowley, Midwestern University CVM 2018. (b) The domestic long-haired cat as example of a cat with a long coat length. Source: Courtesy of Emily Dodge.

country that are unseasonably hot for prolonged periods, such as the Southwest. Cats who undergo this particular style of grooming have their torso shaved, and only the face, mane, legs, and tail tip remain in their original plush form (Figure 2.15).

In addition to coat length, coat odor is an important consideration. Every patient has its own unique smell from apocrine and sebaceous gland secretions and by-products of resident bacterial populations. However, there are times when the veterinarian will be overtaken by an odor that is clearly abnormal. When this occurs, closer inspection is warranted. Sometimes the odor is a "red herring" – it may be a by-product of the environment in which the patient has been living, for example, the smell of smoke on the coat of a cat who lives with a smoker. However, when the smell is acrid, it should not be overlooked – it is a clue to look deeper. Skin lesions, metabolic disease, or both may be to blame.

2.5 Identifying Coat Colors and Coat Patterns

Coat colors and coat patterns, which refer to combinations of colors, are additional patient-specific characteristics that should be documented within the medical record

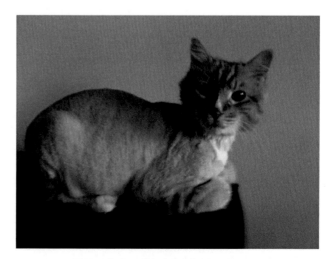

Figure 2.14 The short-haired face along with the extensive mane makes it difficult to identify this cat definitively as being medium- or long-haired. Source: Courtesy of Bianca J. Hartrum.

Figure 2.15 The typical appearance of a long-haired cat with a lion cut. Source: Courtesy of Karen Burks, DVM.

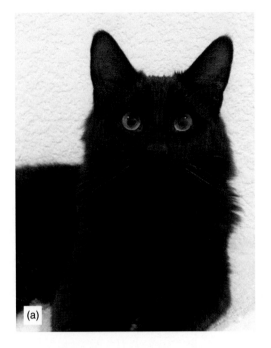

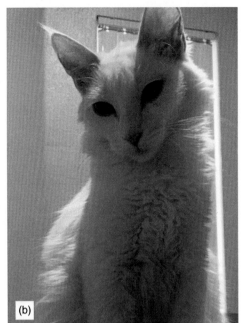

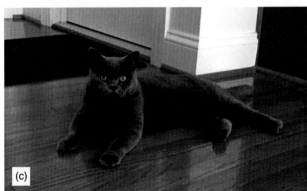

Figure 2.16 (a) An example of a solid black cat. Source: Courtesy of Amanda Coleman. (b) An example of a solid white cat. Source: Courtesy of Kelly Chappell. (c) An example of a solid blue cat. Source: Courtesy of Richard and Jill Englar.

any time the veterinary team is meeting a patient for the first time. There are six basic cat coat color patterns:

1) solid;
2) tabby;
3) bicolor;
4) tricolor;
5) tortoiseshell;
6) color-point.

Solid cats are characterized as having coats with only one color. Black, white, and blue ("gray") are three examples of solid coat colors (Figure 2.16).

Note that black coats may develop rusty tinges over time, especially those with intense sunlight exposure. Black-coated cats may also have concurrent underlying tabby coat color patterns. White-coated cats with blue eyes tend to be deaf. This combination of solid coat color and eye color is genetically linked to apoptosis of the hair cells in the inner ear, resulting in hearing impairment shortly after birth [27–34].

The tabby pattern involves two types of colored fur. The "background" fur of a tabby cat consists of agouti hairs: these are banded, with several different colors along their length. The second colored fur is typically darker and, when "stamped" against the lighter background fur, creates distinct contrast [35]. Tabby coats also are characterized as having an "M" on the forehead and bold "eyeliner" (Figure 2.17).

There are four sub-variations of the tabby coat pattern [28, 35–37]:

1) Striped tabby: this is sometimes referred to as the Mackerel tabby because the pattern looks very similar to what one would imagine if fish bones were painted on the coat (Figure 2.18a). In the wild, the best example of a big cat with this coat pattern is the tiger.
2) Classic tabby: this is sometimes referred to as the Blotched or Marbled tabby because the pattern looks more swirled, and there is typically a bull's-eye pattern along the lateral aspect of the coat (Figure 2.18b).

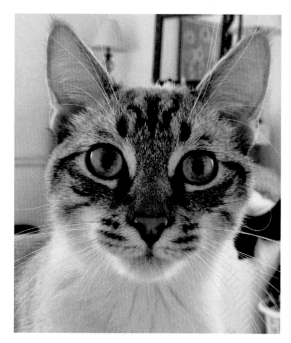

Figure 2.17 The characteristic "M" on the forehead of a cat with a tabby coat pattern. Note also the prominent "eyeliner."
Source: Courtesy of Emily Denning.

3) Ticked tabby: the tabby "M' on the forehead is present, but otherwise there is no contrast throughout the coat. There is only agouti fur (Figure 2.18c). A purebred cat with this coat pattern is the Abyssinian. In the wild, the best example of a big cat with this coat pattern is the lion.
4) Spotted tabby: the darker fur appears in spots all over the body rather than as stripes (Figure 2.18d). In the wild, the best example of a big cat with this coat pattern is the leopard.

Bicolor cats are characterized as having coats with two colors. Black and white, also known as the "tuxedo" color combination, and blue ("gray") and white are classic examples of this coat pattern. Tuxedo cats can be primarily black or primarily white (Figure 2.19a and b). Tuxedo cats are also not all short-haired (Figure 2.19c). Similarly, blue and white bicolor cats may be short-haired (Figure 2.19d), medium-haired, or long-haired [35].

Tricolor cats are characterized as having coats with three colors. Typically this assortment consists of white, black (blue, if diluted [38]), and orange (cream, if diluted). The more white there is within the coat, the more defined the patches of orange and black become. A cat with this patchy coat is typically referred to as a calico (Figure 2.20). Calico cats are typically female [28, 35, 39, 40]. Anecdotally, calico cats are said to possess "catitude" and are thought to be less tolerant, as reported by their owners [41].

A "tabico" is a cat that is both calico and a tabby (Figure 2.21).

A tortoiseshell, affectionately referred to as the "tortie," is like a calico cat without the white (Figure 2.22). In other words, the tortie is a hodgepodge of black (blue, if diluted [38]) and orange (cream, if diluted). As with calicos, they tend to be female [39]. When male torties do occur, they tend to be sterile [39, 40, 42, 43]. Like calicos, torties are said to possess "tortitude" and are also reported to be less tolerant by their owners [41].

A "torbie" is a cat that is both tortie and tabby (Figure 2.23).

A color-point coat pattern is one in which the face of the cat and its extremities (ears, paws, and tail) are said to be "pointed" – in other words, these regions are darker than other areas of the body such as the torso. Points develop in affected cats due to a mutation of the albino gene. Ordinarily, the enzyme tyrosinase plays a role in melanin formation, which determines pigmentation of the skin and coat. When there is a mutation of the albino gene, tyrosinase is active only at lower temperatures. This allows for areas of the body that are cooler than core body temperature to become darkened by points. However, the same mutation of the albino gene causes tyrosinase to be inactivated by higher temperatures. Therefore, areas of the body such as the trunk that register at core body temperature remain under-pigmented [27, 28, 44, 45].

Color-point coat patterns are most notably seen in the Siamese, Burmese, Tonkinese, Balinese, and Himalayan breeds [27, 46]. Each breed has breed-specific terminology to identify various colors of points. Siamese cats are typically referred to as seal points (brown), flame points (red–orange), blue points (gray), and lilac (lavender) points (Figure 2.24) [24]. By contrast, the equivalent of a seal point Siamese would be a so-called champagne mink Tonkinese. A platinum mink Tonkinese would appear visually to be a blend between a blue and lilac point Siamese, with more of a creamy latte-colored base (Figure 2.25).

Note that color-point cats can also have an underlying tabby coat pattern. For example, seal point cats can also be tabbies (Figure 2.26).

In color-point cats, points are not present at birth, but develop as the kitten ages. By 4 weeks of age, color points are obvious (Figure 2.27). Geography plays a role in how dark the points will ultimately become. Adult color-point cats that live in warm climates tend to have lighter coats than those in cool climates.

2.6 Assessing Coat Quality

Coat quality should always be assessed and documented. Following every physical examination on every patient,

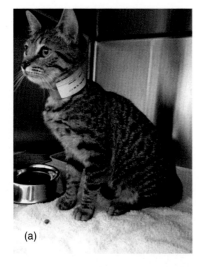
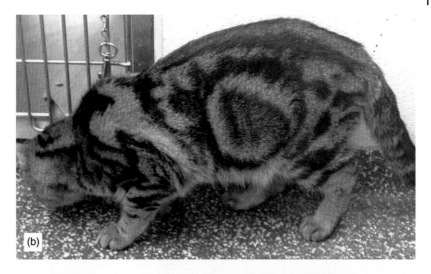
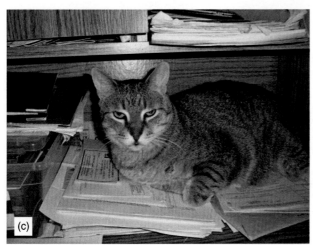
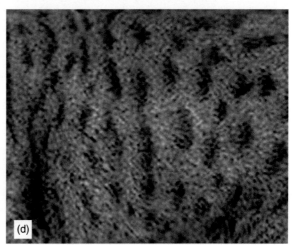

Figure 2.18 (a) An example of a striped or mackerel tabby. (b) An example of a classic tabby. Source: Courtesy of Karen Burks, DVM. (c) An example of a ticked tabby. Source: Courtesy of Carmela Berton. (d) An example of a spotted tabby.

the veterinarian should be able to answer the following questions:

- Is the coat displaying piloerection?
- Is the coat well groomed or unkempt?
- Is the coat shiny or dull?
- Is the coat full or are there regions of hypotrichosis or alopecia?

Piloerection refers to when an animal's fur stands on end due to activation of the sympathetic nervous system [47]. The "fight or flight" reflex causes the bristling of fur that leads observers to say that the cat is "fluffed up." This "fluffed" appearance is most prominent when a cat is startled. The effect is such that the cat appears bigger to its enemies. The "fluffed" cat may be perceived as a threat.

Sometimes piloerection is particularly prominent in the tail and not so much in the rest of the body (Figure 2.28). Sometimes the tail is less affected; however, the fur along the dorsum will be raised (Figure 2.29).

If the coat quality is poor, then the veterinarian should inquire as to whether this has always been the case or whether it is a new finding. Unkempt cats that were previously fastidious about their appearance should raise a red flag. The location of the matted or soiled fur may provide insight as to the source of the problem. For instance, a geriatric cat that suddenly starts to look disheveled in the hindquarters may be unsuccessfully coping with the onset of osteoarthritis that makes it challenging to groom the most caudal regions of the body. On the other hand, a cat that suddenly begins to over-groom is equally concerning. Cats with idiopathic cystitis, for example, often over-groom their ventrum, specifically their ventrocaudal abdomen, during flare-ups as if to indicate that this region of the body is irritating to them. Similarly, cats with carpal arthritis may over-groom their forelimbs.

If there is thinning of or absence of fur, the location is important to note. The veterinarian must remind himself that bilaterally symmetrical peri-aural alopecia is normal

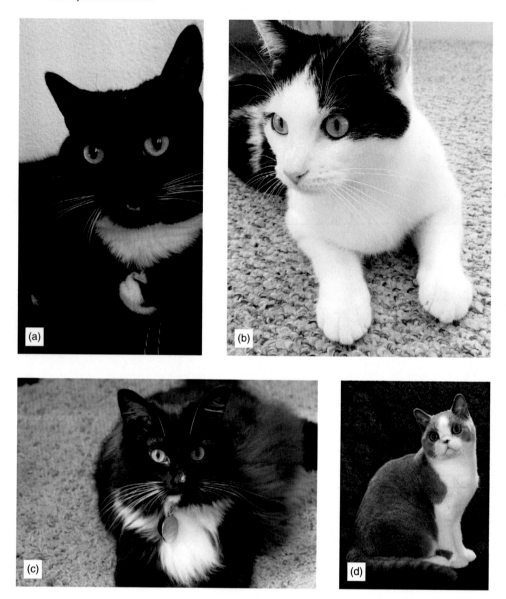

Figure 2.19 (a) An example of a bicolor tuxedo cat that is primarily black. Source: Courtesy of Abby Rife. (b) An example of a bicolor tuxedo cat that is primarily white. Source: Courtesy of Kelly Chappell. (c) An example of a bicolor tuxedo cat that has a longer coat than would be classified as a DSH. Source: Courtesy of Marissa Haglund, Midwestern University CVM 2019. (d) An example of a blue and white bicolor cat. Source: Courtesy of Cheryl A. Kelly.

in cats (Figure 2.30) whereas peri-ocular alopecia is not (Figure 2.31).

If there is evidence of hypotrichosis or alopecia in other areas of the body, the location should be noted, and also whether or not there is a bilaterally symmetrical distribution. Loss of fur with hairs that are easily epilated can reflect an underlying endocrine disorder. The classic example is bilaterally symmetrical flank alopecia in the hypothyroid dog [48]. If the shafts of the epilated fur were viewed under the light microscope, they would appear normal and unbroken. By contrast, shafts that are damaged may have become that way through

self-trauma: the cat may have intentionally scratched, chewed, or over-groomed the fur in such a way that it is thinning or absent altogether [48]. This is sometimes referred to as "fur-mowing."

Fur-mowing can be triggered by an underlying dermatological condition such as parasites. For example, in the presence of fleas, cats typically chew heavily at the base of their tail. The result is tail base hypotrichosis or alopecia, depending upon the severity of the pruritus and the motivation of the cat to chew [48]. Early on in this condition, fur loss may be minimal but there may be two other concurrent physical

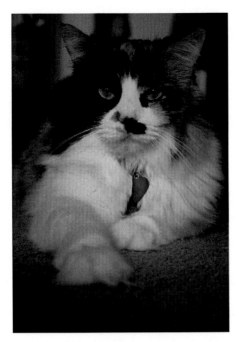

Figure 2.20 An example of a tricolor calico cat. Source: Courtesy of Marissa Haglund, Midwestern University CVM 2019.

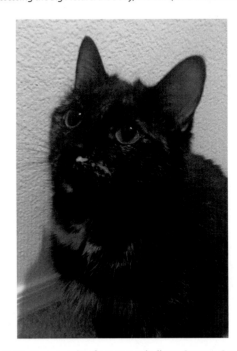

Figure 2.22 An example of a tortoiseshell cat. Source: Courtesy of Amanda D. Schellinger.

examination findings that may help in the diagnosis of this dermatopathy:

1) rusty brown discoloration of the fur at the tail base due to salivary staining;
2) the presence of flea dirt.

Flea dirt is essentially flea feces, which consist of dried digested blood. In order to look for flea dirt, the fur often needs to be parted (Figure 2.32). If debris is identified when the fur is parted, but the veterinarian is uncertain whether or not the debris is flea dirt and no live fleas are

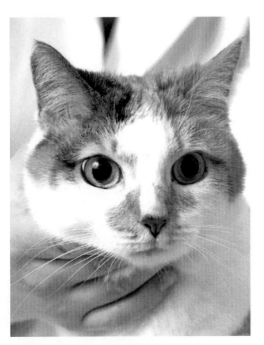

Figure 2.21 An example of a tabico cat. Source: Courtesy of the Media Resources Department at Midwestern University.

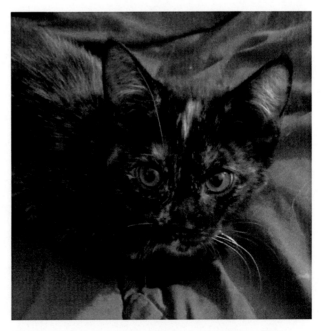

Figure 2.23 An example of a torbie. Source: Courtesy of Brian Collins, DVM, DABVP (Canine and Feline Practice)

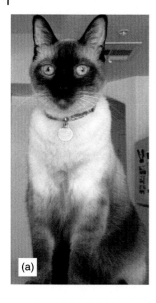

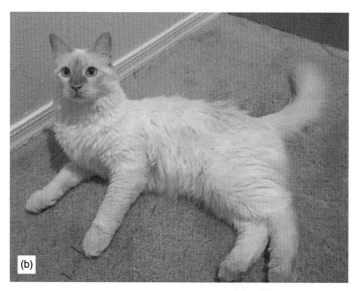

Figure 2.24 (a) An example of a seal point Siamese. Source: Courtesy of Kyley Olson. (b) An example of a flame point Siamese. Source: Courtesy of Amanda Schellinger. (c) An example of a blue point Siamese. Source: Courtesy of Lydia T. McDaniel. (d) An example of a lilac point Siamese. Source: Courtesy of Lydia T. McDaniel.

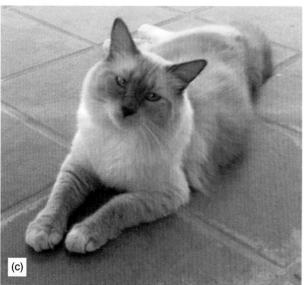

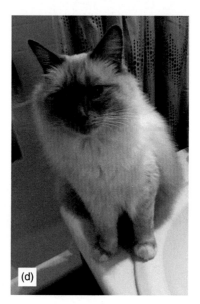

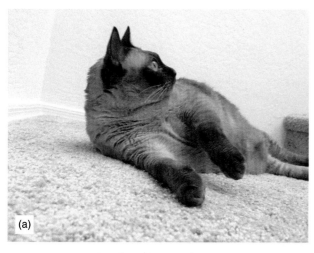

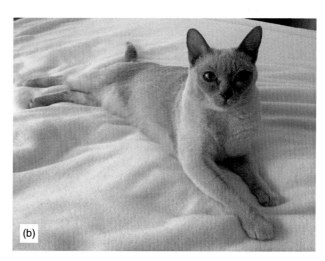

Figure 2.25 Examples of (a) a champagne mink Tonkinese and (b) a platinum mink Tonkinese.

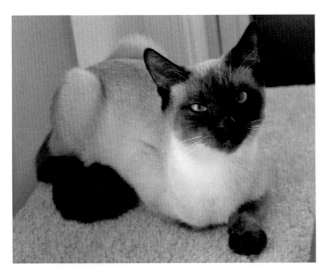

Figure 2.26 An example of a cat that is both a seal point and a tabby. Source: Courtesy of Erika Olney.

present to corroborate his suspicions, he can perform the following table-side test:

- Sprinkle the debris on a paper towel.
- Add a few drops of water or alcohol to the debris.
- Fold the paper towel.
- Rub vigorously.

If the debris is in fact flea dirt, the veterinarian will notice a rusty brown pigment that forms on the paper towel as the dried blood is moistened.

However, fleas are not the only ectoparasite that can cause fur-mowing. Feline demodicosis, notoedric mange, and cheyletiellosis may also induce varying degrees of pruritus that can then lead to fur loss. In these cases, other abnormalities on the physical examination may lead the clinician to suspect an underlying parasitic dermatopathy. For instance, patients that are infested with *Cheyletiella* mites classically exhibit excessive scale on their coat. This classic appearance, localized to the topline of the cat, led to the condition being referred by laymen as "walking dandruff" [48]. When it is suspected, "walking dandruff" needs to be differentiated from ordinary dandruff, which also frequently localizes to the topline (Figure 2.33). This is easily achieved through the gross observation of mites when the "dandruff" is combed out onto dark paper and the "dandruff" appears to move freely or via microscopy: the evaluation of "scale" under the light microscope will allow for detection of *Cheyletiella* mites.

Fur-mowing can also be psychogenic in origin, meaning that the skin condition is self-induced without an underlying primary dermatologic disease [48–50]. These so-called psychocutaneous disorders may stem from anxiety or compulsion, and are typically diagnoses of exclusion. It is important not to label fur-mowing as psychogenic

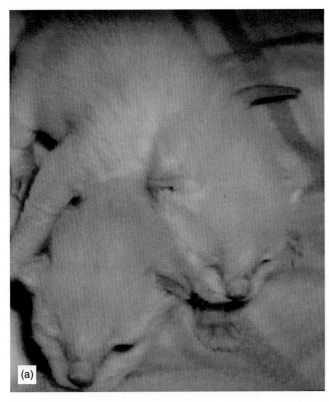

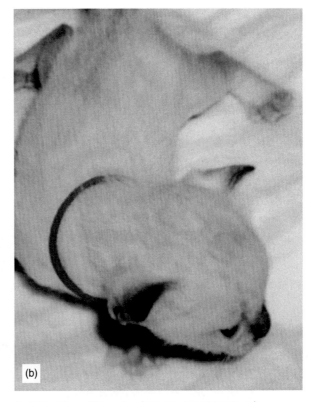

Figure 2.27 (a) A 1-week old Tonkinese kitten, without points; (b) 2–3-week old Tonkinese kitten, developing points; (*Continued*)

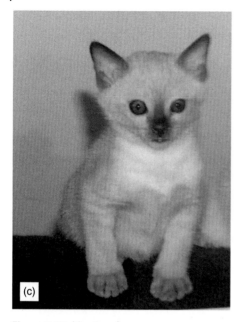

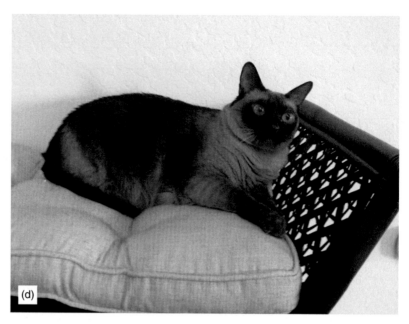

Figure 2.27 (*Continued*)
(c) 2-month-old Tonkinese, developing points; (d) 10-year-old Tonkinese, with points established.

until other primary dermatologic disease is effectively ruled out. Differential diagnoses for fur-mowing include bacterial, parasitic, or fungal folliculitis, ectoparasite infestation, endocrinopathy, paraneoplastic syndromes, eosinophilic granuloma complex, and atopy [49].

Fur-mowing may or may not be obvious. Sometimes it requires a very thorough inspection of the coat to identify very small lesions (Figure 2.34).

2.7 Inspecting the Skin

The skin should be thoroughly examined in order to make an assessment of whether or not it is normal for the patient. This evaluation should consider skin integrity, skin color, and other skin lesions.

Skin integrity refers to whether or not the skin is abraded and, if so, to what extent. Disrupted skin integrity is often the result of external trauma; however, it may also be self induced (Figure 2.35).

A thorough assessment of the skin as a whole should also take into account what is considered normal pigmentation for the patient versus abnormal discoloration. In particular, the clinician should screen for any areas of active bruising, as this is reflective of either an injury to the underlying soft tissues or coagulopathy. In the case of the former, it is important to recognize that the sustained injury can be from an underlying disease process or can be iatrogenic (Figure 2.36).

In addition to bruising, another form of discoloration to the skin that should be identified on physical examination is icterus. Icterus is the yellowish

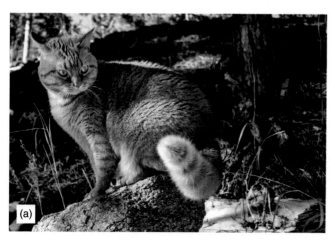

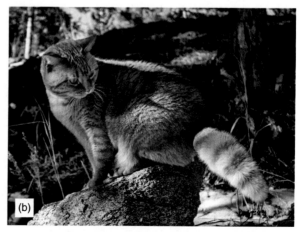

Figure 2.28 (a) Orange tabby demonstrating piloerection of the tail. Note what the ear carriage says about the patient's tolerance of the situation. (b) Second view of the orange tabby demonstrating piloerection of the tail. The ears are now pointing toward the perceived threat and the situation is de-escalating, although the tail will take time to reverse the piloerection. Source (a), (b): Courtesy of Jesse Hartlein.

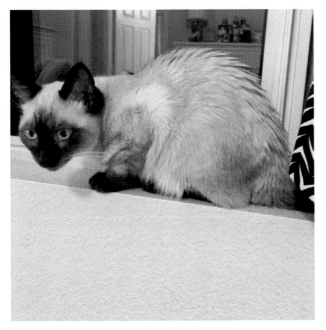

Figure 2.29 Young Siamese cat demonstrating piloerection along its topline after being startled. Source: Courtesy of Natalie Reeser.

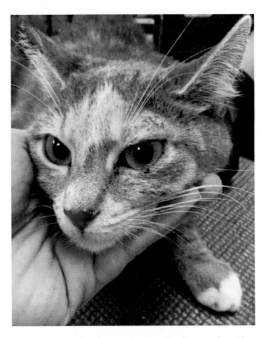

Figure 2.31 Peri-ocular alopecia in a cat is abnormal until proven otherwise.

discoloration of the body. In human medicine, it is sometimes referred to as jaundice. Unlike bruising, which is caused by damaged vessels that lead to blood accumulation under the skin, icterus is the result of excessive bilirubin. Icterus may be present due to increased hemolysis, liver disease, or biliary tract obstruction. On the skin of a cat, the easiest location in which to identify icterus is the peri-aural region owing to its naturally alopecic state. However, icterus can be identified elsewhere when the underlying disease process is advanced (Figure 2.37).

Another pigmentary abnormality that should be identified if present on physical examination is lentigo. Lentigo is a benign condition that occurs in both dogs and cats in which there is "freckling" of black pigment on the skin. In dogs, this is a common occurrence, especially along the ventrum. By contrast, lentigo is infrequently seen in cats. When it does occur in cats, it tends to be

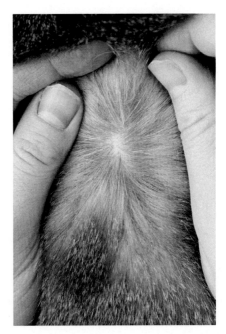

Figure 2.32 This patient does not have flea dirt, but the process of parting the fur to look for evidence of it helps to confirm its absence.

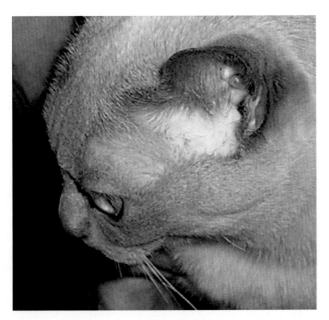

Figure 2.30 Normal peri-aural alopecia in a cat.

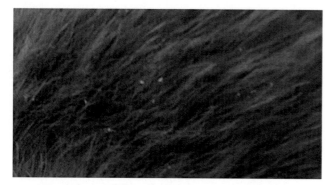

Figure 2.33 This patient has dandruff along the topline due to dry skin as opposed to "walking dandruff"; however, it may be initially challenging upon gross inspection to tell the two apart.

associated with orange coat colors and the freckles appear to be concentrated on the eyelids, lips, gingiva, or pinnae (Figure 2.38) [48]. Lentigo is one example of a primary skin lesion called a macule, a flat area that is different in color from the surrounding skin.

There are several other types of primary skin lesions that should be identified if present on the physical examination [51, 52]:

- *Papule:* a small elevation of the skin, typically less than 0.25 cm (Figure 2.39a).
- *Nodule:* a papule that is large, typically measuring up to 1 cm in diameter (Figure 2.39b).
- *Tumor:* a nodule that is large, typically measuring greater than 1 cm in diameter (Figure 2.39c).
- *Pustule:* a pus-filled papule ("a pimple").
- *Vesicle:* an elevation that is fluid filled but devoid of purulent material.
- *Bullae:* a large vesicle, typically greater than 0.5 cm.
- *Wheal:* a focal allergic reaction.

- *Plaque:* an elevation with a flat rather than rounded top.

Secondary skin lesions should also be identified if present on physical examination and include [51, 52]:

- *Scale:* loose flakes of skin ("dandruff").
- *Collarette:* what is left after a pustule ruptures.
- *Crust:* dried exudate and keratin that forms over the skin's surface.
- *Scab:* dried fibrin and platelet plug that caps the surface of a wound, under which a new layer of skin begins to form (Figure 2.40).
- *Comedone:* a plug of oil and dead skin cells at the surface of a pore ("a blackhead").
- *Lichenification:* abnormally thick, leathery skin that typically signifies chronic skin irritation, inflammation, and/or infection.
- *Hyperpigmentation:* dark gray to black discoloration of the skin that typically signifies chronic skin irritation, inflammation, and/or infection.

When lesions are identified and recorded in the medical record, the veterinarian should be as descriptive as possible and should take care to document the following:

- the number of lesions;
- the size of the lesions;
- the location of the lesions;
- the configuration of the lesions;
- the progression of the lesions, either as reported by the history or as observed if this is a recheck examination.

A "skin map" may be used to keep track of lesions as they develop, progress, and/or resolve. When recording the size of the lesions, be accurate. Always measure with calipers rather than "guesstimating." The location

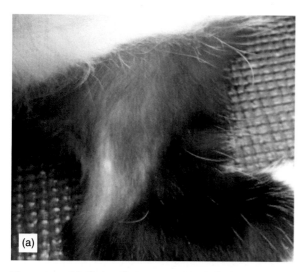
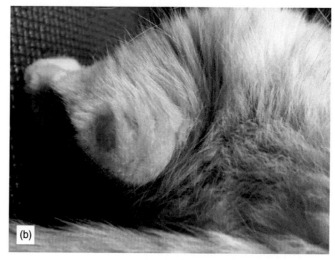

Figure 2.34 (a) Obvious fur-mowing along the left medial thigh of this feline patient. Source: Courtesy of Elizabeth Robbins, DVM. (b) Obvious fur-mowing distal to the left hock of this feline patient. (*Continued*)

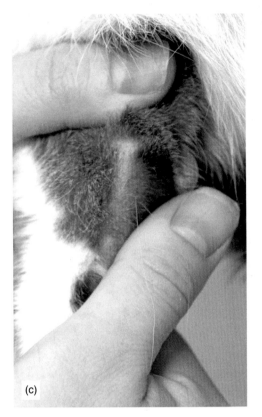

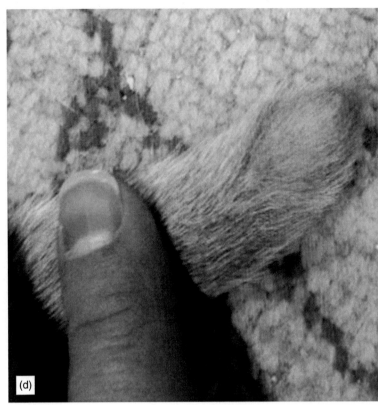

Figure 2.34 (*Continued*) (c) Fur-mowing extending from the left hock to the metacarpal pad. Source: Courtesy of the Media Resources Department at Midwestern University. (d) Fur-mowing of the tail tip.

of lesions is especially important because it can lead the clinician to pursue certain differential diagnoses and may prompt them to expand the history-taking portion of the examination in order to solidify the list of differentials. For instance, the presence of papules, pustules, and/or comedones at the chin of a cat may be consistent with chin acne [53, 54].

The head, neck, and torso are relatively easy to remember when evaluating the skin, but paws and claws are often forgotten. It is important to examine both in order to evaluate for abrasions and other evidence of wear and tear.

Start by examining the paws with the claws in their retracted state (Figure 2.41). Once the paws have been thoroughly examined, including both dorsal and palmar/plantar surfaces, extend the claws. Applying firm, yet gentle pressure to the base of each toe will facilitate this process. With the claws extended, the veterinarian can

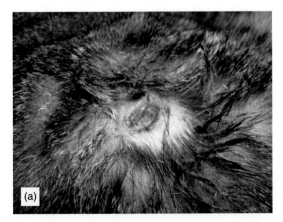

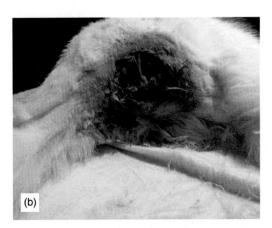

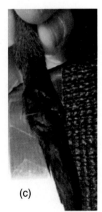

Figure 2.35 (a) Full-thickness traumatic skin injury located along the right lateral thorax of a cat. Source: Courtesy of Patricia Bennett, DVM. (b) Open perineal wound with multiple draining tracts. Note the bruising discoloration around the periphery of the wound. Source: Courtesy of Daniel Foy, MS, DVM, DACVIM, DACVECC. (c) Open wound located mid-shaft along the tail. (*Continued*)

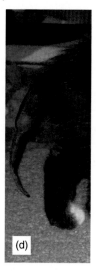
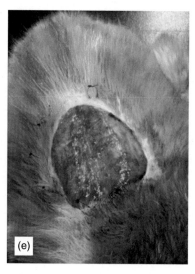
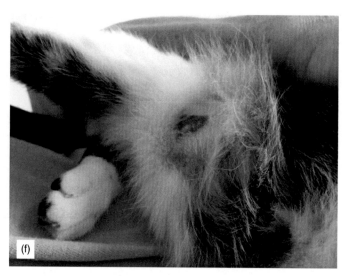

Figure 2.35 (*Continued*) (d) De-gloving injury to the tail. The distal half of the tail is leathery in texture and non-viable. It will likely require amputation. Source: Courtesy of Juliane Daggett, MBS. (e) Chronic non-healing wound on the dorsum of a cat. Source: Courtesy of Andrew Weisenfeld, DVM. (f) Self-induced superficial abrasion located along the cat's ventrum. This patient had been over-grooming and created this disruption in skin integrity. Source: Courtesy of Elizabeth Robbins, DVM.

assess whether or not they are brittle and flaky, or abnormally thickened. The latter is common in many geriatric and hyperthyroid patients (Figure 2.42).

If there are overgrown claws growing directly into the digital pads, these need to be addressed. Identify the vessel that runs down the center of each claw. This is the vessel that clients often nick when trimming claws too close. When the vessel is nicked, the claw bleeds. Clients who want to learn how to trim their cats' claws should be advised to avoid this vessel (Figure 2.43).

Another important aspect of the examination is counting the claws: are there too many? Polydactyl cats have extra toes (Figure 2.44). There are often extra claws in addition to the extra toes. These cats are most at risk of having their claws overgrow into the digital pads because there are more toes and claws crammed into the same amount of paw space as there is in a non-polydactyl cat.

The paw pads should also be examined (Figure 2.45). Check for burns. Cats that are countertop "surfers" may walk on a hot stove, burn their pads, and present for lameness.

Check for paw pad cracks and associated sensitivities to palpation. Cracks could be the result of "normal" wear-and-tear, but certain autoimmune diseases such as pemphigus foliaceus can cause these fissures [48, 52].

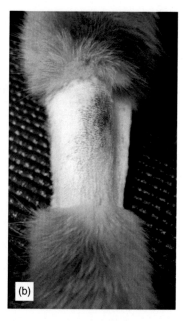

Figure 2.36 (a) Peri-anal erythema and bruising over the left anal gland due to the traumatic rupture of an anal gland abscess. (b) Iatrogenic bruising over the cephalic vein in the forearm of a cat due to unsuccessful IV catheter placement.

Some cats have excess fur between their toes (Figure 2.46). This is normal. However, it is important to examine these "feathers" because the excess fur could be a site that attracts clumping litter, burrs, and matts.

Finally, the mammary chain tends to be ignored when completing a "thorough" physical examination. This is likely because many of our feline patients undergo pre-pubescent ovariohysterectomy and therefore do not have prominent nipples to cue the veterinarian's attention to the ventrum. As a result, the mammary chain very often becomes an afterthought. That being said, mammary neoplasia is a significant concern in both female and

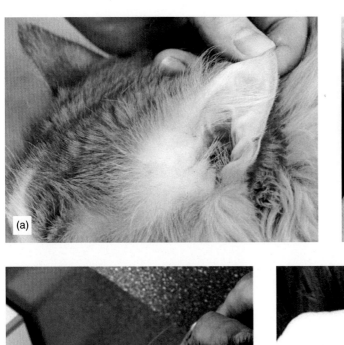
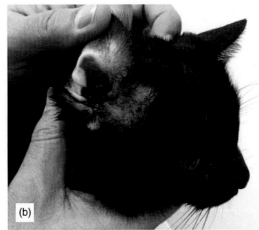
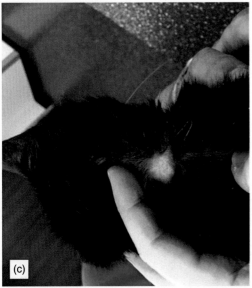
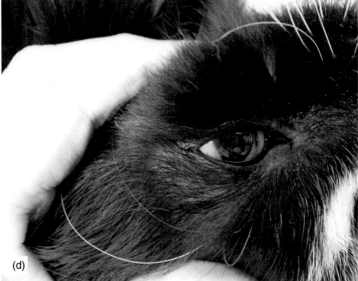

Figure 2.37 (a) This patient is non-icteric in the peri-aural region. Source: Courtesy of the Media Resources Department at Midwestern University. (b) This patient is icteric in the peri-aural region. (c) This patient has generalized icterus that is apparent at the base of the neck when fur has been parted to the side to allow the clinician to visualize the skin. (d) This patient has peri-ocular icterus. Source: Courtesy of Samantha Thurman, DVM.

male cats in that when it occurs, the chance of malignancy is between 85 and 93% [55].

Cats typically have four sets of mammary glands for a total of eight glands and their associated nipples [51]. The integrity of the nipples should be appreciated, taking care to note any peri-areolar abrasions, and both mammary chains (the left and the right side of the ventrum) in males and females should be palpated along their entire length. Note that it is difficult to see the nipples because cats, unlike dogs, tend to have a ventral abdomen full of fur (Figure 2.47). In order to visualize each nipple in a prepubescent female cat or a cat that has not had multiple litters, the fur must be parted (Figure 2.48). When a cat has had several litters of kittens, the nipples become much more prominent and the fur no longer requires parting in order to visualize them (Figure 2.49).

It is also important to evaluate each nipple for peri-areolar dermatitis (Figure 2.50). This can be a clinical sign of autoimmune disease in cats. It can also be a sign of compulsive self-mutilation as from over-grooming.

Additionally, in the lactating female cat, the veterinarian should assess each mammary gland for asymmetry, swelling, redness, discharge, or heat on palpation. The presence of one or more of these findings may indicate mastitis. If the patient is tolerant, the clinician may also take care to express each gland to make sure that the patient is producing milk and to evaluate the milk's consistency [51, 56].

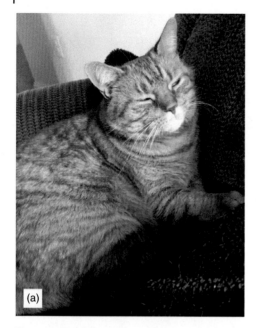
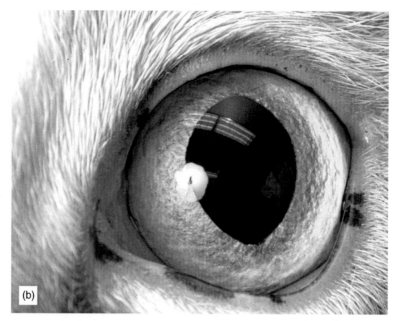

Figure 2.38 (a) Cats with an orange coat color are more likely to develop lentigo. (b) Lentigo associated with the eyelids. Source: Courtesy of the Media Resources Department at Midwestern University.

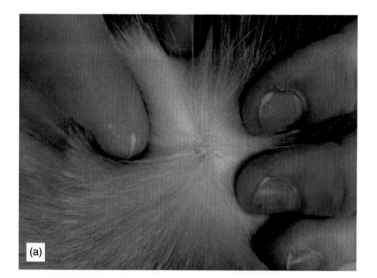
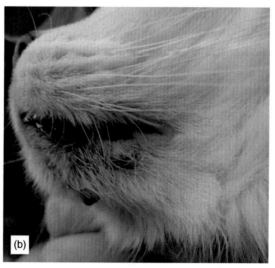

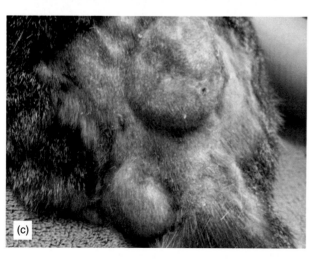

Figure 2.39 (a) Example of an inter-scapular papule. Source: Courtesy of Patricia Bennett, DVM. (b) Example of several ventral chin nodules. Source: Courtesy of Elizabeth Robbins, DVM. (c) Example of multiple cutaneous tumors along the dorsum and to the left of the tail base that were subsequently diagnosed as apocrine ductular adenomas. Source: Courtesy of Samantha Thurman, DVM.

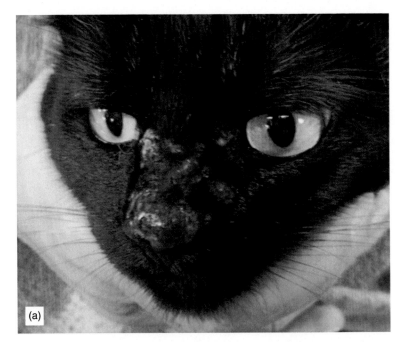
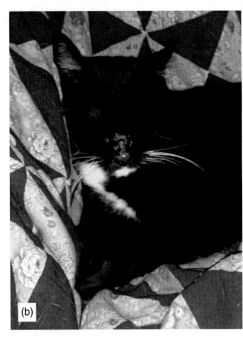

Figure 2.40 (a) Fresh wound with scabs over the bridge of the nose of a cat with mosquito bite hypersensitivity. Source: Courtesy of Elizabeth Robbins, DVM. (b) This cat also has mosquito bite hypersensitivity but is further along in the healing process. Note that there are still a number of scabs on the nasal planum. Source: Courtesy of Julianne Daggett.

Figure 2.41 (a) Lateral view and (b) aerial view of forepaw with claws retracted. Source (a), (b): Courtesy of the Media Resources Department at Midwestern University.

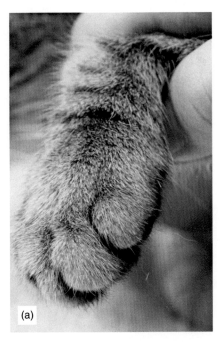
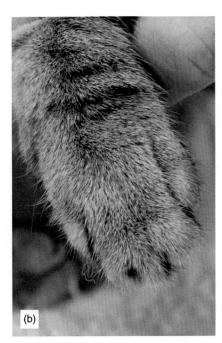

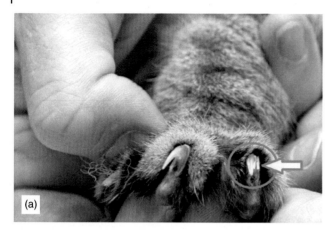

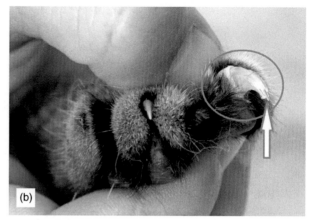

Figure 2.42 (a) Extending the claws reveals that one claw is frayed at the lateral margin. (b) Lateral view of the frayed claw. This could easily become snagged on something in the environment and should be trimmed. Source (a), (b): Courtesy of the Media Resources Department at Midwestern University.

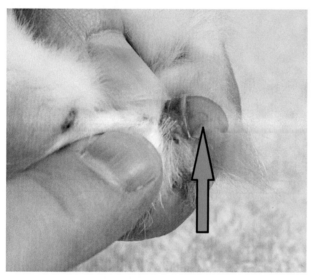

Figure 2.43 Lateral view of cat claw demonstrating central vessel. Source: Courtesy of the Media Resources Department at Midwestern University.

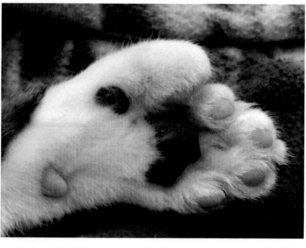

Figure 2.44 Plantar aspect of the hind paw of a polydactyl cat. Rather than having four toes on each hind limb, this patient has five. The additional toe has a claw that is retracted and therefore out of view. Source: Courtesy of Karen Burks, DVM.

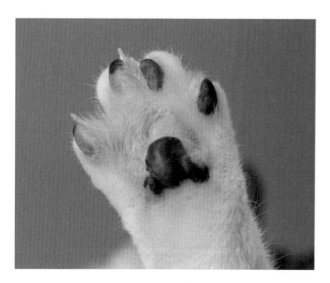

Figure 2.45 Plantar aspect of the cat's hind paw, demonstrating digital and tarsal paw pads. Note the mottled paw pad pigmentation, which is normal for this particular patient. Source: Courtesy of the Media Resources Department at Midwestern University.

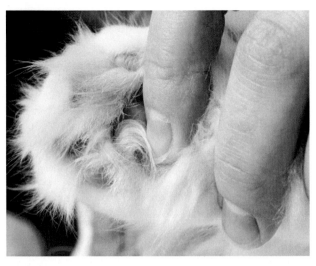

Figure 2.46 Ventral aspect of the paw, demonstrating a variation of normal in medium- to long-haired cats that have tufts of fur between their toes. Source: Courtesy of the Media Resources Department at Midwestern University.

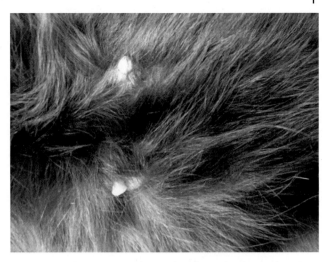

Figure 2.49 Prominent nipples in a female cat that has had multiple litters in the past. Source: Courtesy of the Media Resources Department at Midwestern University.

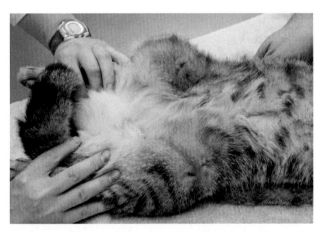

Figure 2.47 The ventrum of a feline patient. Note how the furred abdomen obscures the nipples from view. Source: Courtesy of the Media Resources Department at Midwestern University.

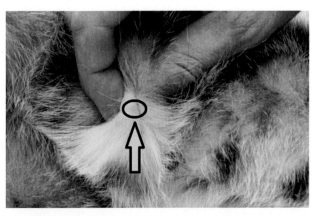

Figure 2.48 Parting the fur on the ventrum brings the nipples into view. Source: Courtesy of the Media Resources Department at Midwestern University.

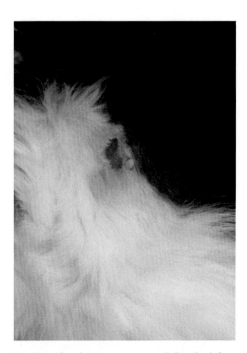

Figure 2.50 Note the abrasion cranio-medial to the left mammary chain due to excessive licking by a cat without evidence of any underlying primary skin disease. Source: Courtesy of the Media Resources Department at Midwestern University.

References

1 Weiss, E., Slater, M., and Lord, L. (2012) Frequency of lost dogs and cats in the United States and the methods used to locate them. *Animals*, **2** (2), 301–315.

2 Humane Society of the United States (2016) *Pets by the Numbers: U.S. Pet Ownership, Community Cat and Shelter Population Estimates*, http://www.humanesociety.org/issues/pet_overpopulation/facts/pet_ownership_statistics.html (accessed 11 April 2016).

3 Lord, L.K., Griffin, B., Slater, M.R., and Levy, J.K. (2010) Evaluation of collars and microchips for visual and permanent identification of pet cats. *Journal of the American Veterinary Medical Association*, **237** (4), 387–394.

4 Lord, L.K., Wittum, T.E., Ferketich, A.K. *et al.* (2007) Search and identification methods that owners use to find a lost cat. *Journal of the American Veterinary Medical Association*, **230** (2), 217–220.

5 Lord, L.K. (2008) Attitudes toward and perceptions of free-roaming cats among individuals living in Ohio. *Journal of the American Veterinary Medical Association*, **232** (8), 1159–1167.

6 Lord, L.K., Ingwersen, W., Gray, J.L., and Wintz, D.J. (2009) Characterization of animals with microchips entering animal shelters. *Journal of the American Veterinary Medical Association*, **235** (2), 160–167.

7 Dingman, P.A., Levy, J.K., Rockey, L.E., and Crandall, M.M. (2014) Use of visual and permanent identification for pets by veterinary clinics. *Veterinary Journal*, **201** (1), 46–50.

8 Bjornvad, C.R., Nielsen, D.H., Armstrong, P.J. *et al.* (2011) Evaluation of a nine-point body condition scoring system in physically inactive pet cats. *American Journal of Veterinary Research*, **72** (4), 433–437.

9 Scarlett, J.M. and Donoghue, S. (1998) Associations between body condition and disease in cats. *Journal of the American Veterinary Medical Association*, **212** (11), 1725–1731.

10 Shoveller, A.K., DiGennaro, J., Lanman, C., and Spangler, D. (2014) Trained vs untrained evaluator assessment of body condition score as a predictor of percent body fat in adult cats. *Journal of Feline Medicine and Surgery*, **16** (12), 957–965.

11 Michel, K. and Scherk, M. (2012) From problem to success: feline weight loss programs that work. *Journal of Feline Medicine and Surgery*, **14** (5), 327–336.

12 Lund, E., Armstrong, P.J., Kirk, C. *et al.* (2005) Prevalence and risk factors for obesity in adult cats from private US veterinary practices. *International Journal of Applied Research in Veterinary Medicine*, **3** (2), 88–96.

13 German, A.J. (2006) The growing problem of obesity in dogs and cats. *Journal of Nutrition*, **136** (7 Suppl.), 1940S–1946S.

14 Doria-Rose, V.P. and Scarlett, J.M. (2000) Mortality rates and causes of death among emaciated cats. *Journal of the American Veterinary Medical Association*, **216** (3), 347–351.

15 Freeman, L.M. (2012) Cachexia and sarcopenia: emerging syndromes of importance in dogs and cats. *Journal of Veterinary Internal Medicine*, **26** (1), 3–17.

16 Mallery, K.F., Freeman, L.M., Harpster, N.K., and Rush, J.E. (1999) Factors contributing to the decision for euthanasia of dogs with congestive heart failure. *Journal of the American Veterinary Medical Association*, **214** (8), 1201–1204.

17 Laflamme, D. (1997) Development and validation of a body condition score system for cats: a clinical tool. *Feline Practice*, **25** (5–6), 13–18.

18 Burkholder, W.J. (2000) Use of body condition scores in clinical assessment of the provision of optimal nutrition. *Journal of the American Veterinary Medical Association*, **217** (5), 650–654.

19 Sandoe, P., Palmer, C., Corr, S. *et al.* (2014) Canine and feline obesity: a One Health perspective. *Veterinary Record*, **175** (24), 610–616.

20 Kienzle, E. and Bergler, R. (2006) Human–animal relationship of owners of normal and overweight cats. *Journal of Nutrition*, **136** (7 Suppl.), 1947S–1950S.

21 Singh, R., Laflamme, P., and Sidebottom-Nielsen, M. (2002) Owner perceptions of body condition score. *Journal of Veterinary Internal Medicine*, **16**, 362.

22 DiBartola, S.P. and Bateman, S. (2006) Introduction to fluid therapy, in *Fluid, Electrolyte, and Acid–Base Disorders in Small Animal Practice*, 3rd edn. (ed. S.P. DiBartola), Saunders Elsevier, St. Louis, pp. 325–344.

23 Genovese, D.W., Johnson, T.L., Lamb, K.E., and Gram, W.D. (2014) Histological and dermatoscopic description of sphynx cat skin. *Veterinary Dermatology*, **25** (6), 523–529, e89–e90.

24 Siegal, M. and Richards, J.R. (1997) *The Cornell Book of Cats: A Comprehensive and Authoritative Medical Reference for Every Cat and Kitten*, 2nd edn., Villard Books, New York.

25 Edwards, A. (2004) *The Ultimate Encyclopedia of Cats, Cat Breeds and Cat Care*, Lorenz Books, New York.

26 Gandolfi, B., Alhaddad, H., Affolter, V.K. *et al.* (2013) To the root of the curl: a signature of a recent selective sweep identifies a mutation that defines the Cornish Rex cat breed. *PLoS One*, **8** (6), e67105.

27 Stokking, L.B. and Campbell, K.C. (2004) Disorders of pigmentation, in *Small Animal Dermatology Secrets* (ed. K.C. Campbell), Hanley & Belfus, Philadelphia, pp. 352–355.

28 Cat Fanciers Association (2016) *Cat Colors FAQ: Cat Color Genetics*, http://www.fanciers.com/other-faqs/color-genetics.html (accessed 12 April 2016).

29 Cvejic, D., Steinberg, T.A., Kent, M.S., and Fischer, A. (2009) Unilateral and bilateral congenital sensorineural deafness in client-owned pure-breed white cats. *Journal of Veterinary Internal Medicine*, **23** (2), 392–395.

30 Strain, G.M. (1999) Congenital deafness and its recognition. *Veterinary Clinics of North America: Small Animal Practice*, **29** (4), 895–907, vi.

31 Luttgen, P.J. (1994) Deafness in the dog and cat. *Veterinary Clinics of North America: Small Animal Practice*, **24** (5), 981–989.

32 Strain, G.M. (2007) Deafness in blue-eyed white cats: the uphill road to solving polygenic disorders. *Veterinary Journal*, **173** (3), 471–472.

33 Geigy, C.A., Heid, S., Steffen, F. et al. (2007) Does a pleiotropic gene explain deafness and blue irises in white cats? *Veterinary Journal*, **173** (3), 548–553.

34 Bergsma, D.R. and Brown, K.S. (1971) White fur, blue eyes, and deafness in the domestic cat. *Journal of Heredity*, **62** (3), 171–185.

35 Griffin, B. (2011) *Cat Identification*, http:// sheltermedicine.vetmed.ufl.edu/files/2011/11/ identification-and-coat-colors-patterns.pdf (accessed 12 April 2016).

36 Lomax, T.D. and Robinson, R. (1988) Tabby pattern alleles of the domestic cat. *Journal of Heredity*, **79** (1), 21–23.

37 Kaelin, C. and Barsh, G. (2010) Tabby pattern genetics – a whole new breed of cat. *Pigment Cell and Melanoma Research*, **23** (4), 514–516.

38 Prieur, D.J. and Collier, L.L. (1981) Morphologic basis of inherited coat-color dilutions of cats. *Journal of Heredity*, **72** (3), 178–182.

39 University of Miami (2016) *The Genetics of Calico Cats*, http://www.bio.miami.edu/dana/dox/calico.html (accessed 12 April 2016).

40 The Tech Museum of Innovation (2005) *Other Genetic Principles*, http://genetics.thetech.org/ask/ask141 (accessed 12 April 2016).

41 Stelow, E.A., Bain, M.J., and Kass, P.H. (2016) The relationship between coat color and aggressive behaviors in the domestic cat. *Journal of Applied Animal Welfare Science*, **19** (1), 1–15.

42 Centerwall, W.R. and Benirschke, K. (1975) An animal model for the XXY Klinefelter's syndrome in man: tortoiseshell and calico male cats. *American Journal of Veterinary Research*, **36** (9), 1275–1280.

43 Pedersen, A.S., Berg, L.C., Almstrup, K., and Thomsen, P.D. (2014) A tortoiseshell male cat: chromosome analysis and histologic examination of the testis. *Cytogenetic and Genome Research*, **142** (2), 107–111.

44 Lyons, L.A., Imes, D.L., Rah, H.C., and Grahn, R.A. (2005) Tyrosinase mutations associated with Siamese and Burmese patterns in the domestic cat (*Felis catus*). *Animal Genetics*, **36** (2), 119–126.

45 Ye, X.C., Pegado, V., Patel, M.S., and Wasserman, W.W. (2014) Strabismus genetics across a spectrum of eye misalignment disorders. *Clinical Genetics*, **86** (2), 103–111.

46 Gebhardt, R.H., Pond, G., and Raleigh, I. (1979) *A Standard Guide to Cat Breeds*, McGraw-Hill, New York.

47 Overall, K.L. (1997) *Clinical Behavioral Medicine for Small Animals*, Mosby, St. Louis.

48 Medleau, L. and Hnilica, K.A. (2006) *Small Animal Dermatology: A Color Atlas and Therapeutic Guide*, 2nd edn., Saunders Elsevier, St. Louis.

49 Patterson, A.P. (2004) *Psychocutaneous Disorders. Small Animal Dermatology Secrets*, Hanley & Belfus, Philadelphia, pp. 324–332.

50 Schaer, M. (2011) *Clinical Medicine of the Dog and Cat*, 2nd edn., Manson, London.

51 Rijnberk, A. and van Sluijs, F.J. (eds.) (2009) *Medical History and Physical Examination in Companion Animals*, 2nd edn. Saunders Elsevier, St. Louis.

52 Miller, W.H., Griffin, C.E., Campbell, K.L. et al. (2013) *Muller & Kirk's Small Animal Dermatology*, 7th edn., Elsevier, St. Louis.

53 Jazic, E., Coyner, K.S., Loeffler, D.G., and Lewis, T.P. (2006) An evaluation of the clinical, cytological, infectious and histopathological features of feline acne. *Veterinary Dermatology*, **17** (2), 134–140.

54 Moriello, K.A. (2012) *Feline skin diseases, in The Cat: Clinical Medicine and Management* (ed. S.E. Little), Saunders, St. Louis, pp. 398–399.

55 Lana, S.E., Rutteman, G.R., and Withrow, S.J. (2007) *Tumors of the mammary gland, in Withrow & MacEwen's Small Animal Clinical Oncology*, 4th edn. (eds. S.J. Withrow and D.M. Vail), Saunders, St. Louis, p. 629.

56 Johnston, S.D. and Hayden, D.W. (1980) Non-neoplastic disorders of the mammary glands, in *Current Veterinary Therapy VII* (ed. R.W. Kirk), Saunders, Philadelphia, pp. 1224–1226.

3

Examining the Head of the Cat

3.1 Skull Shape and Facial Symmetry

The skull serves two main functions: its rostral aspect is the foundation upon which the face is built, and the caudal aspect protects the central nervous system [1, 2]. Skull shapes evolved to match structure to function [3]. Accordingly, skull shape varies between species [1]. The skull of the modern cat is adapted to support predation by providing the infrastructure that allows for a bite that kills with precision [3–5] (Figure 3.1). However, there is great variety in skull shape that has led to breed-specific traits and predispositions to disease [6, 7].

Two phenotypically distinct skull types in the domestic cat have been recognized, namely mesocephalic and brachycephalic, of which the Persian cat is a prime example [8]. The European Shorthairs are considered to be sandwiched somewhere in between [6] (Figure 3.2).

The brachycephalic skull has a shortened face of decreased width, a reduced brain case, and open orbits [7, 9]. This creates a child-like face that is extremely popular among cat enthusiasts of the Persian and Exotic Shorthair breeds [9]. However, extreme facial distortion is required to achieve this appearance. The anatomical implications of this skull shape are vast: the brachycephalic breeds of cat are medically predisposed to a number of health conditions, which range in severity from minor to life-threatening [10].

The foreshortened face prevents the nasolacrimal duct from staying on course. The more severe the brachycephaly, the more likely it is that the nasolacrimal duct does not line up with the lacrimal foramen, hindering tear drainage [9, 11]. Epiphora with facial dermatitis is commonplace in Persians and other brachycephalic cats [9, 12]. Furthermore, the orbits are open and shallow, which predisposes the brachycephalic cat to exophthalmos [10], exposure keratitis, and the formation of corneal sequestra [13].

The abnormal eruption of teeth, the dorsal displacement of maxillary teeth, and the development of extreme underbites adversely impact prehension of food, leading to increased risk of periodontal disease [10], and brachycephalic cats often have impaired breathing through their stenotic nares. They may also be predisposed to airway obstruction due to other structural components of brachycephalic syndrome [12], and their incidence of dystocia is increased compared with mesocephalic cats [14].

It is the responsibility of the veterinary team to recognize the link between skull shape and breed-associated medical concerns, and to anticipate the level of care that such a patient may require. This then needs to be articulated to the client so that breeders and cat-owners may anticipate the care necessary to maintain good quality of life [9].

Once skull shape has been identified and recorded, the veterinarian should shift focus to assess for facial symmetry. Facial symmetry can be a challenge if the patient's posture is such that it is crouched or tucking up the head and neck into its body (Figure 3.3); keep in mind that it is not uncommon for a scared cat to hunch or tuck up its head and neck.

When it is possible to view the cat from the front without it perceiving the clinician to be a direct threat, the clinician should evaluate for asymmetry of the head (Figure 3.4).

The presence of a head tilt may indicate compromised neurologic status. Similarly, drooped lips, ears, and eyelids, especially when assymetrical, are concerning and should be noted in the medical record.

A deviated nasal philtrum may indicate the presence of primary neoplasia (Figure 3.5a) or trauma (Figure 3.5b). In the case of the latter, there are likely to be additional physical examination clues, such as cuts or scrapes, bite wounds, and the presence of blood, fresh or dried.

3.2 The Eyes and Accessory Visual Structures

3.2.1 A Systematic Approach to the Eye Examination

Examination of the eyes and their adnexa should be performed in every patient using a systematic approach, even in the absence of an ocular presenting complaint. In the event that a unilateral ocular concern is raised by the client, the examination should still include both eyes to be thorough. It may be that the contralateral eye is also

Performing the Small Animal Physical Examination, First Edition. Ryane E. Englar.
© 2017 John Wiley & Sons, Inc. Published 2017 by John Wiley & Sons, Inc.

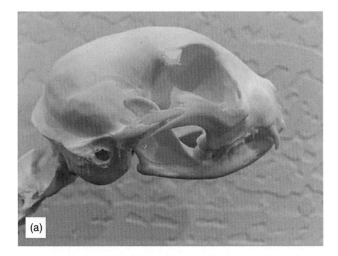

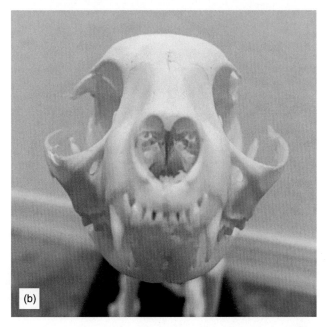

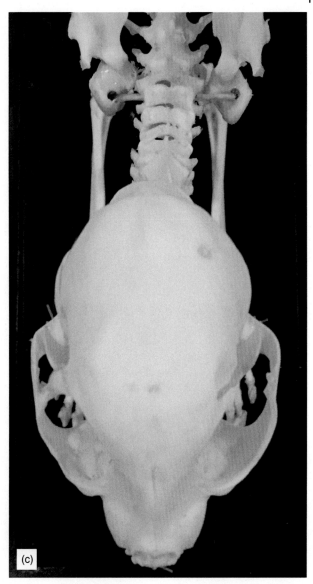

Figure 3.1 (a) Lateral aspect, (b) head-on view, and (c) aerial view of a skull model of the domestic cat.

affected, but that there has been a lag phase in demonstrating sufficient clinical signs to flag the attention of the client [15–18].

When clients do present cats for an ophthalmologic complaint, one or more of the following symptoms are classically reported [19–21]:

- "red eye";
- "cloudy eye";
- "bulging eye";
- vision loss;
- ocular discharge;
- blepharospasm (squinting);
- photophobia (light sensitivity);
- pawing at one or both eyes;
- rubbing one or both sides of the face on the carpet.

When taking a history, the clinician should question the client about duration (how long has the issue been present?) and progression (is the issue getting worse?). It is also important to understand what, if anything, led up to the issue, and whether the patient is indoor-only, indoor–outdoor, or outdoor-only, as lifestyle assists with an assessment of to what or to whom the patient may have been exposed. Finally, the veterinarian should inquire as to whether the presenting issue is a new complaint, a recurrent issue, or one that has persisted, meaning that it has never resolved [19].

3.2.2 Evaluating the Adnexa of the Eye

After taking a thorough history, the "eye exam" may commence. Before evaluating the globes themselves, the

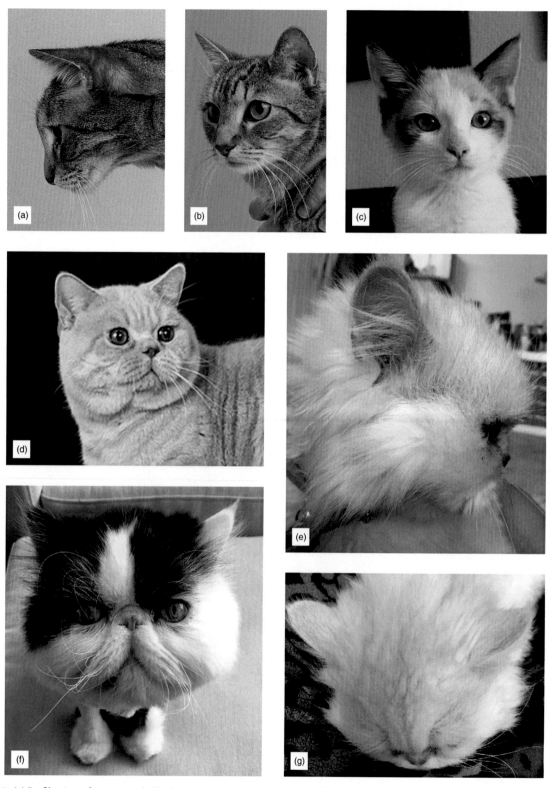

Figure 3.2 (a) Profile view of a mesocephalic domestic shorthaired cat. Source: Courtesy of the Media Resources Department at Midwestern University. (b) Three-quarter view of a mesocephalic domestic shorthaired cat. Source: Courtesy of the Media Resources Department at Midwestern University. (c) Head-on view of a mesocephalic cat. Source: Courtesy of Arielle Hatcher. (d) Three-quarter view of a British Shorthair cat. Note how the facial structure is rounder than in the domestic shorthaired cat. However, it is not as foreshortened as in the brachycephalic cats pictured in parts (e), (f), and (g). Source: Courtesy of Cheryl A. Kelly. (e) Profile view of a brachycephalic Persian cat. Source: Courtesy of Madison Lea Skelton. (f) Head-on view of a brachycephalic Persian cat. Source: Courtesy of Lai-Ting Torres. (g) Aerial view of a brachycephalic Persian cat. Source: Courtesy of Madison Lea Skelton. Note the foreshortened face.

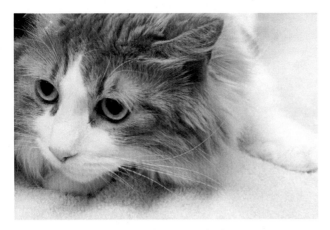

Figure 3.3 The patient is in a frozen, hunched position, most likely attributable to fear. It is difficult to assess facial symmetry in this state because the patient is strongly motivated to lean away and avert eye contact. Source: Courtesy of the Media Resources Department at Midwestern University.

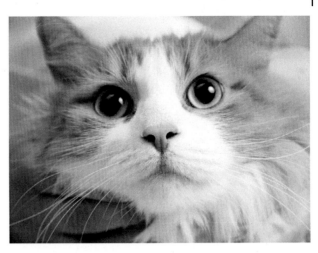

Figure 3.4 Evaluating the head and face for symmetry. There is no apparent facial asymmetry in this patient. Source: Courtesy of the Media Resources Department at Midwestern University.

adnexa of the eye should first be examined. The adnexa include the eyelids, lacrimal apparatus, the nictitating membrane, and the conjunctiva (Figure 3.6).

With regard to the eyelids, the veterinarian should note whether they are present, partially present, or absent [21] (Figure 3.7). If present, do they roll inward (entropion) or do they curl out (ectropion)? [18, 21, 22]. The eyelids should be also evaluated for redness (Figure 3.8).

Further, is there blepharospasm of the eyelids that may suggest light sensitivity or ocular pain? (Figure 3.9). If blepharospasm is present, is it associated with ocular discharge? When noting ocular discharge, one must take care to differentiate what is normal for the patient from what is pathologic. For some patients, epiphora is "normal" and they have experienced tear overflow for their entire life. These patients may have "tear stripes" – a

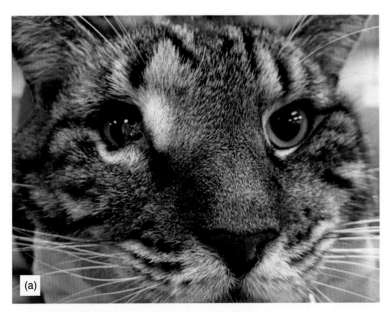

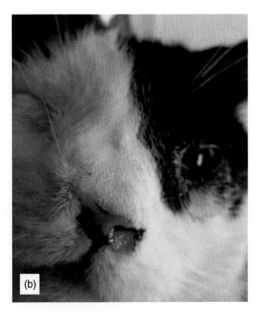

Figure 3.5 (a) Facial asymmetry due to neoplasia. Note the extreme distortion of the face along the bridge of the nose, particularly the right lateral aspect. In this case, the mass is growing into the conjunctiva associated with the right eye. (b) Facial asymmetry in a trauma patient with a previously enucleated right eye. This patient had been bitten in the face by a dog. Source (a), (b): Courtesy of Patricia Bennett, DVM.

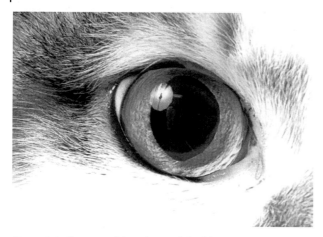

Figure 3.6 Close-up of the adnexa of the feline eye.
Source: Courtesy of the Media Resources Department at
Midwestern University.

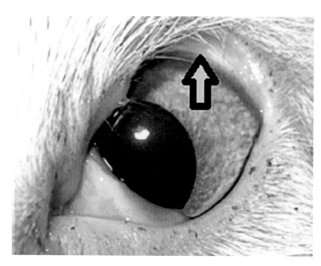

Figure 3.7 Partial eyelid agenesis of the right eye in a feline
patient. Note where the upper eyelid is absent (arrow).

dark discoloration of fur that starts at the medial canthus and tracks ventrally (Figure 3.10). For other patients, a recent onset of epiphora may indicate a plugged nasolacrimal duct or ocular irritation.

How the discharge is colored, its consistency, and whether it is unilateral or bilateral matter. Clear ocular discharge may indicate irritation, inflammation, allergies, or viral infection. If ocular discharge becomes more opaque and takes on a color such as white, yellow, or green, it may be indicative of an underlying bacterial infection (Figure 3.11).

The conjunctiva should be evaluated for color and symmetry: is the conjunctiva associated with both eyes colored pink and of equal intensity or is the conjunctiva of one eye hyperemic (reddened), as from an increased blood supply? [22]. The conjunctiva should also be evaluated for chemosis: is the conjunctiva edematous? Conjunctiva that is swollen tends to be prominent and takes on a "puffy" appearance [22]. Further, the conjunctiva should be evaluated for pathologic adherence to the eye itself. For instance, in cases of symblepharon, the palpebral conjunctiva partially or completely adheres to the bulbar conjunctiva of the eye. This is usually the result of trauma. As a result, the eyelid of the affected eye is effectively "locked" in place. There is great risk for exposure keratitis. Concurrent corneal discoloration typically

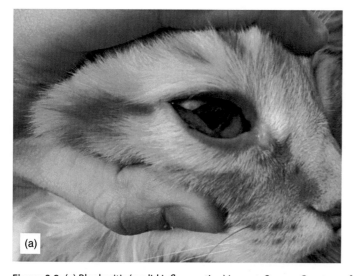

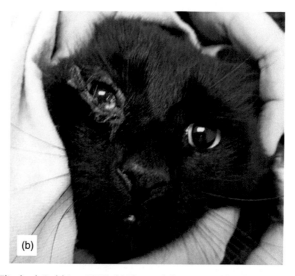

Figure 3.8 (a) Blepharitis (eyelid inflammation) in a cat. Source: Courtesy of Elizabeth Robbins, DVM. (b) The eyelids associated with the right eye of this patient were damaged in a cat fight. They are heavily crusted with discharge and will likely require surgical repair of underlying lid lacerations. Source: Courtesy of Patricia Bennett, DVM.

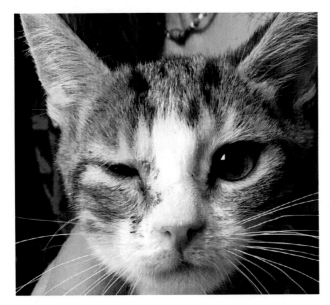

Figure 3.9 Unilateral blepharospasm of the right eye.
Source: Courtesy of Frank Isom, DVM.

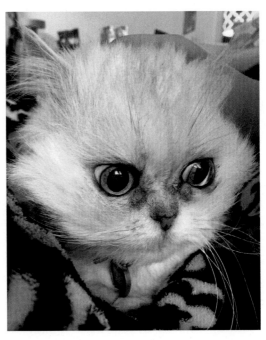

Figure 3.10 Epiphora (tear-overflow), which is considered "normal" for this patient. Chronic epiphora is associated with rusty brown discoloration of peri-ocular fur as seen here.
Source: Courtesy of Madison Lea Skelton.

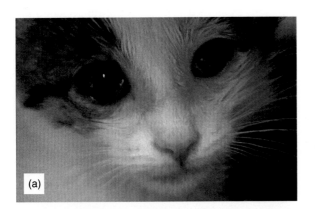

(a)

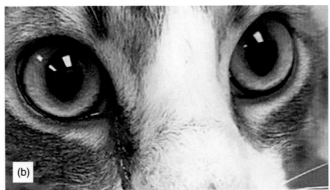

(b)

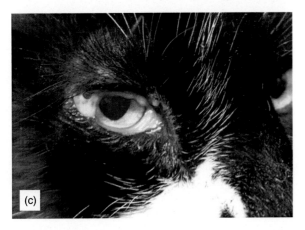

(c)

Figure 3.11 (a) Serous ocular discharge in a cat. Source: Courtesy of Karen Burks, DVM. (b) Rusty brown ocular discharge from the right eye (OD) in a cat. Note that the discharge is not transparent like that in (a). The ocular discharge that is depicted here is semi-opaque. (c) Note the extensive mucopurulent discharge that is associated with the right eye of this patient. Source: Courtesy of Patricia Bennett, DVM.

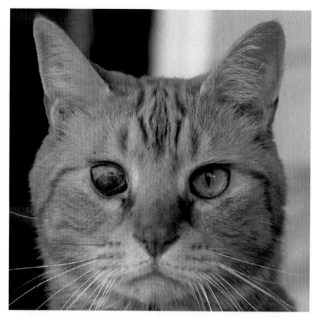

Figure 3.12 Symblepharon associated with the right eye. Note the resultant corneal disease and discoloration. Source: Courtesy of Jackie Kucskar, DVM.

is present and indicates that the corneal surface is not healthy (Figure 3.12) [21, 22]. The conjunctiva should also be evaluated for masses (Figure 3.13).

The nictitating membrane associated with each orbit should be evaluated. To do so, the veterinarian must manipulate the soft tissue over each orbit to get the nictitating membrane to come into view. Pushing down gently, but firmly, over the upper palpebra will facilitate visualization of this structure (Figure 3.14).

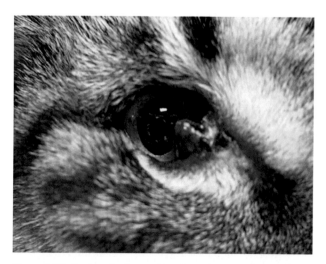

Figure 3.13 Conjunctival mass. Note how the mass distorts the normal anatomy of the adnexa and how the mass is contacting the globe of the right eye. Source: Courtesy of Patricia Bennett, DVM.

Patients that present with ocular complaints may have prominent nictitating membranes that do not require as much effort on the veterinarian's part to extrude them completely. They may already be out and exposed. Their prominence may indicate general malaise or systemic poor health. In some instances, their prominence has been linked to heavy gastrointestinal parasite burden. More often, the prominent nictitating membrane reflects ocular pain or irritation as from a corneal ulcer [22].

Nictitating membranes may also be prominent if there is a foreign body in the orbit. Plant material, especially seeds, can become lodged beneath the nictitating membrane and is a common source of corneal abrasion and ulceration. Topical ophthalmic anesthetics such as proparacaine must be used to numb the affected eye. This allows for the insertion of a cotton tip applicator, moistened with saline, under the nictitating membrane to see if there is indeed a foreign body trapped underneath. Because topical ophthalmic anesthetics delay corneal healing, these are inappropriate for use on an outpatient basis to maintain comfort of the eye. However, their one-time use is necessary in this instance [22].

3.2.3 Evaluating the Globe

Once the adnexa has been thoroughly examined, the globes can be evaluated next. Systematic evaluation is important so as to prevent one from missing abnormalities that may have implications for patient wellness, care, and comfort. In particular, the following should be assessed [22]:

- globe location within the orbit;
- globe shape;
- globe retropulsion;
- presence or absence of strabismus;
- sclera;
- cornea;
- iris;
- pupil;
- lens;
- fundus.

The globe should be well seated within the orbit. It should not be caudally displaced within the orbit, a condition that is referred to as enophthalmos. Enophthalmos may occur as a result of loss of orbit fat or loss of function of the orbitalis muscle. Barring breed-specific conformations due to skull shape, as was discussed earlier with regard to brachycephalic breeds, the globe should also not be rostrally displaced from the orbit, as is the case with exophthalmos. When unrelated to cat breed, exophthalmos typically is the result of a disease process at the back of the orbit such as a mass effect pushing the globe forward [21, 23]. This can be due to neoplasia or simply inflammation secondary to trauma [23]. If severe

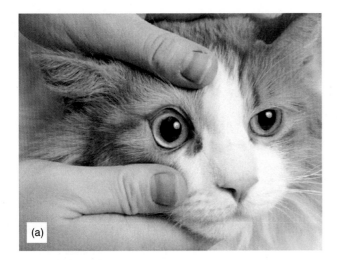
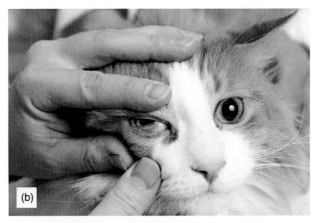
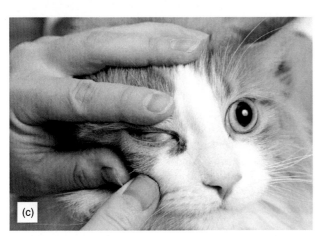
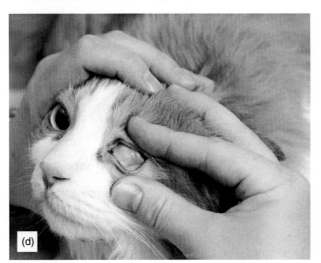

Figure 3.14 (a) Demonstrating hand placement in preparation for exposing the nictitating membrane. (b) Pushing down with firm pressure over the right globe to expose the nictitating membrane. (c) The nictitating membrane is now fully exposed. (d) It is important to repeat the process of exposing the nictitating membrane on the contralateral side. Source (a)–(d): Courtesy of the Media Resources Department at Midwestern University.

enough, exophthalmos can prevent eyelid closure. When lids do not close as they ought to, the cornea is at risk of drying out. Exposure keratitis with subsequent corneal ulceration is a significant concern (Figure 3.15) [22].

In Figure 3.15a and b, exophthalmos is obvious and should alert the clinician to the presence of intra-ocular or retro-orbital disease. However, when the patient is in the early stages of disease, exophthalmos may be less overt. Retropulsion of each globe can help to identify retro-orbital disease before there is gross pathology that is visible. Retropulsion is a technique that requires the clinician to apply even, firm pressure to the globe through closed eyelids. An orbit that is devoid of disease should allow for some "give": the globe should be able to be balloted gently because there is nothing to obstruct the globe's movement in the retro-orbital space. By contrast, the presence of a retro-orbital mass will create an obstruction that hinders the ability of the globe to be balloted. In this case, there will be resistance to

retropulsion. The ability of both eyes to be retropulsed should be evaluated at each visit, and both eyes should be equal in their response. If one eye retropulses easily and the other does not, there is either an orbital mass or severe orbital inflammation. Ultrasonography of the retrobulbar region can be a helpful diagnostic tool [22].

Another gross observation that is important to make is whether or not there is strabismus and, if so, in which direction. Strabismus is colloquially referred to as being "cross-eyed." In reality, it encompasses several forms of misalignment between the eyes so that the eyes are prevented from directing their gaze at the same point in space at the same time. Binocular vision is compromised as a result, and depth perception may be hindered [18, 21, 24, 25].

In human medicine, the presence of strabismus indicates that the extraocular eye muscles are uncoordinated [24, 25]. By contrast, its presence in veterinary medicine typically is indicative of an underlying neuropathy. The

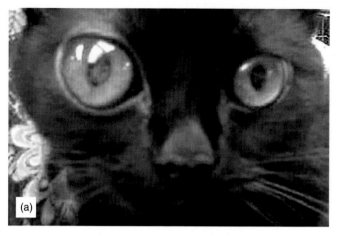
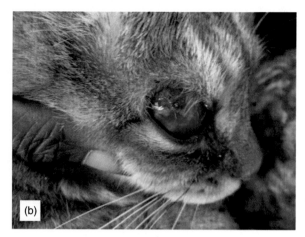

Figure 3.15 (a) Extreme exophthalmos of the right globe due to severely increased ocular pressure (glaucoma). (b) Moderate exophthalmos of the right globe due to glaucoma. Note the extreme corneal discoloration that indicates corneal disease secondary to exophthalmos. Source: Courtesy of Patricia Bennett, DVM.

direction of the strabismus confers which cranial nerve is impacted:

- Ventrolateral strabismus involves cranial nerve III – the oculomotor nerve.
- Medial strabismus involves cranial nerve VI – the abducens nerve.
- Rotatory strabismus involves cranial nerve IV – the trochlear nerve.

Strabismus can occur in one or both eyes. It is common in Siamese cats [19, 26–28] (Figure 3.16).

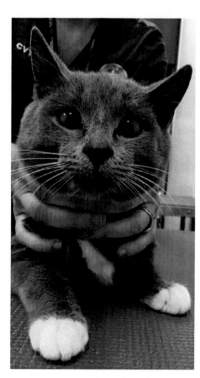

Figure 3.16 Bilateral ventromedial strabismus in a Siamese cat.

Another clinically relevant observation to record is whether or not there is nystagmus. Nystagmus refers to involuntary eye movement of one or both eyes. It may be physiologic or pathologic, congenital or acquired. When acquired, nystagmus may be the result of systemic disease [29], central nervous system disease, toxicosis [30], or pharmacotherapy [31–35]. It may also be the result of idiopathic vestibular disease in cats [36].

Nystagmus may be defined based on the direction of the eye movement [33]:

- horizontal;
- vertical;
- rotatory.

Nystagmus may also be defined based on the speed of the rhythmic oscillation [33]:

- When phasic nystagmus is observed, two phases of eye movement are observed: there is a slow movement in one direction, followed by a rapid movement in the other. The result is rhythmic oscillation.
- When pendular nystagmus is observed, there is no difference in speed between directions.

Finally, nystagmus may be defined based on when it occurs [33]:

- Spontaneously nystagmus is ever-present.
- Positional nystagmus is present only when the head is in a particular position.
- Positional-change nystagmus is present only immediately after head position has changed.

3.2.4 Evaluating the Sclera

Moving on in terms of the eye examination, the sclera should be inspected for hyperemia, abnormal vasculature, evidence of hemorrhage, and icterus (Figure 3.17).

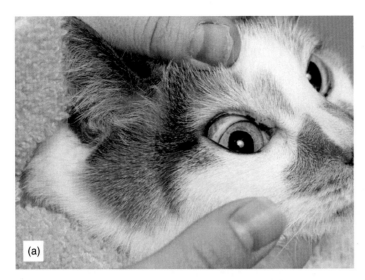
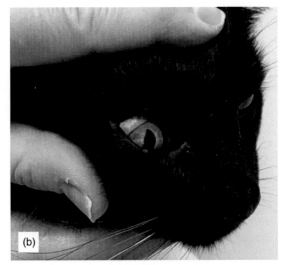

Figure 3.17 Examining the sclera in (a) a non-icteric and (b) an icteric cat.

Icterus develops from an excess of bilirubin. Just like the peri-aural region of the body, the sclera is an easy place to identify icterus in cats.

3.2.5 Evaluating the Cornea

In addition to the sclera, the cornea should be evaluated for integrity, transparency, and reflectivity. Some corneal defects are so catastrophic that they are visible with the naked eye without additional diagnostic tests (Figure 3.18). Other corneal defects are invisible to the eye without the use of sodium fluorescein stain and a cobalt blue light. Certain types of corneal defects are classic for feline infectious disease: dendritic, or branching, linear ulcers are typical of feline herpesvirus [21, 37–40].

The cornea should also be transparent so that light can pass freely through the eye to fall upon the retina. Traumatic injuries to the eye or underlying uveitis can transiently or permanently impact this transparency [41, 42] (Figure 3.19).

3.2.6 Evaluating the Iris

The iris tends to be most recognizable as the colored part of the eye. Even in patients in whom it does not contain pigment due to albinism, it still appears colored pink to red because of its extensive vasculature. This blood supply is also what gives it a slightly irregular surface.

The color of the iris should be documented along with any defects or embryonic remnants [22]. Iris color ranges immensely in companion animals. In the cat it tends to range from coppery yellow to green, although Siamese as a breed tend to boast brilliant blue eyes [43] (Figure 3.20).

Iris color is important to note because it may be linked to increased risk of certain diseases: it has been said that copper-eyed cats tend to have a greater chance of developing portosystemic shunts [44–46]. Iris color is equally important because changes in this characteristic may indicate pathology. For instance, an iris that acutely takes on a gray appearance may be a reflection of underlying uveitis.

Irises may also develop "freckles" of deep brown to black pigmentation. These are benign iris nevi (Figure 3.21). However, these can bear a striking resemblance

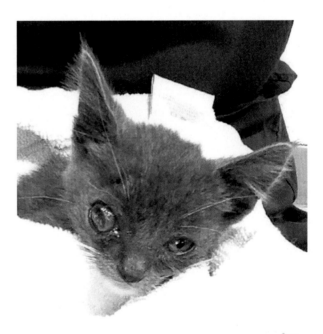

Figure 3.18 The corneal defect in the right eye (OD) of this patient is both visible without sodium fluorescein staining and is occurring in combination with exophthalmos. This patient sustained traumatic injury to the OD, which is in danger of rupturing. Source: Courtesy of Molly Klein, BS.

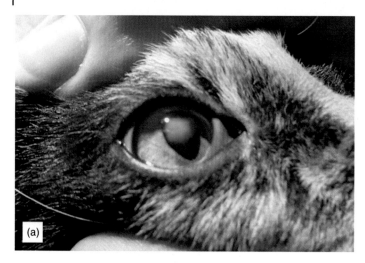
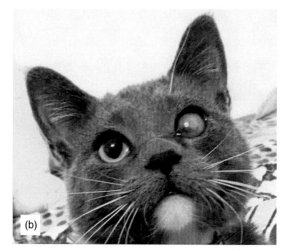

Figure 3.19 (a) There is a scar on the surface of the cornea that has caused the cornea to take on a semi-opaque appearance. This makes the cornea look cloudy where previously there had been an ulcer. (b) This patient sustained extensive injury to its left eye. As a result, there is a widespread change in the translucency of the cornea.

to aggressive, malignant melanoma [47–53]. Sometimes the only difference between the two is that melanomas tend to grow into focal elevations as opposed to remaining flat [21, 22].

Defects in the iris may be congenital, as in the case of a coloboma. This usually appears as a visible slit in the edge of the iris. Defects in the iris may also be acquired; for instance, the iris may atrophy with age [19, 21].

The iris may also appear to have one or more strands crossing from the iris over the pupil to another part of the iris; alternatively, when viewed from the side with a slit lamp, there may be one or visible strands crossing from the iris to the cornea. These are remnants of the pupillary membrane, which in embryonic life is a normal structure that blankets over the pupil. By the time the patient is 1 month of age, this membrane should have dissolved. When this fails to happen, threads remain behind like a web. They do not create intraocular inflammation [21, 22].

3.2.7 Evaluating the Pupils

The pupil is an intentional defect in the iris, the muscles of which control its size and shape. Different species have different pupil shapes at rest. Dogs, for instance, have round pupils. By contrast, cats should have a vertical slit that is apparent during complete miosis (pupillary constriction) (Figure 3.22).

As ambient lighting dims, pupils dilate in order to increase the amount of light that enters the eye. Pupils also dilate in response to activation of the sympathetic nervous system such as occurs during "fight or flight." This is why it is important to consider where the cat is examined relative to the level of ambient lighting when attempting to determine why a patient's pupils are dilated.

A cat that is examined in a dark room would be expected to have enlarged, bilaterally symmetrical pupils. By contrast, a cat that is examined in a well-lit room yet has saucer-like pupils should be approached cautiously and handled with care: the patient is likely fearful and may be prompted to attack defensively if it feels threatened.

Note that as cats' pupils dilate, their shape changes: rather than retaining their vertical slit, they become increasingly rounded (Figure 3.23).

Note that when pupils are mydriatic, especially when in the clinic setting as a result of the "fight or flight" response, they do not always constrict in response to weak light sources such as a penlight. A stronger light source is often required to obtain a pupillary light reflex (PLR) [54].

Pupils should be bilaterally symmetrical. Anisocoria refers to having asymmetric pupils. The presence of anisocoria may indicate underlying neurologic dysfunction (Figure 3.24a). That being said, cats are extraordinarily sensitive to ambient light. Depending on the location of the light source, cats may have anisocoria without neurologic dysfunction. For example, a cat that is sitting on a window ledge in broad daylight may have anisocoria yet be neurologically normal. In this situation, as a result of the light source and location, the pupil closest to the window may be slightly smaller (Figure 3.24b) [54].

3.2.8 Assessing Ocular Reflexes

The pupillary light reflex (PLR) is designed to test cranial nerves II (optic nerve) and III (oculomotor nerve). A bright light is directed at each eye. The eye at which the light is directed should constrict its pupil rapidly and remain small as long as the light source is persistent. This tests the direct PLR. The indirect or consensual PLR

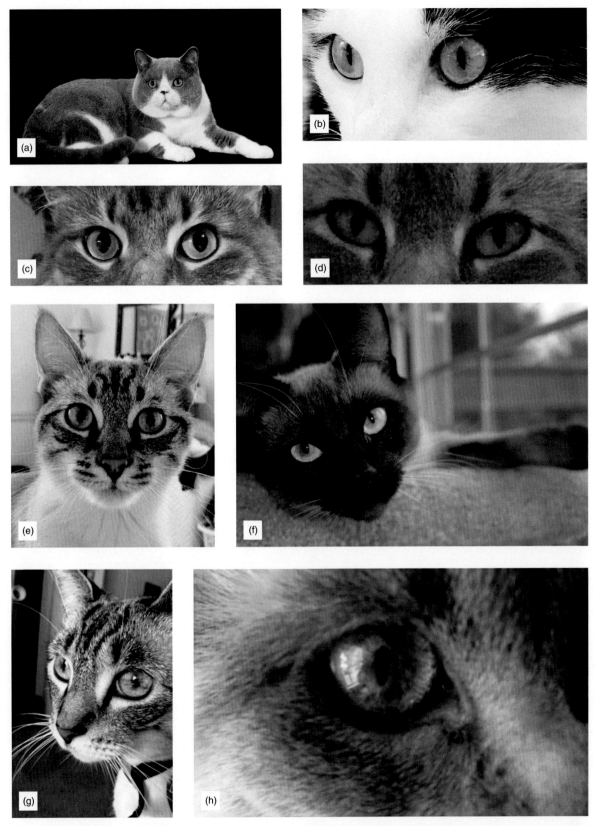

Figure 3.20 (a) Copper eyes in a British Shorthair cat. Source: Courtesy of Cheryl A. Kelly. (b) Coppery yellow cat eyes. Source: Courtesy of Kelly Chappell. (c) Yellow–green cat eyes. Source: Courtesy of Garrett Rowley (Midwestern University DVM 2018). (d) Green cat eyes. Source: Courtesy of Rozalyn Donner. (e) Green–blue cat eyes. Source: Courtesy of Emily Denning. (f) Light blue eyes in a Siamese cat. Source: Courtesy of Erika Olney. (g) Medium blue cat eyes. Source: Courtesy of Samantha Rudolph. (h) Brilliant Caribbean blue cat eyes.

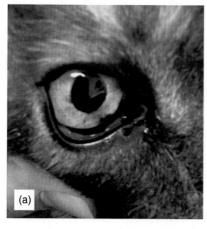 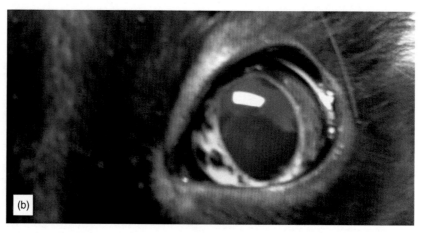

Figure 3.21 (a) Presumptive iris nevus located at the ventral-most portion of the iris. Source: Courtesy of Patricia Bennett, DVM. (b) Multiple focal dark areas of pigmentation in the iris of a cat with presumptive iris melanoma.

evaluates the contralateral eye; for instance, if a bright light is directed at the left eye, the right eye should also exhibit miosis. Note that positive PLRs do not guarantee that the patient is visual. Normal PLRs will be present in a patient who is cortically blind [19, 54].

The palpebral reflex tests cranial nerves V (trigeminal nerve) and VII (facial nerve). The medial canthus of each eyelid is touched. Doing so in a neurologically normal cat with this reflex intact will cause the cat to blink as a result of the tactile stimulus [19, 54].

The menace response tests cranial nerves II (optic nerve) and VII (facial nerve). The clinician makes a

menacing gesture toward each eye. A patient who has this response intact must first see the threat and then blink as a protective function. It is important to take care not to touch the eyelids themselves in the process or to create excessive air currents because although the outcome may be the same (the patient blinks), it will be due to touch as a stimulus rather than vision [19, 54].

3.2.9 Assessing the Anterior Chamber

The anterior chamber of the eye represents the space between the cornea and the lens. It is not an empty

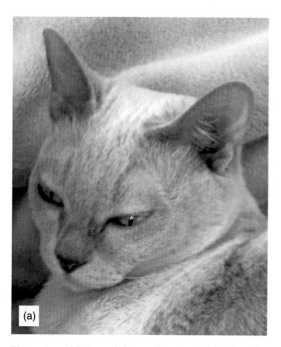 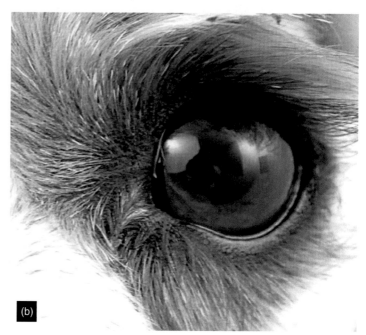

Figure 3.22 (a) Normal shape of a cat pupil. (b) Normal rounded shape of a dog pupil. Source: Courtesy of the Media Resources Department at Midwestern University.

Figure 3.23 (a) When the patient is not in "fight or flight" mode and when it is exposed to adequate ambient lighting, the pupil takes on its normal shape: a vertical slit. Source: Courtesy of Leigh Ann Howard. (b) As lighting or stress response is altered, the cat's pupil becomes increasingly rounded. Note the progression from this patient to those in (c) and (d). Source: Courtesy of Bianca Hartrum. (c) Elliptical to rounded pupils in a cat. Source: Courtesy of Abby Rife. (d) Fully rounded pupils in cat. Source: Courtesy of Lydia T. McDaniel.

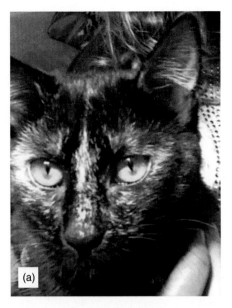
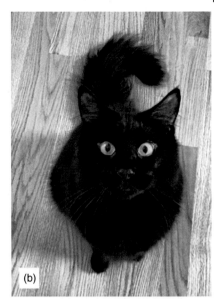
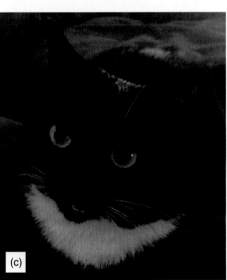
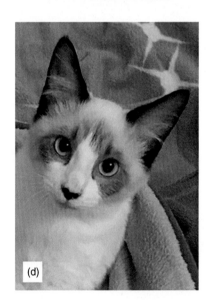

space: it is filled with aqueous humor. This is a clear fluid – it should not be cloudy or hazy. When the slit lamp is used to shine a light beam through the anterior chamber, the space should appear transparent. Any opacities typically indicate underlying pathology. Traumatic events such as blunt force trauma to the eye may cause hyphema, blood within the anterior chamber [55]. In the case of uveitis, purulent material may accumulate in the anterior chamber – this is referred to as hypopion [41, 42]. Uveitis may also cause residual adhesions, anterior synechiae, between the cornea and the iris [19, 21, 22, 41, 42].

3.2.10 Assessing the Lens

The lens sits at the rostral aspect of the posterior chamber, suspended by the ciliary body. The lens is transparent also, like aqueous humor, avascular, and without innervation. It cannot be appreciated without a light source – and even then, a normal lens is invisible. A portion of, if not all of, the lens becomes visible in the face of physiologic or pathologic change. Physiologic change comes about through the normal aging process. As the center of the lens ages, the structure of its fibers changes in such a way as to create central haziness within the lens. Cataracts also cause cloudiness of the lens; however, unlike nuclear sclerosis, cataracts are considered a disease process rather than part of the aging process. Also, cataracts may form anywhere within the lens itself rather than being limited to a central location [19, 22].

Cataracts may be named based on their location within the eye. Nuclear cataracts are centrally located whereas equatorial cataracts arise at the lens periphery. Cortical

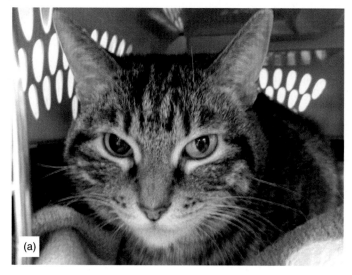
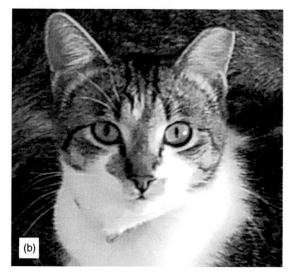

Figure 3.24 (a) This patient presented to the clinic with anisocoria. Note that the right eye (OD) is larger than the left eye (OS). Primary neurologic disease was suspected. (b) Note the asymmetry in pupil size. The right pupil is larger than the left pupil. In this patient, anisocoria was not due to underlying neuropathy. Anisocoria was induced by the angle of the camera and the position of the light source, which came from the patient's left side. Source: Courtesy of Kyndel Lann.

cataracts arise at the periphery but work their way to the interior to the lens like spokes on a wheel. Cataracts may be anteriorly or posteriorly located, and may be capsular or subcapsular [21, 22].

Cataracts may also be named based on their stage of development. Incipient cataracts are those that have been caught early. They only take up 10–15% of the volume of the lens, and do not prevent visualization of the fundus through direct or indirect ophthalmoscopy. Immature cataracts create a cloudier appearance within the lens; however, like incipient cataracts, immature cataracts still allow for fundoscopy. Mature cataracts are advanced usually to the extent that the entire lens in involved and tapetal reflection is hidden from view. The lens may be unstable. Lens fibers break down and release protein. Over time, the lens volume is reduced. Eventually, the cataract becomes hypermature: the lens capsule wrinkles and the cortex becomes milky white and opaque [19, 22].

Cataracts tend to be seen more commonly in dogs than cats, and they are especially seen more acutely in dogs that have been diagnosed with diabetes mellitus due to an accumulation of sorbitol within the lens [56–59].

The lens relies upon glucose as its primary energy source [60]. In non-diabetic companion animal patients, the majority of glucose is metabolized via the glycolytic pathway [60]. However, as the concentration of glucose rises in the blood, the glycolytic enzyme hexokinase is saturated [61, 62]. The result is that glucose is shunted into a different metabolic pathway: it is converted by aldose reductase into sorbitol. The problem with sorbitol is that it is impermeable to cell membranes [61]. As

such, its concentration builds within the cells, drawing water in along the concentration gradient [60]. When this occurs in the lens, the lens swells, setting the stage for diabetic cataract development.

Lenses should be evaluated in cats for the presence or absence of cataracts and also for subluxations. Traumatic injuries such as blunt force trauma to the head can lead to lens displacement. If severe enough, a luxation can cause the lens to obstruct the outflow tract of aqueous humor [18].

3.2.11 Introduction to Fundoscopy

Fundoscopy refers to the evaluation of the most caudal layers of the globe. The retina is the innermost layer, and is transparent. In a healthy eye, the pigmented portion of the choroid shines through as the tapetum nigrum and the retina is invisible. Only in the face of retinal pathology such as hemorrhage or detachment is the retina visible [19, 21].

In addition to visualizing the choroid during the fundic exam, it is also possible to see where the nerve fibers of the retina pool together. This pink–white, triangular-to-round region is referred to as the optic disc. A depression may be visible at the center of the optic disc – this is normal, and is where the previous hyaloid vessel had emerged. Dorsal to the optic disc, there is a hemispherical zone called the tapetum lucidum. The tapetum lucidum increases what light is available to photoreceptors, which creates "eyeshine": the pupils appear to glow when light is directed at a patient with a tapetum lucidum (Figure 3.25) [18, 19, 21].

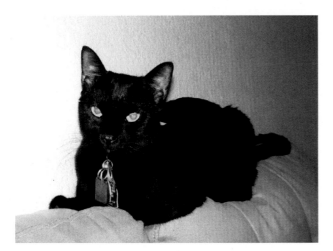

Figure 3.25 Note the strength of the "eyeshine" or tapetal reflection in this patient. Source: Courtesy of Alexandra Aczona-Velasquez.

The tapetum lucidum varies in color from blue-green to orange-yellow. The colors are produced by light scatter caused by the crystalline structures that are contained within. These are absent at birth and take weeks to develop. As a result, this zone is purple–blue in kittens and puppies less than 2–4 months of age [18, 19, 21].

Choroidal vessels are hidden from view because of the tapetum lucidum. The only vessels that are typically seen on the fundic examination are the thinner retinal arteries and the darker red veins of greater diameter [18, 19]. In a patient with albinism, there is no pigment to make up the tapetum nigrum and tapetum lucidum, so the choroidal vessels are visible coursing to and from the optic disc.

When examining the fundus, the clinician should take note of the retinal vasculature relative to its [18, 21]

- presence;
- thickness;
- tortuosity.

Dogs typically have three to five retinal veins and several smaller retinal arteries. The former may course over the optic disc; the latter may partially join a ring near its center. By contrast, cats typically have three retinal veins, and both the veins and the arteries disappear at the perimeter of the optic disc [21].

It is important to note vessel thickness. Vessels that are thinner than expected may be the result of congenital or acquired retinal atrophy [21]. Vessels should not be tortuous. Tortuosity likely reflects underlying pathology such as systemic hypertension [21].

3.2.12 Fundoscopy and Direct Ophthalmoscopy

Fundoscopy requires direct or indirect ophthalmoscopy. Both are tools that require manipulating light through lenses to bring an image of the fundus into view [63]. Of the two methods, direct ophthalmoscopy is most commonly performed by general practitioners. This method creates a view of the fundus that is upright and magnified. However, the resultant image paints a very narrow picture of the fundus: the veterinarian can see only about 10 mm in diameter of the fundus using direct ophthalmoscopy. When the patient's eyes are miotic, this limited view is even further narrowed. As a result, generalists will often turn to topical mydriatic agents such as short-acting tropicamide or longer-acting atropine to dilate the pupil prior to fundic examination [63, 64].

A direct ophthalmoscope has a built-in light source and the ability to shift the clinician's focus rostrally or caudally within the globe by adjusting the diopters, the optical power of the lens:

- As the clinician turns the diopter setting to numbers that are colored green, the lens acquires more converging power, allowing him or her to focus rostrally within the globe.
- As the clinician turns the diopter setting to numbers that are colored red, the lens acquires more diverging power, allowing him or her to focus caudally within the globe.

Within the eye, a distance of 3 diopters equals 1 mm, so the diopter setting allows the clinician to make very fine adjustments in focus.

To initiate a fundic examination using the direct ophthalmoscope, the clinician should begin with the diopter setting at zero. The clinician should stand at a flexed arm's length from the patient and direct the light into the patient's eye. They may then look through the viewing aperture to catch the tapetal reflection. Once this reflection is captured, he should move in with the ophthalmoscope until approximately 5 cm from the patient's eye [63–65] (Figure 3.26). A fraction of the fundus should be visible: typically the central fraction including the optic disc. As needed, the clinician may adjust the diopters dial 1–3 diopters each way from zero to crisp up the view [63, 64].

For safety purposes, the clinician should get used to evaluating the patient's right eye with his right eye and the patient's left eye with his left eye. This minimizes "nose to nose" contact, which increases the chance of a clinician sustaining a bite to the face.

3.2.13 Fundoscopy and Indirect Ophthalmoscopy

Indirect ophthalmoscopy is an alternative method of performing the eye exam. It uses a light source and a hand-held convex lens. This lens is placed between the patient's eye and the veterinarian's eye – the resultant image is upside down and backwards, and is also less

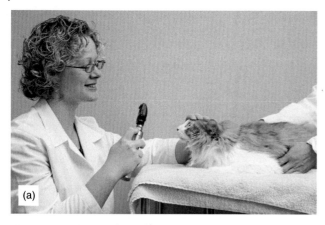
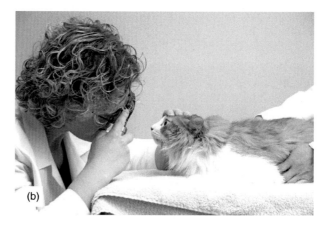

Figure 3.26 (a) Using direct ophthalmoscopy to begin the eye exam. Note that the clinician starts the examination at a distance from the patient and directs the light source into the patient's eye from a distance. (b) Once the tapetal reflex is captured, it is appropriate for the clinician to move in toward the patient with the ophthalmoscope. Ultimately, the clinician will be standing cheek-to-cheek with the patient with the ophthalmoscope in between. Good restraint is important to protect the clinician from injury in the event that the patient becomes spooked. *Source (a), (b): Courtesy of the Media Resources Department at Midwestern University.*

magnified. However, a distinct advantage of indirect ophthalmoscopy is that it provides the clinician with a larger field of view. This allows the clinician to perform a more thorough examination of the fundic periphery. Another advantage is that does not require such close proximity to the patient, meaning that the patient may be less likely to feel threatened and the clinician is more likely to be safe [63, 65].

Indirect ophthalmoscopy is more often performed by specialists than generalists. To perform it with consistency, practice is important. The author finds this to be much more technically challenging than direct ophthalmoscopy, although the rewards of the indirect approach are greater in terms of the ability to visualize the fundus [63].

To perform indirect ophthalmoscopy, the clinician begins by standing at a flexed arm's length from the patient. The clinician then places a strong light source at eye level alongside his head. With the light source maintaining its position alongside his head, the clinician should direct the light at the patient's eye to catch the tapetal reflection. Once the tapetal reflection is captured, the clinician must bring the lens in between himself and the patient. For stability, the clinician may rest the hand that is holding the lens against the patient's brow [63, 65]. With the lens in place and perpendicular to the light source, the fundic image should be visible, albeit inverted [63]. The clinician may then adjust his view by moving the lens toward and away from the eye until the eyelids and iris disappear from view, allowing the fundic image to fill the lens [63].

3.3 The Ears

Just as the eyes are an important sensory organ in the visual pathway, the ears are important structures in

the auditory system. The ears consist of the pinnae, the external ear canal, which encompasses the vertical and horizontal ear canals, the tympanic membrane, and the middle and inner ears [19, 66, 67]. Together, these work in concert with the central nervous system through a series of intricate signaling pathways to confer the special sense of hearing [66, 67].

Among mammals, the cat has one of the broadest ranges for hearing, from 48 Hz to 85 kHz [68]. Cats are able to appreciate high-frequency sounds without sacrificing their ability to hear low-frequency sounds [68]. Hearing is a critical special sense for an obligate carnivore such as a cat to possess: it facilitates hunting. It also influences feline vocalization through auditory feedback that occurs primarily during neonatal and juvenile development. Such feedback helps to determine volume, frequency, and duration of vocalizations [69, 70].

The clinician's ability to detect hearing loss in a cat based on physical examination alone is limited. The clinician may note the cat's reaction or lack thereof to a loud, sudden, human-made sound such as a clap of the hands, a stomp of the foot, or even a whistle. If the cat responds, it may be said to have heard the sound. However, the cat could also simply have been responding to the visual stimulus: the rapid motion of hands slapping together or the foot against the floor.

The clinician will probably have more success in determining if the cat is likely to be hearing impaired if he elicits the owner's perspective. Clients may report that their cat no longer startles at the sound of a vacuum or a door slamming shut, or that their cat no longer responds to the garage door opening or their voice in the same room. This history is more beneficial than any assessment that the clinician could make without the patient undergoing electrodiagnostic testing such as brain-stem auditory evoked response (BAER) [19, 71–74].

The use of BAER to diagnose deafness in cats is infrequent. When it comes to the physical examination, cats are typically presented more with the chief complaint of external ear disease. Clients may report a change in ear position that is unilateral or bilateral, or that the cat has developed an ear twitch or flick. Cat owners may also notice focal pruritus: scratching at the ear with a hind foot or rubbing one or both ears excessively with a forepaw. Clients may notice hair loss over the ears secondary to pruritus or over-grooming, abnormal discharge in one or both ears, and/or an aural odor. Any of these findings may prompt a client to present a cat for a physical examination with an emphasis on the affected ear(s). Regardless of what the client has reported, both ears should be evaluated even if only ear has been concerning the patient [19].

The examination of the external ear should begin with observation of ear carriage: how is each pinna positioned relative to the other? If the two ears are not symmetrical, is positioning likely the result of the cat communicating a visual cue such as uncertainty [75], as was outlined in Chapter 1, or is positioning more likely the result of an underlying condition? An ear that is itchy or painful may not be as erect as an ear that is without disease.

Other than ear carriage, the structure of each pinna should be noted. Is the pinna intact or is it lacerated? In the latter case, is the injury fresh or is the pinnal structure reflective of an old wound. Some changes to ear structure and shape are intentional. Specifically, tipped or notched left ears are commonly the result of patient participation in a trap–neuter–release (TNR) program to convey visually from afar that the patient is no longer intact.

Other changes are unintended and reflect underlying pathology. For instance:

- One ear may be "puffed up" if there is a hematoma or an abscess in between the auricular cartilage [76] (Figure 3.27a).
- One ear may be thickened due to scarring associated with past injury. For example, long after an aural hematoma has resolved, the ear may retain a "cauliflower" or "crinkle" shape (Figure 3.27b).

Each pinna should also be palpated to assess for warmth. If one ear is palpably warmer than the other, then the warmer ear may be inflamed as from an underlying infection.

Loss of fur on the dorsal pinnae or scratch marks in the peri-aural region may also provide clues to the practitioner as to underlying ear pathology (Figure 3.28). The dorsal aspects and margins of both pinnae should also be evaluated for crusting, which may indicate fungal or parasitic diseases such as ringworm and sarcoptic mange, respectively [77, 78].

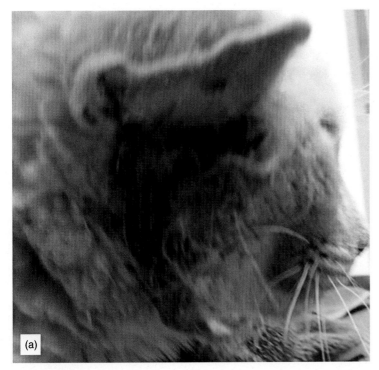 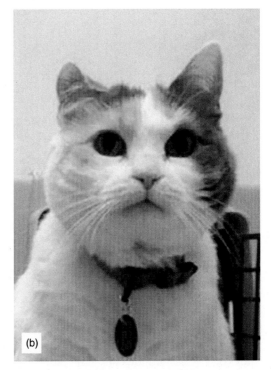

Figure 3.27 (a) Aural hem the right ear (AD). Source: Courtesy of Patricia Bennett, DVM. (b) Chronic scarring secondary to a resolved aural hematoma of the right ear.

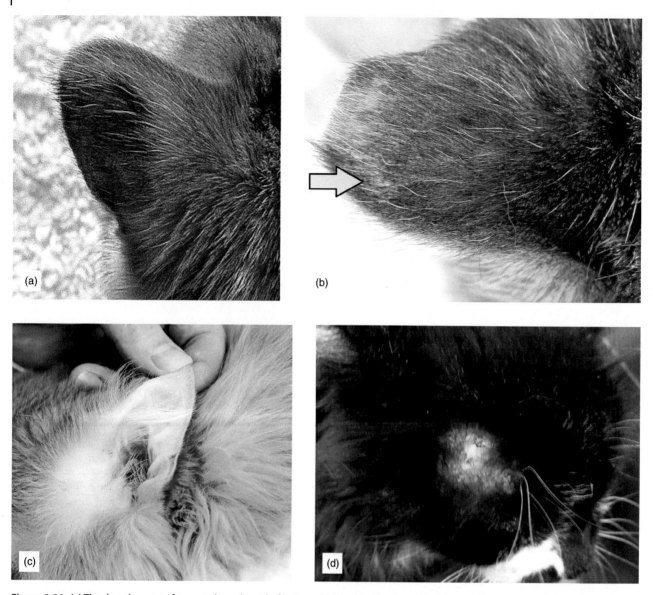

Figure 3.28 (a) The dorsal aspect of a normal ear, devoid of lesions. (b) The dorsal aspect of an abnormal ear, demonstrating fur loss and subtle erythema. (c) Evaluating the peri-aural region of a normal ear, devoid of lesions. Source (a)–(c): Courtesy of the Media Resources Department at Midwestern University. (d) Peri-aural excoriations secondary to self-trauma. Source: Courtesy of Patricia Bennett, DVM.

Once the pinnae have been sufficiently examined, the clinician should grossly inspect the external ear canal (Figure 3.29). In cats, the entrance to the external ear canal tends not to be obstructed by hair, as is the case for certain dog breeds such as the Poodle and Schnauzer [19]. What can be observed is true narrowing of the entrance to the external ear canal as from inflammation or perceived narrowing due to the presence of copious, obstructive discharge. Small amounts of cerumen can be normal. Certain breeds are known for excessive ceruminous discharge, such as the Sphynx [79]. What should not be observed is purulent material or dark brown, "coffee-ground" debris. The former may

be indicative of an underlying infection and the latter may be suggestive of parasitic ear disease as from *Otodectes cynotis*, the ear mite. If ear mites are suspected, the clinician can take an ear swab, roll it in mineral oil on a glass slide, and examine it under the microscope (Figure 3.30) [80, 81].

The clinician should get in the habit of smelling each ear even if it looks clean. In so doing, he may begin to appreciate the subtle differences in scent between different types of infection. For instance, some describe yeast otitis as smelling slightly sweet yet characteristically pungent. Others associate bacterial otitis externa with rod-shaped organisms with a rancid aroma.

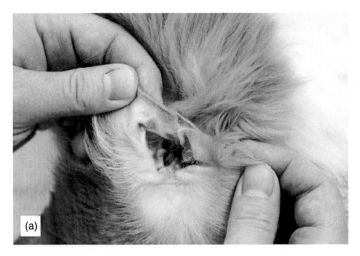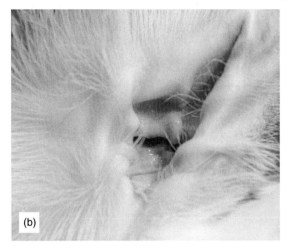

Figure 3.29 (a) Evaluating the external ear canal of a normal ear. (b) Close-up view of the external ear canal of a normal ear. Source (a), (b): Courtesy of the Media Resources Department at Midwestern University.

The vertical ear canal should be palpated to assess for erythema, pain, and compressibility. A normal vertical canal should not be painful on palpation and it should be slightly compressible, without eliciting a squishing or sloshing sound. If the vertical canal is not compressible, it may indicate the presence of a space-occupying mass. If compression of the vertical canal elicits a whooshing sound, then there is likely excessive fluid within the ear canal [19].

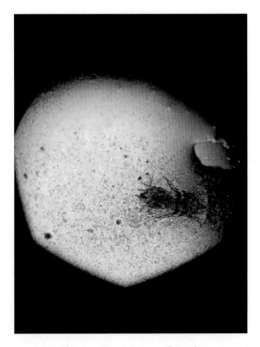

Figure 3.30 Confirming the presence of *Otodectes cynotis* on an ear swab. Source: Courtesy of Samantha Thurman, DVM.

It is impossible to examine the horizontal ear canal without an otoscope. There is an approximately 75° bend between the vertical and horizontal ear canals that leads to the tympanic membrane [82]. The ultimate goal of the otoscopic examination is to view this membrane to assess its integrity and whether or not it is bulging, as from a build-up of fluid in the middle ear. One may also be able to appreciate the presence of a nasopharyngeal polyp if it extends to the external ear canal [63, 67, 76].

To perform the otoscopic examination successfully, the cat must be restrained effectively by the veterinary team so that the it is looking straight ahead. The restrainer should avoid the tendency to tilt the head and neck to the side, because doing so can "crimp" the external ear canal, in effect obstructing the view. The pinna should be gently lifted cranio-dorso-laterally to straighten artificially the bend between the vertical and horizontal ear canals. At that point, an otoscope can be placed into the entrance to the external ear canal, taking care to have it equipped with a cone of the correct tip diameter and length. The patient should be given a moment to acclimate. At that point, the otoscope can be advanced while continuing to maintain gentle but firm traction on the pinna [63, 67] (Figure 3.31).

Performing the otoscopic examination allows the clinician to visualize both the horizontal ear canal and the tympanic membrane. As with the vertical ear canal, the horizontal ear canal can be assessed for the presence of discharge, erythema, pain, and narrowing such as may occur in otitis externa. The tympanic membrane, the ear drum, should be transparent and intact. It consists of a grayish blue pars tensa and a more dorsal, pinkish, elastic pars flaccida [63, 67].

In cases of chronic otitis media, the tympanic membrane may take on a more opaque, cloudy white

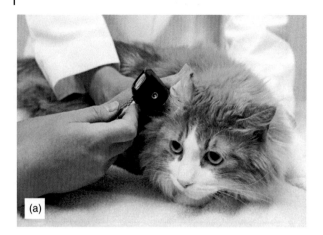
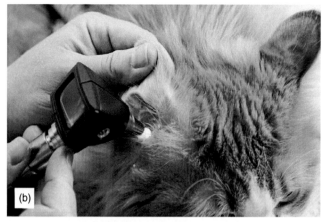

Figure 3.31 (a) Lifting the pinna and placing the otoscope near the opening of the ear canal. (b) Gently applying traction on the pinna to straighten the ear canal. Source (a), (b): Courtesy of the Media Resources Department at Midwestern University.

appearance. If fluid has built up in the middle ear, the tympanic membrane may also bulge forward into the horizontal ear canal. A ruptured ear drum is visible as an overt tear in the tympanic membrane [67, 83].

The novice may have difficulty visualizing the tympanum by means of the otoscopic examination. This may occur due to inexperience or to overt ear canal disease. For example:

- The clinician may not have taken care to straighten out the bend between the vertical and horizontal ear canals. This causes the tip of the cone to be pressed against the wall of the ear canal rather than up against the tympanum.
- The clinician may not have sized the cone appropriately. If the ear cone is too short, the ear drum may be too far away to see.
- The ear canal may be narrowed due to excessive inflammation or abnormal architecture. In this case, regardless of how the clinician attempts to manipulate the otoscope, he often cannot insert the cone far enough to see.
- The ear canal may be filled with debris that acts like dirt on a window screen. In this case, the clinician cannot see through the debris. The ear has to be cleaned first before the clinician reattempts the otoscopic examination.
- The ear drum could be ruptured. In this case, the clinician may actually see ragged edges of tissue that was once the intact ear drum. More often, the clinician just sees a black hole where the ear drum used to be.

If ear cleaning is required in order to visualize better the architecture of the ear canal and the tympanic membrane, the clinician should take care to collect any and all ear samples (swabs for ear cytology and swabs for ear culture) prior to cleaning. If the ear drum could not be

visualized prior to cleaning, sterile saline should be used as a cleaning agent because it is safe to come into contact with the middle or inner ear in the event that the tympanic membrane has ruptured.

3.4 The Nose

The nose is the external opening to the respiratory system. It is also an important structure in the olfactory pathway. As such, it ought to be evaluated at each visit, beginning with the external nares.

Each patient should have two nares, and these should be evaluated for symmetry (Figure 3.32). Regardless of pigmentation, the nasal planum should have a cobblestone appearance (Figure 3.33).

A palpably moist nose is considered normal. However, the nares themselves should be evaluated for gross discharge. The presence of serous discharge can be normal or abnormal, unilateral or bilateral. Serous discharge may be the result of allergic rhinitis. Bilaterally symmetrical serous discharge could also indicate the development of volume overload in a hospitalized patient that is receiving an excess of intravenous fluids. It is abnormal to see mucoid, mucopurulent, and hemorrhagic nasal discharges (Figure 3.34).

Airflow through each nostril should be assessed by placing a glass slide in front of the nose. Because cats are nasal breathers, the breath should fog up the slide in two concentric circles: one per nare. If one side lacks a circle of fog on the slide, then airflow is minimal to non-existent through that side of the upper respiratory tract. Alternatively, the clinician may hold a tuft of cotton in front of each nostril and assess for movement of the cotton.

The bridge of the nose should be assessed for swelling or other lesions (Figure 3.35; see also Figure 3.5).

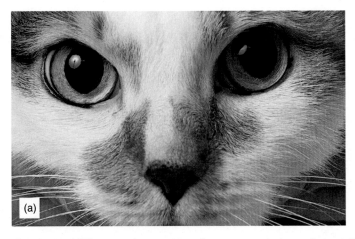
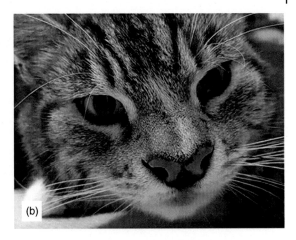

Figure 3.32 (a) The normal appearance of two symmetrical nares in a cat. Source: Courtesy of the Media Resources Department at Midwestern University. (b) This patient has a rare congenital defect that has resulted in three nares. Source: Courtesy of Derek Calhoon, DVM, MSc.

The clinician should also take care to evaluate the mucocutaneous junction where the nasal planum meets the bridge of the nose. Any depigmentation, abrasion, or ulceration should be noted. Solar dermatosis, especially in white cats, along with squamous cell carcinoma, pemphigus, systemic and discoid lupus erythematosis, and dermatophytosis can cause changes in this location.

3.5 The Extra-Oral Examination

It is tempting to equate the oral examination with opening the patient's mouth. However, the oral examination should be broken into two components: the extra-oral and the intra-oral examination. Because it is less invasive, the extra-oral should precede the intra-oral examination. The extra-oral examination provides important information about the stability and integrity of structures that comprise the oral cavity that may not always be obvious from the intra-oral examination [84].

The clinician begins the extra-oral examination by assessing the face for symmetry, as reviewed in Section 3.1, with emphasis on the maxilla and mandible (Figure 3.36). In addition to assessing the symmetry of the bones that form the oral cavity, the clinician should also assess the symmetry of the muscles of mastication: the masseter and temporal muscles.

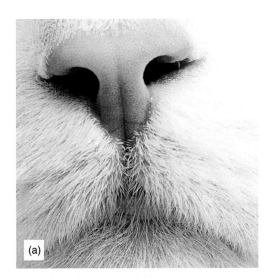
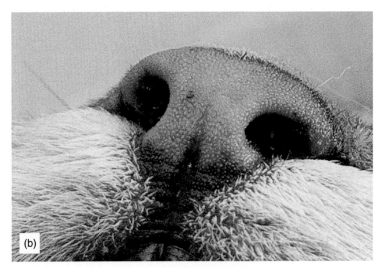

Figure 3.33 (a) This pink nasal planum has a natural cobblestone appearance. (b) This pigmented nasal planum also has a natural cobblestone appearance. Source (a), (b): Courtesy of the Media Resources Department at Midwestern University.

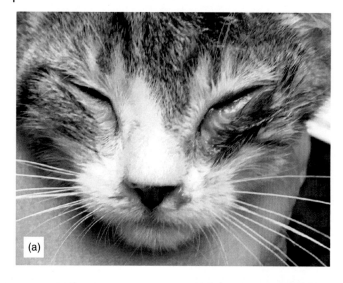

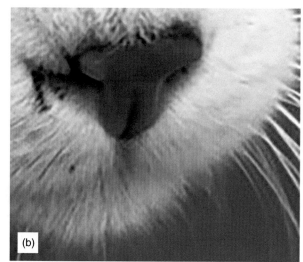

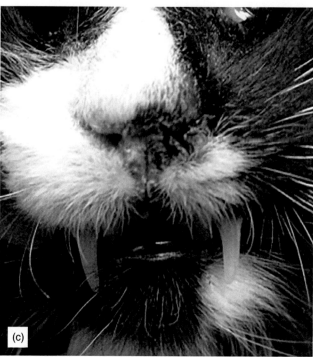

Figure 3.34 (a) Serous to mucoid left nasal discharge with concurrent serous left ocular discharge in a kitten with an upper respiratory tract infection. Source: Courtesy of Frank Isom, DVM. (b) Dried rust brown right nasal discharge in an adult cat. This may or may not be normal for this patient. (c) Yellow mucopurulent discharge is abnormal. It is also heavily crusting the nares of this patient. Source: Courtesy of Samantha Thurman, DVM.

The clinician should also determine structural stability. To do so, the clinician should:

- palpate over the maxilla;
- palpate over the zygomatic arches;
- palpate over the temporomandibular joints;
- palpate the angular processes of the mandible;
- palpate the ventral aspect of the left and right bodies of the mandible for fractures and/or symphyseal instability;
- palpate the intermandibular space.

In addition, the clinician should palpate the submandibular lymph nodes and the mandibular salivary gland

[84]. The submandibular lymph nodes are caudoventral to the angle of the mandible. In order to feel them, the clinician should slide his fingers down the angle of the mandible to the ventrolateral neck. Grasping a generous amount of skin bilaterally between the thumb and index fingers, the clinician should then slide his fingers from deep to superficial. This should allow the submandibular lymph nodes to "slip" through his fingers (Figure 3.37).

There are normally two submandibular lymph nodes on each side. In the cat, each is about the size of a pea, and they are located cranial to the mandibular salivary gland, which is also palpable in the normal cat. Finding

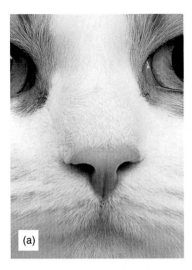
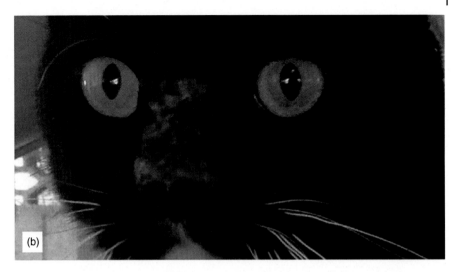

Figure 3.35 (a) The bridge of the nose of this patient is normal. There is no swelling associated with it. There are also no excoriations. Source: Courtesy of the Media Resources Department at Midwestern University. (b) The bridge of the nose of this patient is crusted over as a result of a mosquito bite hypersensitivity reaction. Source: Courtesy of Juliane Daggett, MBS.

one or more enlarged submandibular lymph nodes may raise the clinician's index of suspicion that there is underlying dental disease.

Like the submandibular lymph nodes, the mandibular salivary gland should be discrete, smooth, and supple. Changes in size, texture, and consistency, especially when asymmetric, should be a red flag that underlying disease is probable. Changes may be subtle, but they can also present in quite a dramatic fashion (Figure 3.38).

Other important extra-oral findings to note include upper or lower lip swellings, erosions, ulcerations, or ptyalism. Some cats will hypersalivate when stressed or in response to something aversive, especially substances

that taste bitter; however, ptyalism may also be a response to oral pain or other oral pathology (Figure 3.39).

Only after all of the above has been evaluated and documented is the clinician ready to lift the cat's lips and dive into the intra-oral examination.

3.6 The Intra-Oral Examination

3.6.1 Assessing Mucous Membrane Color

The intra-oral examination is designed to assess mucous membranes, the dentition, the gingiva, the mucosa, the

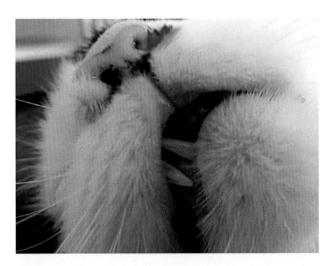

Figure 3.36 This patient sustained bite wounds to the face and extensive facial trauma that led to luxation of the mandible. The result is grossly visible misalignment between the maxilla and mandible. Source: Courtesy of Patricia Bennett, DVM.

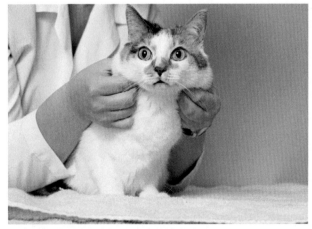

Figure 3.37 Standing behind the patient, grasping skin folds caudoventral to the angle of the mandible on either side allows the submandibular lymph nodes to "slip" through the examiner's fingers. Source: Courtesy of the Media Resources Department at Midwestern University.

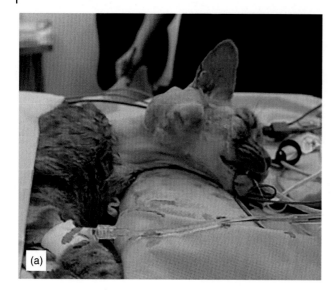
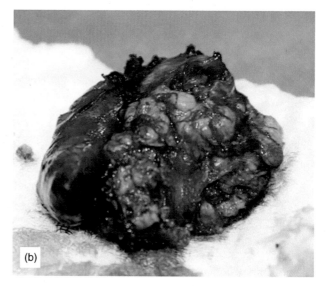

Figure 3.38 (a) Grossly visible right mandibular salivary gland tumor. Note its multi-nodular appearance. (b) Gross inspection of the salivary gland tumor in (a) after surgical excision. Source (a), (b): Courtesy of Stephanie Shaver, DVM, DACVS-SA.

tongue, the sublingual space, the palate, and the oropharynx.

Mucous membrane color is an important tool by which to assess circulatory status. Normal mucous membranes are a healthy pink; however, some patients with lentigo have mottled black pigment throughout – this is also considered normal. By contrast, white or pale mucous membranes indicate that the patient may be experiencing shock

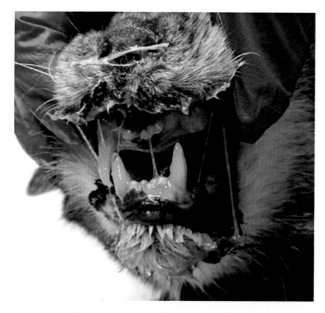

Figure 3.39 This is a patient with extensive extra-oral lesions, including an abundance of thick, ropy saliva and necrotic margins of the upper lips. The odor was rancid, and an extensive sublingual tumor was identified on intra-oral examination.

or is significantly anemic. Cyanotic mucous membranes typically confer hypoxia. Cherry red mucous membranes are classic for carbon monoxide toxicosis, and icteric mucous membranes reflect underlying hyperbilirubinemia as from intravascular hemolysis or hepatopathy. If there are petechiations or ecchymoses within the mucous membranes, coagulopathies are a potential concern.

Mucous membranes should be moist. If they are tacky or stick to the clinician's fingers, then the patient is likely dehydrated, as was discussed in Section 2.3.

Depending on the patient's temperament, the clinician may use fingers or a tongue depressor to lift the lip folds in order to assess mucous membrane color and moistness (Figure 3.40).

3.6.2 Assessing Capillary Refill Time

In addition to evaluating the mucous membranes for color and moisture, the clinician should assess the capillary refill time (CRT). The CRT is a means by which a patient's circulatory status is assessed. The clinician uses a finger or the end of a tongue depressor to press down on an area of the gumline firmly, which forces blood out of the capillaries at that site. When the clinician then releases his finger or the tongue depressor, the blood should return to the capillaries, thereby refilling them, within one to two seconds on average. If a patient is in shock or dehydrated, blood is slower to refill, which results in a prolonged CRT.

3.6.3 Examining the Mucosa

After assessing the patient's CRT, the clinician should assess the buccal and alveolar mucosa for redness, erosions, ulcerations, masses, and other abnormalities (Figure 3.41).

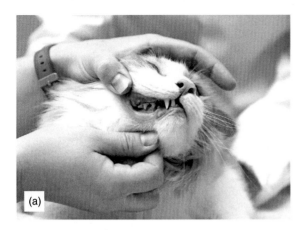
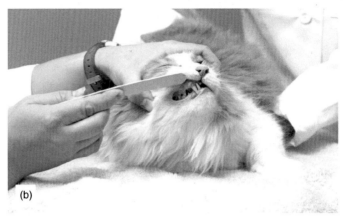

Figure 3.40 (a) Lifting the lips with fingertips in order to view buccal mucosa, gingiva, and a significant portion of the upper right dental arcade. One can obtain a good amount of information using this approach before even attempting to open the mouth! (b) Lifting the lips with a tongue depressor in a cat of unknown temperament. This is an easy way to spare fingertips from being nipped if this patient objects to having its gums assessed. Source (a), (b): Courtesy of the Media Resources Department at Midwestern University.

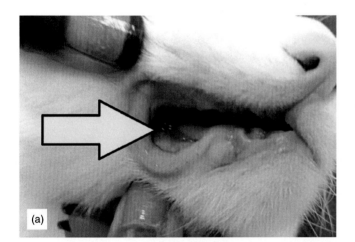
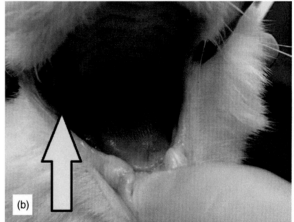
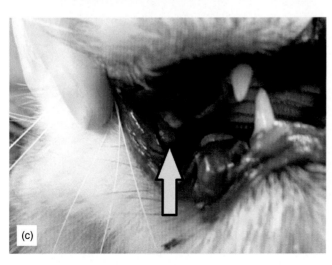

Figure 3.41 (a) This patient previously underwent a total mouth extraction to manage severe gingivostomatis. Even so, it is experiencing an acute flare characterized by buccal mucosal irritation and associated bleeding. (b) The same patient as in (a), when asked to open its mouth. Note the buccal mucosal irritation. (c) This patient has a buccal mucosal nodule. Source (a)–(c): Courtesy of Patricia Bennett, DVM.

3.6.4 Examining the Gingiva

In addition to assessing the buccal and alveolar mucosa, the clinician should evaluate the gingiva and ask the following (Figure 3.42):

- Is there gingivitis?
- If so, is it focal or diffuse?
- Is there gingival bleeding with or without the clinician touching the gum line?
- Is there gingival recession?
- Is there gingival hyperplasia or other "mass effect"?

During an intra-oral examination, gingivitis is typically classified as focal versus generalized. However, during dental charting under general anesthesia, each individual tooth can be assigned a gingival index (GI) score. There is no universal standardization in veterinary medicine with regard to the gingival index score; however, the author has adapted the following based upon others' approaches that have been documented in the human and veterinary medical literature [85, 86]:

- GI 0: Normal gingiva.
- GI 1: Mild inflammation. Slight color change and edema. No bleeding on probing.
- GI 2: Moderate inflammation. Redness. Moderate edema. Bleeding on probing.
- GI 3: Severe inflammation, marked redness, edema and ulceration. Tendency for spontaneous bleeding.

Note that assigning the GI score requires probing of and around the gum line surrounding each tooth. Because this is not a procedure that awake patients will tolerate, the GI score is typically reserved for dental charting, to provide a score for each individual tooth. This will allow the veterinary team to keep track of trends, progress, and how at-home and in-clinic interventions are working.

3.6.5 Assessing the Dentition

The clinician should also assess the dentition. In order to evaluate the dentition properly, the clinician needs first to understand the dental formula for the feline patient [8, 87, 88]:

- The dental formula for an immature cat, meaning one with deciduous dentition, is

$$2 \times (I3/3, C1/1, P3/2) = 26 \text{ teeth total}$$

- The dental formula for an adult cat, meaning one with permanent dentition, is

$$2 \times (I3/3, C1/1, P3/2, M1/1) = 30 \text{ teeth total}$$

Deciduous teeth tend to be smaller than permanent teeth. In the cat, the deciduous incisors erupt at between 2 and 3 weeks of age, followed by the deciduous canines (at 3–4 weeks of age) and the deciduous premolars (at 3–6 weeks of age). Eruption of permanent teeth begins with the permanent incisors between 3 and 4 months

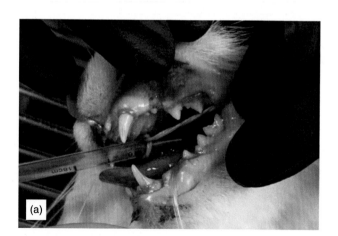

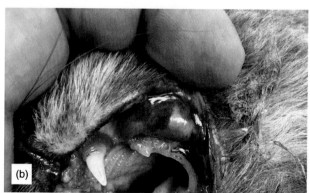

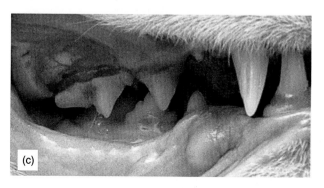

Figure 3.42 (a) Note the presence of focal gingivitis that is primarily associated with the left maxillary and mandibular canine tooth. Source: Courtesy of Elizabeth Robbins, DVM. (b) Note the severity of the gingivitis that was localized to this patient's left maxillary dental arcade and corresponded to dental disease. Source: Courtesy of Frank Isom, DVM. (c) Note the presence of focal gingivitis along the right maxillary dental arcade. By contrast, there is no apparent gingivitis along the right mandibular dental arcade. Source: Courtesy of the Media Resources Department at Midwestern University.

of age. Eruption of permanent teeth is complete by 5–6 months of age [19]. Because eruption of permanent teeth is gradual, it is typical for kittens to exhibit age-appropriate mixed dentition, meaning that deciduous and permanent teeth can both be present in the mouth simultaneously (Figure 3.43). Typically, the molars are the last to erupt [87, 89].

To facilitate the identification of teeth in veterinary medicine, the modified Triadan system of nomenclature was developed [8, 88–90]. Each tooth is given a three-digit identification number. The dental arcade that the tooth is in dictates what the first digit in the three-digit identification number will be:

- Every tooth in the right maxillary arcade has an identification number that starts with 1.
- Every tooth in the left maxillary arcade has an identification number that starts with 2.
- Every tooth in the left mandibular arcade has an identification number that starts with 3.
- Every tooth in the right mandibular arcade has an identification number that starts with 4.

The teeth are then numbered beginning from midline. For instance, each arcade has three incisors. So, in the right maxillary arcade, the incisor nearest midline is given the identification number 101; the middle incisor is 102; and the third incisor from midline is 103.

The canine teeth are always number 4. So, in the right maxillary arcade, the canine tooth is given the identification number 104; the canine tooth in the left maxillary arcade is 204; the canine tooth in the left mandibular arcade is 304; and the canine tooth in the right mandibular arcade is 404.

The last tooth in each arcade for the cat is given the number 9. So, in the right maxillary arcade, the one and only molar is 109; in the left maxillary arcade, the one and only molar is 209; in the left mandibular arcade, the one and only molar is 309; and in the right mandibular arcade, the one and only molar is 409.

The remaining teeth (the premolars) are filled in numerically, counting down from 9, when moving caudal to midline. Because cats have fewer teeth than dogs and the modified Triadan system was built around dogs, cats are missing teeth 105, 205, 305, 306, 405, and 406 (Figure 3.44).

The modified Triadan system allows the clinician to identify lesions in specific teeth, and provides for more thorough notations during dental charting under general anesthesia. The system also helps the clinician to keep track of teeth in the mouth and to identify when a tooth is missing, fractured, extracted, or in the process of resorption. Clinicians can also identify if there are supernumerary teeth such as retained deciduous teeth [8, 84].

3.6.6 Assessing the Occlusion

In addition to numbering the dentition, the clinician should assess the occlusion by asking whether or not the bite is normal [8, 84, 88]. A "scissors bite" represents normal occlusion: there is a space between the upper canines and the adjacent incisor into which the lower canines should naturally fit [87, 88] (Figure 3.45).

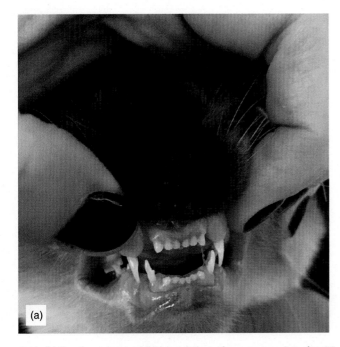
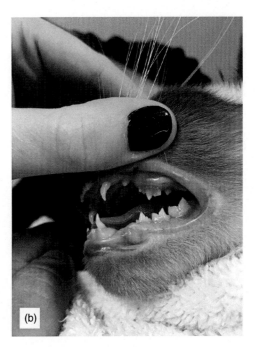

Figure 3.43 (a) Head-on view and (b) lateral view of age-appropriate dentition in a kitten. Note that all four canine teeth are deciduous. Source (a), (b): Courtesy of Natalie Reeser.

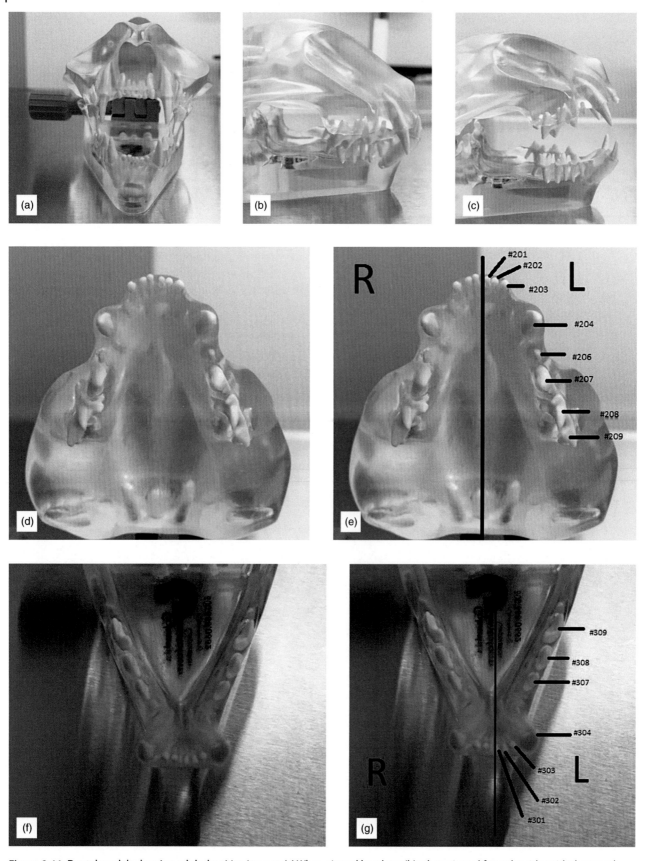

Figure 3.44 Dental models showing adult dentition in a cat. (a) When viewed head-on; (b) when viewed from the side, with the mouth closed; (c) when viewed from the side, with the mouth open; (d) in the maxillary arcades only; (e) in the maxillary arcades only, with the teeth labeled using the modified Triadan system; (f) in the mandibular arcades only (g) in the mandibular arcades only, with the teeth labeled using the modified Triadan system.

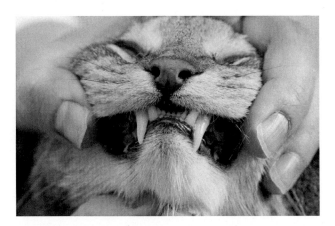

Figure 3.45 Normal occlusion: the classic "scissors bite." Source: Courtesy of the Media Resources Department at Midwestern University.

A malocclusion occurs when there is misalignment of the teeth. This may be a primary dental issue or may be due to a primary skeletal issue. Class I malocclusions are the result of the former whereas Class II and III malocclusions are due to the latter [8, 91].

The most commonly identified types of Class I malocclusions include the following:

- Mesioversion: the tooth is anatomically in the correct location, but its angle is mesial compared with the norm, meaning that the tooth points toward the front midline [87]. When this involves the maxillary canine teeth, the canine teeth are said to be spearing or lancing tusks. This condition is commonly seen in Persians [8, 91].
- Distoversion: the tooth is anatomically in the correct location, but its angle is distal compared with the norm, meaning that the tooth points away from the front midline [8, 87, 91].

A less commonly seen Class I malocclusion occurs when a tooth is anatomically in the correct location, but its angle is lingual compared with the norm, meaning that the tooth points toward the tongue [87]. This condition is called linguoversion [8, 91].

Class I malocclusions also include crossbites:

- A rostral crossbite occurs when a mandibular incisor is labial to the maxillary incisor of the same number, where labial refers to the tooth protruding toward the lip. For example, this would occur if #401 were labial to #101 [88, 91].
- A caudal crossbite occurs when the mandibular cheek teeth are buccal to the maxillary cheek teeth of the same number, where buccal refers to pointing toward the cheek [87]. For example, this would occur if #407 were buccal to #107 [88, 91].

When the mandible is shorter than expected, the patient is said to have a Class II malocclusion. This

results in the appearance of an overbite, characterized by the maxillary dental arcades protruding beyond the mandibular arcades. This is sometimes referred to as "parrot mouth." If this is severe, the mandibular canine teeth may come into contact with the hard palate. Irritation or ulceration may result. In worst-case scenarios, an oronasal fistula may develop due to penetration of the mandibular canines through the hard palate [8, 88, 91].

A Class III malocclusion occurs when the mandible is too long (mandibular prognathism) or the maxilla is too short (maxillary brachygnathism). This results in the appearance of an underbite, characterized by the mandibular dental arcades protruding beyond the maxillary dental arcades. This is sometimes referred to as "monkey mouth." Persian cats often have this type of malocclusion [10, 88, 91].

3.6.7 Assessing for Calculus

A further aspect of the intra-oral examination is to assess for the presence of calculus, otherwise known as tartar. Calculus is a hardened deposit of dead microorganisms encased in calcium salts. Calculus forms when plaque, a sticky substance that intra-oral bacteria produce, binds to the teeth. Like gingivitis, calculus distribution may be non-existent, focal, or generalized (Figure 3.46).

Just as each individual tooth can be assigned a gingival index (GI) score during dental charting under general anesthesia, each individual tooth can also be assigned a calculus index (CI) score. As with the GI score, there is no universal standardization in veterinary medicine with regard to the CI score; however, the author has adapted the following based upon others' approaches that have been documented in the human and veterinary medical literature [84, 92–96]:

- CI 0: No observable calculus present.
- CI 1: Scattered calculus covering less than one-third of the buccal surface of the tooth.
- CI 2: Calculus covering between one- and two-thirds of the buccal surface of the tooth with minimal subgingival calculus.
- CI 3: Calculus covering more than two-thirds of the buccal surface of the tooth and extending subgingivally.

3.6.8 Opening the Mouth

Note how much information the clinician is able to acquire without opening the cat's mouth. Only after all of the above data have been gathered is it essential to complete the final step of the intra-oral examination, opening the mouth. When opening a cat's mouth, it is best that

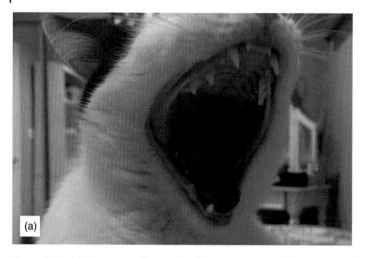 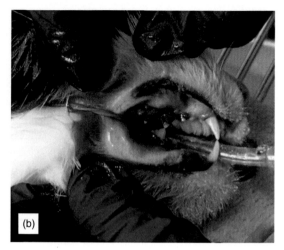

Figure 3.46 (a) Cat opening its mouth wide on its own, providing an exceptional view of the oral cavity. Note that calculus distribution is scant to non-existent. Source: Courtesy of Kelly Chappell. (b) Cat undergoing dentistry prophylaxis under general anesthesia. Note the presence of heavy, yet focal tartar distribution on the maxillary and mandibular premolars and molars. The right maxillary and mandibular canines are minimally involved by comparison. Source: Courtesy of Elizabeth Robbins, DVM.

the clinician position themself relative to the cat using one of the following three approaches:

1) If the cat is on an examination room table, the clinician may stand behind the cat and press up against the table. Often when a cat's mouth is opened, the cat will try to back up to escape the maneuver. In this approach, the clinician's body serves as a wall to block the escape route.
2) If the cat is on the floor and the clinician is kneeling, the clinician should squeeze his knees together to create a similar wall through which the cat cannot back up and escape.
3) Alternatively, the clinician may stand directly in front of the patient, provided that the restrainer stands immediately behind the patient to block it from backing up.

Using the non-dominant hand, the clinician may cup the patient's head such that the thumb and index finger grasp the zygomatic arches. With the non-dominant hand in place, the clinician may then raise the cat's head to the sky. This often causes the cat to weaken or drop its lower jaw. Using the index finger or the middle finger of the dominant hand, the clinician may then push down on the mandibular incisors to open the mouth (Figure 3.47).

Once the patient's mouth is open, the clinician should be able to smell the patient's breath [84] and ask:

- Does it smell like ketones, indicating an underlying metabolic pathology?
- Does it smell fetid as if there is appreciable oral disease or necrotic tissues?

With the patient's mouth open, the clinician should also be able to evaluate the hard palate for clefts, masses, or asymmetry (Figure 3.48).

The clinician should evaluate the pharyngeal region as far back as possible for masses and other lesions (Figure 3.49). Using an otoscope or ophthalmoscope to illuminate the region can be very helpful. Sedation may be required.

3.6.9 Examining the Tongue

In addition, the tongue's surface should be assessed for normal anatomy and also for erosions or ulcerations [84] (Figure 3.50). These could result from:

- calicivirus;
- electrocution burns, as from a cat biting a wire;
- uremic syndrome in a patient with kidney disease.

The clinician should always remember to look under the tongue for string foreign bodies [19]. When cats eat string, it easily gets caught around the frenulum.

Looking underneath the tongue in a cat's mouth requires coordination, patience, and dexterity. The clinician should use his thumb to apply firm pressure to the inter-mandibular space from the ventral aspect while the cat has its mouth open. At the same time, the clinician must use the index finger of the same hand to flip the tongue up and over (Figure 3.51). It is equally important to identify sublingual masses (Figure 3.52).

3.6.10 Assessing for Periodontal Disease

The peridontium refers to the supporting structures that surround the teeth: the gingiva, which were discussed previously, the periodontal ligament, and the alveolar bone. Periodontal disease refers to inflammation and/or infection of one or more of these structures. At its earliest stages, periodontal disease

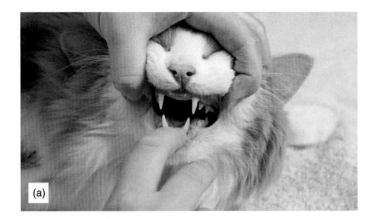
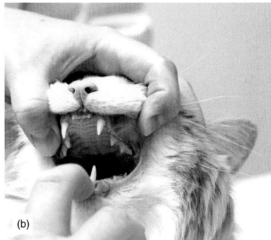
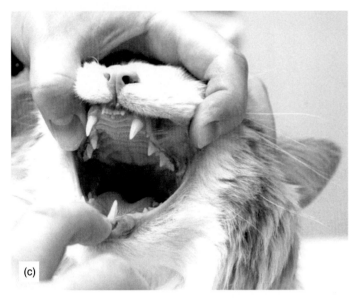
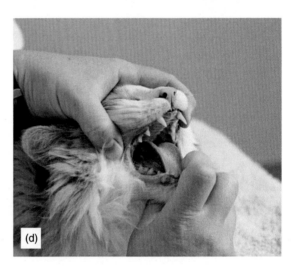

Figure 3.47 (a) Proper technique for cupping the cat's head with one hand while placing the index finger of the opposite hand over the mandibular incisors in preparation for opening the mouth. (b) Extending the cat's head and neck toward the ceiling while using the index finger to push down on the jaw over the mandibular incisors. (c) Opening the cat's mouth wider so that the clinician has a good view of the palatal and pharyngeal regions. (d) Side view demonstrating that the patient has been coaxed into opening its mouth wide. Source (a)–(d): Courtesy of the Media Resources Department at Midwestern University.

is characterized by gingivitis, which is visible to the naked eye. However, what is seen above the gum line may or may not reflect what is occurring beneath. Bacteria can also get up under the gum line, where they secrete plaque and stimulate the immune system to react with an inflammatory response. As white cells migrate to their target location in an attempt to manage focal infection, damage may be done to the structures surrounding the tooth. The gingiva recedes and tooth roots become visible. When teeth have multiple roots, one or more can be exposed. As this occurs, there is progressive loss of the periodontal ligament and alveolar bone. Without this support, affected teeth may become mobile, and surgical extraction may be indicated [8, 84, 87, 89].

Assessing cats and dogs for periodontal disease requires a more extensive oral examination than is allowed by an awake patient, even a patient that is tolerant. Assessing for periodontal disease involves extensive dental charting, probing around each tooth to determination class of furcation exposure, and radiographic determination of the health of the alveolar bone. Periodontal disease cannot be definitively staged without whole-mouth radiographs to augment gross physical examination findings [8, 87, 97].

When periodontal disease is diagnosed, the diagnosis may pertain to a single tooth or multiple teeth. Different teeth can be at different stages of periodontal disease, which is yet another reason why dental charting is so important. It allows the veterinary team to track the

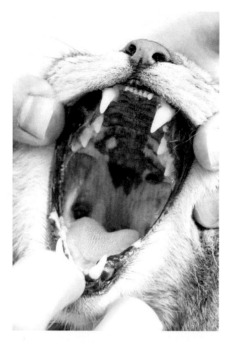

Figure 3.48 Examining the hard palate. This represents a variation of normal in terms of pigmentation. Not every hard palate is mottled pink and black like the one depicted here, which is a variation of normal. Source: Courtesy of the Media Resources Department at Midwestern University.

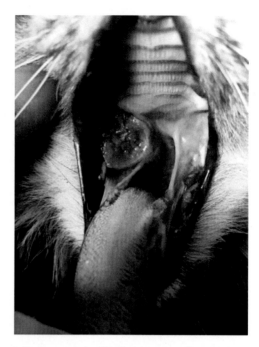

Figure 3.49 An example of oral squamous cell carcinoma. Source: Courtesy of Amanda Maltese, DVM.

progression of disease and identify patient-appropriate areas of intervention.

In order to standardize the language that is used to describe periodontal disease, the American Veterinary Dental College (AVDC) developed a classification system [8, 87, 91, 98]. This system allows for the staging of periodontal disease in a way that is universally understood among the veterinary profession and minimizes confusion:

- PD 0: Negative for gingivitis, with radiographically normal peridontium.
- PD 1: Gingivitis is present as the only indication of periodontal disease. The peridontium is radiographically normal.
- PD 2: Gingivitis is present, and radiographic signs of periodontal disease are present: at most there is 25% loss of periodontal attachment.
- PD 3: Gingivitis is present, and radiographic signs are progressive: there is between 25% and 50% loss of periodontal attachment.
- PD 4: Periodontal disease is advanced, with greater than 50% loss of periodontal attachment.

3.6.11 Feline-Specific Dentistry

The importance of evaluating the oral mucosa was discussed in Section 3.6.3; however, feline gingivostomatitis

as a diseased state of the oral cavity was not discussed. Feline gingivostomatitis is a feline-specific diagnosis: *gingivo*, referring to the gingiva, and *stomatitis*, referring to inflammation of the oral cavity's mucous membranes. Stomatitis can be widespread or focal. In the latter case, its name is expanded to include its location in the oral cavity. For example, caudal stomatitis is the

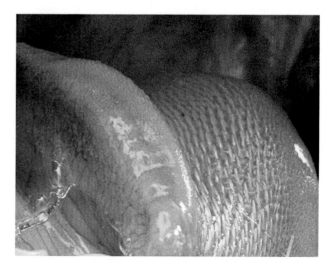

Figure 3.50 Visually inspecting the dorsal aspect of a cat's tongue. Note the sharp spines, otherwise referred to as papillae. These are backward-facing "hooks" that assist with grooming. Source: Courtesy of the Media Resources Department at Midwestern University.

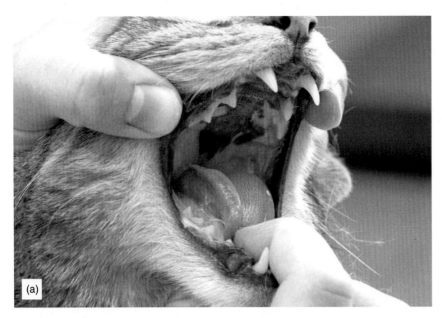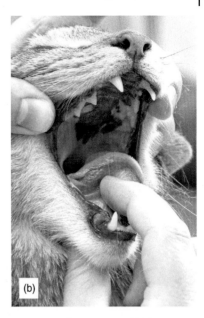

Figure 3.51 (a) Preparing to flip up the tongue in order to visualize its ventral aspect. (b) Putting pressure on the inter-mandibular space with the thumb while flipping the tongue up and over with the index finger of the same hand to see if anything is trapped underneath the tongue. There is no string foreign body in this patient. Source (a), (b): Courtesy of the Media Resources Department at Midwestern University.

condition by which stomatitis extends to the lateral palatine folds.

Feline gingivostomatitis has a raw hamburger-like appearance in the oral cavity. When present, it can be

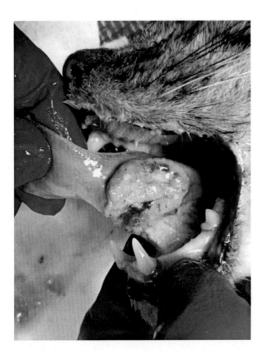

Figure 3.52 Sublingual mass in a patient that was humanely euthanized due to perceived poor quality of life.

quite extensive and inflammatory, with raspberry red color to the affected tissue, spontaneous bleeding, and a nodular or cobblestone appearance. On gross inspection, it cannot be definitely differentiated from oral cancer due to its characteristically aggressive appearance. Biopsies are required to rule out squamous cell carcinoma, among other types of oral neoplasia, and also feline eosinophilic granulomas [84, 87, 98] (Figure 3.53).

Feline gingivostomatitis is thought to be an inappropriate immune response to a number of triggers. Underlying viral infections such as feline calicivirus, feline immunodeficiency virus (FIV) and feline leukemia virus (FeLV) may aggravate it. The same may be said of certain bacterial populations in the mouth, such as *Bartonella* and *Pasteurella*. It is also thought that these cats over-react to plaque and to their own teeth as if their teeth were foreign objects requiring an immune attack. As a result, whole-mouth extraction is considered to be the standard of care to remove any potential trigger that could incite a flare-up. However, not every patient is responsive to whole-mouth extraction, and flare-ups may still occur even without any overt stimulation in the oral cavity. As a result, clients should expect chronic medical management even in patients that have had all teeth extracted, to include antibiotic and immunosuppressant therapy as indicated [8].

In addition to feline gingivostomatitis, feline odotoclastic resorptive lesions (FORLS) or, simply put, tooth resorption, are a common dental finding in feline practice

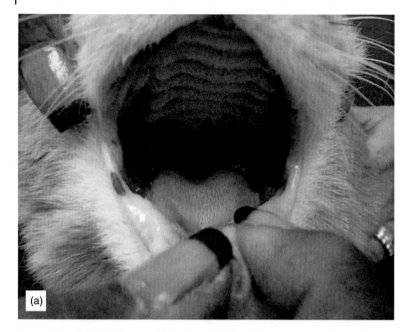
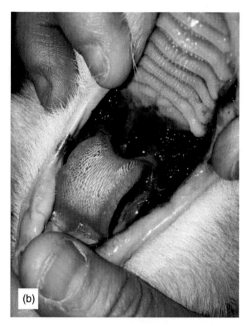

Figure 3.53 (a) Caudal stomatitis. Note the brick red appearance to the caudalmost aspect of the oropharynx. (b) Close-up view of caudal stomatitis in the same patient as in (a). Note the friability of the tissue. Source (a), (b): Courtesy of Patricia Bennett, DVM.

[87]. It is thought that nearly half of the cat population is grossly affected by this condition [8]. When assessed radiographically, the incidence may be nearer 75% [8, 97, 99]. Young Burmese and Siamese cats (less than 12 months of age) appear to be at increased risk [84, 100]. Other breeds tend to be predisposed when over 6 years of age [84, 100].

The definitive cause of these lesions is unknown [97]. Past theories have included that FORLS were the result of hairballs being vomited up, causing stomach acid to bathe and ultimately dissolve the teeth. An underlying nutritional cause has also been suspected, given that tooth resorption in laboratory rats can be induced by vitamin D toxicosis [8].

When tooth resorption occurs, it may involve the crown only, the root only, or both. The earliest sign of its development may be focal gingivitis (Figure 3.54).

To help identify lesions, the AVDC developed the following classification system [8, 91, 97, 98]:

- TR 0: Negative for gross or radiographic signs of tooth resorption.
- TR 1: Mild loss of cementum or cementum plus enamel.
- TR 2: Moderate loss of cementum or cementum plus enamel; however, dentin loss does not extend into the pulp cavity.
- TR 3: Moderate loss of cementum or cementum plus enamel, and dentin loss extends into the pulp cavity. Structurally, the tooth appears to retain its integrity.

- TR 4: Extensive loss of cementum or cementum plus enamel, and dentin loss extends into the pulp cavity. Structurally, the tooth has lost its integrity.
- TR 5: Only remnants of the tooth are visible radiographically. Grossly, there appears to be no tooth, only gingiva [84].

There is debate as to whether or not tooth resorption progresses in stages like periodontal disease [98]. What is agreed upon is that stages 2–4 require extraction [8].

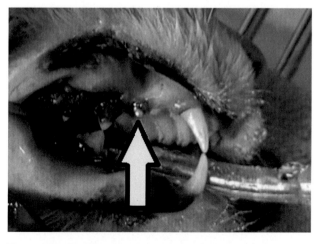

Figure 3.54 Significant gingivitis surrounding #106. This may be the beginning of tooth resorption. Source: Courtesy of Elizabeth Robbins, DVM.

References

1 Sisson, S., Grossman, J.D., and Getty, R. (1975) *Sisson and Grossman's The Anatomy of the Domestic Animals*, 5th edn., Saunders, Philadelphia.

2 Uddin, M., Sarker, M.H.R., Hossain, M.E. *et al.* (2013) Morphometric investigation of neurocranium in domestic cat (*Felis catus*). *Bangladesh Journal of Veterinary Medicine*, **11** (1), 69–73.

3 Christiansen, P. (2008) Evolution of skull and mandible shape in cats (Carnivora: Felidae). *PLoS One*, **3** (7), e2807.

4 Biknevicius, A.R. and Van Valkenburgh, B. (1996) Design for killing: craniodental adaptations of predators, in *Carnivore Behavior, Ecology, and Evolution, 2* (ed. J.L. Gittleman), Cornell University Press, Ithaca, NY, pp. 393–428.

5 Christiansen, P. and Wroe, S. (2007) Bite forces and evolutionary adaptations to feeding ecology in carnivores. *Ecology*, **88** (2), 347–358.

6 Kunzel, W., Breit, S., and Oppel, M. (2003) Morphometric investigations of breed-specific features in feline skulls and considerations on their functional implications. *Anatomia, Histologia, Embryologia*, **32** (4), 218–223.

7 Monfared, A.L. (2013) Anatomy of the Persian cat's skull and its clinical value during regional anesthesia. *Global Veterinaria*, **10** (5), 551–555.

8 Holmstrom, S.E. (2013) *Veterinary Dentistry: A Team Approach*, 2nd edn., Saunders Elsevier, St. Louis.

9 Schlueter, C., Budras, K.D., Ludewig, E. *et al.* (2009) Brachycephalic feline noses: CT and anatomical study of the relationship between head conformation and the nasolacrimal drainage system. *Journal of Feline Medicine and Surgery*, **11** (11), 891–900.

10 Malik, R., Sparkes, A., and Bessant, C. (2009) Brachycephalia – a bastardisation of what makes cats special. *Journal of Feline Medicine and Surgery*, **11** (11), 889–890.

11 Breit, S., Kunzel, W., and Oppel, M. (2003) The course of the nasolacrimal duct in brachycephalic cats. *Anatomia, Histologia, Embryologia*, **32** (4), 224–227.

12 Hobson, H.P. (1995) Brachycephalic syndrome. *Seminars in Veterinary Medicine and Surgery*, **10** (2), 109–114.

13 Featherstone, H.J. and Sansom, J. (2004) Feline corneal sequestra: a review of 64 cases (80 eyes) from 1993 to 2000. *Veterinary Ophthalmology*, **7** (4), 213–227.

14 Gunn-Moore, D.A. and Thrusfield, M.V. (1995) Feline dystocia: prevalence, and association with cranial conformation and breed. *Veterinary Record*, **136** (14), 350–353.

15 Harvey, A. and Tasker, S. (2013) *BSAVA Manual of Feline Practice: A Foundational Manual*, 2nd edn., British Small Animal Veterinary Association, Gloucester.

16 Gould, D. and McLellan, G. (2015) *BSAVA Manual of Canine and Feline Ophthalmology*, 2nd edn., British Small Animal Veterinary Association, Gloucester.

17 Gelatt, K.N. (2014) *Essentials of Veterinary Ophthalmology*, 3rd edn., Wiley-Blackwell, Ames, IA.

18 Maggs, D.J., Miller, P.E., and Ofri, R. (2013) *Slatter's Fundamentals of Veterinary Ophthalmology*, 5th edn., Saunders Elsevier, St. Louis.

19 Rijnberk, A. and van Sluijs, F.S. (2009) *Medical History and Physical Examination in Companion Animals*, 2nd edn., Saunders Elsevier, St. Louis.

20 Dziezyc, J. and Millichamp, N.J. (2004) *Color Atlas of Canine and Feline Ophthalmology*, Saunders Elsevier, St. Louis.

21 Ketring, K.L. and Glaze, M.B. (2012) *Atlas of Feline Ophthalmology*, 2nd edn., Wiley-Blackwell, Ames, IA.

22 Lim, C.C. (2015) *Small Animal Ophthalmic Atlas and Guide*, Wiley-Blackwell, Ames, IA.

23 Betbeze C. (2015) Management of orbital diseases. *Topics in Companion Animal Medicine*, **30** (3), 107–117.

24 Gunton, K.B., Wasserman, B.N., and DeBenedictis, C. (2015) Strabismus. *Primary Care*, **42** (3), 393–407.

25 Campos, E.C. (2008) Why do the eyes cross? A review and discussion of the nature and origin of essential infantile esotropia, microstrabismus, accommodative esotropia, and acute comitant esotropia. *Journal of AAPOS*, **12** (4), 326–331.

26 Rengstorff, R.H. (1976) Strabismus measurements in the Siamese cat. *American Journal of Optometry and Physiological Optics*, **53** (10), 643–646.

27 Blake, R. and Crawford, M.L. (1974) Development of strabismus in Siamese cats. *Brain Research*, **77** (3), 492–496.

28 Hyde, J.E. (1962) Cross-eyedness: a study in Siamese cats. *American Journal of Ophthalmology*, **53**, 70–75.

29 Forrester, S.D., Greco, D.S., and Relford, R.L. (1992) Serum hyperviscosity syndrome associated with multiple-myeloma in 2 cats. *Journal of the American Veterinary Medical Association*, **200** (1), 79–82.

30 Fitzgerald, K.T., Bronstein, A.C., and Newquist, K.L. (2013) Marijuana poisoning. *Topics in Companion Animal Medicine*, **28** (1), 8–12.

31 Oliver, J.A. and Bradbrook, C.A. (2013) Suspected brainstem anesthesia following retrobulbar block in a cat. *Veterinary Ophthalmology*, **16** (3), 225–228.

32 Mettens, P., Godaux, E., and Cheron, G. (1990) Effects of ketamine on ocular movements of the cat. *Journal of Vestibular Research: Equilibrium & Orientation*, **1** (4), 325–338.

33 Rossmeisl, J.H., Jr. (2010) Vestibular disease in dogs and cats. *Veterinary Clinics of North America: Small Animal Practice*, **40** (1), 81–100.

34 Thomas, W.B. (2000) Vestibular dysfunction. *Veterinary Clinics of North America: Small Animal Practice*, **30** (1), 227–249, viii.

35 Kornegay, J.N. (1991) Ataxia, head tilt, nystagmus. Vestibular diseases. *Problems in Veterinary Medicine*, **3** (3), 417–425.

36 Burke, E.E., Moise, N.S., de Lahunta, A., and Erb, H.N. (1985) Review of idiopathic feline vestibular syndrome in 75 cats. *Journal of the American Veterinary Medical Association*, **187** (9), 941–943.

37 Stiles, J. (2000) Feline herpesvirus. *Veterinary Clinics of North America: Small Animal Practice*, **30** (5), 1001–1014.

38 Andrew, S.E. (2001) Ocular manifestations of feline herpesvirus. *Journal of Feline Medicine and Surgery*, **3** (1), 9–16.

39 Hartley, C. (2010) Aetiology of corneal ulcers assume FHV-1 unless proven otherwise. *Journal of Feline Medicine and Surgery*, **12** (1), 24–35.

40 Thiry, E., Addie, D., Belak, S. *et al.* Feline herpesvirus infection. ABCD guidelines on prevention and management. *Journal of Feline Medicine and Surgery*, **11** (7), 547–555.

41 Townsend, W.M. (2008) Canine and feline uveitis. *Veterinary Clinics of North America: Small Animal Practice*, **38** (2), 323–346, vii.

42 Colitz, C.M. (2005) Feline uveitis: diagnosis and treatment. *Clinical Techniques in Small Animal Practice*, **20** (2), 117–120.

43 Kaas, J.H. (2005) Serendipity and the Siamese cat: the discovery that genes for coat and eye pigment affect the brain. *ILAR Journal*, **46** (4), 357–363.

44 Tillson, D.M. and Winkler, J.T. (2002) Diagnosis and treatment of portosystemic shunts in the cat. *Veterinary Clinics of North America: Small Animal Practice*, **32** (4), 881–899, vi–vii.

45 Center, S.A. and Magne, M.L. (1990) Historical, physical examination, and clinicopathologic features of portosystemic vascular anomalies in the dog and cat. *Seminars in Veterinary Medicine and Surgery*, **5** (2), 83–93.

46 Lamb, C.R., Forster-van Hijfte, M.A., White, R.N. *et al.* (1996) Ultrasonographic diagnosis of congenital portosystemic shunt in 14 cats. *Journal of Small Animal Practice*, **37** (5), 205–209.

47 Acland, G.M., McLean, I.W., Aguirre, G.D., and Trucksa, R. (1980) Diffuse iris melanoma in cats. *Journal of the American Veterinary Medical Association*, **176** (1), 52–56.

48 Patnaik, A.K. and Mooney, S. (1998) Feline melanoma: a comparative study of ocular, oral, and dermal neoplasms. *Veterinary Pathology*, **25** (2), 105–112.

49 Dubielzig, R.R. (1990) Ocular neoplasia in small animals. *Veterinary Clinics of North America: Small Animal Practice*, **20** (3), 837–848.

50 Morgan, G. (1969) Ocular tumours in animals. *Journal of Small Animal Practice*, **10** (10), 563–570.

51 Schaffer, E.H. and Gordon, S. (1993) Feline ocular melanoma. Clinical and pathologico-anatomic findings in 37 cases. *Tierärztliche Praxis*, **21** (3), 255–264 (in German).

52 Peiffer, R.L., Jr., Seymour, W.G., and Williams, L.W. (1977) Malignant melanoma of the iris and ciliary body in a cat. *Modern Veterinary Practice*, **58** (10), 854–856.

53 Cardy, R.H. (1977) Primary intraocular malignant melanoma in a Siamese cat. *Veterinary Pathology*, **14** (6), 648–649.

54 de Lahunta, A., Glass, E., and Kent, M. (2015) *Veterinary Neuroanatomy and Clinical Neurology*, 4th edn., Saunders Elsevier, St. Louis.

55 Telle, M.R. and Betbeze, C. (2015) Hyphema: considerations in the small animal patient. *Topics in Companion Animal Medicine*, **30** (3), 97–106.

56 Torrance, A.G. and Mooney, C.T. (eds.) (1998) *BSAVA Manual of Small Animal Endocrinology*, 2nd edn., British Small Animal Veterinary Association, Cheltenham.

57 Salgado, D., Reusch, C., and Spiess, B. (2000) Diabetic cataracts: different incidence between dogs and cats. *Schweizer Archiv für Tierheilkunde*, **142** (6), 349–353.

58 Basher, A.W. and Roberts, S.M. (1995) Ocular manifestations of diabetes mellitus: diabetic cataracts in dogs. *Veterinary Clinics of North America: Small Animal Practice*, **25** (3), 661–676.

59 Peiffer, R.L. and Gelatt, K.N. (1974) Cataracts in the cat. *Feline Practice*, **4** (1), 34–38.

60 Richter, M., Guscetti, F., and Spiess, B. (2002) Aldose reductase activity and glucose-related opacities in incubated lenses from dogs and cats. *American Journal of Veterinary Research*, **63** (11), 1591–1597.

61 Chylack, L.T., Jr. and Kinoshita, J.H. (1969) A biochemical evaluation of a cataract induced in a high-glucose medium. *Investigative Ophthalmology*, **8** (4), 401–412.

62 Chylack, L.T., Jr. and Cheng, H.M. (1978) Sugar metabolism in the crystalline lens. *Survey of Ophthalmology*, **23** (1), 26–37.

63 Welch Allyn (2015) *Direct and Indirect Veterinary Eye and Ear Examination Instructions*, Welch Allyn, Skaneateles Falls, NY, https://www.welchallyn.com/content/dam/welchallyn/documents/sap-documents/LIT/80020/80020547LITPDF.pdf (accessed 14 June 2016).

64 Boeve, M.H., Stades, F.C., and Djajadiningrat-Laanen, S.C. (2009) The eyes, in *Medical History and Physical Examination in Companion Animals*, 2nd edn. (eds. A. Rijnberk and F.J. van Sluijs), Saunders Elsevier, St. Louis, pp. 175–201.

65 Eaton, J.S. (2015) *Facing Your Fundic Fears: Examination of the Ocular Fundus*, http://www.cuvs.org/pdf/pdflinks/Examination%20of%20the%20Ocular%20Fundus%20Lab.pdf (accessed 14 June 2016).

66 Heine, P.A. (2004) Anatomy of the ear. *Veterinary Clinics of North America: Small Animal Practice*, **34** (2), 379–395.

67 Cole, L.K. (2004) Otoscopic evaluation of the ear canal. *Veterinary Clinics of North America: Small Animal Practice*, **34** (2), 397–410.

68 Heffner, R.S. and Heffner, H.E. (1985) Hearing range of the domestic cat. *Hearing Research*, **19** (1), 85–88.

69 Hubka, P., Konerding, W., and Kral, A. (2015) Auditory feedback modulates development of kitten

vocalizations. *Cell and Tissue Research*, **361** (1), 279–294.

70 Shipley, C., Buchwald, J.S., and Carterette, E.C. (1988) The role of auditory feedback in the vocalizations of cats. *Experimental Brain Research*, **69** (2), 431–438.

71 Bach, J.P., Lupke, M., and Wefstaedt, P. (2013) Deafness in the dog and cat: aetiology, diagnostics and treatment. *Tierärztliche Praxis. Ausgabe K, Kleintiere/Heimtiere*, **41** (6), 421–427; quiz, 8 (in German).

72 Sims, M.H. (1988) Electrodiagnostic evaluation of auditory function. *Veterinary Clinics of North America: Small Animal Practice*, **18** (4), 913–944.

73 Dijkshoorn, N.A. and van der Wel, T. (1997) Screening for deafness in companion animals. *Tijdschrift voor Diergeneeskunde*, **122** (6), 168–169 (in Dutch).

74 Cook, L.B. (2004) Neurologic evaluation of the ear. *Veterinary Clinics of North America: Small Animal Practice*, **34** (2), 425–435, vi.

75 Overall, K.L. (1997) *Clinical Behavioral Medicine for Small Animals*, Mosby, St. Louis.

76 Lanz, O.I. and Wood, B.C. (2004) Surgery of the ear and pinna. *Veterinary Clinics of North America: Small Animal Practice*, **34** (2), 567–599, viii.

77 Medleau, L. and Hnilica, K.A. (2006) *Small Animal Dermatology: A Color Atlas and Therapeutic Guide*, 2nd edn., Saunders Elsevier, St. Louis.

78 Matousek, J.L. (2004) Diseases of the ear pinna. *Veterinary Clinics of North America: Small Animal Practice*, **34** (2), 511–540.

79 Siegal, M. (1989) *The Cornell Book of Cats: A Comprehensive Medical Reference for Every Cat and Kitten*, 1st edn, Villard Books, New York.

80 Angus, J.C. (2004) Otic cytology in health and disease. *Veterinary Clinics of North America: Small Animal Practice*, **34** (2), 411–424.

81 Rosser, E.J., Jr. (2004) Causes of otitis externa. *Veterinary Clinics of North America: Small Animal Practice*, **34** (2), 459–468.

82 Angus, J.C. (2004) Diseases of the ear, in *Small Animal Dermatology Secrets* (ed. K.L. Campbell), Hanley & Belfus, Philadelphia, pp. 364–384.

83 Gotthelf, L.N. (2004) Diagnosis and treatment of otitis media in dogs and cats. *Veterinary Clinics of North America: Small Animal Practice*, **34** (2), 469–487.

84 Clarke, D.E. and Caiafa, A. (2014) Oral examination in the cat: a systematic approach. *Journal of Feline Medicine and Surgery*, **16** (11), 873–886.

85 Mestrinho, L.A., Runhau, J., Braganca, M., and Niza, M.M. (2013) Risk assessment of feline tooth resorption: a Portuguese clinical case control study. *Journal of Veterinary Dentistry*, **30** (2), 78–83.

86 Silness, J. and Loe, H. (1964) Periodontal disease in pregnancy. II. Correlation between oral hygiene and periodontal condition. *Acta Odontologica Scandinavica*, 22, 121–135.

87 Lobprise, H B. and Wiggs, R.B. (2000) *The Veterinarian's Companion for Common Dental Procedures*, AAHA Press, Lakewood, CO.

88 Shipp, A.D. and Fahrenkrug, P. (1992) *Practitioners' Guide to Veterinary Dentistry*, Dr. Shipp's Laboratories, Beverly Hills, CA.

89 Reiter, A.M. and Soltero-Rivera, M.M. (2014) Applied feline oral anatomy and tooth extraction techniques: an illustrated guide. *Journal of Feline Medicine and Surgery*, **16** (11), 900–913.

90 Floyd, M.R. (1991) The modified Triadan system: nomenclature for veterinary dentistry. *Journal of Veterinary Dentistry*, **8** (4), 18–19.

91 American Veterinary Dental College (2009) *AVDC Nomenclature*, http://www.avdc.org/nomenclature.pdf (accessed 16 April 2016).

92 Logan, E.I. and Boyce, E.N. (1994) Oral health assessment in dogs: parameters and methods. *Journal of Veterinary Dentistry*, **11** (2), 58–63.

93 Hennet, P. (1999) Review of studies assessing plaque accumulation and gingival inflammation in dogs. *Journal of Veterinary Dentistry*, **16** (1), 23–29.

94 Fischman, S.L. (1988) Clinical index systems used to assess the efficacy of mouthrinses on plaque and gingivitis. *Journal of Clinical Periodontology*, **15** (8), 506–510.

95 Gunsolley, J.C., Chinchilli, V.M., Koertge, T.E. *et al.* (1989) The use of repeated measures analysis of variance for plaque and gingival indexes. *Journal of Clinical Periodontology*, **16** (3), 156–163.

96 Fischman, S.L. (1986) Current status of indexes of plaque. *Journal of Clinical Periodontology*, **13** (5), 371–374.

97 Lemmons, M. (2013) Clinical feline dental radiography. *Veterinary Clinics of North America: Small Animal Practice*, **43** (3), 533–554.

98 Holmstrom, S.E. (2012) Veterinary dentistry in senior canines and felines. *Veterinary Clinics of North America: Small Animal Practice*, **42** (4), 793–808, viii.

99 DuPont, G.A. and DeBowes, L.J. (2002) Comparison of periodontitis and root replacement in cat teeth with resorptive lesions. *Journal of Veterinary Dentistry*, **19** (2), 71–75.

100 Lommer, M.J. and Verstraete, F.J. (2000) Prevalence of odontoclastic resorption lesions and periapical radiographic lucencies in cats: 265 cases (1995–1998). *Journal of the American Veterinary Medical Association*, **217** (12), 1866–1869.

4

Examining the Endocrine and Lymphatic Systems of the Cat

4.1 Evaluating the Thyroid Gland

Endocrine organs are not typically palpable, with the exception of the testes in an intact male. Barring extreme medical conditions such as pancreatic adenocarcinoma, the clinician typically cannot access organs such as the abdominally located pancreas, adrenals, and ovaries, the parathyroid, or the pituitary gland. Yet the thyroid glands are accessible to the primary care clinician, who routinely makes a habit of checking for their palpability as a sign of their enlargement [1].

The paired thyroid gland is seated on the ventral aspect of the neck in close apposition to the trachea, distal to the cricoid cartilage. Its right and left lobes are connected by thyroidal tissue called the isthmus. Developmentally, the thyroid gland arises from the pharyngeal floor and may have ectopic tissue that extends through the thoracic inlet into the thoracic cavity [2–4].

Two pairs of parathyroid glands are embedded within thyroidal tissue. In the typical, healthy, euthyroid dog or cat, neither the thyroid nor the parathyroid glands are palpable [3].

The follicular cells of the thyroid gland produce thyroxine (T4) and triiodothyronine (T3), which influence growth and metabolism. Significantly more T4 than T3 is secreted by the thyroid. Once in circulation, the majority of both hormones is protein bound. The 0.2% of each that is free in the circulation is bioactive and can effect changes in metabolism [3, 4].

4.1.1 The Pathophysiology of Hyperthyroidism

Hyperthyroidism is a type of endocrinopathy in which the thyroid hormones are produced in excess [5–8]. In theory, this could arise as a primary disorder (originating from the thyroid gland itself), secondary disorder (originating from unchecked overstimulation of the thyroid gland by the pituitary gland via thyroid-stimulating hormone, TSH), or tertiary disorder (originating from unchecked overstimulation of the thyroid gland indirectly by the hypothalamus via thyrotropin-releasing hormone, TRH). In reality, hyperthyroidism of the

cat is due primarily to the thyroid gland itself, irrespective of its interactions with the pituitary gland and hypothalamus [9].

Primary malignant tumors of the thyroid, such as thyroid carcinoma, are rare in cats [9–11]. Therefore, the majority of tumors that lead to hyperthyroidism in the cat are benign. Depending upon which medical literature is referenced, the overactive neoplastic thyroidal tissue is referred to as adenomatous hyperplasia, adenomas, or multinodular adenomatous goiter [9, 12].

The resultant thyrotoxicosis promotes catabolism. Lean muscle mass is not spared. In addition to encouraging muscle wasting, hyperthyroidism alters neuromuscular and cardiac excitability. Hyperthyroid cats often exhibit generalized muscle weakness and tremors, nervousness, and altered mentation. The excess of thyroid hormone hypersensitizes the heart to catecholamines by increasing the number of cardiac beta-adrenergic receptors. Cardiac myosin concentrations are also increased. The resultant tachycardia and increased stroke volume cause the heart to work harder [4, 9].

In addition, thyrotoxicosis increases oxygen consumption by as much as 200%, based upon observations made in the laboratory. Heat is produced as the mitochondria make use of the oxygen in aerobic metabolism for ATP production and utilization. As a result of these metabolic and physiologic changes, the hyperthyroid cat typically takes on a sarcopenic, underweight, unkempt appearance despite being polyphagic. The hyperthyroid cat is heat intolerant and may become polydipsic as an adaptive mechanism. The hyperthyroid cat tends to have tachycardia with or without dyspnea, and thyroid-induced heart murmurs with or without a gallop rhythm [4, 9].

Clients most often present a mid-aged to senior patient for weight loss in spite of a good appetite. However, owner recognition of clinical signs is often delayed. It is estimated that the diagnosis of hyperthyroidism is postponed by 6–12 months because the onset of disease is insidious and slowly progressive. Because these patients are if anything overactive, clients may misinterpret the other clinical signs as being normal signs of aging rather than the result of underlying pathology [9].

4.1.2 The Etiology of Hyperthyroidism

Hyperthyroidism was first described in cats in the late 1970s [13, 14]. It has since surpassed diabetes mellitus as the top feline endocrine disease in the United States, Canada, United Kingdom, Europe, Australia, New Zealand, and Japan, and its incidence is increasing [8, 14–23]. In North America alone, the prevalence climbed from 0.3% in 1979 to 4.5% in 1985 [17, 24]. In 2002, Japan reported a prevalence of 8.9% [21] compared with Germany's 11.4% in 2006 [23].

Despite the rise in feline hyperthyroidism, the etiology remains unknown [14]. One risk factor is the patient's breed: Siamese and Himalayan cats appear to be least at risk [24–26]. Other relevant risks include the use of commercial litter by the cat and the use of topical flea preventatives [17, 25, 26]. Consumption of a canned diet, especially one that contains fish, liver, and giblets [26, 27], appears to double or even triple the risk of developing hyperthyroidism [25].

Because canned diets increase the risk for development of hyperthyroidism, investigations have been launched to explore whether the content or the container is to blame. With regards to the former, soy isoflavones are abundant in commercial cat food as an inexpensive source of dietary protein [28, 29]. Soy isoflavones are known to disrupt thyroid function through the inhibition of thyroid peroxidase [30–32] and 5′-deiodinase [32]. This ability to block the production of thyroid hormones should stimulate the pituitary gland to secrete additional TSH, with resultant thyroid hyperplasia; indeed, soy consumption has been linked to goiter formation in human infants [33, 34]. However, despite the high content of soy isoflavones in 60–75% of cat foods tested [28, 29], the link between it and goiter formation in cats has not been proven experimentally [15].

Metal cans and pop-top lids contain bisphenol A (BPA) [35–37] to prevent container corrosion and to extend shelf life [15] and, during processing and storage, food becomes contaminated with this chemical residue [38, 39]. This applies both to human-grade canned foods [37–40] and to those destined for the pet food industry [40, 41]. BPA is known to disrupt the thyroid gland by hindering signaling pathways and acting as a thyroid hormone receptor antagonist [35, 42–49]. Although BPA levels in blood or tissue have not been demonstrated in cats that consume canned foods, they are expected to be high [35]. BPA undergoes glucuronidation prior to being eliminated from the body [50], and cats are extraordinarily inefficient at this process because they are deficient in the enzyme glucuronyl transferase [51]. A study by Edinboro *et al.* associated feline hyperthyroidism with

consumption of foods in pop-top cans [35]. It is thought that BPA is responsible for this link.

Dietary iodine has also been implicated as playing a role in the development of feline hyperthyroidism. As iodine is an important constituent of thyroid hormones [52], iodine deficiency can induce goiter formation [53, 54]. The decrease in iodine results in decreased T4 and T3 production by the thyroid. This in turn triggers the release of TRH and TSH by the hypothalamus and the pituitary gland, respectively, to stimulate the thyroid to produce more hormone, not recognizing that the thyroid is unable to produce additional hormone without more iodine. The result is development of thyroid hyperplasia leading to a visible goiter both in people and in animals [15, 52–56].

Initially, it was postulated that iodine excess rather than deficiency was to blame for feline hyperthyroidism [15]. After feline hyperthyroidism was first diagnosed in the late 1970s, it was discovered that the majority of commercial cat foods contained up to 10 times the recommended level of iodine [57], and recommendations for dietary iodine were subsequently reduced [58]. By the early 1990s, only 10% of foods exceeded recommendations; commercial brands were more likely to dip below the lower limit [59]. By 2002, the iodine content in commercial diets was extraordinarily variable, with 30-fold differences between brands [60]. This complicates the veterinary profession's understanding of any potential association between iodine content of food and hyperthyroidism: there is such a broad range of iodine levels based upon manufacturer differences and ingredients that it is unclear whether the profession should cast blame on too much or too little iodine or, rather, rapid fluctuations in iodine levels [61–64].

Synergy between implicated factors is likely [15]. Iodine deficiency can be exacerbated by other micronutrient deficiencies, such as selenium, vitamin A, and zinc [15, 65, 66]. Similarly, iodine deficiency may potentiate the anti-thyroid effects of soy isoflavones [15, 31, 67–69]. The potential for combined effects is real, which makes the task of preventing this condition even more daunting. Altering one risk factor may shift the weight of another factor [15].

Prevention of feline hyperthyroidism focuses on limiting known risks when possible. Eliminating canned diets that use cans lined with BPA is preferred [40, 41]. When it is unknown whether or not the manufacturer uses BPA in the processing of a commercial diet, switching from canned foods to foods in pouches increases the safety of consumption [40].

4.1.3 The Art of Palpating an Enlarged Thyroid Gland

Because the etiology of hyperthyroidism is so complex and because so many questions remain, the focus of hyperthyroidism more commonly shifts to how it can be diagnosed as opposed to how it can be prevented. Given its location in the ventral neck, the thyroid gland of a normal cat or dog is typically too deep to palpate [1, 9]. However, when the thyroid gland is enlarged, it is easy to appreciate on physical examination. As such, the veterinary team should palpate for the thyroid gland at every visit in an adult cat regardless of whether or not the patient is clinical for the disease [70]. Although not every ventral cervical mass is an enlarged thyroid gland [9], over 90% of cats with hyperthyroidism do have a thyroid gland that is evident on palpation [5, 9, 20]. Both lobes are enlarged in 70% of cases. It is significantly less common, but possible, to have unilateral involvement [5, 7, 18, 71].

Whereas the normal thyroid gland sits deeply in the neck, an enlarged thyroid gland is weightier. Gravity causes the thyroid gland to sink nearer to the neck's surface, facilitating its palpation [9].

It is important to remember that not all cats with hyperthyroidism have enlarged thyroids that are palpable: ectopic thyroid tissue may be overactive yet out of reach past the thoracic inlet and within the mediastinum [9]. Similarly, not all cats with palpable thyroid glands are hyperthyroid [70]. For reasons yet to be understood, some cats with enlargement of the thyroid are euthyroid: their total T4 (TT4) is normal, if not low [72].

However, when the thyroid gland is palpable, especially in a patient whose thyroid had never been palpated before, it should raise concern that the patient may be hyperthyroid. If subsequent diagnostic testing is confirmatory, then medical management may be instigated.

To feel for the thyroid gland, the clinician may stand directly behind the patient or immediately in front. The author prefers the former approach. The patient can be seated or standing. Standing behind the patient, the clinician uses his non-dominant hand to gently extend the cat's head and neck. The thumb and index finger of the dominant hand are pinched together as if the clinician were crimping pie crust. Together, the thumb and index finger are then placed in the jugular furrows such that they straddle the trachea. Beginning at the larynx, the thumb and index finger are progressively slid down the throat, applying firm and constant pressure all the way to the thoracic inlet (Figure 4.1). If there is one or more thyroid nodules, the nodule(s) will "slip" through the fingers as a subcutaneous "pop" of tissue that is not typically present on palpation. Rarely is the mass grossly visible without palpation: the largest one to be recorded in the literature measured 4 × 7 × 10 cm [73]. More commonly, the thyroid "slip" will range in size from a lentil to a lima bean [9]. On average, it typically is half the size of a normal popliteal lymph node [9, 70, 74].

Some clinicians prefer to turn the cat's elevated head and neck 45° to the left from the vertical to palpate the right lobe of the thyroid, and 45° to the right from the vertical to palpate the left lobe of the thyroid [70, 74]. Other clinicians prefer to stand face-to-face with the cat and repeat the procedure outlined above (Figure 4.2).

Recall that feeling one or more thyroid nodules is not pathognomonic for hyperthyroidism [70, 72], although

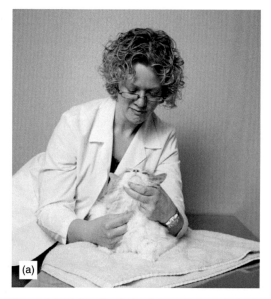
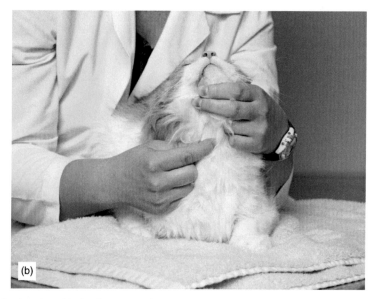

Figure 4.1 (a) Standing behind the patient and crimping the thumb and index finger together in preparation for sliding them down the throat to feel for a thyroid "slip." (b) Close-up of thumb and finger placement as the throat is examined for the presence or absence of a thyroid "slip." Source (a), (b): Courtesy of the Media Resources Department at Midwestern University.

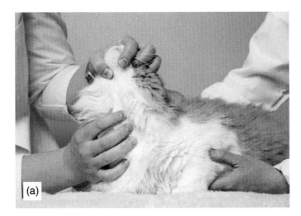
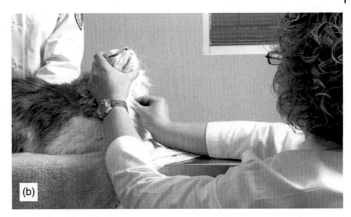

Figure 4.2 (a) An alternative approach is to stand in front of the patient to feel down the throat for a thyroid "slip" with the thumb and index finger. (b) Close-up of thumb and finger placement as the throat is examined for the presence or absence of a thyroid "slip." Source (a), (b): Courtesy of the Media Resources Department at Midwestern University.

it should be considered in a patient with the appropriate signalment and clinical signs. If serum total thyroxine concentration (TT4) and free T4 (fT4) rule out hyperthyroidism, then the palpable nodule(s) may be non-functional [70, 74].

It is also important to take the patient's muscular health into consideration, meaning that it is possible to feel a "slip" in non-hyperthyroid cats with advanced sarcopenia or cachexia. In this case, the thyroid gland is palpable not because it is enlarged but because there is little or nothing for it to hide beneath.

4.2 Assessing the Lymphatic System

Just as the clinician is limited in terms of what he can palpate that comprises the endocrine system, the clinician also has very few opportunities on physical examination to evaluate the lymphatic system.

The lymphatic system is like a neighboring highway of the vasculature: its series of lymphatic vessels serve to collect fluid and proteins that are forced out of blood vessels by hydrostatic pressure. This excess fluid is then returned to the general circulation via lymphatic ducts that drain back into the jugular vein or cranial vena cava. Without lymphatic drainage, edema of the peripheral tissues of the bodies would result [75].

With the exception of lymphatic obstruction, which leads to edematous tissue that is visible on the physical examination, the clinician is unable to evaluate the health of the lymphatic vessels themselves. The only structures of the lymphatic system that the clinician is able to assess at each visit are the lymph nodes. These nexuses are essentially filters of lymph. They also are sites where lymphocytes can proliferate and differentiate as sentinels for the immune system [75].

Lymph nodes are in locations where they interfere the least with mobility and the circulation [75]. The peripheral lymph nodes tend to be paired, and three sets in particular are palpable in the normal patient:

- the submandibular lymph nodes;
- the superficial cervical lymph nodes, otherwise referred to as pre-scapular lymph nodes;
- the popliteal lymph nodes.

These sets of lymph nodes should be palpated at each visit. The clinician should note their size, shape, and consistency, and whether or not contralateral nodes are symmetrical. The clinician should also note if the patient reacts adversely to palpation. Lymph nodes should not be tender to the touch and therefore they should not cause pain upon palpation. Normal lymph nodes should feel rubbery [1], like scallops.

4.2.1 Examining the Submandibular Lymph Nodes

See Section 3.5: The Extra-Oral Examination.

4.2.2 Examining the Superficial Cervical or Pre-Scapular Lymph Nodes

The superficial cervical or pre-scapular lymph nodes are located at the cranial border of each scapula, covered by the cleidocervical and omotransversarius muscles. These nodes are oval and flat, and are paired. There may be as few as one and as many as four on each side, the right and the left. They collectively drain the neck, shoulder, and corresponding forelimb [3, 75].

To palpate the superficial cervical or pre-scapular lymph nodes, the clinician may stand directly behind the patient or immediately in front. The author prefers the former approach, using the left hand to palpate the left nodes and the right hand to palpate the right nodes. Both hands are used simultaneously to appreciate significant differences in symmetry, size, and consistency between sides.

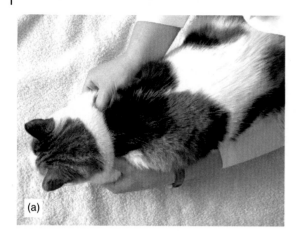 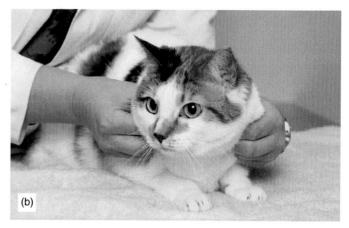

Figure 4.3 (a) and (b) Palpating the superficial cervical lymph nodes by grasping deep to the scapular border at the point of the shoulder. Source (a), (b): Courtesy of the Media Resources Department at Midwestern University.

The patient can be seated or standing for this exercise. The clinician simply moves his fingertips up from the humerus to the point of the shoulder. At the point of the shoulder, the clinician's thumb and index finger should grasp deep to the scapular border. As the clinician then moves his thumb and index finger from deep to superficial, the lymph nodes should "slip" through, much like a thyroid nodule can be felt to "slip" through the fingertips upon ventral neck palpation (Figure 4.3). Note that these nodes may be challenging to feel in an obese patient or one that is tucked up in a ball, trying to escape notice.

4.2.3 Examining the Popliteal Lymph Nodes

The popliteal lymph nodes are located at the caudal aspect of each stifle, sandwiched between the biceps femoris and semitendinosus muscles. These nodes are rounder than the superficial cervical lymph nodes, and in the cat they are often encased in a generous layer of fat. They are paired structures, with typically one on each side, the right and the left. They collectively drain the distal hind limbs [3, 75].

To palpate the popliteal lymph nodes, the clinician should stand behind the patient with the patient facing in the same direction as the clinician. The clinician should pinch the thumb and index finger of each hand together as if crimping pie crust. Together, the thumb and index finger of the left hand are placed over the left caudal thigh, and the thumb and index finger of the right hand are placed over the right caudal thigh. Beginning at the caudal thigh, the thumb and index finger are then progressively slid down the thigh to the caudal stifle, applying firm and constant pressure all the way. At the level of the caudal stifle, the clinician can grasp deep to the skin. As the clinician's fingertips move from deep to superficial, the lymph nodes should "slip" through (Figure 4.4).

Both hands are used simultaneously to appreciate significant differences in symmetry, size, and consistency between sides. Because these lymph nodes are covered in a generous blanket of subcutaneous fat in cats, the popliteal lymph nodes often feel larger in cats than they actually are. Therefore, assessing their symmetry in addition to their size is especially important in the cat.

4.2.4 Feeling for Lymph Nodes That Should Not Be Present

In addition to palpating the submandibular, superficial cervical, and popliteal lymph nodes at every visit, there are also two sets of lymph nodes that the clinician should not feel in the normal patient:

- the axillary lymph nodes;
- the superficial inguinal lymph nodes.

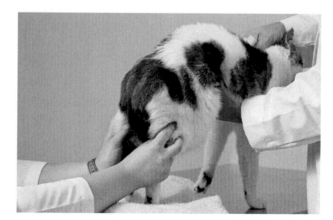

Figure 4.4 Palpating the popliteal lymph nodes. This patient had a tendency to want to sit down, so the restrainer supported the cat's weight to keep the cat standing by placing his hand underneath the cat's caudal chest and cranial abdomen. Source: Courtesy of the Media Resources Department at Midwestern University.

The axillary lymph nodes are located, as their name implies, deep within the arm pit, caudal to the shoulder joint. The teres major muscle forms its lateral boundary and the rectus thoracis muscle forms its medial boundary. The axillary lymph nodes are disc shaped and deeper than expected, which is why they go undetected in the normal patient. They drain the thoracic wall and the thoracic limbs, and also the thoracic and cranial abdominal mammary glands. There may be overlap in drainage of the cranial abdominal mammary glands, in that depending on the patient, the superficial cervical lymph nodes may also play a role. On the other hand, there is no such overlap between the left and right sides of the mammary chain: lymph from the left gland does not cross over to drain through the right set of lymph nodes [3, 75].

To palpate for the axillary lymph nodes, which are only appreciated in diseased states involving lymph drainage, the clinician should stand behind the patient with the patient facing in the same direction as the clinician. The clinician should take flattened hands with fingers pressed together and slide them into the axilla. Using the fingertips as a paddle, the clinician should start by reaching rostrally and then move caudally. The act of strumming one's fingers back and forth should allow the lymph nodes to "blip" past the clinician's fingertips if they are indeed enlarged.

The superficial inguinal lymph nodes are located where the caudalmost, ventrolateral abdominal walls meet the medial thighs. There are one or two nodes per side, and their shape is typically oval. These drain the abdominal and inguinal mammary glands. They also receive drainage from the popliteal nodes, ventral pelvis, tail, and the medial thigh, stifle, and crus. In the male, drainage includes the penis, prepuce, and scrotum [3, 75].

To palpate for the superficial inguinal lymph nodes, which are appreciated only in diseased states involving lymph drainage, the clinician should stand behind the patient with the patient facing in the same direction as the clinician. The clinician should take flattened hands with fingers pressed together and slide them into the crease between the medial thigh and the abdominal wall, with the left palm against the left crease and the right palm against the right crease. Using the fingertips as a paddle, the clinician should feel dorsolateral to the last mammary gland. The act of strumming one's fingers back and forth should allow the lymph nodes to "blip" past the clinician's fingertips if they are indeed enlarged. Alternatively, the clinician may palpate this region one side at a time with the patient in lateral recumbency and its pelvic limb gently abducted. Note that the extensiveness of many patients' abdominal fat pads may make the palpation of these nodes difficult even when enlarged.

References

1 Rijnberk, A. and van Sluijs, F.S. (2009) *Medical History and Physical Examination in Companion Animals*, 2nd edn., Saunders Elsevier, St. Louis.

2 Gilbert, S.G. (1968) *Pictorial Anatomy of the Cat*, University of Washington Press, Seattle.

3 Dyce, K.M., Sack, W.O., and Wensing, C.J.G. (1996) *Textbook of Veterinary Anatomy*, 2nd edn., Saunders, Philadelphia.

4 Eiler, H. (2004) Endocrine glands, in *Dukes' Physiology of Domestic Animals*, 12th edn. (ed. W.O. Reece), Comstock, Ithaca, NY, pp. 621–669.

5 Peterson, M.E., Kintzer, P.P., Cavanagh, P.G. *et al.* (1983) Feline hyperthyroidism: pretreatment clinical and laboratory evaluation of 131 cases. *Journal of the American Veterinary Medical Association*, **183** (1), 103–110.

6 Hoenig, M., Goldschmidt, M.H., Ferguson, D.C. *et al.* (1982) Toxic nodular goitre in the cat. *Journal of Small Animal Practice*, **23** (1), 1–12.

7 Peterson, M.E. and Ward C.R. (2007) Etiopathologic findings of hyperthyroidism in cats. *Veterinary Clinics of North America: Small Animal Practice*, **37** (4), 633–645.

8 Baral, R. and Peterson, M.E. (2012) Thyroid gland disorders, in *The Cat: Clinical Medicine and Management* (ed. S.E. Little), Saunders Elsevier, Philadelphia, pp. 571–592.

9 Feldman, E.C. and Nelson R.W. (2004) *Canine and Feline Endocrinology and Reproduction*, 3rd edn., Saunders, St. Louis.

10 Turrel, J.M., Feldman, E.C., Nelson, R.W., and Cain, G.R. (1988) Thyroid carcinoma causing hyperthyroidism in cats: 14 cases (1981–1986). *Journal of the American Veterinary Medical Association*, **193** (3), 359–364.

11 Hibbert, A., Gruffydd-Jones, T., Barrett, E.L. *et al.* (2009) Feline thyroid carcinoma: diagnosis and response to high-dose radioactive iodine treatment. *Journal of Feline Medicine and Surgery*, **11** (2), 116–124.

12 Carpenter, J.L., Andrews, L.K., and Holzworth, J. (1987) Tumors and tumor like lesions, in *Diseases of the Cat: Medicine and Surgery* (ed. J. Holzworth), Saunders, Philadelphia, pp. 406–596.

13 Peterson, M.E. and Johnson, J.G. (eds.) (1979) *Spontaneous Hyperthyroidism in the Cat*, American College of Veterinary Internal Medicine, Seattle.

14 McLean, J.L., Lobetti, R.G., and Schoeman, J.P. (2014) Worldwide prevalence and risk factors for feline hyperthyroidism: a review. *Journal of the South African Veterinary Association*, **85** (1), 1097.

15 Peterson, M. (2012) Hyperthyroidism in cats: what's causing this epidemic of thyroid disease and can we prevent it? *Journal of Feline Medicine and Surgery*, **14** (11), 804–818.

16 Mooney, C.T. and Peterson, M.E. (2012) Feline hyperthyroidism, in *Manual of Canine and Feline Endocrinology* (eds. C.T. Mooney and M.E. Peterson), British Small Animal Veterinary Association, Gloucester, pp. 92–110.

17 Scarlett, J.M. (1994) Epidemiology of thyroid diseases of dogs and cats. *Veterinary Clinics of North America: Small Animal Practice*, **24** (3), 477–486.

18 Gerber, H., Peter, H., Ferguson, D.C., and Peterson, M.E. (1994) Etiopathology of feline toxic nodular goiter. *Veterinary Clinics of North America: Small Animal Practice*, **24** (3), 541–565.

19 Broussard, J.D., Peterson, M.E., and Fox, P.R. (1995) Changes in clinical and laboratory findings in cats with hyperthyroidism from 1983 to 1993. *Journal of the American Veterinary Medical Association*, **206** (3), 302–305.

20 Thoday, K.L. and Mooney C.T. (1992) Historical, clinical and laboratory features of 126 hyperthyroid cats. *Veterinary Record*, **131** (12), 257–264.

21 Miyamoto, T., Miyata, I., Kurobane, K. *et al.* (2002) Prevalence of feline hyperthyroidism in Osaka and the Chugoku Region. *Journal of the Japanese Veterinary Medical Association*, **55**, 289–292.

22 Olczak, J., Jones, B.R., Pfeiffer, D.U. *et al.* (2004) Multivariate analysis of risk factors for feline hyperthyroidism in New Zealand. *New Zealand Veterinary Journal*, **53**, 53–58.

23 Sassnau, R. (2006) Epidemiological investigation on the prevalence of feline hyperthyroidism in an urban population in Germany. *Tierärztliche Praxis, Ausgabe K, Kleintiere Heimtiere*, **34**, 450–457.

24 De Wet, C.S., Mooney, C.T., Thompson, P.N., and Schoeman, J.P. (2009) Prevalence of and risk factors for feline hyperthyroidism in Hong Kong. *Journal of Feline Medicine and Surgery*, **11** (4), 315–321.

25 Kass, P.H., Peterson, M.E., Levy, J. *et al.* (1999) Evaluation of environmental, nutritional, and host factors in cats with hyperthyroidism. *Journal of Veterinary Internal Medicine*, **13** (4), 323–329.

26 Wakeling, J., Everard, A., Brodbelt, D. *et al.* (2009) Risk factors for feline hyperthyroidism in the UK. *Journal of Small Animal Practice*, **50** (8), 406–414.

27 Martin, K.M., Rossing, M.A., Ryland, L.M. *et al.* (2000) Evaluation of dietary and environmental risk factors for hyperthyroidism in cats. *Journal of the American Veterinary Medical Association*, **217** (6), 853–856.

28 Court, M.H. and Freeman, L.M. (2002) Identification and concentration of soy isoflavones in commercial cat foods. *American Journal of Veterinary Research*, **63** (2), 181–185.

29 Bell, K.M., Rutherfurd, S.M., and Hendriks, W.H. (2006) The isoflavone content of commercially-available feline diets in New Zealand. *New Zealand Veterinary Journal*, **54** (3), 103–108.

30 Divi, R.L., Chang, H.C., and Doerge, D.R. (1997) Anti-thyroid isoflavones from soybean: isolation, characterization, and mechanisms of action. *Biochemical Pharmacology*, **54** (10), 1087–1096.

31 Doerge, D.R. and Sheehan, D.M. (2002) Goitrogenic and estrogenic activity of soy isoflavones. *Environmental Health Perspectives*, **110** (Suppl. 3), 349–353.

32 de Souza dos Santos, M.C., Gonçalves, C.F., Vaisman, M. *et al.* (2011) Impact of flavonoids on thyroid function. *Food and Chemical Toxicology*, **49** (10), 2495–2502.

33 Shepard, T.H., Pyne, G.E., Kirschvink, J.F., and McLean, M. (1960) Soybean goiter – report of 3 cases. *New England Journal of Medicine*, **262** (22), 1099–1103.

34 Kay, T., Kimura, M., Nishing, K., and Itokawa, Y. (1988) Soybean, goiter, and prevention. *Journal of Tropical Pediatrics*, **34** (3), 110–113.

35 Edinboro, C.H., Scott-Moncrieff, J.C., Janovitz, E. *et al.* (2004) Epidemiologic study of relationships between consumption of commercial canned food and risk of hyperthyroidism in cats. *Journal of the American Veterinary Medical Association*, **224** (6), 879–886.

36 Tsai, W.T. (2006) Human health risk on environmental exposure to bisphenol-A: a review. *Journal of Environmental Science and Health. Part C, Environmental Carcinogenesis and Ecotoxicology Reviews*, **24** (2), 225–255.

37 Noonan, G.O., Ackerman, L.K., and Begley, T.H. (2011) Concentration of bisphenol A in highly consumed canned foods on the U.S. market. *Journal of Agricultural and Food Chemistry*, **59** (13), 7178–7185.

38 Goodson, A., Robin, H., Summerfield, W., and Cooper, I. (2004) Migration of bisphenol A from can coatings – effects of damage, storage conditions and heating. *Food Additives and Contaminants*, **21** (10), 1015–1026.

39 Cabado, A.G., Aldea, S., Porro, C. *et al.* (2008) Migration of BADGE (bisphenol A diglycidyl-ether) and BFDGE (bisphenol F diglycidyl-ether) in canned seafood. *Food and Chemical Toxicology*, **46** (5), 1674–1680.

40 Schecter, A., Malik, N., Haffner, D. *et al.* (2010) Bisphenol A (BPA) in U.S. food. *Environmental Science and Technology*, **44** (24), 9425–9430.

41 Kang, J.H. and Kondo, F. (2002) Determination of bisphenol A in canned pet foods. *Research in Veterinary Science*, **73** (2), 177–182.

42 Vandenberg, L.N., Maffini, M.V., Sonnenschein, C. *et al.* (2009) Bisphenol-A and the great divide: a review of controversies in the field of endocrine disruption. *Endocrine Reviews*, **30** (1), 75–95.

43 Boas, M., Main, K.M., and Feldt-Rasmussen, U. (2009) Environmental chemicals and thyroid function: an update. *Current Opinion in Endocrinology, Diabetes, and Obesity*, **216** (5), 385–391.

44 Patrick, L. (2009) Thyroid disruption: mechanism and clinical implications in human health. *Alternative Medicine Review*, **14** (4), 326–346.

45 Diamanti-Kandarakis, E., Bourguignon, J.P., Giudice, L.C. *et al.* (2009) Endocrine-disrupting chemicals: an Endocrine Society scientific statement. *Endocrine Reviews*, **30** (4), 293–342.

46 Meeker, J.D. and Ferguson, K.K. (2011) Relationship between urinary phthalate and bisphenol A concentrations and serum thyroid measures in U.S. adults and adolescents from the National Health and Nutrition Examination Survey (NHANES) 2007–2008. *Environmental Health Perspectives*, **119** (10), 1396–1402.

47 Welshons, W.V., Nagel, S.C., and vom Saal, F.S. (2006) Large effects from small exposures. III. Endocrine mechanisms mediating effects of bisphenol A at levels of human exposure. *Endocrinology*, **147** (6 Suppl.), S56–S69.

48 Moriyama, K., Tagami, T., Akamizu, T. *et al.* (2002) Thyroid hormone action is disrupted by bisphenol A as an antagonist. *Journal of Clinical Endocrinology and Metabolism*, **87** (11), 5185–5190.

49 Kitamura, S., Jinno, N., Ohta, S. *et al.* (2002) Thyroid hormonal activity of the flame retardants tetrabromobisphenol A and tetrachlorobisphenol A. *Biochemical and Biophysical Research Communications*, **293** (1), 554–559.

50 Pottenger, L.H., Domoradzki, J.Y., Markham, D.A. *et al.* (2000) The relative bioavailability and metabolism of bisphenol A in rats is dependent upon the route of administration. *Toxicological Sciences*, **54** (1), 3–18.

51 Chiu, S.H. and Huskey, S.W. (1998) Species differences in *N*-glucuronidation. *Drug Metabolism and Disposition*, **26** (9), 838–847.

52 Soriguer, F., Gutiérrez-Repiso, C., Rubio-Martin, E. *et al.* (2011) Iodine intakes of 100–300 µg/d do not modify thyroid function and have modest anti-inflammatory effects. *British Journal of Nutrition*, **105** (12), 1783–1790.

53 Scott, P.P., Greaves, J.P., and Scott, M.G. (1961) Nutrition of the cat. 4. Calcium and iodine deficiency on a meat diet. *British Journal of Nutrition*, **15**, 35–51.

54 Roberts, A.H. and Scott, P.P. (1961) Nutrition of the cat. 5. The influence of calcium and iodine supplements to a meat diet on the retention of nitrogen, calcium and phosphorus. *British Journal of Nutrition*, **15**, 73–82.

55 Patrick, L. (2008) Iodine: deficiency and therapeutic considerations. *Alternative Medicine Review*, **13** (2), 116–127.

56 Zimmermann, M.B. (2009) Iodine deficiency. *Endocrine Reviews*, **30** (4), 376–408.

57 Mumma, R.O., Rashid, K.A., Shane, B.S. *et al.* (1986) Toxic and protective constituents in pet foods. *American Journal of Veterinary Research*, **47** (7), 1633–1637.

58 Dzanis, D.A. (1994) The Association of American Feed Control Officials Dog and Cat Food Nutrient Profiles: substantiation of nutritional adequacy of complete and balanced pet foods in the United States. *Journal of Nutrition*, **124** (12 Suppl.), 2535S–2539S.

59 Johnson, L.A., Ford, H.C., Tarttelin, M.F., and Feek, C.M. (1992) Iodine content of commercially-prepared cat foods. *New Zealand Veterinary Journal*, **40** (1), 18–20.

60 Ranz, D., Tetrick, M., Opitz, B. *et al.* (2002) Estimation of iodine status in cats. *Journal of Nutrition*, **132** (6 Suppl. 2), 1751S–1753S.

61 Edinboro, C.H., Scott-Moncrieff, J.C., and Glickman, L.T. (2010) Feline hyperthyroidism: potential relationship with iodine supplement requirements of commercial cat foods. *Journal of Feline Medicine and Surgery*, **12** (9), 672–679.

62 Tarttelin, M.F. and Ford, H.C. (1994) Dietary iodine level and thyroid function in the cat. *Journal of Nutrition*, **124** (12 Suppl.), 2577S–2578S.

63 Tarttelin, M.F., Johnson, L.A., Cooke, R.R. *et al.* (1992) Serum free thyroxine levels respond inversely to changes in levels of dietary iodine in the domestic cat. *New Zealand Veterinary Journal*, **40** (2), 66–68.

64 Kyle, A.H., Tarttelin, M.F., Cooke, R.R., and Ford, H.C. (1994) Serum free thyroxine levels in cats maintained on diets relatively high or low in iodine. *New Zealand Veterinary Journal*, **42** (3), 101–103.

65 Hess, S.Y. (2010) The impact of common micronutrient deficiencies on iodine and thyroid metabolism: the evidence from human studies. *Best Practice & Research Clinical Endocrinology & Metabolism*, **24** (1), 117–132.

66 Scott, P.P. (1969) Effect of calcium and vitamin A deficiency on the thyroid gland. *Proceedings of the Royal Society of Medicine*, **62** (3), 240.

67 Kimura, S., Suwa, J., Ito, M., and Sato, H. (1976) Development of malignant goiter by defatted soybean with iodine-free diet in rats. *Gann*, **67** (5), 763–765.

68 Ikeda, T., Nishikawa, A., Imazawa, T. *et al.* (2000) Dramatic synergism between excess soybean intake and iodine deficiency on the development of rat thyroid hyperplasia. *Carcinogenesis*, **21** (4), 707–713.

69 Ikeda, T., Nishikawa, A., Son, H.Y. *et al.* (2001) Synergistic effects of high-dose soybean intake with iodine deficiency, but not sulfadimethoxine or phenobarbital, on rat thyroid proliferation. *Japanese Journal of Cancer Research*, **92** (4), 390–395.

70 Norsworthy, G.D., Adams, V.J., McElhaney, M.R., and Milios, J.A. (2002) Relationship between semi-quantitative thyroid palpation and total thyroxine concentration in cats with and without hyperthyroidism. *Journal of Feline Medicine and Surgery*, **4** (3), 139–143.

71 Birchard, S.J., Peterson, M.E., and Jacobson, A. (1984) Surgical treatment of feline hyperthyroidism – results of 85 cases. *Journal of the American Animal Hospital Association*, **20** (5), 705–709.

72 Chaitman, S.J., Hess, R., Senz, R. *et al.* (1999) Thyroid adenomatous hyperplasia in euthyroid cats. *Journal of Veterinary Internal Medicine*, **13**, 242.

73 Hofmeister, E., Kippenes, H., Mealey, K.L. *et al.* (2001) Functional cystic thyroid adenoma in a cat. *Journal of the American Veterinary Medical Association*, **219** (2), 190–193.

74 Norsworthy, G.D., Adams, V.J., McElhaney, M.R., and Milios, J.A. (2002) Palpable thyroid and parathyroid nodules in asymptomatic cats. *Journal of Feline Medicine and Surgery*, **4** (3), 145–151.

75 Bezuidenhout, A.J. (1993) The lymphatic system, in *Miller's Anatomy of the Dog*, 3rd edn. (eds. H.E. Evans and M.E. Miller), Saunders, Philadelphia, pp. 717–757.

5

Examining the Cardiovascular and Respiratory Systems of the Cat

5.1 The Cardiac Patient

The majority of cats do not present with a known history of cardiac disease. More often, heart murmurs and cardiac arrhythmias are incidental findings on the cardiothoracic component of the physical examination during a wellness visit, auscultation prior to general anesthesia, or evaluation of a different presenting complaint [1].

Kittens may be clinically normal, yet have an innocent, functional, non-pathologic murmur identified on their initial wellness or vaccination follow-up examinations. These murmurs are systolic, low grade, and louder at the left side of the chest. They result from turbulence within the heart and vessels as the heart is still developing, and they tend to resolve by 5 months of age [2].

Congenital heart disease is rare in kittens, with an estimated prevalence of 1.6% in adoption centers [3] and an incidence of 0.2–1 per 1000 hospital admissions [2]. When congenital heart disease occurs in cats, it is most commonly mitral or tricuspid valve dyplasia. Congenital heart disease in the cat may also be related to a defect that over time will cause volume overload, such as ventricular septal defects or patent ductus arteriosus. Alternatively, the congenital cardiac defect may be sub-aortic stenosis, which over time will cause pressure overload. Tetralogy of Fallot will primarily result in clinically evident cyanosis [2].

In the apparently healthy adult cat, systolic murmurs are ausculted in 16% of cats in a hospital population compared with 44% of shelter cats [4–6]. Additional diagnostic testing is required to differentiate structural from functional heart disease. Of those with abnormal echocardiographic findings, 15% had underlying hypertrophic cardiomyopathy (HCM) and 8–16% had non-pathologic dynamic right ventricular outflow tract obstruction [4–10]. HCM is the most common form of cardiomyopathy in the cat [11, 12], especially when the murmur is an incidental finding on examination and the patient is asymptomatic [11].

Like murmurs, most arrhythmias are incidental findings in asymptomatic cats [13]. Even when arrhythmias are linked to known heart disease, the patients are rarely clinical: syncope is uncommonly seen in feline patients [13–16]. More commonly, the cardiac patient presents without cardiac complaint [14]. Silent heart disease is common in cats [8]. Cardiothoracic auscultation is the best non-invasive screening test available to the general practitioner to identify new murmurs and arrhythmias and proactively pursue further diagnostic interventions [1] such as echocardiography [8].

When a feline patient is clinical for heart disease, the presenting complaint is often non-specific. Unlike dogs, cats rarely cough with primary heart disease or the resulting congestive heart failure, even when the left atrium is enlarged [17]. Cats are more likely to display dyspnea with or without open-mouth breathing. When cats are dyspneic, they may decompensate rapidly, making it challenging to differentiate cardiac from respiratory disease without adding to the stress of the patient. Swift *et al.* identified that cardiac disease was present in 38% of 90 dyspneic cats, and that presenting heart rate, the presence of concurrent murmurs, or gallop rhythms assisted with the diagnosis [18]. When dyspnea in cats is heart related, it is typically due to pleural effusion induced by right-sided heart failure- or left-sided heart failure-induced pulmonary edema [17].

Of cats that do not present as overtly dyspneic, owners may report increased sleeping and resting respiratory rates [19]. Generalized weakness and exercise intolerance are rarely reported in cats for obvious reasons, although clients may retrospectively admit to thinking that their cat had been progressively slowing down owing to the normal aging process [17]. Similarly, the owner may have been quick to dismiss weight loss and loss of lean body mass as age-related or arthritis-induced.

Cats with heart disease, typically HCM, may also present acutely for paresis, classically of one or both hind limbs secondary to an embolus of left atrial origin, although emboli can also occlude the forelimbs. In these cases, the paw pads of the associated limb(s) will be cyanotic, the distal limb(s) will be cool to the touch, the patient will show pain, and pulses may be weak to absent [17, 20].

Cats with hypertension may present for visual deficits. On physical examination, these cats typically have reduced pupillary light reflexes, with the potential for retinal hemorrhages and retinal detachments to be diagnosed on the fundic examination [17, 21].

Performing the Small Animal Physical Examination, First Edition. Ryane E. Englar.
© 2017 John Wiley & Sons, Inc. Published 2017 by John Wiley & Sons, Inc.

5.2 Assessing the Cardiovascular System Prior to Auscultation

An assessment of the cardiovascular system begins with observation of the patient in the examination room. The following characteristics should be observed and documented for every physical examination, especially when a patient presents with a cardiac complaint.

5.2.1 Attitude

The clinician should consider the patient's attitude, mentation, and emotional status immediately on entering the examination room. In particular, the following two questions should be asked:

- Is the patient alert and responsive?
- Is the patient visibly distressed?

As discussed in Chapter 1, cats frequently exhibit stress in the veterinary clinic [22–26], and cats that are stressed may go into "fight or flight" or even "fight, flight, or freeze" mode [27]. A "frozen" cat, one that is glued to the floor or hunched against the wall, may be frozen out of fear. However, a cat may also be "frozen" because of respiratory distress: a cat may be so concentrated on breathing to survive that it takes little else into consideration.

Paying attention to the cat's visual cues (ears, eyes, body and tail posture) may help the clinician to decide if the patient is acting out of fear or due to disease [27].

5.2.2 Respiratory Rate

The respiratory rate for a normal cat ranges from 20–40 breaths per minute [28, 29]. The respiratory rate for a stressed cat may be elevated; the respiratory rate for a cat with cardiac disease may also be elevated. Again, the cat's visual cues (ears, eyes, body and tail posture) may help the clinician to decide whether an elevated respiratory rate is due to stress or underlying disease [27].

5.2.3 Respiratory Effort

Inspiration is a mechanical process that is active. It occurs because of the coordinated contraction of the diaphragm and the intercostal muscles that shift the ribs rostrally, ventrally, and laterally to expand the thoracic cavity. By contrast, expiration is passive: the diaphragm and ribcage resume their original positions. This requires the thoracic cage to be flexible and the lungs to be elastic. Together, one round of inspiration and expiration completes the respiratory cycle [28, 30].

Dyspnea occurs when there is difficulty getting air in, getting air out, or both, creating effort on the part of the patient to complete the respiratory cycle [28, 30]. Inspiratory dyspnea results when the upper airway narrows. It takes more effort to draw air into the body, and the body may require the use of the auxiliary respiratory muscles, the scalenus and the sternocephalicus, to complete the process. In addition, the alar folds of the nostrils may flare and the lips may retract to increase airflow [28].

When the lungs are inelastic, the ribcage is non-compliant, or the bronchi are narrowed, expiratory dyspnea results. It takes more effort to push air out of the body. Abdominal pressure is engaged against the diaphragm to expel air forcibly by increasing the intra-thoracic pressure. However, this process may narrow smaller bronchi, exacerbating respiratory distress [28–30].

Increased respiratory effort is grossly visible.

5.2.4 Respiratory Route

A normal cat breathes through its nose – cats are not built to sustain long periods of open-mouth breathing [31]. An open-mouth breathing cat is either significantly stressed or significantly distressed from underlying respiratory or cardiac disease [17, 29, 32]. An open-mouth breathing cat can easily become a respiratory or cardiac emergency [32].

5.2.5 Mucous Membrane Color

See Section 3.6.1.

Recall that the gums are the most commonly used tissue to assess mucous membrane color. However, when the gums are not accessible, an alternative mucous membrane that can be assessed easily in the cat is the conjunctival sac. Evaluating mucous membrane color through examination of the vulva or the prepuce is much less tolerated in the cat than in the dog [28].

5.2.6 Capillary Refill Time (CRT)

See Section 3.6.2.

5.2.7 Jugular Pulse

The jugular vein is the largest vein on either side of the neck. Although it is used frequently to sample blood in cats, the veterinary team often forgets that it is equally useful, if not more so, as an indicator of venous return and central venous pressure [28].

In the normal standing patient that is staring straight ahead, the jugular vein cannot be seen or felt. This does not hold true if venous return to the heart is obstructed [17, 28]. In right-sided heart failure, there is a back-up of blood returning to the right side of the heart because that side of the heart is inefficient, ineffective, or both. This overload of blood distends the jugular veins so that they become visible, palpable, or both. Sometimes the jugular veins become so distended that they may visibly pulse with each heartbeat [17, 28, 33].

Other places to look for evidence of poor venous return are the ventral thorax and abdomen. These areas may "stock up" in situations involving poor venous return, meaning that they may appear rather edematous. Stocking up of the abdomen is often referred to as ascites. This may occur in cats, but does so less frequently than in dogs. In cats, increased central venous pressure is more likely to affect the pleural space than the abdomen. This more typically results in a cat that presents in respiratory distress [17, 28].

5.2.8 Palpating the Ventral Neck

See Section 4.1.3.

The ventral neck of any adult cat should be routinely palpated for evidence of an enlarged thyroid gland. Feline hyperthyroidism is known to induce cardiac pathology. The excess of thyroid hormones exerts positive inotropic and chronotropic effects that cause increased heart contractility and heart rate, respectively. Furthermore, hyperthyroid cats have increased metabolic rates with increased oxygen consumption, and cardiac output must rise to keep up. Over time, this may result in hypertension [21], myocardial hypertrophy, and chamber dilation. Congestive heart failure is a potential outcome [34].

5.2.9 Palpating the Limbs for Warmth and Assessing the Extremities for Color

As already mentioned, cats with overt or subclinical HCM are at risk of thrombus formation within the left atrium or left auricle. Each thrombus has the potential to enter into systemic circulation as an embolus. While being transported in the vasculature, the embolus can occlude a vessel, leading to circulatory compromise of the associated tissue. The most common location for embolus occlusion to occur is at the terminal aorta. The embolus may lodge cranial to the aortic bifurcation, leading to occluded blood flow in both hind limbs, or it may lodge distal to the bifurcation, leading to occlusion of only one hind limb. The affected limb(s) will experience acute paresis or paralysis. The patient typically presents on emergency as acutely painful, with cyanotic paw pads and weak to absent femoral pulses [17, 20, 29, 32].

Of all cats that frequented a veterinary teaching hospital in North America, the occurrence rate was 0.1% [35]. Males are predisposed, with Ragdoll, Birman, Tonkinese, Abyssinian, and Maine Coon cats at increased risk [35].

5.2.10 Assessing Femoral Pulses

The arterial pulse is the palpable wave generated by ventricular systole, whereby blood forcibly passes from the left ventricle of the heart to the aorta. What is felt as the pulse is essentially the stretch of an artery to accommodate the blood [17].

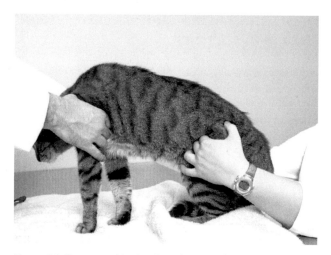

Figure 5.1 Proper positioning for palpation of the femoral pulses. Source: Courtesy of the Media Resources Department at Midwestern University.

The femoral arteries are the most common site of pulse detection in the cat. Every heartbeat should be associated with a pulse [17] (Figure 5.1). To appreciate the femoral pulse, the clinician should position himself behind the patient, with the patient facing away from the clinician. With fingers together and curled palms, the clinician may feel for the femoral arteries, which are located in the groin at the crease where the pelvic limbs attach to the body. Using the fingertips as opposed to the thumbs will increase the clinician's sensitivity in detecting pulses. Using the fingertips will also reduce the chance that the pulse that is felt is not the clinician's own digital pulse and is instead truly the patient's. If there is any doubt, the clinician may auscult the heart at the same time as feeling for the pulse: the patient's pulse and heart rate should match.

Once the clinician has become used to where to feel to appreciate the femoral pulse, he should practice palpating both the left and right femoral arteries at the same time. As the clinician develops sound technical skills, feeling both arteries simultaneously will help in assessing the symmetry of the pulses. The presence of asymmetric pulses may help to facilitate a diagnosis of underlying cardiac compromise.

The following information can be obtained from the pulse:

- pulse rate;
- perfusion;
- pulse quality.

As already mentioned, the pulse rate should match the heart rate – for each heartbeat that is auscted, there should be a corresponding pulse. To determine if the pulse rate matches the heart rate, the clinician should simultaneously auscult the heart and palpate the femoral pulses. If the pulses are not synchronous with heart rate, then there are so-called "dropped beats" of the heart, as can occur with cardiac arrhythmias. When contraction of the heart occurs prematurely owing to the electrical activity of an ectopic focus, the ventricles may not have had a chance to fill such that ventricular output is reduced. The resultant stroke volume may be insufficient to translate into a palpable pulse. The pulse is then absent despite cardiac contraction [14].

Absent pulses can also reflect lack of perfusion. For example, in a cat with an aortic thromboembolism (a so-called "saddle thrombus"), there is a blood clot at the distal end of the aorta at the level of the aortic bifurcation. Distal to this clot, the tissues are unable to receive arterial blood, hence the femoral pulse is reduced to absent. Tissues distal to the clot are cooler to the touch owing to poor perfusion, which is also reflected by cyanosis of tissues such as the digital paw pads [17, 32, 33, 35].

How strong or weak a pulse is depends on the difference between the systolic and diastolic blood pressures. The greater the difference, the stronger is the pulse; the smaller the difference, the poorer is the pulse [17].

- "Bounding" pulses are stronger than normal and result from either a reduced diastolic pressure or an elevated systolic pressure, or both [17].
- "Thready" pulses are weaker than normal and result from either a reduced systolic pressure or an elevated diastolic pressure, or both [17].
- Erratic pulses may reflect underlying atrial fibrillation [17].

Assessing the pulse is an imperfect science, and there are shortcomings in its evaluation. First, it is not easy to feel the femoral pulse in a normal cat, let alone an abnormal one. Another shortcoming is that if the patient is hypotensive but experiences an equal reduction in the systolic and diastolic blood pressures, pulse quality will be unaffected because the net difference between the two blood pressures is unchanged.

5.3 Cardiothoracic Auscultation

When considering the cardiovascular system, it is important to review the pathway of blood through the body, as this is the foundation for understanding cardiac parameters, heart sounds, and the various points in the cycle at which dysfunction can arise.

5.3.1 Recalling the Cardiac Cycle

At its most basic, the cardiac cycle consists of systole (ventricular contraction) and diastole (ventricular relaxation). Imagine a droplet of oxygenated blood seated in the left ventricle of the heart. During systole, this droplet is forced from the left ventricle of the heart, out through the aorta, and from there to the rest of the body. The blood journeys from arteries to arterioles to capillary beds in order to perfuse tissues with oxygen. The deoxygenated blood is then gathered up in venules, which pool into veins, which

return to the right side of the heart, specifically the right atrium. Blood fills the right atrium and right ventricle during diastole. When systole recurs, blood is forced out from the right ventricle to the pulmonary artery to the lungs, where blood is reoxygenated. This reoxygenated blood returns to the heart to fill the left atrium and left ventricle during diastole via the pulmonary vein. When systole recurs, the cycle repeats. Oxygenated blood is now actively pumped from the left ventricle to the body [30].

The heart valves facilitate the cardiac cycle in order for blood to continue to move in a forward direction:

- The atrioventricular (A-V) valves are located precisely where their name implies – at the junction between the atria and the ventricles. The right A-V valve is also referred to as the tricuspid valve and the left A-V valve as the mitral valve.
- The pulmonic valve sits between the right ventricle and the pulmonary artery.
- The aortic valve separates the left ventricle and the aorta.

During systole, the A-V valves close to prevent blood from backing up from the ventricles to the atria. At the end of systole and thus the beginning of diastole, the aortic and pulmonic valves close. In preparation for the next systole, oxygenated blood moves forward from the lungs to fill the left side of the heart; deoxygenated blood moves forward from the periphery to fill the right side of the heart.

5.3.2 Normal Heart Sounds

When we think of what the heart sounds like at its most basic, we tend to recall "lub-dub." The first heart sound, S1, represents the "lub" and the second heart sound, S2, represents the "dub." More specifically, S1 occurs as the A-V valves close and the ventricles contract, whereas S2 occurs as the pulmonic and aortic valves close and the heart fills.

5.3.3 Abnormal Heart Sounds: Murmurs

Murmurs are specific types of cardiac sounds that are not heard in the normal patient and are the result of turbulent blood flow. Whereas S1 and S2 are typically crisp, discrete sounds, murmurs may be described as a "whoosh" as from turbulence [17]. When murmurs are ausculted, they should be described by their location in the cardiac cycle [17]:

- Systolic murmurs occur between S1 and S2.
- Diastolic murmurs occur between S2 and S1.

Murmurs should also be described by their intensity, which is typically described in terms of grade, of which there are six [17]:

- Grade 1 murmurs are low-intensity sounds that are difficult to pick up immediately, often because they are highly focal. They are often indistinct in that they may blend into S1 such that the only indication of their presence is a seemingly prolonged S1.

- Grade 2 murmurs are also soft sounds, but unlike Grade 1 murmurs, they are distinct. They are also more readily identified despite tending to be focal.
- Grade 3 murmurs are of moderate intensity and are easily heard as soon as the stethoscope is applied to the chest.
- Grade 4 murmurs are loud and tend to be more diffuse.
- Grade 5 murmurs are very loud and diffuse, and are characterized by a palpable thrill – that is, turbulence is so great as to create a vibration that is palpable across the chest wall.
- Grade 6 murmurs are very loud and do not require the use of a stethoscope to hear.

Murmurs should further be described by the so-called point of maximal intensity – that is, the valve corresponding to the loudest region of the murmur. This may suggest that the identified valve is dysfunctional, which is why it is so important to auscult the entire chest, including over each valve.

5.3.4 Other Heart Sounds

S1 and S2 are typically both audible on cardiothoracic auscultation of the normal patient. However, in addition to S1 and S2, there are certain heart sounds that are not typically heard in health but that may arise with cardiac pathology [36]:

- S3 occurs on the coattails of S2 as blood flows from the atria into the now relaxed, partially filled ventricles. S3 is heard in pathologic situations involving ventricular dilation such as dilated cardiomyopathy (DCM), rare in cats but secondary to taurine deficiency.

- S4 occurs with atrial contraction, just prior to S1. S4 is heard in pathologic situations involving atrial dilation, such as HCM.

When heard, S3 and S4 result in "gallop rhythms" [36]. When S3 is present, the gallop rhythm that is created is

$$1 \quad 23 \quad 1 \quad 23 \quad 1 \quad 23 \quad 1 \quad 23$$

When S4 is present, the gallop rhythm that is created is

$$41 \quad 2 \quad 41 \quad 2 \quad 41 \quad 2 \quad 41 \quad 2$$

5.3.5 Ausculting the Heart

The cat has a very small thoracic cavity in comparison with the dog (Figure 5.2). The small thoracic cavity of the cat seems even smaller when taking into account how the heart fits into an already tight space. Even so, it is important that the clinician gets into the habit of ausculting over each individual heart valve.

When evaluating the left lateral thorax, the clinician may use the acronym P–A–M to recall the valves that may be auscfrom in this region of the chest (Figure 5.3a and b) [17, 28]:

- The **pulmonic** valve: auscult over the left second to third intercostal space, seated dorsal to the sternum at approximately one-third of the distance between the sternum and vertebral column.
- The **aortic** valve: auscult over the left second to third intercostal space.
- The **mitral** valve: auscult over the left fifth to sixth intercostal space, near the sternum.

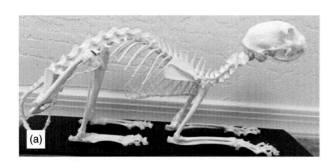
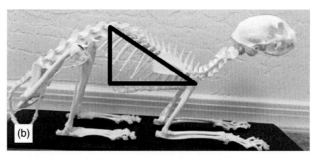
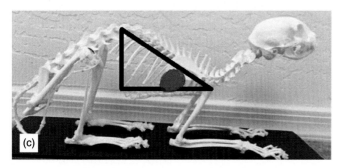
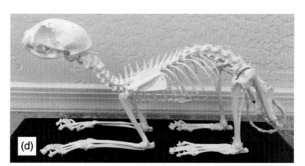

Figure 5.2 (a) Right lateral cat skeleton. (b) Right lateral cat skeleton with thoracic cavity outlined in black. (c) Right lateral cat skeleton with thoracic cavity outlined in black and rudimentary heart drawn in, in red. (d) Left lateral cat skeleton. (*Continued*)

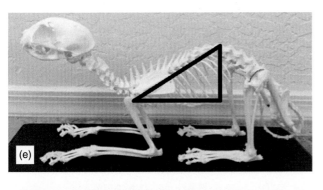

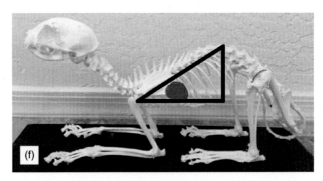

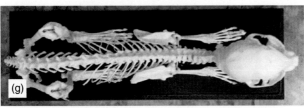

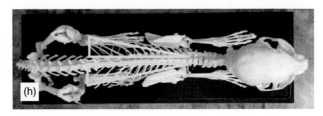

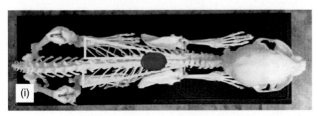

Figure 5.2 (*Continued*)
(e) Left lateral cat skeleton with thoracic cavity outlined in black.
(f) Left lateral cat skeleton with thoracic cavity outlined in black
and rudimentary heart drawn in, in red. (g) Aerial view of cat
skeleton. (h) Aerial view of cat skeleton with thoracic cavity
outlined in yellow. (i) Aerial view of cat skeleton with thoracic
cavity outlined in yellow and rudimentary heart drawn in, in red.

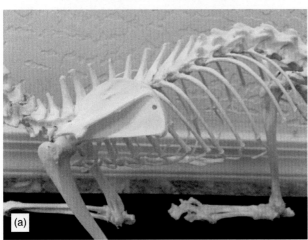

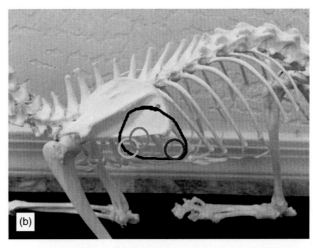

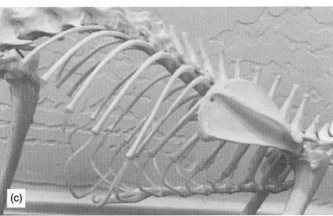

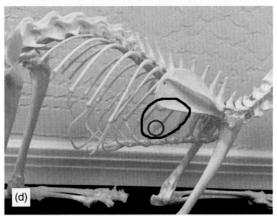

Figure 5.3 (a) Left lateral cat skeleton, close-up. (b) Left lateral cat skeleton, close-up, with rudimentary heart valves drawn in:
pink = pulmonic valve; orange = aortic valve; red = mitral valve. (c) Right lateral cat skeleton, close-up. (d) Right lateral cat skeleton,
close-up, with rudimentary heart valve drawn in: purple = tricuspid.

When evaluating the right lateral thorax, the clinician may use the acronym R–A–T to recall that the **right atrial** valve is the **tricuspid**, which may be ausculted over the fourth to fifth intercostal space near the sternum [17, 28] (Figure 5.3c and d).

To appreciate these landmarks on a live patient, see Figure 5.4. Note that although different body positions are demonstrated in Figure 5.4, the feline patient should ideally be ausculted standing up or sitting as opposed to lying down. This maintains the heart in its anatomically normal position and avoids the potential for a positional murmur, an artifact that may occur when the patient is lying down [17].

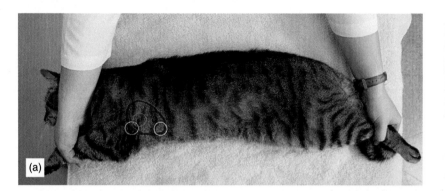
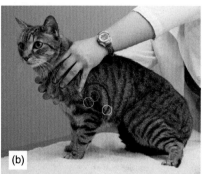
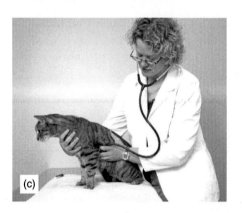
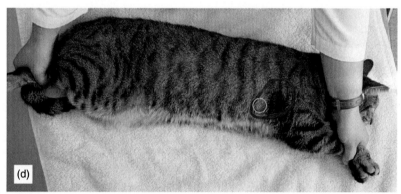
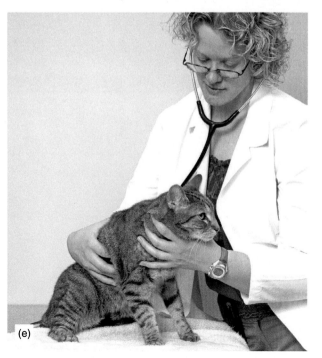

Figure 5.4 (a) Live cat in right lateral recumbency. Appreciate the structures localized to the left lateral thorax in anticipation of auscultation: pink = pulmonic valve; orange = aortic valve; yellow = mitral valve. (b) Live cat, seated. Appreciate the structures localized to the left lateral thorax in anticipation of auscultation: pink = pulmonic valve; orange = aortic valve; yellow = mitral valve. (c) Left lateral thoracic auscultation in a live patient. (d) Live cat, restrained in left lateral recumbency. Appreciate the structures localized to the right lateral thorax in anticipation of auscultation: lavender = tricupsid valve. (e) Right lateral thoracic auscultation in a live patient. Source (a)–(e): Courtesy of the Media Resources Department at Midwestern University.

In addition to the valve-associated areas highlighted above, it is important to auscult the parasternal region. This is a common site of murmurs in cats.

5.3.6 Understanding How the Stethoscope Is Built to Facilitate Auscultation

The stethoscope is the primary tool of cardiothoracic auscultation. It consists of ear pieces, tubing, the bell, and the diaphragm.

The diaphragm preferentially transmits higher frequency sounds (300–1000 cycles per second) to the listener. Both S1 and S2 are heard well with the diaphragm. By contrast, the bell preferentially transmits lower frequency sounds (20–300 cycles per second) to the listener. This facilitates the hearing of S3 and S4.

The majority of stethoscopes have dual-sided chest pieces. The clinician learns to switch between sides of the chest piece depending upon which heart sounds are of interest (Figure 5.5a–c).

When patients are small (under 15 pounds), a pediatric stethoscope is preferred because its smaller chest piece will allow the clinician to hear preferentially over certain valves without the chest piece overlaying the entire heart. Note that the pediatric stethoscope also has a dual-sided chest piece (Figure 5.5d).

Some stethoscopes no longer have a dual-sided chest piece; instead, they incorporate both sides into one. The clinician is able to alternate between low and high frequency sounds by adjusting finger-tip pressure when pressing the chest piece against the thorax (Figure 5.5e). The advantage is that the clinician does not need to switch between the two sides of the chest piece but simply modulates pressure depending upon what is being listened for.

Neither style of stethoscope is superior. Clinician preference dictates which is purchased, then it is up to the clinician to practice in order to be both accurate and efficient.

5.4 The Respiratory Patient

The feline respiratory patient typically has one of three presentations: disease of the upper airway, lower airway, and/or the thoracic cavity.

5.4.1 The Upper Airway Patient

Upper airway disease is common in cats and is especially prevalent among kittens and in communal settings such as shelters and catteries [37–43]. When it strikes shelters, it is costly to manage [39, 42] and, second only to overcrowding, is a leading cause of euthanasia [44].

Infectious causes predominate and include the following [42, 45–54]:

- Viral:
  - Feline herpesvirus (FHV-1);
  - Feline calicivirus (FCV).
- Bacterial:
  - *Chlamydia felis;*
  - *Bordetella bronchiseptica;*
  - *Mycoplasma felis.*

Of these agents, FHV-1 and FCV are the most prevalent worldwide [37]. These viruses most commonly result in nasal discharge, with or within conjunctivitis, and sneezing [43]. Nasal discharge is typically serous but may become mucopurulent once upper airway inflammation is sufficient and/or if opportunistic secondary bacterial infections take root [37, 38, 43]. See Section 3.4 for images of nasal discharge.

Non-infectious causes of upper airway disease include nasopharyngeal polyps (Figure 5.6), which occur primarily in young cats, and neoplasia in older cats [38, 55–57]. Because these conditions tend to cause upper airway obstruction during the inspiratory part of the respiratory cycle, clients may report stertor, a snoring sound. This is typically pronounced when the patient is asleep; however, it may persist when the patient is awake. An oropharyngeal examination under sedation may assist with the diagnosis of a nasopharyngeal polyp by allowing manipulation of the soft palate; however, advanced imaging such as a CT scan may be indicated to evaluate the upper airway sinuses better for turbinate destruction and/or mass effect [38].

Laryngeal disease is markedly less common in cats than dogs; however, it, too, results in upper airway obstruction and typically stridorous breathing in which a harsh, high-pitched sound materializes during inspiration [38].

5.4.2 The Lower Airway Patient

Whereas infectious diseases tend to strike the upper airway, the lower airway patient tends to be plagued by inflammation or neoplasia causing expiratory rather than inspiratory difficulty. The classic feline lower airway patient is a cat with feline bronchial disease, which is similar to recurrent airway obstruction in horses and asthma in people [58, 59]. Because of its striking similarity to asthma in people, feline bronchial disease is sometimes referred to as feline asthma. In the feline asthmatic, the airway is hyper-reactive to airborne particulate matter, causing an exaggerated inflammatory response with resultant airway constriction [59].

Young adult cats are at increased risk of developing feline bronchial disease, and are frequently presented to the veterinary team by owners who are concerned about a developing cough [59]. In addition to a cough,

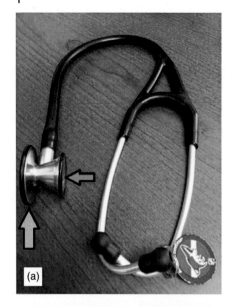

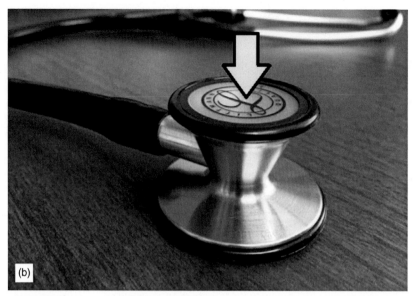

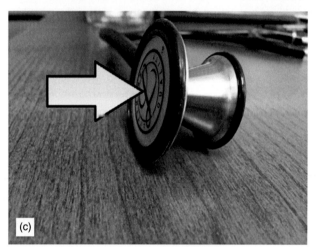

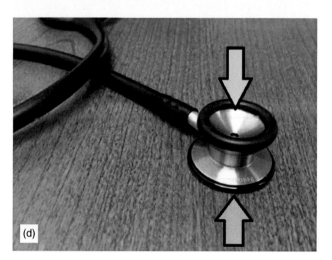

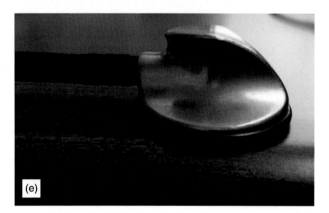

Figure 5.5 (a) Stethoscope with dual-sided chest piece. The blue arrow is pointing to the bell and the pink arrow to the diaphragm. (b) Stethoscope with dual-sided chest piece. The arrow is pointing to the bell. (c) Stethoscope with dual-sided chest piece. The arrow is pointing to the diaphragm. (d) Stethoscope with dual-sided chest piece. The blue arrow is pointing to the bell and the pink arrow to the diaphragm. (e) Stethoscope with touch-sensitive chest piece.

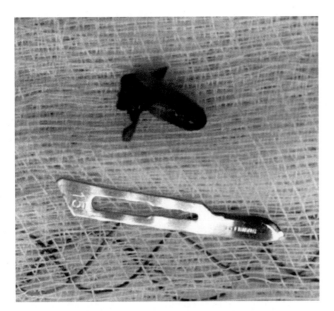

Figure 5.6 Nasopharyngeal polyp after manual extraction.

the patient may present with tachypnea, if not dyspnea, making it challenging to eliminate the potential for underlying cardiac disease without physically examining the patient and initiating a diagnostic work-up. On examination, the patient with feline bronchial disease typically has an expiratory wheeze and harsh lung sounds. A wheeze is unlikely to occur secondary to cardiomyopathy [58, 59].

With the exception of feline bronchial disease, lower airway disease is rare in cats. Only 21 cases of pneumonia over a 5-year period [60] and 39 cases over 10 years [61] have been reported by two different teaching hospitals engaged in retrospective studies, and primary pulmonary neoplasia in cats has been reported even more infrequently [62–64].

Radiography plays an important role in diagnosing lower airway disease. Gadbois *et al.* demonstrated that 37 of 40 cats (92.5%) with bronchial disease had a classic bronchial radiographic pattern [65]. This pattern is characterized by bronchial walls that are accentuated either because of age-related mineralization within the bronchial tree or the abnormal presence of peri-bronchial infiltrate due to bronchial inflammation [66, 67]. On cross-section, each bronchus takes on an altered appearance that some radiologists refer to as the donut pattern: rather than appearing to be outlined by a thin circle of black, each bronchus is rimmed with a thicker circle of black. This signifies bronchial thickening secondary to inflammation [67] (Figure 5.7).

Note that radiography is helpful in identifying that lower airway disease is present; however, it cannot discern the cause of lower airway disease [58]. Feline bronchial disease is a diagnosis of exclusion. The clinician must take care to rule out other causes of a bronchial radiographic pattern such as chronic bronchitis [67–69], pulmonary eosinophilic infiltrates [70, 71], and lungworms [72]. All of these lower airway diseases may look identical on radiographic examination of the thoracic cavity (Figure 5.8).

5.4.3 The Patient with Thoracic Cavity Disease

Thoracic cavity disease results when there is an accumulation of either fluid, air, or solid tissue within the pleural

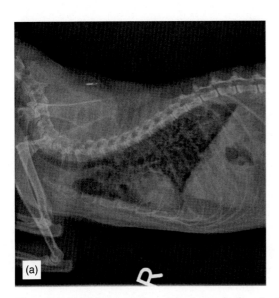
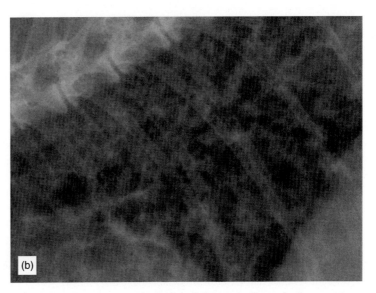

Figure 5.7 (a) Right lateral thoracic radiograph of a cat with feline asthma. (b) Close-up of right lateral thoracic radiograph of a cat with feline asthma. (*Continued*)

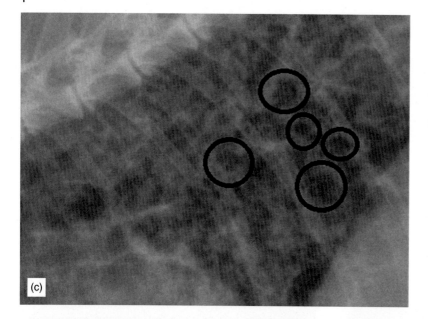

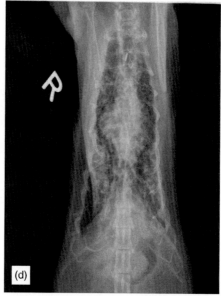

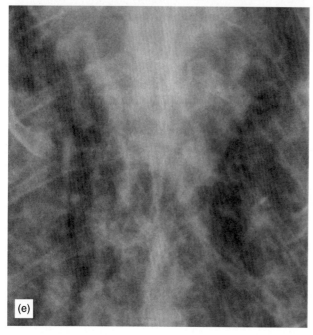

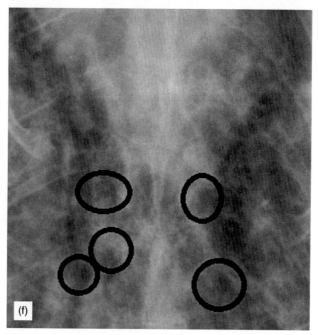

Figure 5.7 (*Continued*)
(c) Close-up of right lateral thoracic radiograph of a cat with feline asthma, with the classic "donut" bronchial pattern identified.
(d) Ventrodorsal (V/D) thoracic radiograph of a cat with feline asthma. (e) Close-up of V/D thoracic radiograph of a cat with feline asthma.
(f) Close-up of V/D thoracic radiograph of a cat with feline asthma, with the classic "donut" bronchial pattern identified.
Source (a)–(f): Courtesy of Daniel Foy, MS, DVM, DACVIM, DACVECC.

space, so the lungs' ability to expand is compromised. The patient typically presents in respiratory distress, with head and neck extended in an attempt to gasp air, with or without open-mouth, rapid, shallow breathing. Unlike cats with feline bronchial disease in which expiratory effort is pronounced, cats with thoracic cavity disease struggle with the inspiratory part of the respiratory cycle [73].

When fluid accumulates within the pleural space, the cat is said to have pleural effusion. This effusion can be secondary to [73]:

- congestive heart failure, in which case the fluid is clear to pale yellow;
- "wet" feline infectious peritonitis, in which case the fluid is straw colored;

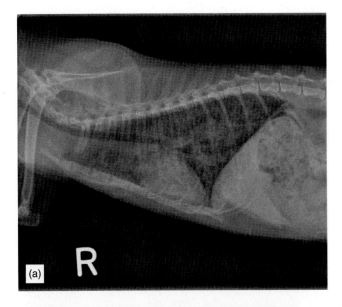
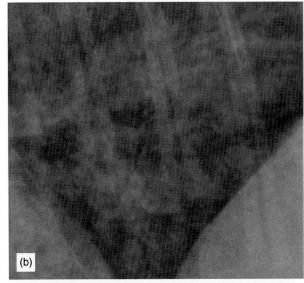
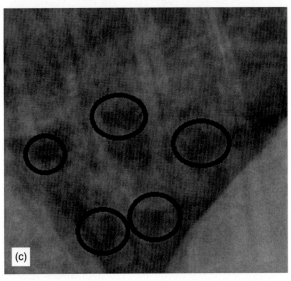
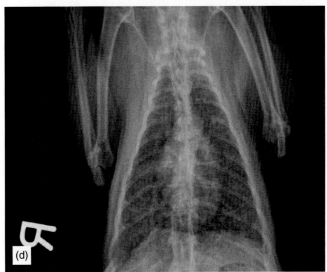

Figure 5.8 (a) Right lateral thoracic radiograph of a cat with lungworms. (b) Close-up of right lateral thoracic radiograph of a cat with lungworms. (c) Close-up of right lateral thoracic radiograph of cat with lungworms, with the classic "donut" bronchial pattern identified. (d) Ventrodorsal (V/D) thoracic radiograph of a cat with lungworms. (*Continued*)

- pyothorax, in which case the fluid is opaque and cream colored;
- hemothorax, in which case the fluid is hemorrhagic; or
- chylothorax, in which case the fluid is milky white to pink [73].

Regardless of the fluid type, its presence causes the lungs to float up to the dorsocaudal margin of the thoracic cavity, resulting in muffled heart and lung sounds cranio-ventrally [73]. This is evident radiographically, although not all cats with pleural effusion are stable enough for diagnostic imaging: many cats are so severely compromised and dyspneic that the stress of radiographs could easily cause them to decompensate into respiratory arrest [73].

When cats with pleural effusion can tolerate a radiographic examination, one can appreciate the rounding or scalloping of lung margins, the separation of the lung from the thoracic wall, the increased haziness of the cardiac silhouette, and classic interlobar fissure lines (Figure 5.9).

By contrast, when free air accumulates within the thoracic cavity, as in cases of pneumothorax, the change in pressure within the thoracic cavity causes the lungs to collapse. When the lungs are collapsed, they cannot expand adequately to preserve tidal volume. As a result, the patient has to work harder to get air in by increasing their respiratory rate [73].

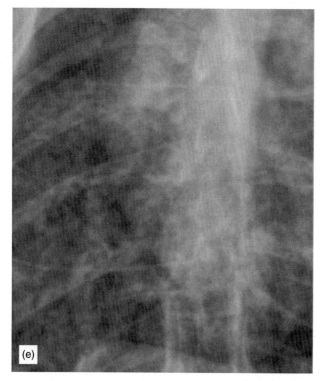

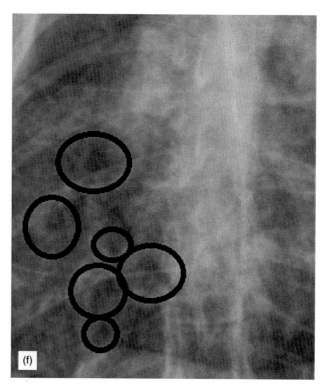

Figure 5.8 (*Continued*)
(e) Close-up of V/D thoracic radiograph of a cat with lungworms. (f) Close-up of V/D thoracic radiograph of a cat with lungworms, with the classic "donut" bronchial pattern identified. Source (a) (f): Courtesy of Daniel Foy, MS, DVM, DACVIM, DACVECC.

Solid tissue within the pleural space could be the result of trauma, as in the case of diaphragmatic hernias [74–76], congenital malformations, as in the case of peritoneopericardial hernias [77], and neoplastic disease, such as thymomas, thymolipomas, and thymic cysts [73, 78, 79]. As with fluid accumulation within the pleural space, tissue accumulation encroaches upon the lung fields, taking away the lungs' ability to expand maximally. The net result is a patient with compromised ability to fully inflate its lungs (Figure 5.10).

5.5 Assessing the Respiratory System Prior to Auscultation

An assessment of the respiratory system begins with observation of the patient in the examination room.

Review the following characteristics from Sections 5.2.1–5.2.6:

- attitude;
- respiratory rate;

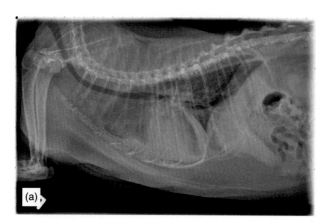

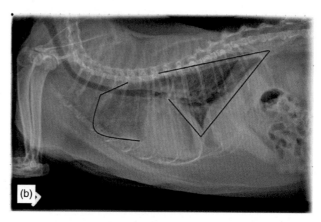

Figure 5.9 (a) Left lateral thoracic radiograph of a cat with acute onset of pleural effusion. (b) Left lateral thoracic radiograph of a cat with acute onset of pleural effusion, with lung fields outlined in blue. Note the rounded lung margins and the pulling away of the lungs from the thoracic wall. (*Continued*)

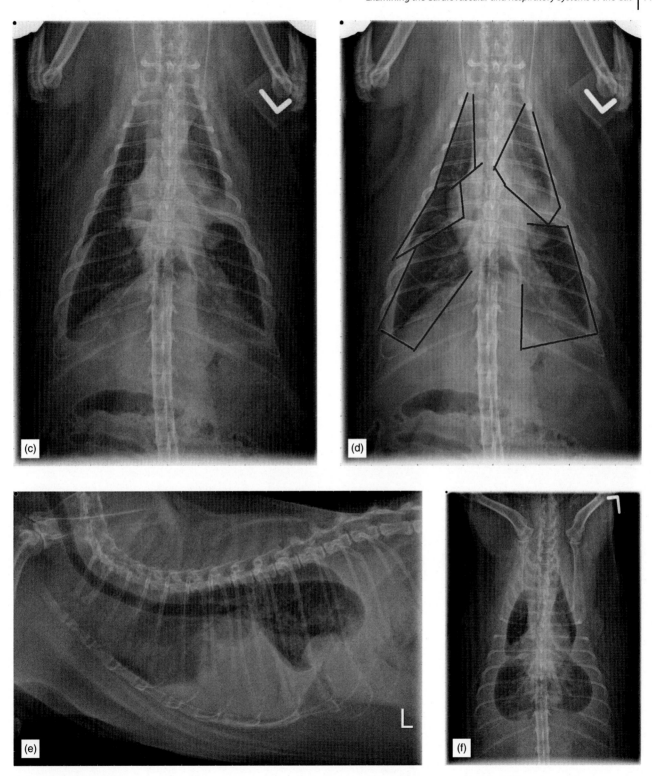

Figure 5.9 (*Continued*)
(c) Ventrodorsal (V/D) thoracic radiograph of a cat with acute onset of pleural effusion. (d) V/D thoracic radiograph of a cat with acute onset of pleural effusion, with lung fields outlined in blue. Note the interlobar fissure lines that make the lung lobes look like individual sails. (e) Left lateral thoracic radiograph of a cat with chronic pleural effusion. Note the rounding of the lung margins. (f) V/D thoracic radiograph of a cat with chronic pleural effusion. Note how far the lungs have pulled away from the thoracic wall. Source (a)–(f): Courtesy of Daniel Foy, MS, DVM, DACVIM, DACVECC.

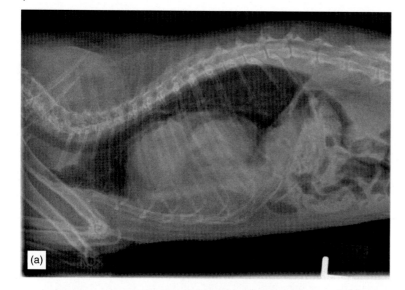

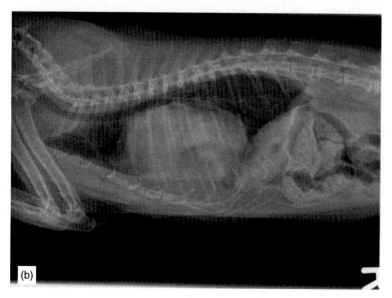

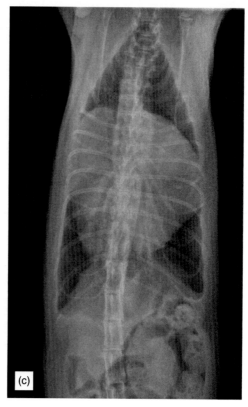

Figure 5.10 (a) Left lateral thoracic radiograph of a cat with peritoneopericardial hernia (PPDH), a congenital abnormality that improperly allows maintained communication between the thoracic and abdominal cavities. (b) Right lateral thoracic radiograph of the same cat with PPDH. (c) Ventrodorsal thoracic radiograph of the same cat with PPDH. Source (a)–(c): Courtesy of Daniel Foy, MS, DVM, DACVIM, DACVECC.

- respiratory effort;
- respiratory route;
- mucous membrane color;
- capillary refill time (CRT).

As when assessing the cardiovascular system, these same characteristics should be observed and documented for every physical examination, especially when a patient presents with a respiratory complaint. In addition, the clinician should observe whether or not the patient sneezes or coughs. If either action is observed, the clinician should follow up with the owner as to duration, frequency, progression, and also if the action, in particular coughing, occurs during a particular time of day or night.

Both sneezing and coughing are non-specific signs involving the respiratory system. Sneezing may be a protective response to allergens or other irritants [28]. Sneez-ing could also be the body's response to inflammation or a foreign body, tumor or otherwise [28]. Coughing is a second protective reflex that may be stimulated by the larynx, trachea, or bronchi. A laryngeal-induced cough tends to be episodic. It may be so harsh as to trigger gagging that may or may not be productive [28].

5.5.1 The Nose

The clinician should note whether or not the patient has nasal discharge. If nasal discharge is present, the clinician should ask:

- Is it unilateral or bilateral?
- Is it fresh or dry?
- Is it copious?
- Is it serous, mucoid, mucopurulent, or hemorrhagic?

See Section 3.4 for images of nasal discharge.

The clinician should also check for airflow. Recall from Section 3.4 that airflow through each nostril can be assessed by placing a glass slide in front of the nose. Because cats are nasal breathers, the breath should fog up the slide in two concentric circles: one per nare. If one side lacks a circle of fog on the slide, then airflow is minimal to non-existent through that side of the upper respiratory tract. Alternatively, the clinician may hold a tuft of cotton in front of each nostril and assess for movement of the cotton.

The clinician should listen for audible upper airway noise. Specifically, the clinician should listen for stridor and stertor, both of which are audible without a stethoscope. Both sounds, if present, are abnormal and are associated with the passage of air through a narrowed airway.

Recall that stridor is a wind-like, high-pitched sound that occurs when air passes over more rigid tissue [38]. When present, stridor typically results from abnormal narrowing of the nasal cavities or laryngeal tissue. By contrast, stertor is a snore-like, low-pitched sound that occurs when loose tissue projects into an airway as from an elongated soft palate. By contrast, stertor is typically pharyngeal in origin.

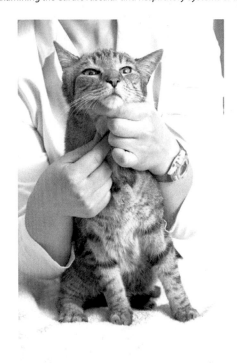

Figure 5.11 Palpating the length of the trachea. Source: Courtesy of the Media Resources Department at Midwestern University.

5.5.2 The Larynx and the Trachea

The larynx should be palpated to assess for symmetry. To facilitate this examination, the clinician may lift the patient's head and neck. Note that the larynx is very sensitive. Firm pressure may elicit a cough in a normal patient.

The trachea should also be palpated, beginning distal to the larynx and ending at the thoracic inlet (Figure 5.11). It is important to note if doing so elicits a reproducible cough. A cough on tracheal palpation is not normal, and typically indicates tracheal sensitivity.

5.5.3 Thoracic Compliance

The thoracic cavity should be assessed for compliance in every feline patient. To assess for thoracic cavity compliance, the clinician should cup his hand underneath the ventral chest of the cat such that the thumb grasps one side of the cat's sternum and the fingers grasp the other side. The clinician should then give the ribcage a firm squeeze.

The thoracic wall in a "normal" cat is adequately compliant and should compress somewhat. If there is no compliance or if the cat's thoracic cavity used to be compliant but is now not, there may be a space-occupying mass within the thorax. Mediastinal lymphoma is one of the more common intra-thoracic malignancies in cats. When it occurs, it tends to be associated with pleural effusion [73].

5.5.4 Thoracic Percussion

When percussion is used in the physical examination, it refers to the clinician tapping against a part of the body. Doing so can help the clinician to determine if a body part is painful or to characterize the resonating sound to understand better the underlying disease process. When percussion is used to assess a body cavity, such as the thoracic cavity, the clinician is percussing to achieve the latter. The technique of acoustic percussion originated in 1761 in Vienna, as a standard component of the human physical examination, and evolved by the early 1800s to improve sound quality through the use of plessimeters. Because companion animals tend to be small, plessimeters are not necessary. When used, if used at all, finger-against-finger percussion is sufficient. To perform this technique, the clinician rests the left hand on one side of the thoracic wall, with the middle finger pressed firmly against the body wall. Then, with the middle finger of the right hand, the clinician strikes the middle finger of the left hand, over its middle phalanx. A single tap is performed and the sound that it produced is appreciated before the tap is repeated. Not only is the tap repeated in the same location to check for consistency, it is also repeated in adjacent tissue to note any changes between neighboring areas of the body [28].

Thoracic percussion is designed to assess the health of the lung fields in addition to evaluating for space-occupying lesions. Hence thoracic percussion should take place on both sides of the chest, left and right. In addition, thoracic percussion should take place dorsally, ventrally, and across an invisible line drawn to bisect the shoulder joint to allow the middle of the chest to be evaluated. The normal lung fields should sound sonorous when percussed. This sound is low and resonant. By contrast, in the presence of a space-occupying mass, the sound would be dull because solid tissue does not contain gas. For example, as percussion nears the caudal border of the lung field on the right side of the thoracic cavity, it is typical to hear a change in resonance that is attributable to the presence of the liver [28].

Not every primary care clinician utilizes percussion as a standard aspect of the physical examination. In fact, some clinicians do not make use of it at all because the smaller the patient, the more difficult it is to distinguish normal from abnormal resonance. However, with practice, percussion can corroborate physical examinaton findings that are suggestive of thoracic cavity disease. For instance, in cases of pneumothorax, percussion should yield increased resonance dorsally, in cases of pyo- or hemothorax, resonance should be decreased ventrally, and in cases of infiltrate within a particular lung lobe, the affected area should be less resonant [28, 73].

5.6 Understanding Normal Airway Sounds

Airway sounds occur when airflow through an air space creates vibrations within that air space. The speed with which the air flows and the degree of turbulence within the air current influence the type of vibrations that can be heard [28]. When airway sounds are ausculted, they can be normal or adventitious (abnormal).

Normal airway sounds include bronchial and vesicular sounds [28]:

- Bronchial sounds arise from the caudal trachea and larger bronchi. These sound harsh, like wind on a stormy day, due to expected turbulence of airflow in these regions.
- Vesicular sounds arise from the periphery of the thoracic cavity. They are soft sounds like leaves rustling on an autumn day. Their presence confirms that there is air-filled lung between the chest wall and the more turbulent larger airways such as the trachea.

Bronchovesicular sounds are sandwiched between bronchial and vesicular in terms of their location, tone, and loudness. Decreases in these sounds may indicate abnormal tissue or fluid accumulation between the chest wall and the airspace [28].

Note that normal airway sounds are dynamic. For example [28]:

- Normal airway sounds tend to be louder on inspiration than expiration.
- Normal airway sounds may also be increased or decreased. For instance, normal airway sounds are accentuated in patients that are tachypneic.

5.7 Ausculting the Airway

The upper and lower airways should be ausculted in every patient to appreciate airway sounds. Ausculting the trachea should yield bronchial sounds; ausculting the lower airway should yield vesicular and bronchovesicular sounds [28].

It is important to auscult the entire lower airway: both the right and left thoracic cavity and also the cranial and caudal borders of the lung fields (Figure 5.12).

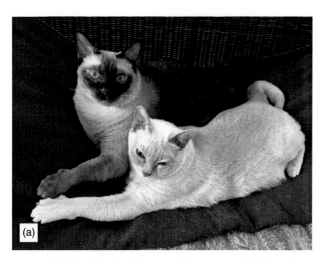
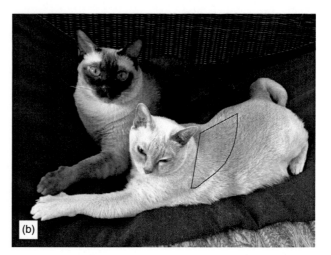

Figure 5.12 (a) Left lateral thorax of a live cat. (b) Left lateral thorax of a live cat with the estimated borders of the lung fields drawn in.

The novice clinician should consider comparing the clinical anatomy in a live cat with what is seen on a lateral thoracic radiograph to broaden their understanding of respiratory anatomy relative to the cardiovascular system (Figure 5.13a and b). The novice clinician might also consider taking it a step further, by attempting to conceptualize the lung field in terms of where one would expect to auscult the normal airway sounds (Figure 5.13c).

5.8 Understanding Adventitious Airway Sounds

Adventitious airway sounds are abnormal. Two examples that are routinely ausculted in general practice are crackles and wheezes:

- Crackles are "popping" sounds that occur when airways that were obstructed finally open. The presence

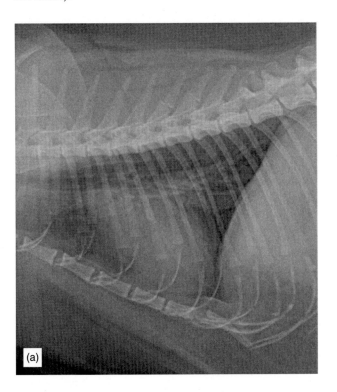

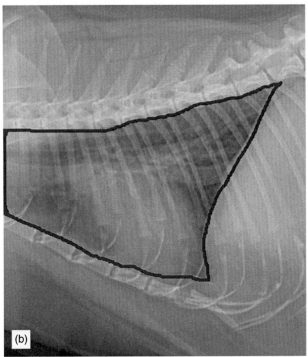

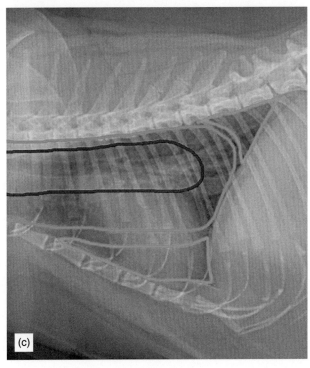

Figure 5.13 (a) Left lateral thoracic radiograph. (b) Left lateral thoracic radiograph with the borders of the lung field outlined in red. (c) Left lateral thoracic radiograph demonstrating rudimentary diagramming of the lung fields based upon where one might expect to auscult normal airway sounds. Bronchial sounds are heard within the region outlined in red. Bronchovesicular sounds are heard within the region bordered by the blue and red lines. Vesicular sounds are heard within the green triangles.

of crackles usually indicates that there is an abundance of airway secretion.

- Wheezes are "musical" sounds that occur when airways that had been collapsed open during inspiration or close during expiration. They result when there is decreased airway lumen diameter, as in reactive airways that have thickened, or airway collapse due to neighboring pulmonary disease.

As before, the clinician should take care to auscult the entire lung field, including the left and right thoracic cavity and the cranial and caudal borders. Respiratory sounds, whether they are normal and adventitious, are not always symmetrical. Unilateral changes in airflow can result in unilateral changes in respiratory sounds.

5.9 Using Airway Sounds to Corroborate Percussive Findings

As was discussed in Section 5.5.4, percussion can provide information about the presence of thoracic cavity disease [73]. Auscultation can confirm percussive findings, increasing clinician confidence. For example, when there is effusive disease, a fluid line may be ausculted. Above the fluid line, normal respiratory sounds are heard. Below the fluid line, respiratory sounds are dull or muted owing to the effusion sinking to the ventral thorax. By contrast, patients with pneumothorax have leakage of air into the pleural space. The air rises to the dorsal thorax, causing dull respiratory sounds dorsally while respiratory sounds ventrally are less unaffected [28].

5.10 Purring as an Obstruction to Auscultation

Purring can be a huge obstacle by obscuring subtle sounds. Stopping a cat from purring is not always possible, but the following may help to deter purring:

- If the owner is petting the cat, the clinician may ask that they momentarily discontinue it: physical contact may encourage purring whereas discontinuing physical contact may have the opposite effect.
- If a cat is purring, the clinician may turn on the faucet in the examination room to run water and stand with the patient near the sink. This may encourage the patient to stop purring. The clinician needs to inform the client prior to attempting this, however, so that the client does not think that the clinician is trying to frighten (or bathe) their cat unnecessarily.
- Only as a last resort should the clinician use alcohol on a cotton ball or gauze square to discourage purring by encouraging the cat to sniff the alcohol. As was discussed in Section 1.6, alcohol is aversive to cats [80]. As a result, the odor has a tendency to squelch purring even if the purring was of nervous origin rather than a display of contentment. Although the use of alcohol may facilitate this veterinary visit, it may complicate subsequent visits because the cat's memory of it will become permanent. The cat will associate the odor of the alcohol with the clinic whether or not alcohol is used in future examination rooms with future client–patient interactions. The net result is a predetermined negative experience so far as the cat is concerned [81–83].

References

1 Cote, E., Edwards, N.J., Ettinger, S.J. *et al.* (2015) Management of incidentally detected heart murmurs in dogs and cats. *Journal of Veterinary Cardiology,* **17** (4), 245–261.

2 Strickland, K.N. (2008) Congenital heart disease, in *Manual of Canine and Feline Cardiology,* 4th edn. (eds. L.P. Tilley, F.W.K. Smith, M.A. Oyama, and M.M. Sleeper), Saunders, Philadelphia, pp. 215–239.

3 Kittleson, M.D. (1998) The approach to the patient with cardiac disease, in *Small Animal Cardiovascular Medicine* (eds. M.D. Kittleson and R.D. Kienle), Mosby, St. Louis, pp. 195–217.

4 Cote, E., Manning, A.M., Emerson, D. *et al.* (2004) Assessment of the prevalence of heart murmurs in overtly healthy cats. *Journal of the American Veterinary Medical Association,* **225** (3), 384–388.

5 Paige, C.F., Abbott, J.A., Elvinger, F., and Pyle, R.L. (2009) Prevalence of cardiomyopathy in apparently healthy cats. *Journal of the American Veterinary Medical Association,* **234** (11), 1398–1403.

6 Wagner, T., Fuentes, V.L., Payne, J.R. *et al.* (2010) Comparison of auscultatory and echocardiographic findings in healthy adult cats. *Journal of Veterinary Cardiology,* **12** (3), 171–182.

7 Bonagura, J.D. (2000) Feline echocardiography. *Journal of Feline Medicine and Surgery,* **2** (3), 147–151.

8 Dirven, M.J., Cornelissen, J.M., Barendse, M.A. *et al.* (2010) Cause of heart murmurs in 57 apparently healthy cats. *Tijdschrift voor Diergeneeskunde,* **135** (22), 840–847.

9 Nakamura, R.K., Rishniw, M., King, M.K., and Sammarco, C.D. (2011) Prevalence of echocardiographic evidence of cardiac disease in apparently healthy cats with murmurs. *Journal of Feline Medicine and Surgery,* **13** (4), 266–271.

10 Rishniw, M. and Thomas, W.P. (2002) Dynamic right ventricular outflow obstruction: a new cause of systolic murmurs in cats. *Journal of Veterinary Internal Medicine,* **16** (5), 547–552.

11 Fuentes, V.L. (2006) Cardiomyopathy: establishing a diagnosis, in *Consultations in Feline Internal*

Medicine, vol. **5** (ed. J.R. August), Saunders Elsevier, St. Louis, pp. 301–310.

12. Ferasin, L., Sturgess, C.P., Cannon, M.J. *et al.* (2003) Feline idiopathic cardiomyopathy: a retrospective study of 106 cats (1994–2001). *Journal of Feline Medicine and Surgery*, **5** (3), 151–159.

13. Gordon, S.G. (2006) Cardiomyopathy – therapeutic decisions, in *Consultations in Feline Internal Medicine*, vol. **5** (ed. J.R. August), Saunders Elsevier, St. Louis, pp. 311–317.

14. Cote, E. and Harpster, N.K. (2009) Feline cardiac arrhythmias, in *Kirk's Current Veterinary Therapy*, vol. XIV (eds. J.D. Bonagura and D.C. Twedt), Saunders Elsevier, St. Louis, pp. 731–739.

15. Laste, N.J. and Harpster, N.K. (1995) A retrospective study of 100 cases of feline distal aortic thromboembolism: 1977–1993. *Journal of the American Animal Hospital Association*, **31** (6), 492–500.

16. Smith, S.A., Tobias, A.H., Jacob, K.A. *et al.* (2003) Arterial thromboembolism in cats: acute crisis in 127 cases (1992–2001) and long-term management with low-dose aspirin in 24 cases. *Journal of Veterinary Internal Medicine*, **17** (1), 73–83.

17. Gompf, R.E. (2008) The history and physical examination, in *Manual of Canine and Feline Cardiology*, 4th edn. (eds. L.P. Tilley, F.W.K. Smith, M.A. Oyama and M.M. Sleeper), Saunders Elsevier, St. Louis, pp. 2–23.

18. Swift, S., Dukes-McEwan, J., Fonfara, S. *et al.* (2009) Aetiology and outcome in 90 cats presenting with dyspnoea in a referral population. *Journal of Small Animal Practice*, **50** (9), 466–473.

19. Ljungvall, I., Rishniw, M., Porciello, F. *et al.* (2014) Sleeping and resting respiratory rates in healthy adult cats and cats with subclinical heart disease. *Journal of Feline Medicine and Surgery*, **16** (4), 281–290.

20. Smith, S.A. and Tobias, A.H. (2004) Feline arterial thromboembolism: an update. *Veterinary Clinics of North America: Small Animal Practice*, **34** (5), 1245–1271.

21. Stepien, R.L. and Henik, R.A. (2009) Systemic hypertension, in *Kirk's Current Veterinary Therapy*, vol. XIV (eds. J.D.Bonagura and D.C.Twedt), Saunders Elsevier, St. Louis, pp. 713–717.

22. Belew, A.M., Barlett, T., and Brown, S.A. (1999) Evaluation of the white-coat effect in cats. *Journal of Veterinary Internal Medicine*, **13** (2), 134–142.

23. Volk, J.O., Thomas, J.G., Colleran, E.J., and Siren, C.W. (2014) Executive summary of phase 3 of the Bayer Veterinary Care Usage Study. *Journal of the American Veterinary Medical Association*, **244** (7), 799–802.

24. Vogt, A.H., Rodan, I., Brown, M. *et al.* (2010) AAFP–AAHA Feline Life Stage Guidelines. *Journal of Feline Medicine and Surgery*, **12** (1), 43–54.

25. Volk, J.O., Felsted, K.E., Thomas, J.G., and Siren, C.W. (2011) Executive summary of phase 2 of the Bayer Veterinary Care Usage Study. *Journal of the American Veterinary Medical Association*, **239** (10), 1311–1316.

26. Greco, D.S. (1991) The effect of stress on the evaluation of feline patients, in *Consultations in Feline Internal Medicine* (ed. J.R. August), Saunders, Philadelphia, pp. 13–17.

27. Overall, K.L. (1997) *Clinical Behavioral Medicine for Small Animals*, Mosby, St. Louis.

28. Rijnberk, A. and van Sluijs, F.S. (2009) *Medical History and Physical Examination in Companion Animals*, 2nd edn., Saunders Elsevier, St. Louis.

29. Cote, E., MacDonald, K.A., Meurs, K.M., and Sleeper, M.M. (2011) *Feline Cardiology*, Wiley-Blackwell, Ames, IA.

30. Dyce, K.M., Sack, W.O., and Wensing, C.J.G. (2010) *Textbook of Veterinary Anatomy*, 4th edn., Saunders Elsevier, St. Louis.

31. Hunt, G.B. and Foster, S.F. (2009) Nasopharyngeal disorders, in *Kirk's Current Veterinary Therapy*, vol. XIV (eds. J.D. Bonagura and D.C. Twedt), Saunders Elsevier, St. Louis, pp. 622–626.

32. Kienle, R.D. (2008) Feline cardiomyopathy, in *Manual of Canine and Feline Cardiology*, 4th edn. (eds. L.P. Tilley, F.W.K. Smith, M.A. Oyama and M.M. Sleeper), Saunders Elsevier, St. Louis, pp. 151–175.

33. Cole, S.G. and Drobatz, K.J. (2008) Emergency management and critical care, in *Manual of Canine and Feline Cardiology*, 4th edn. (eds. L.P. Tilley, F.W.K. Smith, M.A. Oyama and M.M. Sleeper), Saunders Elsevier, St. Louis, pp. 342–355.

34. Smith, F.W.K., Schrope, D.P., and Sammarco, C.D. (2008) Cardiovascular effects of systemic disease, in *Manual of Canine and Feline Cardiology*, 4th edn. (eds. L.P. Tilley, F.W.K. Smith, M.A. Oyama and M.M. Sleeper), Saunders Elsevier, St. Louis, pp. 240–276.

35. Hogan, D.F. (2006) Prevention and management of thromboembolism, in *Consultations in Feline Internal Medicine*, vol. **5** (ed. J.R. August), Saunders Elsevier, St. Louis, pp. 331–345.

36. Stokhof, A.A. and De Rick, A. (2009) Circulatory system, in *Medical History and Physical Examination in Companion Animals*, 2nd edn. (eds. A. Rijnberk, F.J. vanSluijs), Saunders Elsevier, St. Louis, pp. 75–85.

37. Sykes, J.E. (2012) Pediatric feline upper respiratory disease. *Veterinary Clinics of North America: Small Animal Practice*, **44** (2), 331–342.

38. Quimby, J. and Lappin, M.R. (2012) The upper respiratory tract, in *The Cat: Clinical Medicine and Management* (ed. S.E. Little), Saunders Elsevier, St. Louis, pp. 846–861.

39. McManus, C.M., Levy, J.K., Andersen, L.A. *et al.* (2014) Prevalence of upper respiratory pathogens in four management models for unowned cats in the southeast United States. *Veterinary Journal*, **201** (2), 196–201.

40. Dinnage, J.D., Scarlett, J.M., and Richards, J.R. (2009) Descriptive epidemiology of feline upper respiratory tract disease in an animal shelter. *Journal of Feline Medicine and Surgery*, **11** (10), 816–825.

41. Binns, S.H., Dawson, S., Speakman, A.J. *et al.* (2000) A study of feline upper respiratory tract disease with reference to prevalence and risk factors for infection with feline calicivirus and feline herpesvirus. *Journal of Feline Medicine and Surgery*, **2** (3), 123–133.

42. Bannasch, M.J. and Foley, J.E. (2005) Epidemiologic evaluation of multiple respiratory pathogens in cats in animal shelters. *Journal of Feline Medicine and Surgery*, **7** (2), 109–119.

43. Di Martino, B., Di Francesco, C.E., Meridiani, I., and Marsilio, F. (2007) Etiological investigation of multiple respiratory infections in cats. *New Microbiologica*, **30** (4), 455–461.

44. Foley, J.E. and Bannasch, M.J. (2004) Infectious diseases of dogs and cats, in *Shelter Medicine for Veterinarians and Staff* (eds. L. Miller and S. Zawistowski), Iowa University Press, Ames, IA, pp. 235–284.

45. Chandler, F.A., Gaskell, C.J., and Gaskell, R.M. (2004) *Feline Medicine and Therapeutics*, 3rd edn., Blackwell, Oxford.

46. Foley, J.E., Rand, C., Bannasch, M.J. *et al.* (2002) Molecular epidemiology of feline bordetellosis in two animal shelters in California, *USA. Preventive Veterinary Medicine*, **54** (2), 141–156.

47. Hartmann, A.D., Hawley, J., Werckenthin, C. *et al.* (2010) Detection of bacterial and viral organisms from the conjunctiva of cats with conjunctivitis and upper respiratory tract disease. *Journal of Feline Medicine and Surgery*, **12** (10), 775–782.

48. Helps, C.R., Lait, P., Damhuis, A. *et al.* (2005) Factors associated with upper respiratory tract disease caused by feline herpesvirus, feline calicivirus, *Chlamydophila felis* and *Bordetella bronchiseptica* in cats: experience from 218 European catteries. *Veterinary Record*, **156** (21), 669–673.

49. Hoskins, J.D., Williams, J., Roy, A.F. *et al.* (1998) Isolation and characterization of *Bordetella bronchiseptica* from cats in southern Louisiana. *Veterinary Immunology and Immunopathology*, **65** (2–4), 173–176.

50. Ruch-Gallie, R.A., Veir, J.K., Spindel, M.E., and Lappin, M.R. (2008) Efficacy of amoxycillin and azithromycin for the empirical treatment of shelter cats with suspected bacterial upper respiratory infections. *Journal of Feline Medicine and Surgery*, **10** (6), 542–550.

51. Sykes, J.E., Anderson, G.A., Studdert, V.P., and Browning, G.F. (1999) Prevalence of feline *Chlamydia psittaci* and feline herpesvirus 1 in cats with upper respiratory tract disease. *Journal of Veterinary Internal Medicine*, **13** (3), 153–162.

52. Harbour, D.A., Howard, P.E., and Gaskell, R.M. (1991) Isolation of feline calicivirus and feline herpesvirus from domestic cats 1980 to 1989. *Veterinary Record*, **128** (4), 77–80.

53. Cai, Y., Fukushi, H., Koyasu, S. *et al.* (2002) An etiological investigation of domestic cats with conjunctivitis and upper respiratory tract disease in Japan. *Journal of Veterinary Medical Science*, **64** (3), 215–219.

54. Coutts, A.J., Dawson, S., Binns, S. *et al.* (1996) Studies on natural transmission of *Bordetella bronchiseptica* in cats. *Veterinary Microbiology*, **48** (1–2), 19–27.

55. Henderson, S.M., Bradley, K., Day, M.J. *et al.* (2004) Investigation of nasal disease in the cat – a retrospective study of 77 cases. *Journal of Feline Medicine and Surgery*, **6** (4), 245–257.

56. Schmidt, J.F. and Kapatkin, A. (1990) Nasopharyngeal and ear canal polyps in the cat. *Feline Practice*, **18** (4), 16–19.

57. Kapatkin, A.S., Matthiesen, D.T., Noone, K.E. *et al.* (1990) Results of surgery and long-term follow-up in 31 cats with nasopharyngeal polyps. *Journal of the American Animal Hospital Association*, **26** (4), 387–392.

58. Baral, R.M. (2012) Lower respiratory tract diseases, in *The Cat: Clinical Medicine and Management* (ed. S.E.Little), Saunders Elsevier, St. Louis, pp. 861–891.

59. Johnson, L.R. (2006) Bronchial disease, in *Consultations in Feline Internal Medicine*, vol. 5 (ed. J.R. August), Saunders Elsevier, St. Louis, pp. 361–367.

60. Foster, S.F., Martin, P., Allan, G.S. *et al.* (2004) Lower respiratory tract infections in cats: 21 cases (1995–2000). *Journal of Feline Medicine and Surgery*, **6** (3), 167–180.

61. Macdonald, E.S., Norris, C.R., Berghaus, R.B., and Griffey, S.M. (2003) Clinicopathologic and radiographic features and etiologic agents in cats with histologically confirmed infectious pneumonia: 39 cases (1991–2000). *Journal of the American Veterinary Medical Association*, **223** (8), 1142–1150.

62. Mehlhaff, C.J. and Mooney, S. (1985) Primary pulmonary neoplasia in the dog and cat. *Veterinary Clinics of North America: Small Animal Practice*, **15** (5), 1061–1067.

63. Miles, K.G. (1988) A review of primary lung-tumors in the dog and cat. *Veterinary Radiology*, **29** (3), 122–128.

64. Theilin, G.H. and Madewell, B.R. (1979) Tumours of the respiratory tract and thorax, in *Veterinary Cancer Medicine* (eds. G.H. Theilen and B.R. Madewell), Lea & Febiger, Philadelphia, p. 341.

65. Gadbois, J., d'Anjou, M.A., Dunn, M. *et al.* Radiographic abnormalities in cats with feline bronchial disease and intra- and interobserver variability in radiographic interpretation: 40 cases (1999–2006). *Journal of the American Veterinary Medical Association*, **234** (3), 367–375.

66. Berry, C.R., Love, N.E., and Thrall, D.E. (2002) Interpretation paradigms for the small animal thorax, in *Textbook of Veterinary Diagnostic Radiology*, 4th edn. (ed. D.E. Thrall), Saunders Elsevier, Philadelphia, pp. 307–322.

67. Lamb, C.R. (2002) The canine and feline lung, in *Textbook of Veterinary Diagnostic Radiology*, 4th edn. (ed. D.E. Thrall), Saunders Elsevier, Philadelphia, pp. 431–449.

68. Mantis, P., Lamb, C.R., and Boswood, A. (1998) Assessment of the accuracy of thoracic radiography in the diagnosis of canine chronic bronchitis. *Journal of Small Animal Practice*, **39** (11), 518–520.

69. Moise, N.S., Wiedenkeller, D., Yeager, A.E. *et al.* (1989) Clinical, radiographic, and bronchial cytologic features of cats with bronchial disease: 65 cases

(1980–1986). *Journal of the American Veterinary Medical Association,* **194** (10), 1467–1473.

70. Moon, M. (1992) Pulmonary-infiltrates with eosinophilia. *Journal of Small Animal Practice,* **33** (1), 19–23.

71. Corcoran, B.M., Thoday, K.L., Henfrey, J.I. *et al.* (1991) Pulmonary infiltration with eosinophils in 14 dogs. *Journal of Small Animal Practice,* **32** (10), 494–502.

72. Losonsky, J.M., Thrall, D.E., and Prestwood, A.K. (1983) Radiographic evaluation of pulmonary abnormalities after *Aelurostrongylus abstrusus* inoculation in cats. *American Journal of Veterinary Research,* **44** (3), 478–482.

73. Baral, R.M. (2012) The thoracic cavity, in *The Cat: Clinical Medicine and Management* (ed. S.E. Little), Saunders Elsevier, St. Louis, pp. 892–913.

74. Voges, A.K., Bertrand, S., Hill, R.C. *et al.* (1997) True diaphragmatic hernia in a cat. *Veterinary Radiology and Ultrasound,* **38** (2), 116–119.

75. Worth, A.J. and Machon, R.G. (2005) Traumatic diaphragmatic herniation: pathophysiology and management. *Compendium: Continuing Education for the Practicing Veterinarian,* **27** (3), 178–190.

76. Schmiedt, C.W., Tobias, K.M., and Stevenson, M.A. (2003) Traumatic diaphragmatic hernia in cats: 34 cases (1991–2001). *Journal of the American Veterinary Medical Association,* **222** (9), 1237–1240.

77. Fossum, T.W. (2000) Pleural and extrapleural diseases, in *Textbook of Veterinary Internal Medicine* (eds. S.J. Ettinger and E.C. Feldman), Saunders, Philadelphia, p. 1098.

78. Day, M.J. (1997) Review of thymic pathology in 30 cats and 36 dogs. *Journal of Small Animal Practice,* **38** (9), 393–403.

79. Vilafranca, M. and Font, A. (2005) Thymolipoma in a cat. *Journal of Feline Medicine and Surgery,* **7** (2), 125–127.

80. Herron, M.E. and Shreyer, T. (2014) The pet-friendly veterinary practice: a guide for practitioners. *Veterinary Clinics of North America: Small Animal Practice,* **44** (3), 451–481.

81. Mazur, J.E. (2006) Basic principle of classical conditioning, in *Learning and Behavior,* 6th edn., Pearson Education, Upper Saddle River, NJ, pp. 76–81.

82. Yin, S. (2009) Classical conditioning (aka associative learning), in *Low Stress Handling, Restraint, and Behavior Modification of Dogs and Cats,* Cattle Dog Publishing, Davis, CA, pp. 83–84.

83. Bear, M.F., Connors, B.W., and Paradiso, M.A. (2007) The chemical senses, in *Neuroscience: Exploring the Brain,* 3rd edn., Lippincott Williams & Wilkins, Baltimore, pp. 271–272.

6

Examining the Abdominal Cavity of the Cat

6.1 Overview of the Digestive Tract as It Pertains to Presenting Complaints

The gastrointestinal system consists of the upper and lower digestive tracts. The oral cavity, oropharynx, salivary glands, esophagus, stomach, and duodenum together comprise the upper digestive tract, and the ileum, jejunum, ascending, transverse, and descending colons, rectum, and anus comprise the lower. The hepatobiliary system lies in close proximity to the upper digestive tract and engages with the small bowel to create a loop of enterohepatic circulation that is vital to metabolic and biotransformation pathways. Together, the digestive tract functions to metabolize food into absorbable nutrients that can then be used as energy with which to fuel the body [1–3].

Chapter 3 reviewed the components of the digestive tract up to the oropharynx. This chapter covers all aspects of the digestive tract distal to that region. Unlike the cardiovascular and respiratory systems, in which abnormalities tend to be incidental findings on the physical examination [4–6], dysfunction within the digestive tract tends to be symptomatic [1]. Patients with megaesophagus, esophageal stricture, esophageal obstruction, or pyloric stenosis may present for passive regurgitation whereas those with gastritis may present for vomiting, the active retrograde expulsion of stomach contents [7–9].

Diarrhea is yet another frequent presenting complaint in companion animal medicine. Cats may present with small or large bowel diarrhea. In cases of small bowel diarrhea, large amounts of stool are passed infrequently, without mucous, blood, or tenesmus. Concurrent weight loss is common. In cases of large bowel diarrhea, small amounts of stool with a large quantity of colonic water are passed frequently. The patient typically presents for excessive straining associated with defecation and excessive mucous and/or blood passed in the feces [10].

Patients may present for abdominal pain. Clients may describe the "play bow" or "prayer posture," and patients may actively exhibit it in the examination room. The patient stands with its forelimbs extended, while the ventral chest is lowered to the floor, and the rump is elevated. It is thought that this stretch decreases pressure on the abdominal cavity in such a way as to reduce pain. Although this is far more commonly reported in dogs, cats may display it if the abdominal pain is severe enough [1].

Although less commonly seen at teaching hospitals compared with the aforementioned presenting complaints, cats may present for rounded abdominal silhouettes as from effusive abdominal distension. Typically, the peritoneal cavity contains minimal free-floating fluid to allow organs to slide past one another with ease, with minimal friction. However, when an excess of peritoneal fluid accumulates, the patient is said to have ascites. The client may perceive this as bloating or as weight gain [11].

Abdominal effusions can be secondary to infectious disease, as in the case of the so-called "wet" form of feline infectious peritonitis [12, 13], traumatic hemoperitoneum [14, 15] or uroperitoneum [16, 17], right-sided congestive heart failure [18–22], hepatopathy [23–27], or neoplasia [11, 18, 28].

Abdominal distension can also be non-effusive, that is, due to the presence of a space-occupying mass. When these masses involve the liver, they are more typically metastatic than primary hepatic tumors, which are uncommon in cats [29, 30]. Primary hepatocellular tumors include benign hepatocellular adenomas and malignant hepatocellular carcinomas. Primary mesenchymal liver tumors include benign hemangiomas and malignant leiomyosarcomas, hemangiosarcomas, and hepatic fibrosarcomas. All are rare in cats as primary disease. Hepatic neuroendocrine tumors are even rarer primary tumors of cats that arise from neuroectodermal cells. Unlike hepatocellular and mesenchymal tumors, neuroendocrine tumors tend to target younger patients and exhibit more aggressive biologic behavior [29].

By contrast, primary bile duct tumors occur more frequently in cats, comprising more than 50% of all feline hepatobiliary tumors. Benign bile duct tumors, biliary cystadenomas, occur more often than their malignant counterparts, biliary cystadenocarcinomas. Synonyms for biliary cystadenoma are abundant in the veterinary literature and over the years have included bile duct adenoma, cholangiocellular adenoma, cystic cholangioma, and hepatobiliary cystadenoma [29, 31].

Performing the Small Animal Physical Examination, First Edition. Ryane E. Englar.
© 2017 John Wiley & Sons, Inc. Published 2017 by John Wiley & Sons, Inc.

When biliary cystadenomas or cystadenocarcinomas arise, they can take up a significant portion of the abdomen, causing grossly visible abdominal distension (Figure 6.1). Moreover, their prominence within the abdominal cavity compresses neighboring organs, which may cause appetite suppression by pressing on the cranial abdomen, specifically the stomach [32].

Whenever a patient presents for digestive concern, the clinician should take a comprehensive history aimed at elucidating the timeline [1]:

- *When were clinical signs first apparent? Did they develop at or around a particular age?*
  Kittens may be food intolerant whereas young adults and middle-aged cats are more likely to develop true enteritis. Kittens that nursed without complaint yet develop regurgitation following weaning may have a persistent right aortic arch [8].

- *Are clinical signs continuous or episodic?*
  Gastroenteritis typically waxes and wanes whereas exocrine pancreatic insufficiency (EPI) tends to result in continuous symptoms.

- *Are clinical signs associated with a particular time of day?*
  For example, cats may present with vomiting episodes that occur in the morning only, before breakfast, after being fasted overnight.

- *Are clinical signs associated with a particular type of food?*
  Maybe the cat vomits only after ingesting canned food, but can tolerate kibble.

- *Are clinical signs associated with a particular activity?*
  For example, cats may instinctively consume plant material when they are nauseous. Grass eating may therefore be a sign that vomiting is imminent.

- *Are clinical signs progressing? If so, in what way? Frequency? Duration? Severity?*

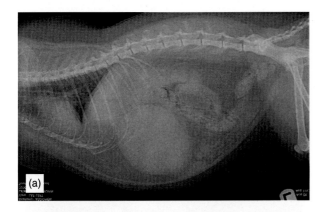

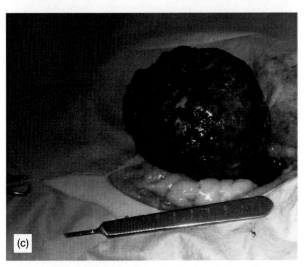

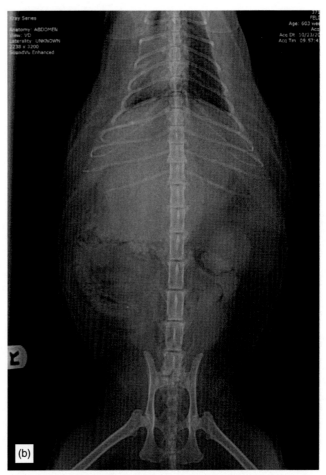

Figure 6.1 (a) Left lateral radiograph of a feline patient with an appreciable biliary cystadenoma as was diagnosed following partial liver lobectomy with histopathology of the excised mass. Note the prominence of the cranial to mid-ventral abdominal mass, causing compression of cranial abdominal structures. (b) Ventrodorsal (V/D) radiograph of a feline patient with an appreciable biliary cystadenoma as was diagnosed following partial liver lobectomy with histopathology of the excised mass. Note the prominence of the cranial to mid-ventral abdominal mass, causing compression of the liver and stomach. (c) Intra-operative depiction of a biliary cystadenoma of a feline patient for size comparison. Appreciate how large these masses can be and how much compression of neighboring organs is possible when they are present intra-abdominally.

The history should precede the physical examination to establish a solid foundation for the patient that may stimulate the clinician's acumen when it comes to his or her diagnostic capabilities.

In the author's experience, the abdominal cavity is often immensely frustrating to preclinical students because its evaluation requires subtle precision and patience, yet cats are not the most tolerant species when it comes to abdominal palpation [33, 34]. It is also difficult for students to appreciate structures that they cannot see [33], especially when they are taught to feel for the absence of normal yet they themselves are largely unconfident as to what normal is and what normal feels like. When students are just learning how to examine the abdominal cavity, it is important to start broad. The author begins by reminding them which organs are typically palpable when they are structurally normal versus those that are not. This provides a starting point to help students identify the "normals" of the abdomen before beginning to search for the more nebulous "abnormals."

To review, the digestive tract offers very few organs that are typically palpable. In every cat, the small and large bowel should be palpated, keeping in mind that the latter is primarily evident when the descending colon is filled with feces. The stomach is typically not palpable unless greatly distended, as from a large meal. The liver is not typically palpated because in its normal position it does not extend past the costal margin, and unless there is a pancreatic mass of sizable proportions, the pancreas is not a structure that is typically appreciated on the physical exam. Although pancreatitis is likely to trigger abdominal pain on palpation of the right, ventromedial cranial abdomen, the structure of the pancreas itself is rarely identified [1, 35, 36].

6.2 The Esophagus

In keeping with the aforementioned trend that most of the digestive tract is not palpable, the same holds true for the esophagus. Distal to the oropharynx, the esophagus is initially seated dorsal to the trachea. As the esophagus tracks down the neck, it takes on a position to the left of midline. In a normal patient, the esophagus is hidden under muscle and is neither visible nor palpable. The esophagus becomes palpable in cases of esophageal obstruction, in which case there may be a visible or palpable bulge at the left entrance to the thoracic inlet. Esophageal obstruction is rare, but possible, in cats [8]. More commonly, it occurs in dogs that bolt their food, leading to obstruction of the esophagus with large chunks of meat or bone. These patients may show pain when asked to extend their neck or when pressure is applied over the left thoracic inlet. These patients may also hypersalivate and unsuccessfully attempt to regurgitate [1, 37].

To feel for the esophagus, the clinician often stands in front of the patient and encourages the patient to raise its head. As the clinician then runs his hand down the ventrolateral left neck, he feels for any bulge at the level of the thoracic inlet that may suggest esophageal dilation. When esophageal obstruction is severe, causing a back-up of food and water orad to the obstruction, the clinician may even be able to feel sloshing of esophageal contents deep to the skin [1].

6.3 Visual Inspection of the Abdomen

Before the clinician lays a hand on the abdominal cavity, he should observe the abdomen visually for size, shape, and symmetry. The abdominal silhouette should be symmetrical when the patient is viewed from behind and also aerially. Bilaterally symmetrical, diffuse enlargement of the abdomen could be physiologic, as in the case of pregnancy (Figure 6.2), or it could be pathologic, as from ascites. Focal enlargement of the abdomen may reflect organ-associated pathology. For example, cranial abdominal enlargement may indicate hepatomegaly [1].

6.4 Superficial Palpation of the Abdomen

After a cursory visual inspection of the abdominal silhouette, it is tempting to dive straight into deep palpation of the abdominal cavity. However, superficial palpation of the abdomen should precede deep palpation in a thorough, comprehensive physical examination. Superficial palpation involves assessing for the presence or absence of a palpable fluid wave and for hernias.

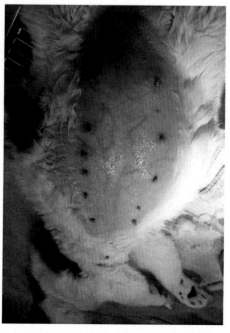

Figure 6.2 Bilaterally symmetrical abdominal distension due to pregnancy in this feline patient who is being prepped to undergo caesarian section. Source: Courtesy of Frank Isom, DVM.

When the clinician evaluates the abdominal cavity for a fluid wave, he is looking to rule in or rule out abdominal effusions. It is especially important to test for a fluid wave in a patient with visible abdominal distension because such distension could be due to peritoneal fluid accumulation or to a mass effect. In the case of the former, a fluid wave should be palpable.

To assess for a fluid wave, the clinician typically stands behind the patient with the patient facing away from him or her. The palm of the left hand is placed flush against the left side of the abdomen and the palm of the right hand is placed loosely against the right side of the abdomen. The clinician then performs ballottement: with the fingertips of his right hand, he taps the right abdominal wall to bounce internal structures off of the opposite wall. He then repeats this by balloting the left abdominal wall to feel for any response against the right abdominal wall. If there is appreciable fluid within the peritoneal cavity, the clinician will feel a wave of fluid against the wall opposite to the one that was tapped. This is not appreciated in a healthy patient, only in a patient with abdominal effusion [1, 11].

If there is a palpable fluid wave, its presence does not diagnose the source of the fluid. Further investigation is required via abdominocentesis to sample and analyze the free-floating peritoneal fluid to determine what it is. It could be frank hemorrhage, bile from a ruptured biliary tract, urine from a ruptured urinary bladder, gastrointestinal contents from a gastrointestinal perforation, or an effusion associated with septic peritonitis [1, 11].

In addition to feeling for a fluid wave, the clinician should feel superficially along the ventral midline for the presence or absence of an abdominal hernia, that is, a defect in the abdominal wall. The abdominal wall is built of the external and internal abdominal oblique and transversus abdominis muscles. At the ventral midline, the aponeuroses of the oblique and transverse abdominal muscles fuse to create the linea alba. From the xyphoid process to the pubis, the linea alba extends as a fibrous, avascular seam through which the abdominal cavity can be entered. Defects in the abdominal wall can occur at any point; however, most common sites of herniation are at the umbilicus along the ventral midline, paracostally at the caudal rib margin, scrotally, and inguinally. These tend to be congenital in origin rather than traumatically induced [38–41].

Hernias vary in size and reducibility. When they occur at the umbilicus, they are often the result of an over-wide linea alba or hypoplastic rectus muscles [38]. Some are visible without palpation: the observant clinician would pick up on it through visual inspection. Others are so small and/or reducible that they require midline palpation to appreciate their presence as a soft swelling at the umbilicus. Some patients may need to be supported so that they are standing upright on their two back feet in order for these small hernias to become apparent visually.

Most umbilical hernias remain soft and contain falciform fat, if anything [38]. The majority that are identified measure less than 2–3 mm and are not rushed to surgery immediately because there is a possibility of spontaneous closure in puppies up to 6 months of age [42]. It is unknown whether the same holds true for cats; however, cats too are postponed in terms of hernia repair surgery until it is convenient for them to undergo routine ovariohysterectomy or orchiectomy.

The primary risk associated with a persistent hernia is that intra-abdominal contents may slip through the defect in the abdominal wall and become trapped between the skin and the muscle layer of the abdominal wall. The most common organs to become entrapped are the intestine, uterus, and urinary bladder. Entrapped tissues may become incarcerated. This is exquisitely painful and can be lethal within hours owing to devitalization of tissues secondary to compromised circulation [38].

When a hernia, umbilical or otherwise, is identified on superficial palpation of the integrity of the abdominal wall, the clinician should note the following:

- *Size of hernia [43]:*
  Hernias that allow one human finger to slip through are at increased risk for bowel entrapment because the small intestine is roughly equal in size [38].
- *Consistency of the hernia [43]:*
  If abdominal contents are palpably poking through the defect in the abdominal wall, they ought to be soft and non-painful to the touch. If abdominal contents ever become firm or tender, there is an increased risk of entrapment [38].
- *Reducibility:*
  Assuming that abdominal contents are palpably poking through the defect in the abdominal wall, are they able to be reduced back into the abdominal cavity or are they entrapped between the skin and the abdominal wall? Non-reducible hernias involve tissue that is poking through the defect in the abdominal wall and cannot readily be replaced within the abdomen. This means that the tissue has become entrapped and, if it is entrapped long enough, adhesions may form. Entrapment and adhesions increase the risk that the patient will present for a surgical emergency because incarcerated tissues are often irreducible [38, 41].

Defects in the abdominal wall are also present caudally; these can present as inguinal hernias. Specifically, an inguinal hernia is a defect in the inguinal ring. The inguinal ring is a normal structure in dogs and cats: it is an opening in the caudoventral abdominal wall through which the genitofemoral nerve, artery, and vein and also the external pudendal vessels pass. In addition, the vaginal process passes through this opening in male cats, containing the spermatic cord. When there is an inguinal hernia, the integrity of the inguinal ring is compromised, allowing for other structures to pass through the same space. This accommodation for other structures is pathologic. If sufficiently large, it is possible for the uterus, urinary bladder, or jejunum to become entrapped. Although it may not be possible to diagnose definitively the entrapped organ by palpation alone, ultrasound can be used to augment the physical examination findings [38, 41, 44].

Hernias are relatively uncommon in cats, yet in spite of their infrequency, the clinician should get into the habit of palpating for a hernia at each new kitten visit. Because hernias vary greatly in terms of risk based upon size, location, and reducibility, superficial palpation of the abdominal wall is an important first step in recognizing that a structural issue exists. This confirmation on physical examination paves the way for a critical conversation between the client and the veterinary team as to if, when, and how to correct the defect surgically. It also raises the issue of genetics: because the bulk of congenital umbilical hernias are believed to be inherited [41], kittens that are born with or subsequently develop umbilical hernias should not be bred once they reach sexual maturity. In particular, the genetics of the Cornish Rex cat have been extensively studied and this breed is said to be predisposed to umbilical hernias [38, 41, 45, 46].

In addition to providing the clinician with important diagnoses, superficial palpation of the abdomen helps to acclimate the patient to what is coming: deep palpation of the abdominal cavity. It is not uncommon for cats to tense or crunch up when the clinician touches the lateral and ventral aspects of their abdomen. Cats typically only allow other members of the same social group to make physical contact [47, 48]. Even then, contact within a social context tends to be limited to the head and neck [47, 48]. When strangers physically touch cats, especially when they make contact with the ventral abdomen, cats may feel threatened and respond accordingly [49]. It is therefore especially important when handling cats to give them time to acclimate to touch, especially given that this is not a particularly favorable part of the body for a stranger such as a clinician to examine. True, a cat may tense its abdomen because it is painful [1], but more likely than not, an adult cat is tense because the action of touch in this region is unfamiliar, unwanted, or both.

Superficial palpation also serves as a good reminder to the clinician to observe the cat for behavioral cues that may suggest fear, aggression, or fearful aggression and to respond accordingly. See Section 1.9 to review feline body language, specifically visual cues.

Finally, superficial palpation reminds the clinician how to make palpation as comfortable as possible for the patient by remembering to use flat hands. This ensures that when the clinician moves on to the deeper portion of abdominal palpation, he is not setting himself up for failure and his patient for discomfort by using

fingers perpendicular to the long axis of the cat to poke and prod [1].

6.5 Deep Palpation of the Abdomen

Deep palpation of the abdomen immediately follows superficial palpation in an attempt to appreciate intra-abdominal architecture. As already mentioned, abdominal palpation is one of the most frustrating aspects of the physical examination for veterinary students. So much of abdominal palpation is geared toward learning what "normal" is: learning not to feel what you shouldn't feel. It is difficult to appreciate "normal" when you cannot visualize what "normal" is. Add to that the potential for patient intolerance of abdominal palpation and the tendency for patients to tense and crunch up, and abdominal palpation becomes a potential recipe for disaster for any novice.

A good way for students to practice abdominal palpation techniques is to perform this examination on every patient of theirs that just so happens to be under general anesthesia. For example, students ought to repeat abdominal palpation on their "sophomore surgery" and "junior surgery" feline and canine spay/neuter patients while these patients are anesthetized. They will be amazed at how much they can appreciate – and with confidence – when the abdominal muscles of their patients are relaxed.

Students can also experiment with different techniques for abdominal palpation to see which works best for them:

- One technique requires the use of both hands at the same time. The clinician can start out with flat hands, one on either side of the abdomen, as when assessing for the presence or absence of a palpable fluid wave. One hand can serve as a "table," against which the other hand can direct abdominal structures (Figure 6.3a).
- An alternative technique is to use one hand only to palpate by cupping the hand, palm up toward the patient (Figure 6.3b).

The author finds the second technique easiest in small cats and kittens whereas the first technique is more effective for her when evaluating overweight and obese patients.

Regardless of which technique the student selects, he should aim for smooth rather than jerky motions. This will improve patient tolerance of the examination. As the student develops confidence in performing deep abdominal palpation in an awake patient, he will also be more apt to believe what it is that he is feeling and will more consistently identify structures that should be present and palpable.

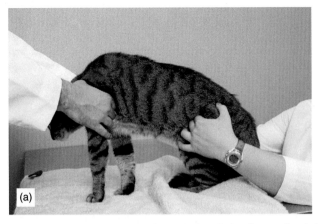 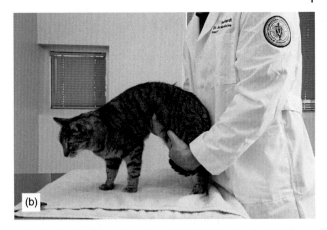

Figure 6.3 (a) Demonstration of the two-handed technique for abdominal palpation. In this patient, the clinician's right hand, which is outside the line of view, is being used, palm down, against the patient's right side to serve as a table against which left-sided organs can be pressed. The clinician uses her left hand to displace left-sided organs toward her right hand in order to make out organ shape and structure. (b) Demonstration of the one-handed technique for abdominal palpation. In this patient, the clinician is using his right hand only to cup up and into the abdomen to appreciate intra-abdominal architecture. He is using his left hand only to stabilize the patient and keep the patient from wandering away. He is not using his left hand to feel the abdomen. Source (a), (b): Courtesy of the Media Resources Department at Midwestern University.

In order to perform a deep abdominal palpation in an awake patient, it is easiest if the patient remains standing. The clinician can then stand behind the patient, with the patient facing away from him, and start the deep abdominal palpation component of the physical examination.

There is no one "right" approach to deep abdominal palpation. The author tends to start cranially and move caudally; other colleagues do the examination in reverse. It is less important which approach is used and more that the clinician develops his own systematic way to be certain that no region of the abdomen is missed.

It may help the novice to break the abdomen into the following three compartments [1] (Figure 6.4a and b):

1) *Cranial abdomen:*
   The cranial abdomen contains the liver, stomach, pancreas, spleen, and kidneys.
2) *Mid-abdomen:*
   The mid-abdomen contains the small intestine, ureters, and the ovaries (females only).
3) *Caudal abdomen:*
   The caudal abdomen contains the urinary bladder, prostate (males only), urethra, descending colon, and rectum.

Once these three compartments of the abdomen can be visualized based upon their location in space, some clinicians further subdivide them into dorsal, medial, and ventral quadrants [1] (Figure 6.4c):

- *Cranio-dorsal abdomen:*
  The cranio-dorsal abdomen contains the kidneys.

- *Cranio-medial abdomen:*
  The cranio-medial abdomen contains the liver and pancreas.
- *Cranio-ventral abdomen:*
  The cranio-ventral abdomen contains the liver, stomach, and spleen.
- *Dorsal mid-abdomen:*
  The dorsal mid-abdomen contains the ureters and ovaries.
- *Medial mid-abdomen:*
  The medial mid-abdomen contains the small intestine.
- *Ventral mid-abdomen:*
  The ventral mid-abdomen contains the small intestine.
- *Dorsal caudal abdomen:*
  The dorsal caudal abdomen contains the descending colon and rectum.
- *Medial caudal abdomen:*
  The medial mid-abdomen contains the urinary bladder and prostate.
- *Ventral caudal abdomen:*
  The ventral caudal abdomen contains the urethra.

Note that there is overlap between some quadrants when this approach to the abdomen is used. For example, the liver falls in both the cranio-medial and cranio-ventral quadrants.

For those who are detail oriented, dividing up the abdomen into quadrants may be effective as a learning tool. For those who are not, dividing up the abdomen in this way may be overwhelming. Student clinicians need to determine for themselves which approach is best and know that compartmentalization of the abdomen is an option, not a requirement.

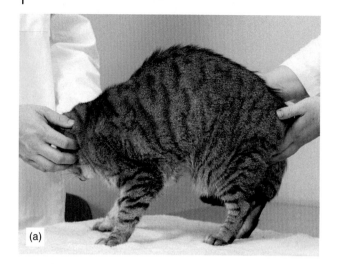

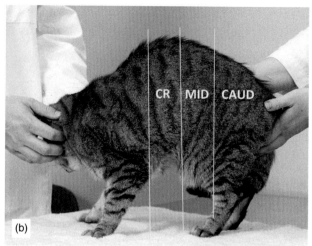

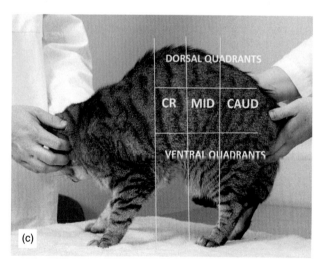

Figure 6.4 (a) Left lateral view of a live feline patient. Note that the patient is standing, albeit hunched up. (b) Left lateral view of a live feline patient, with the abdominal cavity artificially divided into cranial (CR), mid (MID), and caudal (CAUD) compartments. (c) Left lateral view of a live feline patient, with the abdominal cavity artificially divided into cranial (CR), mid (MID), and caudal (CAUD) compartments. In addition, the dorsal and ventral quadrants have been drawn in. Source (a)–(c): Courtesy of the Media Resources Department at Midwestern University.

6.5.1 The Liver

The liver lies within the costal arch [1, 35]. As such, the bulk of the liver is not typically palpable in cats unless it is enlarged, with the exception of its caudal margins [1, 35]. These margins, if palpable, should be distinct and well defined, with sharp rather than rounded edges.

To feel for the liver, it may help to elevate the patient's front end. This allows gravity to work on the organs of the cranial abdomen, in effect causing them to "drop" slightly lower in the abdomen where they may be easier to access.

When the liver is enlarged, typically the right side is more easily appreciated than the left [1]. This is because the liver, although centrally located, is biased slightly to the right of midline as a result of its right-sided caudate process, which cups the right kidney [40].

Hepatomegaly may be the sole finding in a cat with hepatopathy. Cholangitis, hepatic lipidosis, and primary hepatic tumors such as lymphoma are frequently implicated in cases of hepatomegaly. By contrast, a cat with a portosystemic shunt (PSS) would be expected to have microhepatica. Of feline patients with PSS, Himalayans and Persian cats are overrepresented [50].

In addition to changes in liver size, patients may present with non-specific clinical signs: lethargy, decreased appetite, and vomiting. When vomiting occurs, it may be because the enlarged liver is pushing on the upper gastrointestinal tract, inducing nausea, or because toxins are not being efficiently cleared by the liver, causing direct stimulation of the chemoreceptor trigger zone. When diarrhea occurs, it is typically of small bowel origin. If patients are hyperbilirubinemic, they may also display icterus [50]. See Section 2.7 for photographic displays of icterus in feline patients with hepatopathies.

Increased thirst and increased urination are less commonly seen in cats with hepatic disease [50].

Note that because of the liver's enormous potential for regeneration, clinical signs are typically delayed in onset: hepatic disease is often subclinical unless hepatic reserves are exhausted. Even then, when hepatopathy is appreciated on physical examination with corresponding clinical signs, the patient requires a more extensive diagnostic work-up to obtain a definitive diagnosis [50].

6.5.2 The Stomach

The stomach is positioned in the abdominal cavity caudal to the liver. Both the fundus and body of the stomach are predominantly associated with the left side of the cranial abdomen; however, the ventral aspect of the body crosses to the right as it merges with the pylorus [40]. The stomach as a whole is typically not palpable [35].

When the stomach is palpable, it may be either because [1]:

- The liver is enlarged, causing displacement of the stomach caudally.
- The stomach is significantly distended.

When the stomach is distended, it may be the result of a recent ingestion. For example, a kitten that inadvertently gets into a bag of kitten chow is likely to overeat, which will result in an appreciably distended stomach that is palpable, doughy in consistency, and compressible just beyond the costal margins on the left side of the cranial abdomen.

Note that food is not the only item that can distend the stomach. The stomach may also distend as a result of gas and/or fluid accumulation, which occurs in cases of gastric obstruction, regardless of whether the obstruction is a mass, a foreign body, or, rarely, secondary to torsion. In these circumstances, the stomach will also be palpable just beyond the costal margins on the left side of the cranial abdomen. However, typically the stomach will palpate as being tauter in terms of its consistency, and typically painful to the touch.

More commonly, the stomach is not palpable on physical examination; however, the cat may react adversely to deep cranial abdominal palpation as if tender. Alternatively, the cat may respond by licking its lips and/or gagging as if nauseated.

Even more commonly, the stomach is not palpable on physical examination and the cat is non-reactive to deep cranial abdominal palpation; however, the client may provide an extensive history regarding the clinical sign of vomiting. When vomiting is a presenting complaint, the clinician should take care to document the timeframe: see Section 6.1. The development of vomiting, its timing relative to eating, and a description of the vomitus collectively provide insight into gut motility. For example, gut motility is significantly delayed if a cat presents for vomiting undigested food 12 or more hours after eating [51].

6.5.3 The Spleen

In the cat, the spleen is a crescent-shaped organ that is housed within the cranial to mid-abdomen. Its body abuts the left abdominal wall and its tail curls along the ventrolateral abdomen [40, 52, 53]. The spleen is not typically palpable in cats [35].

Splenic disorders are rare in the cat [54, 55]. When they occur, they tend to involve generalized splenomegaly as opposed to focal disease [56]. Generalized splenomegaly can be iatrogenic: the use of sedatives and/or general anesthetic agents can cause splenic congestion [54]. Generalized splenomegaly can also result from increased physiologic demand [54]. For example, massive hemolysis is a stimulus that triggers extramedullary hematopoiesis [54]. In addition, the following infectious diseases can enlarge the spleen through chronic antigenic stimulation: feline leukemia virus, feline immunodeficiency virus, feline infectious peritonitis, ehrlichiosis, and cytauxzoonosis [57].

When generalized splenomegaly is present, its increased weight draws it ventrocaudally beyond the costal arch to the point that it becomes palpable. It can be differentiated from the liver because the liver is relatively fixed in space whereas the spleen can be caudally displaced through palpation [1].

When the spleen is focally enlarged, a regional mass effect may be palpable. This may be the result of a non-neoplastic lesion such as a splenic hematoma as from a traumatic event, an abscess, or nodular hyperplasia. A typical spleen feels smooth. When nodular hyperplasia is present, the surface of the spleen takes on an undulated texture. Less commonly, neoplastic disease effects focal changes in the splenic architecture [54].

When the spleen is palpable, care needs to be taken to avoid rough handling. Diseased spleens tend to be friable. It does not take much force to rupture a splenic mass [54].

6.5.4 The Pancreas

The pancreas is an endocrine and exocrine organ that is seated within the cranial abdomen and consists of two lobes or limbs. The left lobe tracks caudomedially from the neighboring pylorus. It then crosses the median plane behind the stomach to end against the left kidney. The right lobe tracks caudodorsally from the neighboring pylorus and follows the descending duodenum. It is positioned lateral to the ascending colon [40, 58]. Neither limb of the pancreas is palpable in the normal patient [1, 35, 40].

Pancreatic nodular hyperplasia is a commonly observed finding in necropsies of older cats, yet this structural change is not typically evident on the physical examination [59–61]. The diseased pancreas is equally difficult to palpate. Even in cases of pancreatic neoplasia, which is exceedingly rare in cats, pancreatic tumors tend to be identified on post-mortem examinations more so than on the physical examination [59, 62, 63].

Students have asked the author the following question: if the normal and diseased pancreas are so rarely identified on the physical exam, then why should veterinary students be in the habit of feeling for it? Why, when it is so uncommonly appreciated? The answer is that the goal is less about finding the pancreas and more about learning what the normal cranial abdomen feels like, so that on those rare occasions when an abnormal finding exists, a light bulb goes off and the student recognizes pathology.

A secondary goal is to assess for evidence of pancreatic discomfort. Although physical examination findings in cats with pancreatitis tend to be non-specific, abdominal pain is present in up to 19% of cases [59]. Although it is true that cranial abdominal pain is not pathognomonic for pancreatitis, its presence supports it as a potential diagnosis and should encourage the savvy clinician to launch a more extensive diagnostic investigation.

6.5.5 The Small Intestine

The small intestine arises from the pylorus as the duodenum. The duodenum tracks toward the right body wall before it is redirected caudally until it reaches a point between the right kidney and pelvic inlet. From there, it tracks medially, then ascends to enter the mesentery to continue as the jejunum. The jejunum takes up the majority of the ventral mid-abdomen, filling up the space in a series of coils. As the jejunum transitions into the ileum, the ileum passes cranially and to the right into the ascending colon at the level of the first or second lumbar vertebrae [40].

The small intestine is dynamic: it is varied at any given point in time in terms of its contents. While some sections may be filled with ingesta, other segments may be empty and as such transiently flattened by neighboring organs. Peristaltic waves continue to move ingesta aborad to maintain gut transit time and regularity [40].

The clinician is able to examine only a portion of the small bowel – primarily the jejunum owing to its presence in the ventral mid-abdomen. As a result, the clinician is given a snapshot of the health of the intestines. In order to make the most of that snapshot, the clinician should appreciate the thickness of the intestinal loops, the contents of the lumen, and whether or not physical manipulation of the intestines as through palpation is distressing to the patient [64].

The clinician may start by evaluating the texture of the small intestine. A normal cat's intestine has slightly firmer loops than a dog's, and these loops are generally smooth. They should blip through the clinician's fingers with ease [1].

The clinician should then evaluate the general thickness of the intestinal wall by asking whether it is consistently normal, or if it is diffusely or focally thickened [64]. Diffuse thickening commonly occurs in kittens that are overloaded with gastrointestinal parasites such as ascarids. These kittens tend to be bloated and present with a classic "buddha belly" and a doughy feel to their gut. Diffuse thickening of the small bowel may also be the result of food intolerance and/or dietary indiscretion causing enteritis [1, 65].

Inflammatory bowel disease may cause generalized or focal thickening of the small bowel depending upon the patient [66]. Palpation is used to provide a baseline. If the bowel subjectively feels thickened, ultrasonographic investigation is warranted to provide more exact measurements, especially if the patient has presented for chronic vomiting, diarrhea, and/or weight loss [66]. A normal cat's duodenum should measure no more than 2.8 mm in thickness and the same cat's ileum should measure no more than 3.2 mm [67]. It has been postulated that such ultrasonographic evidence of bowel thickening may correlate with histopathologic grade of inflammatory bowel disease [68]. However, it can be difficult to differentiate inflammatory bowel disease from small-cell lymphoma based upon ultrasonographic findings alone [66]. Biopsies are warranted in order to strengthen the diagnosis, yet definitive answers are not always possible because of the overlap between inflammatory and neoplastic infiltrates [66].

It is important that the clinician note focal thickenings in the small bowel because these could indicate a mass effect. About 6% of all tumors in cats are intestinal tumors; of those involving the small bowel, 74% are lymphomas. The second most common small intestinal tumor in the cat is adenocarcinoma, followed by mast cell tumors and leiomyosarcomas [66].

Clinically, cats with inflammatory bowel disease are indistinguishable from cats with small-cell lymphoma. It is up to the astute clinician to recognize that both conditions are potential differential diagnoses and that a more extensive diagnostic work-up is indicated when a patient presents with non-specific clinical signs of vomiting, diarrhea, and/or weight loss [66].

It is equally important to pay attention to focal thickening because this may indicate a foreign body. Historically, discrete foreign bodies were considered far less common in cats than linear foreign bodies [69–71]. As a result, physical examination guides emphasize that the small intestine should be evaluated for overt plication. Bunching of the intestine is abnormal and occurs classically in cases involving a string foreign body [1]. Yet a study by Hayes in 2009 revealed that only one-third of foreign body cases in cats are due to linear foreign bodies [72]. Discrete foreign bodies are a more common occurrence than was once anticipated. They are not always toy related, although this is the trend in young cats less than 2 years of age [66]. No breed predispositions have been reported; however, one might suspect foreign body obstruction to occur more readily in Siamese cats owing to their tendencies toward oral fixation [73]. In long-haired cats, these discrete foreign bodies may actually be trichobezoars [74].

When examining the small bowel, the clinician should also take care to evaluate the luminal contents. Although the clinician cannot actually visualize these contents, he can make use of the sense of touch to appreciate what type of material is likely to be contained within. To begin with, the clinician may ask whether or not the lumen of the small bowel is distended. If it is, then is the bowel distended with fluid? Fluid palpates as being squishy; it sloshes past the clinician's fingers. Alternatively, there may be palpable gas distension [1].

The clinician should also note the patient's reaction to palpation of the intestinal loops. The patient should not react, as if this were a non-event. Palpation of the small bowel should not be painful. A patient that reproducibly tries to bite, claw, or escape, or reproducibly splints the abdomen on palpation over a certain portion of bowel warrants a deeper investigation as these clinical signs could be suggestive of peritonitis or other intestinal disease [1].

Finally, the clinician should auscult the bowel by placing the stethoscope along the ventral abdominal wall and listening for gut sounds. These are classically referred to as borborygmi. In order for borborygmi to be audible, the bowel must contain some fluid and gas, and be motile. If borborygmi are not heard, then either the bowel is empty or not moving, or both. An anorectic patient, for instance, may have absent borborygmi because its digestive tract is empty. Similarly, a patient with bowel stasis as from an obstruction lacks borborygmi because the digestive tract is not moving [1]. By contrast, the auscultation of excessive borborygmi – in terms of both frequency and loudness – may indicate hypermotility of the bowel as may occur with certain types of diarrhea [1].

6.5.6 Mesenteric Lymph Nodes

Cranial mesenteric lymph nodes are dispersed throughout the root of the mesentery; there are also lymph nodes associated with the jejunum, cecum, and colon [40]. None of these nodes are palpable in normal cats [1]. However, because lymph reaches these nodes from jejunal and ileal vessels [58], any underlying inflammatory or neoplastic process can make these nodes prominent and therefore palpable [66]. Palpably prominent mesenteric lymph nodes may be present in 20–50% of intestinal small-cell lymphoma, with a similar incidence in cases of inflammatory bowel disease [66, 75–77]. Enlarged mesenteric lymph nodes may be confirmed via abdominal ultrasonography [66].

6.5.7 The Large Intestine

The ileocolic junction represents the transition between the ileum of the small bowel and the large intestine, comprised of the cecum, ascending, transverse, and descending colons, rectum, and anal canal. Unlike many other species in which the cecum and colon meet end to end, the feline ileum and colon are in line with one another and form a continuous tube [58].

The cecum is comma shaped in the cat. It is palpable in the normal cat by a skilled clinician at the level of the fourth lumbar vertebra; however, it is so firm that it can be mistaken for an intra-abdominal mass [58].

The ascending colon is short and not much wider than the small intestine. It courses cranially along the right abdominal wall, between the duodenum and the root of the mesentery. It then becomes the transverse colon, tracking right to left. The transverse colon then becomes the descending colon, which tracks down the abdominal wall to the left of the mesenteric root. The descending colon is easily palpable in the cat, especially when it contains fecal matter. To differentiate normal fecal matter from a colonic mass, the clinician should try to compress the material. Barring obstipation in a feline patient, fecal matter should be compressible whereas masses tend not to be [40, 58]. Even when the descending colon lacks fecal material, it is palpable and distinguishable from small intestine because the colonic wall is stiffer [40].

Note that the colon is dynamic. It can stretch up to several times its normal diameter due to retained feces. Constipation in cats is not uncommonly seen. It may be the result of diet, as in the ingestion of carcasses or fur, inactivity, dehydration, obesity, pelvic fracture, lumbosacral spinal cord deformity as in certain Manx kittens or lumbosacral spinal cord trauma, and orthopedic disease that compromises the ability to posture in the litter box. When constipation is not resolved expediently and the feces are retained for long periods within the colon, the feces may become impacted, a condition referred to as obstipation [78]. Over time, if obstipation is recurrent, the colonic diameter may not reduce in size after medical resolution of the fecal impaction, leading to megacolon [66, 79].

In human medicine, megacolon is defined as having a colonic diameter greater than 6.5 cm at the pelvic brim

[80]. Although there is no exact guideline in veterinary medicine by which to define megacolon, it has been theorized that the colonic diameter of a cat should be less than the length of the body of L7 [81].

When megacolon occurs, it results in a vicious cycle. When the diameter of the colon increases beyond a certain point, colonic propulsion of the feces is hindered, which encourages fecal retention. As feces are retained, fecal water reabsorption leads to drier, firmer feces that become trapped within the colon. These fecal balls then back up and into each other, further stretching out the colon such that the cycle repeats. The end result is a cat with dyschezia. The cat often presents for persistent straining and occasionally for diarrhea, which occurs when liquid matter shoots around the fecal ball obstruction. These cats are typically nauseated and may present for anorexia, vomiting, or both [66].

If cats strain excessively for long periods, as from megacolon or chronic diarrhea, they are at increased risk of developing rectal prolapse [66]. Minor prolapses of the rectum involve only the mucous membrane; however, as the condition increases in severity, the entire mesorectum may be exteriorized (Figure 6.5) [82]. In this situation, it may initially challenging be to differentiate a rectal prolapse from an ileocolic intussusception: both

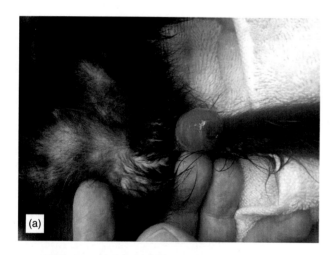

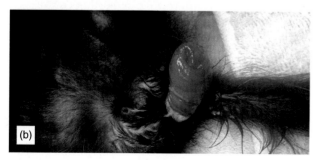

Figure 6.5 (a) Rectal prolapse and (b) progressive rectal prolapse in a cat. Source (a), (b): Courtesy of Frank Isom, DVM.

may look similar to an outside observer [83]. To rule out an ileocolic intussusception, the clinician can attempt to insert a thermometer into the anus alongside the prolapsed tissue. When there is a rectal prolapse, thermometer insertion is possible, which is not so in cases of ileocolic intussusception [66].

Returning now to the digestive anatomy of the normal cat, when the colon reaches the pelvis, it becomes the rectum. At approximately the second or third caudal vertebra, the rectum becomes the anal canal. The anus exits the body dorsal to the urogenital opening in both the cat and dog, but not before paired anal sacs empty into the canal their sebaceous secretions that coat the stool to mark it as a means of interspecies communication [40].

Anal sac secretions in cats were not studied until fairly recently [84], most likely because anorectal disease has not historically been reported in cats in the medical literature with frequency [66]. According to a 2008 study by Frankel, Scott, and Erb [84], normal anal sac secretions in cats vary immensely in color (white, gray, cream, tan, yellow, orange) and thickness (watery to thick). Normal anal sac secretions in cats also tend to be a mixed bag of bacteria with Gram-positive cocci predominating, followed by Gram-negative cocci. Rod-shaped bacteria, although present, are in the minority, as are yeasts. Neutrophils may be present in small numbers, but typically without intracellular bacteria.

Anal sacculitis may be the result of obesity, focal swelling that obstructs the duct, small-diameter fecal material that does not adequately push against the sac to allow for full expression with each bowel movement, or diarrhea. The result of anal sacculitis is a cat that presents with apparent peri-anal irritation. Although cats may be seen to scoot their rear against the floor as would a dog with a similar plight, many cats simply demonstrate attempts to over-groom the perineum. In the author's experience, they may even hike a hind limb up in the air as if to groom the perineum, but redirect their grooming elsewhere such as on the lateral tarsus or dorsal metatarsus (Figure 6.6a and b). The astute client may notice an apparent inability to settle or sit, and in a tolerant cat may even be able to appreciate a peri-anal swelling over the involved sac(s). Without expression of the impacted gland(s), anal sacs may abscess (Figure 6.6c) and rupture outwards.

6.5.8 The Rectal Examination

The rectal examination is not performed in cats at every wellness examination. It is typically reserved for cats that [1]:

- are scooting;
- are presenting for dyschezia or hematochezia;

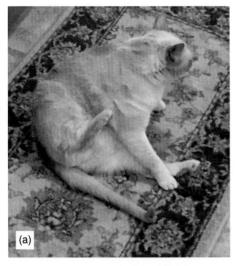
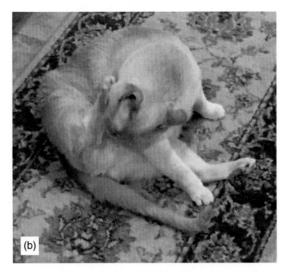
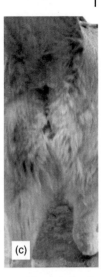

Figure 6.6 (a) Cat with anal gland abscess sitting for long periods of time with hind limb hiked up in the air. (b) Cat with anal gland abscess exhibiting redirected grooming behavior at her hock. (c) Left-sided anal gland abscess in a cat. Note the bruising over the left anal sac.

- have chronic diarrhea, especially large bowel diarrhea;
- have a history of anal sacculitis and/or anal gland abscess;
- have a history of constipation, obstipation, or megacolon;
- have a history of fecal incontinence;
- have sustained trauma to the pelvis and/or pelvic floor.

Vehicular trauma is common in the cat. The pelvic fractures that result from it represent 22% of all fractures seen in cats [85]. Of the types of pelvic fractures, those that involve the ilium and/or the acetabulum are potentially the most detrimental to the cat because they commonly displace axially. This effectively narrows the pelvic canal. When the pelvic canal is narrowed, obstipation and megacolon are frequent outcomes [86].

In addition, the rectal examination is appropriately performed in cats that are members of a breed known for spinal deformities. The Manx cat, for example, is bred for caudal vertebral aplasia. Heterozygotes display variable expression of the tailless trait, which may result in significant myelopathies. In addition to a high incidence of spina bifida with or without meningocele, Manx cats may have urinary and/or fecal incontinence due to reduced perineal or anal tone, if it is present at all [87].

When performing a rectal examination in the cat, sedation is often necessary [66]. That being said, sedation is not a substitute for restraint. A sedated cat still needs to be restrained to prevent injury to the veterinary team.

In anticipation of performing a rectal examination, the veterinary team should be prepared. The hand that will be examining the patient should be gloved and generously lubricated. With a gloved forefinger, the clinician may apply some lubricant to the anal rim also. The

clinician should give the patient a few moments to acclimate rather than just "diving in" [1].

Prior to advancing the gloved forefinger, the clinician should appreciate the perineum (Figure 6.7). While inspecting the perineum, the clinician should consider the following:

- Is the perineum clean or is there adhered fecal matter?
- Are mats of fur adhered to the perineum that may indicate a lack of grooming?

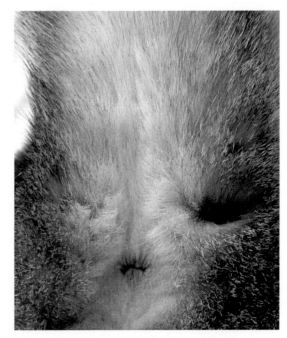

Figure 6.7 Assessing the perineum, which is grossly normal in this patient.

- Are tapeworm segments adhered to the perineum?
- Is there perianal dermatitis?
- Are there perianal fistulas?
- Are there perianal tumors?
- Are the anal sacs enlarged and externally palpable ventrolateral to the anus at the 4 and 8 o'clock positions?

Normal anal sacs are not palpable externally. However, enlarged or obstructed sacs may be palpable as a firm swelling or nodule.

The clinician should also assess if there is anal tone. To determine this, the clinician can take his gloved forefinger and touch the anal rim. An anus with normal tone will "wink" as the anal sphincters close. Decreased or absent tone suggests a problem with the innervation of the anus.

When the clinician is ready to advance a forefinger, he should do so gently, without force and without rapid turning or grinding motions. His motion should be smooth and fluid [1]. The clinician should note whether or not there is appropriate tone: the sphincters of a normal cat should clamp down against the finger. If tone to the anus is reduced or absent, then anal innervation may be compromised [1].

As the clinician advances, the anal canal should easily accommodate the palpating forefinger. Initially, the clinician should consider the rectal wall and the rectal mucosa. He should feel for thickening of the rectal wall and irregularities of the surface of the rectal mucosa, which in a normal patient is supple and uniform [1].

Next, the clinician should appreciate the muscles that border the rectal canal laterally: the coccygeal and levator ani muscles. A defect in these muscles will disrupt the integrity of the canal, resulting in a perineal hernia [1].

Dorsally, the clinician should feel for the internal iliac lymph nodes. These nodes are not palpable unless enlarged. When enlarged, they are palpable dorsally through the rectal wall, and may even displace the rectum ventrally [1].

The clinician should feel ventrally through the rectal wall for pelvic bone abnormalities including old fractures that could explain obstipation or even megacolon. The urethra also lies on the floor of the pelvis and can be palpated through the rectal wall in some patients by an astute clinician. By this same approach, a clinician would be able to appreciate a uretholith [1].

As the clinician backtracks through the anal canal on the way out, he should feel for the left and right anal sacs to gain an appreciation for their shape and size. He should ask the following [1]:

- Are the anal sacs symmetrical?
- Are the anal sacs enlarged?

- Are the anal sacs painful?
- Are the anal sacs easy to express?

If anal sac expression is performed, the clinician should grossly evaluate the secretions of the anal sacs. If the secretions are bloody or purulent, the clinician should create a slide imprint of his gloved finger post-expression to evaluate the contents of both anal sacs microscopically [1, 84].

Finally, as the clinician exits the anal canal, he should remember to appreciate the rim of the rectal canal. It is possible to miss a mass that is close to the mucocutaneous junction because one is too focused on feeling deep inside.

6.6 The Upper Urinary Tract

The upper urinary tract consists of the kidneys and the ureters as conduits to transport urine to the urinary bladder for storage prior to voiding. The kidneys are bilateral, bean-shaped structures that are located in the retroperitoneal space, ventral to the sublumbar muscles. The right kidney is located more cranially than the left: the right kidney sits opposite the first three lumbar vertebrae compared with the left kidney, which spans the second through fifth. The right kidney is cupped cranially by the caudate process of the liver and as such is slightly more anchored in its location; however, both kidneys are mobile in cats compared with dogs and both should be palpable [40, 88, 89].

The ureters are not palpable; however, there is potential to nick them during routine ovariohysterectomy, which is why their location is being addressed here [1, 40].

There is one adrenal gland medial to each kidney. The left gland is more easily accessible during surgical exploration; the right gland is more challenging owing to its position between the kidney, the caudate process of the liver, and the vena cava. Neither adrenal gland is palpable on physical examination [40].

Of those structures in the upper urinary tract, only the two kidneys are palpable on physical examination. In the cat, the skilled clinician should be able to gain an appreciation for the size of each and also the surface texture. In health, the surface of each kidney should feel smooth on examination. As the kidney becomes chronically diseased, its surface may develop undulation that causes it to feel "lumpy bumpy."

Keep in mind that renal size may be overestimated in obese patients owing to a heavy deposition of peri-renal fat [40, 89]. Renal size can be confirmed via imaging studies. Historically, renal size has been evaluated radiographically, with and without excretory urograms [90, 91]. When approached in this manner, the kidneys are compared with the length of the second lumbar vertebra to establish the patient's renal length ratio [88]. Depending upon which study is referenced, normal renal length ratios in the cat have been cited as 2.0–3.0 [91–95].

The sexual status of the cat appears to play a role in renal size. A study by Shiroma *et al.* in 1999 demonstrated that neutered cats have a smaller renal length ratio of 1.9–2.6 compared with 2.1–3.2 in intact cats [93]. Although this distinction was known to be true in laboratory rodents as early as the 1930s, it had not been widely recognized or acknowledged until more recently in cats [93, 96–98]. The presence of testosterone stimulates renal hypertrophy and hyperplasia of cells that line the proximal and distal convoluted tubules [98, 99]. The role of estrogen has been more heavily debated because of conflicting reports in the literature on whether estrogen is stimulatory or inhibitory toward renal size [96, 97, 100, 101].

More recently, abdominal ultrasonography has become a preferred method by which to assess renal length because it can also provide information about intra-renal architecture [102–104]. Depending upon which study is referenced, the normal renal length varies between 3.8 and 4.4 cm, but can reach as high as 5.3 cm [90, 92, 102, 105, 106].

Even though imaging studies provide a more exact means of assessing renal size, the clinician should still take the time to develop and refine technical skills that enable him to appreciate renal architecture by the physical examination alone. The clinician's ability to palpate each patient at every visit allows him to document trends. It also may be the one and only indicator on the physical examination that the upper urinary tract requires more extensive investigation.

The clinician can estimate kidney length by measuring the width of his second through fourth fingers, beginning with the index finger, when they are adjacent to each other, in centimeters, prior to performing the physical examination. In that way, if the length of a cat's kidney spans the width of three of his fingers, and he knows in advance how wide his fingers are, he can estimate the length in centimeters of that kidney.

There are several ways to isolate kidneys in the cat (Figure 6.8):

- One technique involves a patient that is on all fours on the examination room table facing away from the clinician:
  - The clinician can take his left hand and place it flattened against the left body wall.
  - The clinician can then apply firm pressure as if pushing into the abdomen with his left hand. What he is doing is creating a "table" against which organs from the opposite side can be pushed.
  - Now, with his right hand, he can curl his fingers slightly and push deeply into the right side of the cranial abdomen caudal to the last rib.
  - Applying firm pressure, he can then move his right hand caudally to catch the right kidney.
  - He can then repeat the same technique for the contralateral side, using his flattened right hand as a table, with the left hand curled to "catch" the left kidney.
- Another technique involves lifting the cat with one hand and supporting it at the level of its sternum so that it is "standing" on his hind limbs:
  - This posture helps the kidneys sink into a more accessible location.

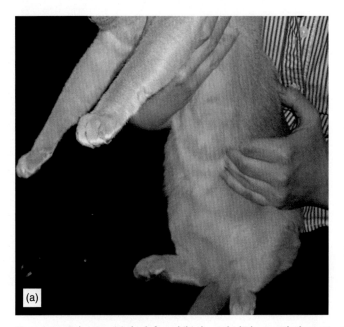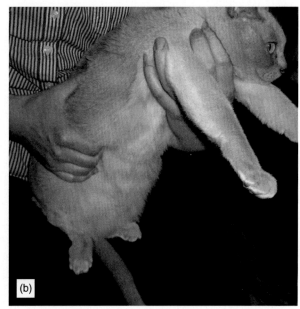

Figure 6.8 Palpating (a) the left and (b) the right kidney with the patient standing.

– The clinician can use his other hand to cup the abdomen to "catch" each kidney.

– In order to evaluate both kidneys, the clinician will have to switch hands.

By estimating kidney length on palpation, the clinician is able to determine whether or not the kidneys are symmetrical or aymmetrical, enlarged or reduced in size:

- If both kidneys are symmetrical, but enlarged, the patient may be experiencing acute kidney failure, as from lily toxicosis [88].
- If both kidneys are symmetrical, but shrunken and small, the patient may be experiencing chronic kidney disease [88].
- Asymmetry between kidneys could indicate a unilateral renal mass, obstruction, or infarction. The most common neoplasia to affect the feline kidney is lymphoma [88].

The clinician can also assess whether or not the kidneys are painful. Palpation of normal kidneys in healthy cats is not painful; however, palpation of a patient with pyelonephritis is [89].

6.7 The Lower Urinary Tract

The lower urinary tract includes the urinary bladder, into which the ureters empty, and the urethra, the tube by which urine exits the body [40].

The urinary bladder is typically palpable. It is critical that the feline practitioner becomes familiar with how a urinary bladder typically feels within the abdominal cavity, because urinary tract obstructions (UTOs) will occur and the patient presenting with a UTO has a very classic feel to its urinary bladder.

In the author's experience, students who have never before felt a UTO panic that they will miss one in clinical practice. However, provided that the students have mastered an understanding of what is normal, they will easily recognize abnormal when it occurs.

The typical empty urinary bladder feels like a wad of balled up tissue: soft, supple, and non-tender to the touch. As the urinary bladder fills a small amount, it feels like a very small water balloon: fluid surrounded by a stable, yet soft and pliable wall. Even when the bladder is moderately full, it still retains that water balloon-like quality, that is, it is compressible [89].

By contrast, a cat with a UTO has a rock-hard bladder that is not compliant, not compressible, and is exceedingly painful. When such a bladder is identified on physical examination, care should be taken not to be forceful with palpation because urinary bladder rupture is possible [107].

When UTO occurs, it is typically due to a urethral plug, a protein-rich mixture of inflammatory cells and urinary crystals [108, 109]. Males are more commonly affected than females because the male's urethra is narrower than the female's [107]. However, there is no correlation between urethral diameter and the age at castration, so pediatric neutering does not increase the risk of UTO [110].

UTO represents one extreme of feline lower urinary tract disease (FLUTD). In 2001, Lekcharoensuk, Osborne, and Lulich reported that UTO occurred in 18% of 22,000 cats that presented to veterinary teaching hospitals with urinary signs [111]. However, non-obstructive FLUTD is also prevalent. Over half of the cases of non-obstructive FLUTD are due to non-infectious feline idiopathic cystitis (FIC) [107–109, 112]. Non-medical, behavioral issues represent roughly one-tenth of all cases of FLUTD, whereas urinary bladder neoplasia and urinary tract infection are implicated the least [107].

Although it is impossible to determine the cause of non-obstructive FLUTD based upon physical examination findings alone, the astute clinician should be on the look-out for physical examination findings that may be suggestive of FLUTD. For example, a cat that presents with bilateral ventrocaudal abdominal and/or inguinal alopecia may be over-grooming due to underlying cystitis. A cat with bloody discharge on and around the perineal fur may be experiencing hematuria. It is also possible to visualize stranguria in male cats with partial or full UTO because on physical examination they display penile pulsing. The owner may also report the following atypical "behaviors" at home: dysuria, pollakiuria, vocalization during urination, and over-grooming of the perineum. As a result, it is important to pair history with physical examination findings to paint a more complete picture of the patient's current health status and to know when further diagnostic investigation is indicated.

In order to palpate the urinary bladder, the clinician must examine the caudoventral abdominal cavity. The urinary bladder is usually seated between the ventral body wall and the descending colon. However, if the descending colon is full, the colon can be displaced so that it sits lateral to the urinary bladder.

As was the case with renal palpation, there is no one "right" way to palpate the urinary bladder. The clinician can appreciate the urinary bladder with the patient positioned in several different ways depending upon patient comfort and clinician preference:

- The patient can be standing and facing away from the clinician.
- The patient can be facing away from the clinician with the front half of its body elevated in the same manner as was performed for kidney palpation.
- The patient can be examined in lateral recumbency. In this position, the clinician cups his hand so that his thumb is on one side of the caudal abdomen and his fingers are on the other. The clinician then firmly

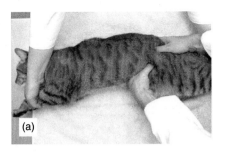
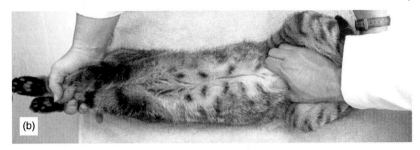

Figure 6.9 Palpating the urinary bladder with the patient in (a) right lateral recumbency and (b) dorsal recumbency. Source (a), (b): Courtesy of the Media Resources Department at Midwestern University.

brings his fingers and thumb together so that they practically touch, with the patient's body in between them. The clinician can now slide his hand cranially and then caudally, then back again, until the urinary bladder "blips" through his hand (Figure 6.9a).

- The patient can be examined in dorsal recumbency (Figure 6.9b).

In cases of urolithiasis, it is possible, although uncommon, to feel stones within the urinary bladder. If there is more than one stone, they may grind together and feel like marbles rolling around in a sack.

6.8 The Male Reproductive Tract

The reproductive tract of the tom cat consists of both internal and external structures. Of the internal structures, the prostate is rarely palpable per rectum and neither the paired bulbourethral glands, which are located near the bulb of the penis, nor the ductus deferens can be appreciated on physical examination [113]. The physical examination of the male feline reproductive tract is therefore restricted to the external anatomy, the penis and the testes.

Unlike the dog, in which the penis is located between the thighs, the cat penis retains its embryonic position: its apex is directed caudoventrally [40]. Because the cat penis is not located in the groin and because it can only be viewed head on from behind the patient in the same way that one would view the vulva of a female cat, sexual determination of kittens can be especially challenging for the veterinary student. Male and female kittens have a tendency to look alike, especially shortly after birth. Male kittens are differentiated from females primarily by understanding that the ano-genital distance in males is greater than that in females. This greater distance in male cats allows for their testes to sit dorsal to the genital opening (Figure 6.10). The difference in ano-genital distance between male and female cats persists into adulthood (Figure 6.11).

As is also demonstrated by Figure 6.11a and b, the penis of the cat is entirely sheathed by the prepuce except

during erection, in which case the penis curves downward and forward [113].

An important distinguishing feature between tom cats and neutered males is that the glans of the penis of the former is characterized by 120–150 caudally directed

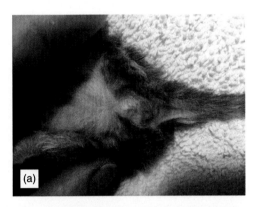

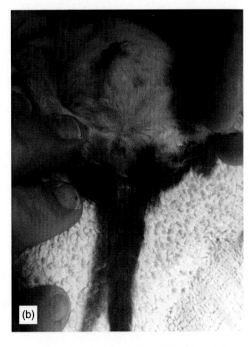

Figure 6.10 Sexing kittens: (a) a male and (b) a female kitten. Source (a), (b): Courtesy of Frank Isom, DVM.

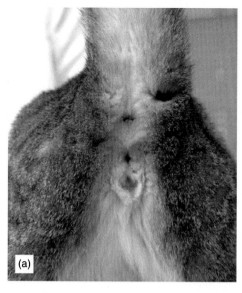
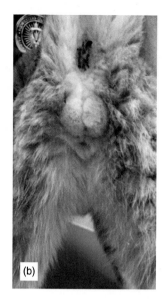
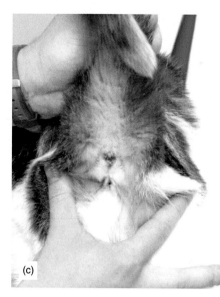

Figure 6.11 Appreciating (a) the greater ano-genital distance in an adult neutered male cat, (b) the greater ano-genital distance in an adult intact tom cat, and (c) the lesser ano-genital distance in a female cat. Source (a)–(c): Courtesy of the Media Resources Department at Midwestern University.

keratinized papillae (Figure 6.12). These spines are testosterone dependent: they begin to develop on the glans at 12 weeks of age and are fully present by puberty. Their function is stimulate the female cat upon intromission. The queen is an induced ovulator: she will not release oocytes without sexual stimulation [40, 113].

When cats are neutered, the sources of testosterone that are so important to maintaining these papillae are removed. As a result, the papillae regress. It may take up to 6 weeks after castration for the papillae to

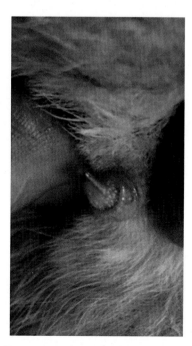

Figure 6.12 Testosterone-dependent spines on the glans of the penis in an intact male cat. Source: Courtesy of Frank Isom, DVM.

disappear [40, 113]. It is very important that the clinician be aware that these papillae exist in the tom cat and under what circumstances they regress, so that if ever presented with a stray that has no scrotal testes, the clinician can more accurately assess whether the stray is in fact already neutered or whether he is bilaterally cryptorchid. In the case of the former, the stray should have no papillae, assuming that he was neutered more than 6 weeks prior to presentation. In the case of the latter, his intra-abdominal testicles will produce enough testosterone to maintain the papillae. Testosterone assays may be used as follow up confirmatory testing: a baseline serum testosterone is compared with the level of sex hormone following administration of gonadotropin-releasing hormone; however, the presence or absence of papillae is very accurate for determining sexual status [113].

The presence of scrotal testicles should also be examined in any intact male, especially at new kitten visits, to establish whether or not testicular descent has occurred and, if not, whether the patient is unilaterally or bilaterally cryptorchid.

During embryonic development, the testes originate near the caudal pole of each kidney. The testes are spurred into migration toward the inguinal canal by the gubernaculum, tissue that spans from the caudal pole of each testis into the inguinal canal. Initially, as the gubernaculum enlarges and itself migrates toward the scrotum, it dilates the inguinal canal, paving the way for testicular descent. At birth, the gubernaculum is often present scrotally, where it is in prime position to encourage the testes to descend through the inguinal canal and into the scrotum. Sometimes the gubernaculum is even mistaken for scrotal testicles. The reality is that in most kittens and puppies, the testes are still abdominal at birth. The testes may make it through the inguinal canal and into the scrotum within 3–4 days after birth. However, the testes may continue to pass in and out of the scrotum through the open inguinal canal until 10–14 weeks of age. A kitten should not be considered unilaterally or bilaterally cryptorchid until 4–6 months old, when the inguinal canal closes, at which point the testes are either scrotally located or not [114, 115].

Testicular disorders in cats are uncommon. Of these, cryptorchidism is the most frequently seen congenital defect in clinical practice. Depending on the study referenced, the prevalence ranges from 1.3 to 3.8% [116–120]. When cats present as being cryptorchid, the majority are only unilaterally affected [113, 118, 119]. Of those, the majority of the retained testes are inguinal as opposed to abdominal [113, 118, 119]. Historically, Persian cats have been over-represented [114, 116, 118]. However, in a 10-year review of 4140 cats that presented to Little's practice in Ottawa, Canada, Ragdolls were implicated as having the highest incidence of 18.75% [113].

Cryptorchidism is passed down through the generations via a recessive mode of inheritance [118]. Because it is inherited, cryptorchid tom cats should not be bred [113]. Only one-fifth of clients identify their cats as being cryptorchid [119]. Therefore, it is the veterinary team's responsibility to evaluate the sexual status of the patient at initial presentation and to convey associated recommendations to the client.

6.9 The Female Reproductive Tract

The reproductive tract of the queen consists of both internal and external structures. Of the internal structures, the normal ovaries are never palpable in the cat, nor is the non-pregnant uterus [121].

Ovaries could potentially be palpable when pathologically enlarged due to ovarian cysts or ovarian tumors [121]. However, the latter are rare and the former are more often identified at the time of ovariohysterectomy as incidental findings such as anovulatory functional follicular cysts [122] (Figure 6.13).

The uterus is palpable during the physiologic state of pregnancy [121, 123]. From mating to parturition, the gestation length in a cat is 56–69 days [124]. Individual spherical balls are palpable as discrete developing fetuses as early as day 14–17 [123, 124]. These so-called "beads on a string" are easiest to feel on abdominal palpation between days 21 and 25 of gestation, at which point the enlarged uterus is also palpable [121, 123]. From day 35 to day 45 of gestation, it may be difficult to appreciate the individual fetuses on abdominal palpation because of placental size: at this point, the placentas are so large that the uterus is palpable as one tubular structure rather than as individual sausage links [123] (Figure 6.14).

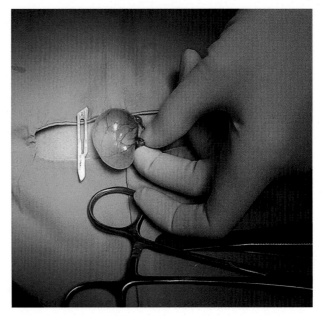

Figure 6.13 Incidental finding of an anovulatory ovarian cyst during routine ovariohysterectomy. Source: Courtesy of Shannon Carey, DVM.

Beyond day 45, it may be possible to discern individual fetal skeletons, especially the rib cages and the skulls [121, 123] (Figure 6.15).

The uterus is also palpable during the pathologic state of pyometra. Pyometra occurs in 2.2% of intact queens by the time they reach 13 years of age. Oriental and exotic purebreds such as the Siamese, Korat, Ocicat, and Bengal appear to be predisposed, with pyometra occurring younger in life than it does within the general population [125].

In cases where there is an open pyometra, meaning that the cervix remains open, allowing for the outflow of hemorrhagic to purulent reproductive tract discharge, the enlarged uterus is less easy to appreciate on abdominal palpation. However, when cats present with a closed pyometra, the closed cervix results in the retention of all reproductive tract discharge such that the uterus becomes very pronounced. Care should be taken during palpation of the enlarged uterus. Just as is the case with an enlarged spleen, rupture of the uterus is possible [126].

Stump pyometras may also be seen in spayed cats if ovarian remnants are inadvertently left behind at the time of ovariohysterectomy. Palpation of a tubular swelling in the caudal abdomen of a recently spayed cat needs to be investigated as a potential stump pyometra until proven otherwise [127, 128].

The physical examination of the female feline reproductive tract should also include a cursory evaluation of the external anatomy, the vulva. The astute clinician should take care to inspect the vulva for discharge. When cats are in proestrus, they may have mucoid vulvar discharge [121, 123]. When cats are actively in heat, they

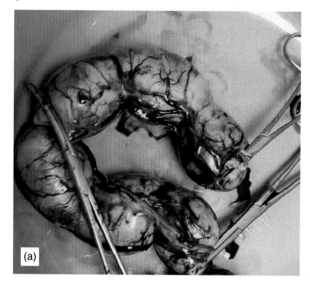
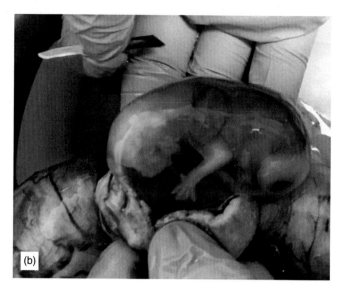

Figure 6.14 (a) Ovariohysterectomy of a pregnant cat between days 35 and 45 of gestation. At this point, identification of individual fetuses would be challenging. Note that the uterus appears as one giant tubular structure. It has lost the "beads on a string" appearance that would have made individual fetal palpation possible. (b) Opening up the uterus of the cat in (a) to appreciate fetal development at this stage of gestation. Source (a), (b): Courtesy of Shannon Carey, DVM.

may or may not have serous to mucoid vulvar discharge, and they tend to exhibit lordosis: the lumbar region is intentionally curved inward like a horse with sway back, causing a forward pelvic tilt. The front legs hunch near to the ground and the tail tilts to one side to display receptivity to the male [123].

Cats should not have hemorrhagic, purulent, or hemopurulent vulvar discharge, and vulvar discharge should not be odorous to the veterinary team. If it is, then the patient needs to be assessed further to rule out pyometra, endometritis, or, in pregnant queens, macerated fetuses [121].

In addition, the clinician should assess for the presence of perivulvar dermatitis and/or a strong urine odor. In obese cats especially, the caudal thigh skin folds often have a tendency to roll inwards and obscure the vulva. This can lead to moist dermatitis that is perpetuated by urine scald and urine crusting of perivulvar fur.

6.10 Being Presented with a Female of Unknown Sexual Status

If, on initial presentation, the patient is acknowledged to be a stray and its sexual status is unknown, the clinician should first look for a left ear notch or tip that would suggest that the cat had undergone sterilization as part of a community Trap–Neuter–Release (TNR) program. If there is no left ear notch or tip, then the clinician may ask for owner permission to shave the abdomen to look for a "spay scar." The presence of a "spay scar" increases the likelihood that the patient was spayed. The presence of a "spay scar," however, is not a guarantee of sterilization: the patient could have been operated on at that location for something else. For example, the patient could have undergone a cystotomy for urolithiasis.

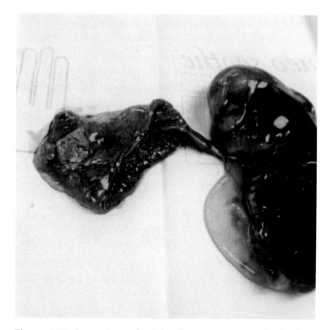

Figure 6.15 Appreciating fetal development after ossification has taken place. This fetus would be palpable on abdominal palpation in late pregnancy (after day 45). Source: Courtesy of Shannon Carey, DVM.

6.11 Neonates

Unexpected litters are common in cats. In a 2006 study by Wallace and Levy that evaluated data from 103,643

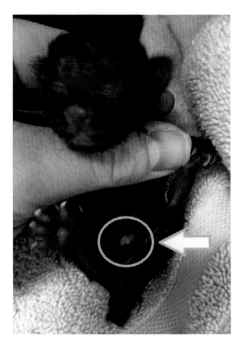

Figure 6.16 Note the stump of the umbilical cord in this 2-hour-old kitten.

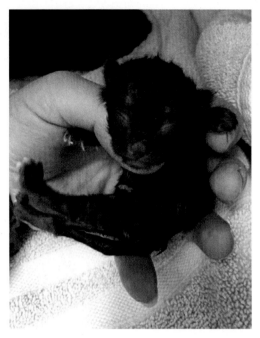

Figure 6.17 Note how flexor tone predominates and the 2-hour-old kitten tends to curl its body.

feral cats that were presented to TNR programs between 1993 and 2004, 15.9% of female cats were pregnant at the time of ovariohysterectomy, with an average of 4.1 fetuses per litter [120]. Cats typically come into heat for the first time between 5 and 9 months of age; however, the earliest reported heat cycle in a cat was at 3.5 months [129]. Therefore, it is not uncommon for kittens to have kittens.

Kittens are born inside the amniotic sac, which the queen bites through, and also the umbilical cord, to free the kitten and lick it, stimulating breathing [123] (Figure 6.16).

Newborn kittens typically weigh 100 g (3.5 oz) at birth [130]. Until 2 weeks of age, their heart rate routinely exceeds 200 beats per minute and their respiration is typically 15–35 breaths per minute [130–132]. They are not able to themoregulate reliably until they reach 4 weeks of age: their core temperature is initially 96–97 °F (35.5–36 °C) [43, 133].

Until 4 days of age, flexor tone predominates (Figure 6.17). This creates a comma shape that is characteristic of newborns. It also allows newborns to be flaccid and curled when they are scruffed by their mother [43, 133].

Eyelids do not separate and ear canals do not open until 5–14 days after birth [43, 133] (Figure 6.18). The menace and pupillary light reflexes are present by 10–21 days old, and vision is normal by 4 weeks of age [43].

The neonate should have a strong rooting reflex and suckle response [43, 133], and the queen should be monitored to make certain that she is allowing the kittens to nurse (Figure 6.19).

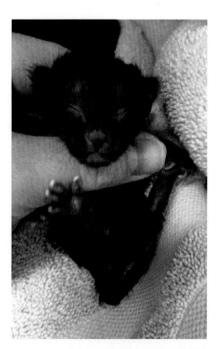

Figure 6.18 Note how the upper and lower eyelids are closed in a normal neonate. They do not separate from one another until 5–14 days of age.

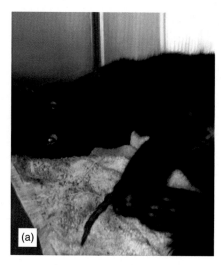
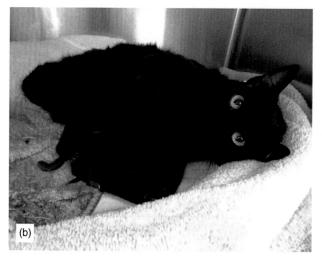

Figure 6.19 (a) The firstborn of a litter of four is nursing less than 1 hour after birth as the queen continues to experience contractions to continue the delivery of its littermates. (b) The queen has completed delivery of all four of her kittens and is allowing all to nurse.

References

1 Rijnberk, A. and van Sluijs, F.S. (eds.) (2009) *Medical History and Physical Examination in Companion Animals*, 2nd edn., Saunders Elsevier, St. Louis.

2 Dyce, K.M., Sack, W.O., and Wensing, C.J.G. (2010) *Textbook of Veterinary Anatomy*, 4th edn., Saunders Elsevier, St. Louis.

3 Dukes, H.H., Swenson, M.J., and Reece, W.O. (1993) *Dukes' Physiology of Domestic Animals*, 11th edn. Comstock, Ithaca, NY.

4 Cote, E., Edwards, N.J., Ettinger, S.J. *et al.* (2015) Management of incidentally detected heart murmurs in dogs and cats. *Journal of the American Veterinary Medical Association*, **246** (10), 1076–1088.

5 Fuentes, V.L. (2006) Cardiomyopathy: establishing a diagnosis, in *Consultations in Feline Internal Medicine*, vol. 5 (ed. J.R. August), Saunders Elsevier, St. Louis, pp. 301–310.

6 Gordon, S.G. (2006) Cardiomyopathy – therapeutic decisions, in *Consultations in Feline Internal Medicine*, vol. 5 (ed. J.R. August), Saunders Elsevier, St. Louis, pp. 311–317.

7 Baral, R.M. (2012) Approach to the vomiting cat, in *The Cat: Clinical Medicine and Management* (ed. S.E. Little), Saunders Elsevier, St. Louis, pp. 426–441.

8 Little, S.E. (2012) Diseases of the esophagus, in *The Cat: Clinical Medicine and Management* (ed. S.E. Little), Saunders Elsevier, St. Louis, pp. 441–450.

9 Willard, M.D. (2014) Clinical manifestations of gastrointestinal disorders, in *Small Animal Internal Medicine*, 5th edn. (eds. R.W. Nelson and C.G. Couto), Mosby Elsevier, St. Louis, pp. 367–389.

10 Baral, R.M. (2012) Approach to the cat with diarrhea, in *The Cat: Clinical Medicine and Management* (ed. S.E. Little), Saunders Elsevier, St. Louis, pp. 459–466.

11 Baral, R.M. (2012) Approach to the cat with ascites and diseases affecting the peritoneal cavity, in *The*

Cat: Clinical Medicine and Management (ed. S.E. Little), Saunders Elsevier, St. Louis, pp. 538–546.

12 Kennedy, M. and Little, S.E. (2012) Viral diseases, in *The Cat: Clinical Medicine and Management* (ed. S.E. Little), Saunders Elsevier, St. Louis, pp. 1029–1063.

13 Sparkes, A.H., Gruffydd-Jones, T.J., and Harbour, D.A. (1991) Feline infectious peritonitis: a review of clinicopathological changes in 65 cases, and a critical assessment of their diagnostic value. *Veterinary Record*, **129** (10), 209–212.

14 Culp, W.T.N., Weisse, C., Kellogg, M.E. *et al.* (2010) Spontaneous hemoperitoneum in cats: 65 cases (1994–2006). *Journal of the American Veterinary Medical Association*, **236** (9), 978–982.

15 Mandell, D.C. and Drobatz, K.J. (1995) Feline hemoperitoneum – 16 cases (1986–1993). *Journal of Veterinary Emergency and Critical Care*, **5** (2), 93–97.

16 Aumann, M., Worth, L.T., and Drobatz, K.J. (1998) Uroperitoneum in cats: 26 cases (1986–1995). *Journal of the American Animal Hospital Association*, **34** (4), 315–324.

17 Kyles, A.E., Hardie, E.M., Wooden, B.G. *et al.* (2005) Management and outcome of cats with ureteral calculi: 153 cases (1984–2002). *Journal of the American Veterinary Medical Association*, **226** (6), 937–944.

18 Wright, K.N., Gompf, R.E., and DeNovo, R.C., Jr. (1999) Peritoneal effusion in cats: 65 cases (1981–1997). *Journal of the American Veterinary Medical Association*, **214** (3), 375–381.

19 Closa, J.M. and Font, A. (1999) Traumatic tricuspid insufficiency in a kitten. *Journal of the American Animal Hospital Association*, **35** (1), 21–24.

20 Harvey, A.M., Battersby, I.A., Faena, M. *et al.* (2005) Arrhythmogenic right ventricular cardiomyopathy

in two cats. *Journal of Small Animal Practice*, **46** (3), 151–156.

21 Harjuhahto, T.A., Leinonen, M.R., Simola, O.T. *et al.* (2011) Congestive heart failure and atrial fibrillation in a cat with myocardial fibro-fatty infiltration. *Journal of Feline Medicine and Surgery*, **13** (2), 109–111.

22 Saxon, B., Hendrick, M., and Waddle, J.R. (1991) Restrictive cardiomyopathy in a cat with hypereosinophilic syndrome. *Canadian Veterinary Journal*, **32** (6), 367–369.

23 Dimski, D.S. (1997) Feline hepatic lipidosis. *Seminars in Veterinary Medicine and Surgery (Small Animal)*, **12** (1), 28–33.

24 Lucke, V.M. and Davies, J.D. (1984) Progressive lymphocytic cholangitis in the cat. *Journal of Small Animal Practice*, **25** (5), 249–260.

25 Prasse, K.W., Mahaffey, E.A., Denovo, R., and Cornelius, L. (1982) Chronic lymphocytic cholangitis in 3 cats. *Veterinary Pathology*, **19** (2), 99–108.

26 Gores, B.R., Berg, J., Carpenter, J.L., and Ullman, S.L. (1994) Chylous ascites in cats – 9 cases (1978–1993). *Journal of the American Veterinary Medical Association*, **205** (8), 1161.

27 Blaxter, A.C., Holt, P.E., Pearson, G.R. *et al.* (1998) Congenital portosystemic shunts in the cat – a report of 9 cases. *Journal of Small Animal Practice*, **29** (10), 631–645.

28 Tasker, S. and Gunn-Moore, D. (2000) Differential diagnosis of ascites in cats. *In Practice*, **22** (8), 472–479.

29 Liptak, J.M., Dernell, W.S., and Withrow, S.J. (2004) Liver tumors in cats and dogs. *Compendium: Continuing Education for the Practicing Veterinarian*, **26** (1), 50–57.

30 Hoskins, J.D. (2005) Liver disease in the geriatric patient. *Veterinary Clinics of North America: Small Animal Practice*, **35** (3), 617–634.

31 Nyland, T.G., Koblik, P.D., and Tellyer, S.E. (1999) Ultrasonographic evaluation of biliary cystadenomas in cats. *Veterinary Radiology and Ultrasound*, **40** (3), 300–306.

32 Witzelben, C.L. (1990) Cystic diseases of the liver, in *Hepatology: a Textbook of Liver Disease*, 2nd edn. (eds. D. Zakim and T.D. Boyer), Saunders. Philadelphia, pp. 1395–1411.

33 Parkes, R., Forrest, N., and Baillie, S. (2009) A mixed reality simulator for feline abdominal palpation training in veterinary medicine. *Studies in Health Technology and Informatics*, **142**, 244–246.

34 Williamson, J.A., Hecker, K., Yvorchuk, K. *et al.* (2015) Development and validation of a feline abdominal palpation model and scoring rubric. *Veterinary Record*, **177** (6), 151.

35 Defarges, A. (2015) The physical examination. *Clinician's Brief, September*, 73–80.

36 Ettinger, S.J. (2010) The physical examination of the dog and cat, in *Textbook of Veterinary Internal Medicine* (eds. S.J. Ettinger and E.C. Feldman), Saunders Elsevier, St. Louis, pp. 1–9.

37 Sack, W.O., Wensing, C.J.G., and Dyce, K.M. (1996) *Textbook of Veterinary Anatomy*, 2nd edn., Saunders, Philadelphia.

38 Smeak, D.D. (2012) Abdominal wall reconstruction and hernias, in *Veterinary Surgery: Small Animal* (eds. K.M. Tobias and S.A. Johnston), Saunders Elsevier, St. Louis, pp. 1353–1379.

39 Hermanson, J.W. and Evans, H.E. (1993) The muscular system, in *Miller's Anatomy of the Dog*, 3rd edn. (ed. H.E. Evans), Saunders Elsevier, Philadelphia, pp. 258–384.

40 Dyce, K.M., Sack, W.O., and Wensing, C.J.G. (1996) *Textbook of Veterinary Anatomy*, 2nd edn., Saunders, Philadelphia.

41 Pratschke, K.M. (2014) Abdominal wall hernias and ruptures, in *Feline Soft Tissue and General Surgery* (eds. S.J. Langley-Hobbs, J.L. Demetriou, and J.F. Ladlow), Saunders Elsevier, St. Louis, pp. 269–280.

42 Read, R. (1985) Cranial abdominal hernias, in *Textbook of Small Animal Surgery* (ed. D.H. Slatter), Saunders Elsevier, Philadelphia, p. 853.

43 Hoskins, J.D. and Partington, B.P. (2001) Physical examination and diagnostic imaging procedures, in *Veterinary Pediatrics: Dogs and Cats from Birth to Six Months*, 3rd edn. (ed. J.D. Hoskins), Saunders Elsevier, Philadelphia, pp. 6–7.

44 Baker, T.W. and Davidson, A.P. (2011) Ultrasonography of the young patient, in *Small Animal Pediatrics: The First 12 Months of Life* (eds. M.E. Peterson and M.A. Kutzler), Saunders Elsevier, St. Louis, p. 197.

45 Robinson, R. (1997) Genetic aspects of umbilical hernia incidence in cats and dogs. *Veterinary Record*, **100** (1), 9–10.

46 Klein, M.D. and Hertzler, J.H. (1981) Congenital defects of the abdominal wall. *Surgery, Gynecology and Obstetrics*, **152** (6), 805–808.

47 Rodan, I., Sundahl, E., Carney, H. *et al.* (2011) Feline focus: AAFP and ISFM feline-friendly handling guidelines. *Compendium: Continuing Education for the Practicing Veterinarian*, **33** (12), E3.

48 Rodan, I. (2010) Understanding feline behavior and application for appropriate handling and management. *Topics in Companion Animal Medicine*, **25** (4), 178–188.

49 Heath, S. (2009) Aggression in cats, in *BSAVA Manual of Canine and Feline Behavioural Medicine*, 2nd edn. (eds. D. Horwitz and D.S. Mills), British Small Animal Veterinary Association, Gloucester, p. 233.

50 Meyer, H.P. and Rothuizen, J. (2013) The liver: history and physical examination, in *Canine and Feline Gastroenterology* (eds. R.J. Washabau and M.J. Day), Saunders Elsevier, St. Louis, pp. 856–863.

51 Spohr, A. (2013) The stomach: diagnostic evaluation, in *Canine and Feline Gastroenterology* (eds. R.J. Washabau and M.J. Day), Saunders Elsevier, St. Louis, pp. 609–613.

52 Miller, M.E., Evans, H.E., and Christensen, G.C. (eds.) (1979) *Miller's Anatomy of the Dog*, 2nd edn., Saunders, Philadelphia.

53 Bezuidenhout, A.J. (1993) *The lymphatic system, in Miller's Anatomy of the Dog*, 3rd edn. (ed. H.E. Evans), Saunders Elsevier, Philadelphia, pp. 749–753.

54 Javinsky, E. (2012) Hematology and immune-related disorders, in *The Cat: Clinical Medicine and Management* (ed. S.E. Little), Saunders Elsevier, St. Louis, pp. 685–688.

55 Culp, W.T. and Aronson, L.R. (2008) Splenic foreign body in a cat. *Journal of Feline Medicine and Surgery*, **10** (4), 380–383.

56 Marino, D. (2000) Diseases of the spleen, in *Kirk's Current Veterinary Therapy XIII – Small Animal Practice* (ed. R.W. Kirk), Saunders, Philadelphia, p. 520.

57 Autran de Morais, H. and O'Brien, R. (2005) *Non-neoplastic diseases of the spleen, in Textbook of Veterinary Internal Medicine*, 6th edn. (eds. S.J. Ettinger and E.C. Feldman), Saunders Elsevier, St. Louis, p. 1944.

58 Evans, H.E. (1993) The digestive apparatus and abdomen, in *Miller's Anatomy of the Dog*, 3rd edn. (ed. H.E. Evans), Saunders Elsevier, Philadelphia, pp. 385–461.

59 Baral, R.M. (2012) Diseases of the exocrine pancreas, in *The Cat: Clinical Medicine and Management* (ed. S.E. Little), Saunders Elsevier, St. Louis, pp. 513–520.

60 Steiner, J.M. and Williams, D.A. (1999) Feline exocrine pancreatic disorders. *Veterinary Clinics of North America: Small Animal Practice*, **29** (2), 551–575.

61 Duffell, S.J. (1975) Some aspects of pancreatic disease in the cat. *Journal of Small Animal Practice*, **16** (6), 365–374.

62 Seaman, R.L. (2004) Exocrine pancreatic neoplasia in the cat: a case series. *Journal of the American Animal Hospital Association*, **40** (3), 238–245.

63 Priester, W.A. (1974) Data from eleven United States and Canadian colleges of veterinary medicine on pancreatic carcinoma in domestic animals. *Cancer Research*, **34** (6), 1372–1375.

64 Rijnberk, A. and van Sluijs, F.J. (eds.) (2009) *Medical History and Physical Examination in Companion Animals*, 2nd edn., Saunders Elsevier, St. Louis.

65 Datz, C. (2011) Parasitic and protozoal diseases, in *Small Animal Pediatrics: The First 12 Months of Life* (eds. M.E. Peterson and M.A. Kutzler), Saunders Elsevier, St. Louis, pp. 154–160.

66 Baral, R.M. (2012) *Diseases of the intestines, in The Cat: Clinical Medicine and Management* (ed. S.E. Little), Saunders Elsevier, St. Louis, pp. 466–477.

67 Goggin, J.M., Biller, D.S., Debey, B.M. *et al.* (2000) Ultrasonographic measurement of gastrointestinal wall thickness and the ultrasonographic appearance of the ileocolic region in healthy cats. *Journal of the American Animal Hospital Association*, **36** (3), 224–228.

68 Baez, J.L., Hendrick, M.J., Walker, L.M., and Washabau, R.J. (1999) Radiographic, ultrasonographic, and endoscopic findings in cats with inflammatory bowel disease of the stomach and small intestine: 33 cases (1990–1997). *Journal of the American Veterinary Medical Association*, **215** (3), 349–354.

69 Basher, A.W. and Fowler, J.D. (1987) Conservative versus surgical management of gastrointestinal linear foreign bodies in the cat. *Veterinary Surgery*, **16** (2), 135–138.

70 Bebchuk, T.N. (2002) Feline gastrointestinal foreign bodies. *Veterinary Clinics of North America: Small Animal Practice*, **32** (4), 861–880, vi.

71 Felts, J.F., Fox, P.R., and Burk, R.L. (1984) Thread and sewing needles as gastrointestinal foreign bodies in the cat: a review of 64 cases. *Journal of the American Veterinary Medical Association*, **184** (1), 56–59.

72 Hayes, G. (2009) Gastrointestinal foreign bodies in dogs and cats: a retrospective study of 208 cases. *Journal of Small Animal Practice*, **50** (11), 576–583.

73 Beaver, B.V. (1994) *Disorders of behavior, in The Cat: Diseases and Clinical Management* (ed. R.G. Sherding), Churchill Livingstone, New York, p. 191.

74 Barrs, V.R., Beatty, J.A., Tisdall, P.L. *et al.* Intestinal obstruction by trichobezoars in five cats. *Journal of Feline Medicine and Surgery*, **1** (4), 199–207.

75 Evans, S.E., Bonczynski, J.J., Broussard, J.D. *et al.* (2006) Comparison of endoscopic and full-thickness biopsy specimens for diagnosis of inflammatory bowel disease and alimentary tract lymphoma in cats. *Journal of the American Veterinary Medical Association*, **229** (9), 1447–1450.

76 Carreras, J.K., Goldschmidt, M., Lamb, M. *et al.* (2003) Feline epitheliotropic intestinal malignant lymphoma: 10 cases (1997–2000). *Journal of Veterinary Internal Medicine*, **17** (3), 326–331.

77 Lingard, A.E., Briscoe, K., Beatty, J.A. *et al.* (2009) Low-grade alimentary lymphoma: clinicopathological findings and response to treatment in 17 cases. *Journal of Feline Medicine and Surgery*, **11** (8), 692–700.

78 Sherding, R. (1994) Diseases of the intestines, in *The Cat: Diseases and Clinical Management*, 2nd edn. (ed. R. Sherding), Churchill Livingstone, New York, p. 1211.

79 Bertoy, R.W. (2002) Megacolon in the cat. *Veterinary Clinics of North America: Small Animal Practice*, **32** (4), 901–915.

80 Preston, D.M., Lennard-Jones, J.E., and Thomas, B.M. (1985) Towards a radiologic definition of idiopathic megacolon. *Gastrointestinal Radiology*, **10** (2), 167–169.

81 O'Brien, T.R. (1978) *Radiographic Diagnosis of Abdominal Disorders in the Dog and Cat: Radiographic Interpretation, Clinical Signs, Pathophysiology*, Saunders, Philadelphia.

82 Holt, P. (1985) Anal and perianal surgery in dogs and cats. *In Practice*, **7** (3), 82–89.

83 Demetriou, J.L. and Welsh, E.M. (1999) Rectal prolapse of an ileocaecal neoplasm associated with intussusception in a cat. *Journal of Feline Medicine and Surgery*, **1** (4), 253–256.

84 Frankel, J.L., Scott, D.W., and Erb, H.N. (2008) Gross and cytological characteristics of normal feline anal-sac secretions. *Journal of Feline Medicine and Surgery*, **10** (4), 319–323.

85 Langley-Hobbs, S.J., Sissener, T.R., and Shales, C.J. (2007) Tension band stabilisation of acetabular physeal fractures in four kittens. *Journal of Feline Medicine and Surgery*, **9** (3), 177–187.

86 Harasen, G.L.G. and Little, S.E. (2012) *Musculoskeletal diseases, in The Cat: Clinical Medicine and Management* (ed. S.E. Little), Saunders Elsevier, St. Louis, pp. 704–733.

87 Barone G. (2012) Neurology, in *The Cat: Clinical Medicine and Management* (ed. S.E. Little), Saunders Elsevier, St. Louis, pp. 734–767.

88 Scherk, M. (2012) The upper urinary tract, in *The Cat: Clinical Medicine and Management* (ed. S.E. Little), Saunders Elsevier, St. Louis, pp. 935–979.

89 van Dongen, A.M. and L'Eplattenier, H.F. (2009) Kidneys and urinary tract, in *Medical History and Physical Examination in Companion Animals*, 2nd edn. (eds. A. Rijnberk and F.J. van Sluijs), Saunders Elsevier, St. Louis, pp. 101–107.

90 Barrett, R.B. and Kneller, S.K. (1972) Feline kidney mensuration. *Acta Radiologica, Supplementum*, **319**, 279–280.

91 Lee, R. and Leowijuk, C. (1982) Normal parameters in abdominal radiology of the dog and cat. *Journal of Small Animal Practice*, **23** (5), 251–269.

92 Walter, P.A., Feeney, D.A., Johnston, G.R., and Fletcher, T.F. (1987) Feline renal ultrasonography: quantitative analyses of imaged anatomy. *American Journal of Veterinary Research*, **48** (4), 596–599.

93 Shiroma, J.T., Gabriel, J.K., Carter, R.L. *et al.* (1999) Effect of reproductive status on feline renal size. *Veterinary Radiology and Ultrasound*, **40** (3), 242–245.

94 Owens, J. (1982) The genitourinary system, in *Radiographic Interpretation for the Small Animal Clinician* (ed. D. Biery), Ralston Purina, St. Louis, p. 175.

95 Biery, D. (1981) Upper urinary tract, in *Radiographic Diagnosis of Abdominal Disorders in the Dog and Cat* (ed. T.R. O'Brien), Covel Park Veterinary Co., Davis, CA, pp. 484–485.

96 Huang, K.C. and McIntosh, B.J. (1955) Effect of sex hormones on renal transport of *p*-aminohippuric acid. *American Journal of Physiology*, **183** (3), 387–390.

97 Freudenberger, C.B. and Howard, P.M. (1937) Effects of ovariectomy on body growth and organ weights of the young albino rat. *Proceedings of the Society for Experimental Biology and Medicine*, **36** (2), 144–148.

98 Selye, H. (1939) The effect of testosterone on the kidney. *Journal of Urology*, **42** (4), 637–641.

99 Jean-Faucher, C., Berger, M., Gallon, C. *et al.* (1987) Sex-related differences in renal size in mice: ontogeny and influence of neonatal androgens. *Journal of Endocrinology*, **115** (2), 241–246.

100 Selye, H. (1940) Interactions between various steroid hormones. *Canadian Medical Association Journal*, **42** (2), 113–116.

101 Li, J.J., Kirkman, H., and Hunter, R.L. (1969) Sex difference and gonadal hormone influence on Syrian hamster kidney esterase isozymes. *Journal of Histochemistry and Cytochemistry*, **17** (6), 386–393.

102 Debruyn, K., Paepe, D., Daminet, S. *et al.* (2013) Renal dimensions at ultrasonography in healthy Ragdoll cats with normal kidney morphology: correlation with age, gender and bodyweight. *Journal of Feline Medicine and Surgery*, **15** (12), 1046–1051.

103 Walter, P.A., Feeney, D.A., Johnston, G.R., and Fletcher, T.F. (1987) Feline renal ultrasonography – quantitative-analyses of imaged anatomy. *American Journal of Veterinary Research*, **48** (4), 596–599.

104 Barr, F.J. (1990) Evaluation of ultrasound as a method of assessing renal size in the dog. *Journal of Small Animal Practice*, **31** (4), 174–179.

105 Yeager, A.E. and Anderson, W.I. (1989) Study of association between histologic features and echogenicity of architecturally normal cat kidneys. *American Journal of Veterinary Research*, **50** (6), 860–863.

106 Park, I.C., Lee, H.S., Kim, J.T. *et al.* (2008) Ultrasonographic evaluation of renal dimension and resistive index in clinically healthy Korean domestic short-hair cats. *Journal of Veterinary Science*, **9** (4), 415–419.

107 Little, S.E. (2012) The lower urinary tract, in *The Cat: Clinical Medicine and Management* (ed. S.E. Little), Saunders Elsevier, St. Louis, pp. 980–1015.

108 Gerber, B., Boretti, F.S., Kley, S. *et al.* (2005) Evaluation of clinical signs and causes of lower urinary tract disease in European cats. *Journal of Small Animal Practice*, **46** (12), 571–577.

109 Kruger, J.M., Osborne, C.A., Goyal, S.M. *et al.* (1991) Clinical evaluation of cats with lower urinary-tract disease. *Journal of the American Veterinary Medical Association*, **199** (2), 211–216.

110 Root, M.V., Johnston, S.D., Johnston, G.R., and Olson, P.N. (1996) The effect of prepuberal and postpuberal gonadectomy on penile extrusion and urethral diameter in the domestic cat. *Veterinary Radiology and Ultrasound*, **37** (5), 363–366.

111 Lekcharoensuk, C., Osborne, C.A., and Lulich, J.P. (2001) Epidemiologic study of risk factors for lower urinary tract diseases in cats. *Journal of the American Veterinary Medical Association*, **218** (9), 1429–1435.

112 Buffington, C.A., Chew, D.J., Kendall, M.S. *et al.* (1997) Clinical evaluation of cats with nonobstructive urinary tract diseases. *Journal of the American Veterinary Medical Association*, **210** (1), 46–50.

113 Little, S.E. (2012) Male reproduction, in *The Cat: Clinical Medicine and Management* (ed. S.E. Little), Saunders Elsevier, St. Louis, pp. 1184–1194.

114 Kutzler, M.A. (2011) The reproductive tract, in *Small Animal Pediatrics: The First 12 Months of Life* (eds. M.E. Peterson and M.A. Kutzler), Saunders Elsevier, St. Louis, pp. 405–417.

115 Christensen, B.W. (2012) Disorders of sexual development in dogs and cats. *Veterinary Clinics of*

North America: Small Animal Practice, **42** (3), 515–526, vi.

116 Millis, D.L., Hauptman, J.G., and Johnson, C.A. (1992) Cryptorchidism and monorchism in cats: 25 cases (1980–1989). *Journal of the American Veterinary Medical Association*, **200** (8), 1128–1130.

117 Meyers-Wallen, V.N. (2012) Gonadal and sex differentiation abnormalities of dogs and cats. *Sexual Development*, **6** (1–3), 46–60.

118 Richardson, E.F. and Mullen, H. (1993) Cryptorchidism in cats. *Compendium: Continuing Education for the Practicing Veterinarian*, **15** (10), 1342–1345.

119 Yates, D., Hayes, G., Heffernan, M., and Beynon, R. (2003) Incidence of cryptorchidism in dogs and cats. *Veterinary Record*, **152** (16), 502–504.

120 Wallace, J.L. and Levy, J.K. (2006) Population characteristics of feral cats admitted to seven trap–neuter–return programs in the United States. *Journal of Feline Medicine and Surgery*, **8** (4), 279–284.

121 Schaefers-Okkens, A.C. and Kooistra, H.S. (2009) Female reproductive tract, in *Medical History and Physical Examination in Companion Animals*, 2nd edn. (eds. A. Rijnberk and F.J. van Sluijs), Saunders Elsevier, St. Louis, pp. 108–116.

122 Ortega-Pacheco, A., Gutierrez-Blanco, E., and Jimenez-Coello, M. (2012) Common lesions in the female reproductive tract of dogs and cats. *Veterinary Clinics of North America: Small Animal Practice*, **42** (3), 547–559, vii.

123 Little, S.E. (2012) Female reproduction, in *The Cat: Clinical Medicine and Management* (ed. S.E. Little), Saunders Elsevier, St. Louis, pp. 1195–1227.

124 Feldman, E.C. and Nelson, R.W. (2004) *Canine and Feline Endocrinology and Reproduction*, 3rd edn., Saunders, St. Louis.

125 Hagman, R., Strom Holst, B., Moller, L., and Egenvall, A. (2014) Incidence of pyometra in Swedish insured cats. *Theriogenology*, **82** (1), 114–120.

126 Hollinshead, F. and Krekeler, N. (2016) Pyometra in the queen: to spay or not to spay? *Journal of Feline Medicine and Surgery*, **18** (1), 21–33.

127 Demirel, M.A. and Acar, D.B. (2012) Ovarian remnant syndrome and uterine stump pyometra in three queens. *Journal of Feline Medicine and Surgery*, **14** (12), 913–918.

128 Johnston, S.D., Kustritz, M.V.R., and Olson, P.N.S. (2001) Disorders of the feline ovaries, in *Canine and Feline Theriogenology*, 1st edn. (eds. S.D. Johnston, M.V.R. Kustritz, and P.S. Olson), Saunders, Philadelphia, pp. 193–205.

129 Griffin, B. (2001) Prolific cats: the estrous cycle. *Compendium: Continuing Education for the Practicing Veterinarian*, **23** (12), 1049–1057.

130 Hoskins, J.D. and Partington, B.P. (2001) *Physical examination and diagnostic imaging procedures, in Veterinary Pediatrics: Dogs and Cats from Birth to Six Months*, 3rd edn. (ed. J.D. Hoskins), Saunders, Philadelphia, pp. 1–21.

131 Mosier, J.E. (1978) The puppy from birth to six weeks. *Veterinary Clinics of North America*, **8** (1), 79–100.

132 Small, E. (1980) Pediatrics, in *Current Veterinary Therapy. VII. Small Animal Practice* (ed. R.W. Kirk), Saunders, Philadelphia, p. 77.

133 Kustritz, M.V.R. (2011) History and physical examination of the neonate, in *Small Animal Pediatrics: the First 12 Months of Life* (eds. M.E. Peterson and M.A. Kutzler), Saunders Elsevier, St. Louis, pp. 20–27.

7

Examining the Musculoskeletal System of the Cat

7.1 Muscle Condition Score (MCS)

Obesity within the companion animal population in the United States is on the rise [1]. Many cats present to veterinary clinics with an estimated 50% body fat, if not higher [2, 3] (Figure 7.1). Yet overweight patients may lose lean body mass that is not accounted for by any current body condition score (BCS), including the nine-point scale introduced by Nestlé Purina PetCare [4, 5] (Figure 7.2).

Underweight patients are also at risk of the veterinary team failing to identify and characterize lean body mass loss [5]. Weight loss in lean patients may be documented as loss of body fat alone when in fact lean body mass has been reduced.

Loss of lean body mass may be age-related, in which case it is referred to as sarcopenia, or it may be the result of disease [6]. In particular, chronic kidney disease, congestive heart failure, and neoplasia induce cachexia in human and veterinary patients alike [6]. Such disease-induced loss of lean body mass has been linked to higher morbidity and mortality in people [6–9]. Poor conditioning has also been linked to decreased survival in veterinary patients [10–12]. Given that veterinary patients may live longer owing to improved medical management options that maintain quality of life, the burden is on the veterinary team to recognize loss of lean muscle mass early. Only through early diagnosis can the veterinary–client partnership address and counter the potential for the deleterious effects of sarcopenic or cachexic weight loss.

Assessing BCS is a valuable component of nutritional screening for every patient; however, the BCS alone paints an incomplete picture. BCS and muscle mass are not always related; therefore, each patient should also receive a muscle mass score (MMS) or muscle condition score (MCS) [13].

As with BCS, the determination of MCS requires gross observation and palpation. In particular, medium- and

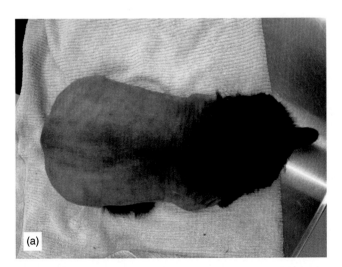 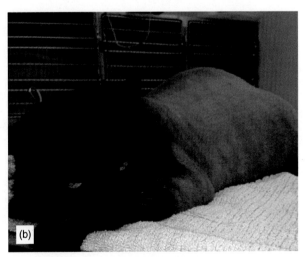

Figure 7.1 (a) Aerial view and (b) lateral view of an obese feline patient. Source: Courtesy of Paola Bazan Steyling, DVM.

Performing the Small Animal Physical Examination, First Edition. Ryane E. Englar.
© 2017 John Wiley & Sons, Inc. Published 2017 by John Wiley & Sons, Inc.

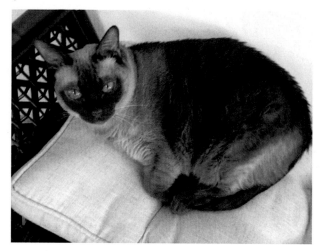

Figure 7.2 Obese feline patient with a BCS of 7/9 and age-related mild to moderate, bilaterally symmetrical muscle atrophy in both caudal thighs. Without an additional scoring system to document this loss of lean body mass, this patient may be inappropriately considered to be leaner at her next veterinary visit when in fact weight loss in this patient is not the result of loss of body fat but loss of muscle reserves.

long-coated patients are most at risk of being over-scored without palpation. The plushness of their coats can mask mild to moderate muscle atrophy that can only be appreciated with a hands-on approach [13] (Figure 7.3).

The easiest areas on the body on which to appreciate muscle mass and recognize muscle wasting are the

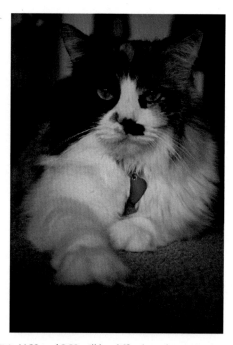

Figure 7.3 MCS and BCS will be difficult to determine based upon observation of this plush-coated cat. Palpation is required to be accurate in one's determination of both scores. Source: Courtesy of Marissa Haglund, Midwestern University CVM 2019.

bony prominences over which there are rarely fat stores to complicate a determination of muscle mass as being adequate or inadequate [13]. The prominence of the temporal bones, scapulae, transverse processes of the lumbar vertebrae, and wings of the ilia are the most common locations on the body that factor into a determination of MCS [13–17] (Figure 7.4).

Based upon muscle mass assessment at these locations, cats are ranked on a four-point scale [5, 17]:

- MCS of 3 equates to normal muscle mass. There is no muscle wasting.
- MCS of 2 equates to mild wasting of muscle mass.
- MCS of 1 equates to moderate wasting of muscle mass.
- MCS of 0 equates to severe wasting of muscle mass.

A 2011 study by Michel *et al.* demonstrated an adequate correlation between this system of scoring cats' true lean body mass as determined by dual-energy X-ray absorptiometry (DEXA) [5].

In addition to numerically providing each patient with an MCS, the clinician should note whether muscle wasting is focal or generalized, and symmetrical or asymmetrical. These details can provide the astute clinician with clues as to the underlying cause of the wasting. For example, a cat with a prior orthopedic injury to the right hind limb may have residual focal muscle wasting of the caudal thigh from disuse; a cat with osteoarthritis of both hind limbs may have bilaterally symmetrical caudal thigh muscle atrophy due to decreased range of motion and mobility; and a cat with a prior amputation of the left forearm is likely to have focal muscle wasting of the muscles that would have been important components of the thoracic girdle.

Because loss of muscle mass is associated with adverse outcomes in human medicine, early recognition of muscle wasting is emphasized so as to allow for earlier medical interventions that may expand the patient's quantity and quality of life [6, 7, 9, 13].

7.2 The Skeleton as a Whole

The skeleton can be divided into two important parts that work together to make the locomotor system functional. There is the axial skeleton, which can be thought of as the skeleton's core: it functions to protect the central nervous system from harm through its vertebral column. In addition, the axial skeleton provides core balance and stability. By contrast, the appendicular skeleton is composed of the extremities and functions to provide mobility, while connecting to the axial skeleton through the thoracic and pelvic girdles [18] (Figure 7.5).

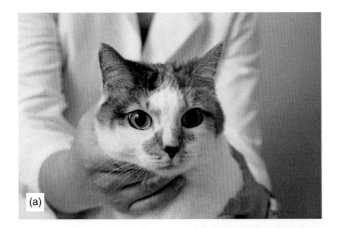
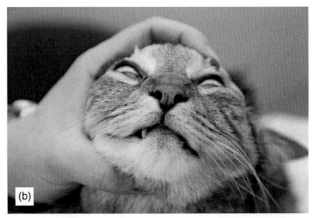
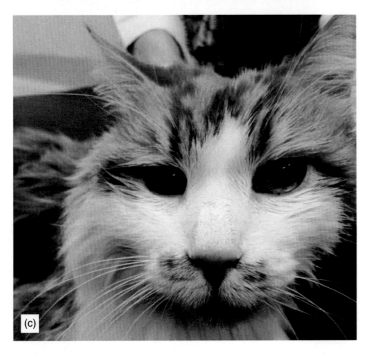
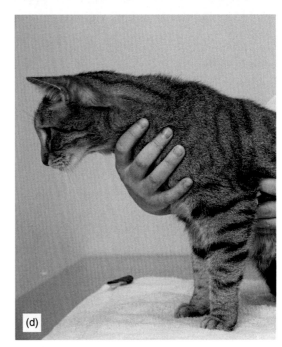
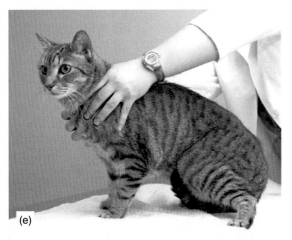
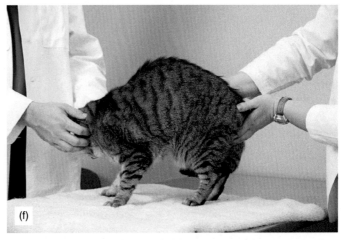

Figure 7.4 (a) The temporal muscles appear to be bilaterally symmetrical based upon gross visual examination. (b) Appreciating the symmetry of the temporal muscles via palpation. (c) This senior patient has asymmetric temporal muscles due to underlying neurologic disease. The right temporal muscles palpate as being mildly wasted compared with the left. (d) Appreciating muscle mass associated with the point of the shoulder through gross visualization. (e) Appreciating muscle mass associated with the transverse processes of the lumbar vertebrae. (f) Appreciating muscle mass associated with the wings of the ilia as well as the caudal thigh muscles. Source (a)–(f): Courtesy of the Media Resources Department at Midwestern University.

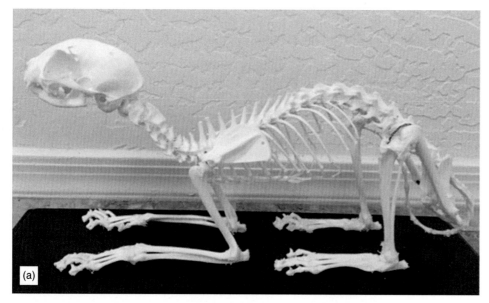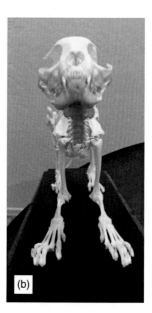

Figure 7.5 The cat skeleton when viewed (a) from the side and (b) from the front.

Both aspects of the skeleton should be assessed in each patient as part of a wellness examination. This is important in new patients to establish a baseline. However, examining the skeleton is particularly critical in new kitten visits in which the clinician may be asked to provide a health certificate or some statement to suggest that the kitten is fit for sale [18].

7.2.1 Key Components of the Axial Skeleton to Appreciate on Physical Examination

In any new kitten, the examination of the axial skeleton should begin with an assessment of the cranium and facial bones.

In fetal life, the skull bones originate from cartilage or membrane. Their ossification occurs throughout prenatal development, beginning with the maxilla and mandible around 35 days of gestation [19, 20]. Where skull bones meet, they create fibrous joints known as sutures [21]. These allow for the growth of different aspects of the skull at different rates [21]. There is a normal prenatal gap between the frontal and parietal bones that is referred to as a fontanelle [19, 21]. This structure should close before birth or shortly thereafter [19, 21, 22]. Although open fontanelles are more likely to occur in toy breeds of dogs rather than in cats, their presence or absence should be confirmed by direct palpation on any new kitten examination [22]. A persistently open fontanelle may be solely a structural defect: one-third of dogs with open fontanelles do not have concurrent neuropathy such as enlarged ventricles within the central nervous system [23]. However, depending on the fontanelle's size, it may be a risk factor for cerebral trauma

or may require further investigation into the possibility of ventriculomegaly. Studies are lacking in cats to determine the incidence of both open fontanelles and their sequelae. However, client communication is just as critical to owners of cats with open fontanelles to convey that the condition may or may not reflect an underlying brain defect.

In addition to feeling for an open fontanelle, the structure of the facial bones should be appreciated for symmetry and breed-specific traits. As discussed in Chapter 3, Persian and Exotic Shorthair breeds are characterized by a brachycephalic skull with a classically shortened face of decreased width, reduced brain case, and open orbits [24, 25]. This facial distortion, although variable in extent from cat to cat, is considered to be the breed standard and creates the classic "smushed face" appearance that is "normal" for the breed (Figure 7.6).

The astute clinician should also note the posture and carriage of the neck. Specifically, he should appreciate when there is torticollis, a twisted or so-called wry-neck, or whether the neck is ventroflexed. A cat is said to be exhibiting ventroflexion of the neck when the chin is tucked in nearer to the chest in a way that gives the illusion that the cat is bowing its head.

Ventroflexion of the neck can be due to fear: the cat hunches as if in an attempt to disappear. However, more often when ventroflexion occurs, it is the result of generalized muscle weakness [26]. Because cats do not have a nuchal ligament, muscle weakness is relatively easy to identify in the neck, which simply droops [26].

Muscle weakness severe enough to cause cervical ventroflexion in a cat typically stems from an underlying genetic, metabolic, neoplastic, nutritional, infectious, or

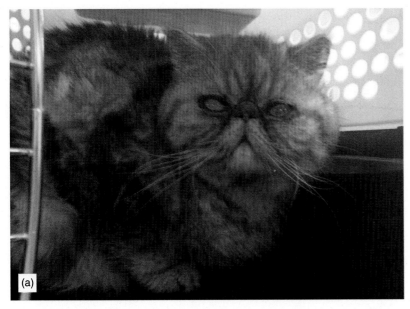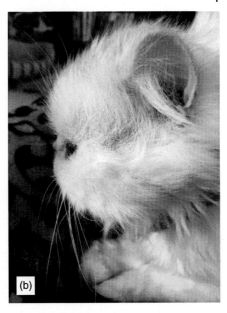

Figure 7.6 (a) Head-on view and (b) lateral view of a brachycephalic cat with the classic "smushed face" appearance due to distorted facial bone structure. Source (a), (b): Courtesy of Madison Lea Skelton.

immune disease. There is a homozygote recessive hereditary condition in Burmese cats, for example, that causes periodic hypokalemic myopathy [26–28]. This condition is caused by rapid, sporadic shifts in extracellular potassium to the intracellular space, causing acute hypokalemia. This electrolyte imbalance leads to an overall loss of excitability because cells become persistently depolarized [26]. The result is muscle weakness.

Hypokalemia is not unique to Burmese cats. There are a host of other conditions that, although not genetic, lead to hypokalemic myopathy that could present as cervical ventroflexion in cats. For example, chronic renal failure leads to potassium wasting in the urine. This is also true of cats with post-obstructional diuresis. The net result is the same. Low serum potassium leads to decreased excitability, which causes muscle weakness [26, 29].

Cervical ventroflexion from hypokalemia has also been appreciated in hyperthyroid cats [30]. Hyperthyroidism creates a hyperadrenergic state. This encourages the release of insulin, which causes intracellular translocation of potassium. Similarly, when diabetic cats are inadvertently administered an overdose of insulin, they too experience an intracellular shift in potassium that leads to hypokalemic myopathies including cervical ventroflexion [26].

Toxoplasmosis causes polymyositis, generalized muscle pain and weakness; myasthenia gravis can cause exercise-induced, generalized muscle weakness [31, 32]; and Devon Rex myopathy can cause generalized weakness that is exacerbated by stress [26].

Vegetarian diets that are deficient in potassium can cause cervical ventroflexion [33]. Thiamine deficiency due to an all-fish diet can also cause ventroflexion, although the neck ventroflexion that results tends to be active rather than passive as is the case in aforementioned conditions [26].

As is evident from the preceding discussion, the presence of cervical ventroflexion is not pathognomonic for one specific form of pathology. A cat that is presenting with a ventroflexed neck may have one or more underlying conditions that could result in the clinical sign. However, recognizing that the symptom exists is the first step to helping the client understand the need for a more extensive work-up so that the clinician is able to make a diagnosis.

In addition to noting the carriage of the neck, the clinician should evaluate its range of motion. Specifically, the clinician should encourage the cat to flex and extend the head and neck in a dorsoventral plane and also rotate the head and neck in a lateral plane. In particular, the clinician needs to determine whether there is reluctance to move the head and neck in one or more directions and also whether movement results in overt pain. The clinician's manipulations of the neck should be repeated to identify patterns in mobility, and the patient's results should be reproducible if they are to be believed [34].

The clinician should then continue to examine the remainder of the vertebral column through superficial palpation over the dorsal spinous processes of the vertebrae (Figure 7.7). This is then followed by deep palpation over the same regions and also in the spaces between the dorsal spinous processes to assess for pain. Pain could be vocalized by the patient or sometimes it is far more subtle: the patient may attempt to retreat

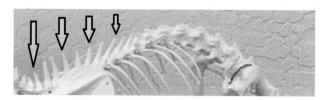

Figure 7.7 Lateral view of the cat skeleton highlighting the dorsal spinous processes of the vertebrae, which should be palpated on physical examination of any live cat.

from touch by dropping its spine away from the pressure exerted by the clinician's fingertips [34].

In addition to palpating the vertebral column for pain, the clinician should identify if there are any structural deviations from the norm. More often, these changes are subtle and identified only through radiography; however, sometimes it is possible to appreciate kyphosis, lordosis, or scoliosis on physical examination alone. These may indicate congenital or acquired spinal deformities as from automobile trauma. They may also increase the patient's risk of developing disc compression: the abnormal architecture of the vertebral column may predispose the patient to pinching of the spinal cord with resultant neuropathy.

7.2.2 Key Components of the Appendicular Skeleton to Appreciate on Physical Examination

The appendicular skeleton includes the forelimbs and the hind limbs, all four of which work together as one cohesive unit to create functional mobility.

Before each limb is examined in isolation, there are several key points that the clinician should examine pertaining to the appendicular skeleton as a whole:

- skeletal conformation;
- stance;
- weight-bearing status;
- gait.

It may seem unusual to discuss conformation when it comes to the cat. More typically, conformation is used in the equestrian world given how structure impacts function: a horse's conformation may enhance or hinder performance. The majority of feline patients are companions rather than show cats, so conformation is often forgotten. However, it is important to consider it because it may predispose the patient to structural wear and tear or create structural disease. Conformation refers to how body parts are proportioned in relation to one another, and how the skeleton as a foundation impacts the supporting architecture of muscles and connective tissue.

As an example of dwarfism, the Munchkin cat breed exhibits distinct conformational changes compared

to the domestic short-haired cat owing to its genetic shortening of the limbs (Figure 7.8). Although further research is indicated to assess the implications of dwarfism that are associated with the Munchkin cat breed [35], some clinicians have raised concerns that Munchkin cats may experience similar orthopedic maladies to their short-limbed canine "cousins," the Dachshunds and Corgis.

Another cat breed that may present with altered conformation is the Scottish Fold. The Scottish Fold was popularized for the ear fold phenotype that occurs as a result of an inherited defect in cartilage [35]. However, the same defect that is so marketable is not limited exclusively to the pinnal cartilage. Cartilage elsewhere throughout the body is also impacted, resulting in malformed joints that may make a patient reluctant to move. There is indeed a higher incidence of musculoskeletal disease in the Scottish Fold breed [36]. Depending upon the patient, orthopedic disease may be subtle and evident only as slight changes in conformation when compared with a "normal" cat.

Another aspect of conformation that should be considered when observing a cat is its stance. Cats should look like they are walking on "high heels," not as if they are walking flat-footed in "flip-flops" (Figure 7.9).

It is abnormal for cats to develop a plantigrade stance, meaning that the ventral aspect of their hind limb distal to the hock comes into contact with the surface of the floor. Cats with this stance should be evaluated for diabetic neuropathy or for rupture of the common calcaneal tendon [37, 38].

In addition to stance, limb deviations from the norm should be noted and documented. Varus deformities are characterized as having a deviation in one or more limbs toward the median line, in the sagittal plane. For example, a patient that presents with carpal varus will have a limb that, distal to the "wrist," angles toward the median line. By contrast, a patient with carpal valgus will have an angular limb deformity in which the limb distal to the "wrist" angles away from the median line. In the author's experience, varus and valgus deformities are more often seen in dogs; however, it is possible for them to be appreciated in cats also.

In addition to evaluating for angular limb deformities, the clinician should note if the patient is weight bearing and, if so, if there are any stipulations to record. For example, a patient may be apparently weight bearing at rest, but not at a walk; or at a walk, but not at a trot.

Lameness examinations in cats can be a challenge because they require the clinician to assess the patient both at rest and at an active gait, and it is a rare cat that will walk and trot on command. Most cats remain hunched or frozen throughout the entire physical

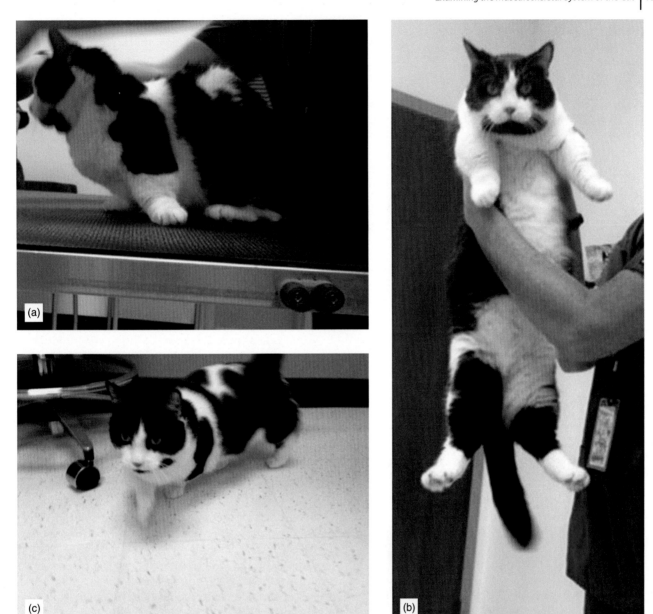

Figure 7.8 (a) Side view of the Munchkin cat on the examination room table. Note the genetic shortening of all four limbs that is associated with this cat breed. Note how evident this Munchkin cat's limb shortening is when (b) it is held and (c) it walks.

examination (Figure 7.10). Cats can also be exceptionally stoic when they perceive it to be in their best interest to hide an underlying medical concern [39, 40].

Cats may be encouraged to walk in the examination room if they are extracted from their hide-out and placed at the opposite end of the room. This may motivate them to return to their hide-out, giving the veterinary team a glimpse of their gait in the process. The treat-motivated cat may be encouraged to migrate from one side of the examination room to the other by

offering a trail of treats. Laser pointers may also entice a young or adolescent cat to exhibit play behavior, which may be sufficient for the clinician to analyze the gait. Owners may also volunteer audiovisual footage taken from their own video-recording devices to document abnormal gait witnessed in the home environment [40, 41].

If the patient is visibly lame, the clinician should attempt to answer the following questions, understanding that not all will be able to be answered given the

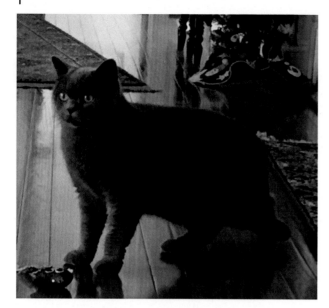

Figure 7.9 Assessing this patient's stance, which is normal. Source: Courtesy of the Media Resources Department at Midwestern University.

cat's tolerance or lack thereof toward this portion of the examination [18, 39]:

- Is the lameness a new finding or a recurrent concern?
- Was there a known inciting factor that triggered the lameness?

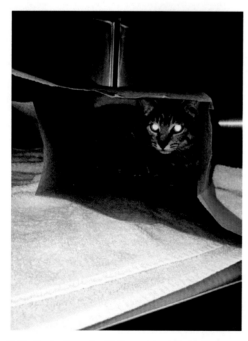

Figure 7.10 Typical hunched feline patient that is doing everything in its power to escape from view. Source: Courtesy of Breanne Craigen, CVT.

- Is the patient partially bearing weight or not bearing any weight at all? A patient that is non-weight bearing may hold up the affected limb(s). The patient may also reproducibly lean against the examination room wall to take pressure off of the affected limb(s).
- Is the lameness persistent or does it come and go?
- Does the patient exhibit shifting leg lameness? That is, does the lameness originate in one limb only to "jump" to another during the course of the examination?
- Does the patient exhibit difficulty or discomfort when standing up or sitting down?
- Is the patient's lameness worse after inactivity or is it worse after activity, such as faster gaits or stepping up and down, on and off a curb?
- Does the lameness progressively worsen with continued movement?

Grading the lameness is helpful in outlining progression of disease [18, 42, 43]. That being said, there is not one universal, standard scoring system for lameness. It is up to the individual clinician or clinic to determine how best to approach defining lameness so that it is consistently understood, recognized, and documented among team members.

If numerical grades are used to distinguish degrees of severity of lameness, an attempt should be made to use words to expand upon what each grade means. This is especially helpful for the referring veterinarian so that if the orthopedist receives a case history detailing "grade 2 lameness" of 2 weeks' duration, he is able to know precisely what that means. By having a solid picture of that clinic's scoring system and by comparing his physical examination findings with those outlined in previous reports, he can easily determine if the lameness is progressively worsening or improving.

The author's clinic has decided upon the following scoring system:

- Grade 1: Shifts weight off affected leg when at rest or standing, but does not exhibit lameness at a walk or trot.
- Grade 2: Mild lameness at trot, none at walk.
- Grade 3: Mild to moderate lameness at walk and trot.
- Grade 4: Carries limb when trotting, although may place leg when standing.
- Grade 5: Non-weight bearing.

This is in contrast to the four-point system outlined by Hazewinkel *et al.* in 2009 [18]. Again, it is less important whether one adopts the author's exact method or Hazewinkel *et al.*'s method – it is more important that each practice relies upon what works best for them, provided that it is practical and user-friendly, understandable to every member of the veterinary team.

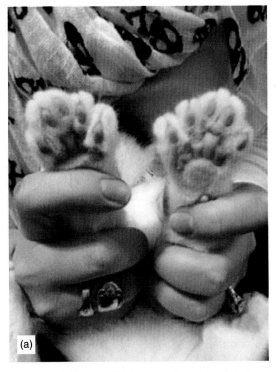
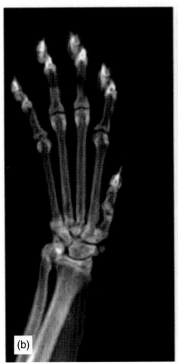
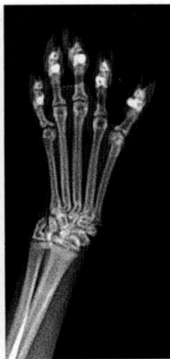

Figure 7.11 (a) Cat with bilateral polydactyly of the forepaws. (b) Radiographic demonstration of polydactyly. Compare the polydactyl forepaw in the image on the right with the normal, non-polydactyl forepaw in the image on the left to appreciate the developmental deformity of the phalanges associated with the first digit. Source (a), (b): Courtesy of Kat Mackin.

7.2.3 Additional Components of the Skeleton to Appreciate on Physical Examination

Prior to examining the forelimbs and hind limbs in depth, the astute clinician should note the presence of any other dysostoses, congenital developmental disorders of bone. One of the more common dysostoses that is seen in feline patients is polydactyly. Polydactyly is a dominant trait with variable expression that results in a patient having one or more additional digits. These digits may or may not be associated with extra claws [38, 44] (Figure 7.11). Regular nail trimming is an important aspect of maintenance for these patients because they are at increased risk of claws over-growing, potentially to the point that they drive into digital pads [38].

Another dysostosis is the congenital loss of a tail, as seen in Manx cats (Figure 7.12). Manx cats are designed to have caudal vertebral aplasia for aesthetic reasons. However, the tailless trait may occur in combination with lumbosacral spinal cord deformity. Clients need to be aware that Manx cats may exhibit reduced perineal or anal tone, if it is present at all, and that fecal and/or urinary incontinence may be chronic medical issues [45, 46].

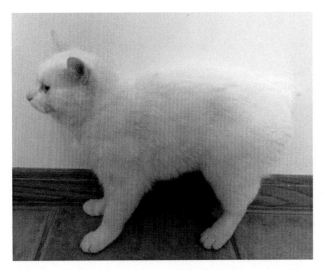

Figure 7.12 Tailless cat. Source: Courtesy of Jule Schweighoefer.

7.3 The Appendicular Skeleton: The Forelimb

The appendicular skeleton may be examined in a cat as part of a comprehensive physical examination or because there is a limb-related presenting complaint.

Owner-reported lameness is rare in cats, ranging from 4 to 16% in cats that ultimately were diagnosed with orthopedic disease by radiography [40, 41, 47–49]. Owners are 2.8 times more likely to identify and report lameness in overweight cats and 5.4 times more likely to identify and report lameness in the obese [11, 41].

Owners are more likely to report a perceived change in their cat's ability to jump and their activity level [40], although both are often attributed to the normal aging process and are therefore not always identified as true "problems." Other cats with musculoskeletal disease may present to the clinic for decreased grooming behavior [40], without the owner making the connection that joint disease could be preventing the cat from maintaining good hygiene.

Because lameness is so infrequently reported in cats, by the time that owners do recognize it, significant clinical disease is usually present. Yet many clinicians feel uncomfortable with the prospect of completing an orthopedic examination on a feline patient when it is commonplace to do the same in canine medicine. The feline orthopedic examination is not only doable, it is essential. Although it may need to be staged on account of patient tolerance and although it may require a comparison of palpation in a sedated versus an awake patient, it can facilitate the development of a list of differential diagnoses and can solidify the next steps in terms of medical management, namely "where to go from here" [40].

Section 7.2.2 touched on gait analysis relative to the whole patient. When considering gait analysis relative to the forelimbs, there are two classic gait abnormalities for the clinician to watch out for [40]:

- Unilateral forelimb lameness may cause the cat to have a head bob when bearing weight on the painful limb.
- Bilateral forelimb lameness may cause the cat to abbreviate its stride by taking short, choppy steps.

When lameness occurs, it may originate from developmental disease, trauma, as from a cat bite or fracture, degenerative joint disease, infectious disease, or neoplasia [41]. The purpose of gait analysis is not to identify the cause of the lameness, but rather the source. Owners are not always certain on presentation which limb(s) represent(s) problem areas.

Standing palpation follows gait analysis as an attempt to localize injury further and/or to appreciate normal structures, as in the case of performing a comprehensive wellness examination. Standing palpation assesses for [40]:

- Symmetry between the forelimbs in terms of bone contour: specifically, palpation concentrates on feeling for continuity of bone: are there open fractures?

- Symmetry between the forelimbs in terms of muscle mass: specifically, palpation concentrates on feeling for the supraspinatus, infraspinatus, triceps, antebrachial flexors, and antebrachial extensors [40].
- Symmetry between the forelimbs in terms of joints: specifically, palpation concentrates on joint diameter, the presence or absence of joint effusion, and the presence or absence of joint heat.

There is not one "right" way to palpate the forelimbs: where to palpate and in what order are matters of clinician preference. Some clinicians prefer to start distal and work their way up proximally, from the digits to the scapulae [39]; others work preferentially in reverse. The author tends to perform standing palpation from proximal to distal because she finds that cats tend to resent manipulation of their feet and toes.

It matters less the order of the examination, and more that the clinician is systematic with the approach that makes the most sense to them so as to cover all of the following structures:

- the thoracic girdle, which includes the scapulae and the clavicles [50, 51];
- the humerus, which comprises the brachium or arm [50, 51];
- the radius and ulna, which compose the antebrachium or forearm [50, 51];
- the carpus or wrist [50, 51];
- the metacarpals;
- the phalanges.

Each of these regions should be palpated superficially, followed by deep palpation and any associated range of motion manipulations through joints. It is common to begin this portion of the examination with the patient standing. However, by the time that range of motion manipulations are required, it is easiest to transition the patient into lateral recumbency. If one forelimb is known to be sensitive, then the author tends to examine that forelimb last [39].

When examining the thoracic girdle, only the scapulae are palpable. The clavicles are only apparent radiographically [18, 50]. The scapulae palpate as large, flat bones of the shoulder. Their outline was described by Evans in 1993 as forming "an imperfect triangle having two surfaces, three borders, and three angles" [50, p. 182].

The lateral surface of each scapula is divided by the spine of the scapula, which is prominent and palpable on a cat of ideal BCS. The supraspinous fossa containing the supraspinatus muscle is dorsal to the spine of the scapula and the infraspinous fossa, containing the infraspinatus muscle, sits ventrally. These two muscles are palpable. They should be symmetrical on comparing left and right forelimbs, and both should be non-painful on manipulation [18, 50]. The acromion is the

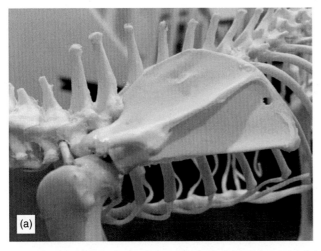 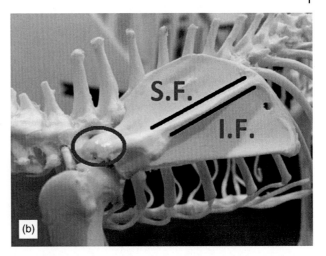

Figure 7.13 (a) Lateral view of the left scapula from a plastic model of the cat skeleton and (b) with key structures identified: the spine of the scapula is outlined with parallel black lines and the acromion is circled in blue. The supraspinous fossa is labeled S.F. and the infraspinous fossa I.F.

widest portion of the distal spine of the scapula. The acromion should be palpable as an important landmark from which muscles such as the deltoid originate [18, 50] (Figure 7.13).

Another important landmark of the scapula is the supraglenoid tubercle, from which the biceps brachii tendon originates. [50] (Figure 7.14).

The shoulder joint is formed by the articulation of the scapula and the proximal humerus. The greater tubercle of the proximal humerus, which is palpable, is where the supraspinatus muscle inserts [50] (Figure 7.15). The shoulder joint should be assessed for swelling, palpable heat that could indicate active inflammation, crepitus, pain, and tolerance of range of motion. In the normal

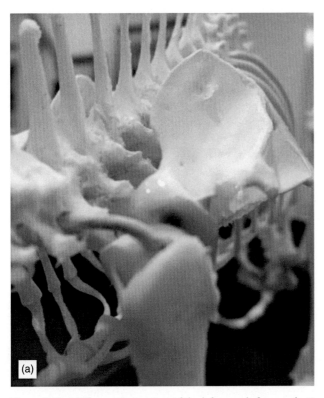 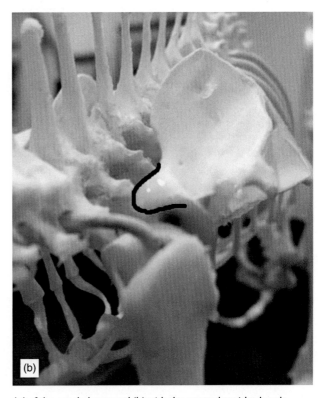

Figure 7.14 (a) Three-quarter view of the left scapula from a plastic model of the cat skeleton and (b) with the supraglenoid tubercle outlined in black.

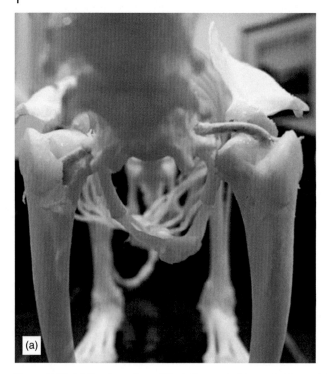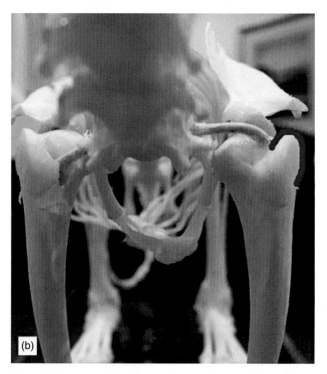

Figure 7.15 (a) Head-on view of the left scapula from a plastic model of the cat skeleton and (b) with the greater tubercle of the humerus outlined in red.

cat, the shoulder joint can be maintained at 32° in flexion and 163° in extension as determined by goniometry [52].

The body of the humerus should be palpated for angular limb deformities, swelling, asymmetry between the left and right forelimb, and pain [18]. The medial and lateral epicondyles are palpable at the distal humerus [50] (Figure 7.16). On the medial aspect of the distal humerus of the cat, but not the dog, there is a supracondylar foramen. Although this structure is not palpable, it should be noted because it allows for the passage of the median nerve and brachial artery. If a fracture were to occur in this location, compression of the nerve and/or artery could result [53].

The distal humerus of the cat also differs from canine anatomy in that the cat does not have an opening at the olecranon fossa. Again, this is not palpable; however, it is important to note because the radiographic appearance of the distal humerus in the cat will appear to be different from that of the dog [53].

Distally, the radius and ulna articulate with the humerus to form the elbow joint. The elbow joint is a common site of osteoarthritis in the cat [53, 54]. Although most of the time elbow osteoarthritis in the cat is an incidental finding on the physical examination, it is being identified with greater frequency [41, 55]. It has been hypothesized that elbow dysplasia may be an inciting factor for elbow osteoarthritis in cats, but there are few case reports on

elbow dysplasia in cats in the medical literature [53]. In general practice, congenital elbow disease such as elbow luxation is rare, yet more prevalent than elbow dysplasia [53, 56, 57]. The flexor muscles can also become avulsed from the medial epicondyle, causing feline epicondylitis that mirrors the same condition in the canine patient, although the dog is more frequently affected [53].

The elbow should be assessed for swelling, palpable heat that could indicate active inflammation, crepitus, pain, and tolerance of range of motion. In the normal cat, the elbow joint can be maintained at 22° in flexion and 162° in extension as determined by goniometry [53].

Moving distally to the antebrachium, the radius is the primary weight bearer. It is shorter than the ulna, which serves primarily as a means of muscle attachment. Proximally, its caudal surface articulates with the ulna; distally, its lateral border articulates with the ulna. Distally, the radius also articulates with the carpus to form the radiocarpal joint [50].

On palpation of the proximal antebrachium, it is possible to appreciate the radial head laterally and the caudally directed protrusion of the ulna, the olecranon. The olecranon plays an important role as a lever for the extensor muscles of the elbow [50].

The radius and ulna crisscross such that on palpation of the distal antebrachium, the radius is now the more medial of the two bones. The styloid process of the distal

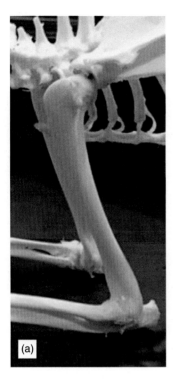

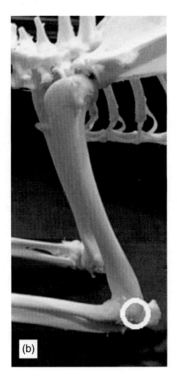

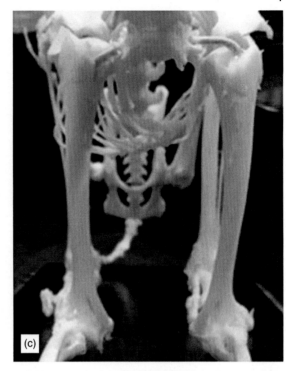

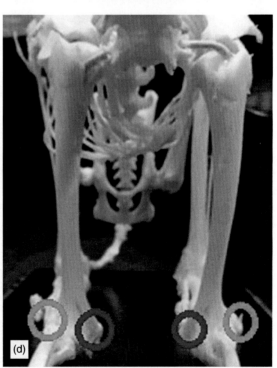

Figure 7.16 (a) Lateral view of the left humerus from a plastic model of the cat skeleton and (b) with the lateral epicondyle of the humerus outlined with a white circle. (c) Head-on view of the left and right humerus from a plastic model of the cat skeleton and (d) with the lateral epicondyles outlined with blue circles and the medial epicondyles with red circles.

ulna is palpable laterally, where it articulates with the accessory carpal bone [50] (Figure 7.17).

The carpus has seven bones arranged in two rows. (Figure 7.18). The distal row of carpal bones articulates with five metacarpal bones. The second through fifth metacarpal bones each bear three phalanges to form the second

through fifth digits; the first metacarpal bone, located medially, bears only two phalanges [50] (Figure 7.19).

Given the size of a cat's forepaw, it is very difficult to identify the individual carpal bones through palpation alone, with the exception of the accessory carpal bone. Therefore, the clinician's goal in examining the carpus

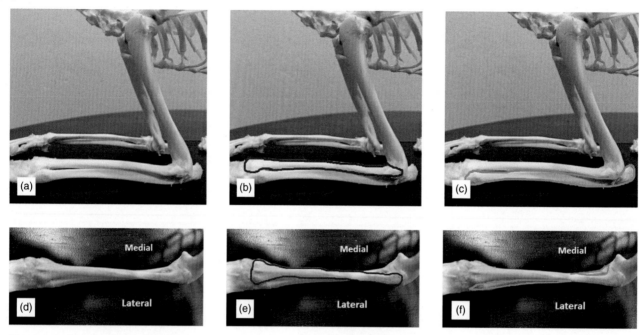

Figure 7.17 (a) Lateral view of the left radius and ulna from a plastic model of the cat skeleton, (b) with the radius outlined in red – note how the proximal radius is lateral and the distal radius is medial relative to the ulna, and (c) with the ulna outlined in blue. (d) Aerial view of the left radius and ulna from a plastic model of the cat skeleton, (e) with the radius outlined in red – note how the proximal radius is lateral and the distal radius is medial relative to the ulna, and (f) with the ulna outlined in blue.

is less to identify individual bones and more to identify any abnormalities such as swelling, heat, crepitus, asymmetry between the left and right forepaws, and pain (Figure 7.20).

The clinician should also assess carpal range of motion. In the normal cat, the carpal joint can be maintained at 22° in flexion and 198° in extension as determined by goniometry [52]. The individual metacarpal bones can be palpated, as can the digits, taking care to manipulate them in such a way as to test for the ability to extend and retract the associated claws. However, the reality is that size is a huge limitation when it comes to examination of the forepaw, and fractures of carpal and metacarpal bones and phalanges can be missed when evaluated based on the physical examination alone [39]. Radiographs provide confirmation regarding the presence or absence of fractures and should be encouraged any time pain, swelling, or lameness is localized to the distal forelimb.

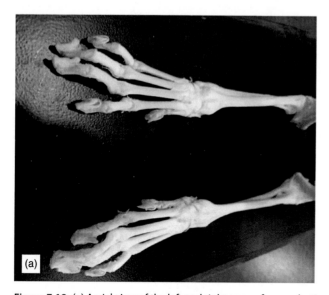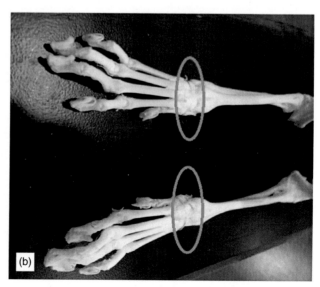

Figure 7.18 (a) Aerial view of the left and right carpus from a plastic model of the cat skeleton and (b) with the carpi outlined in blue.

Figure 7.19 (a) Aerial view of the right forepaw from a plastic model of the cat skeleton, (b) with the metacarpal bones labeled 1–5 – note that the most medial metacarpal bone is considered 1 and the most lateral metacarpal bone is considered 5, (c) with the metacarpal bones labeled 1–5 and the phalanges labeled P1, P2, and P3 – note that P1 is the most proximal phalanx and P3 is the most distal, and (d) with the metacarpal bones labeled 1–5 and the phalanges labeled P1, P2, and P3 – note that there are only two phalanges arising distal to the first metacarpal bone; these are P2 and P3.

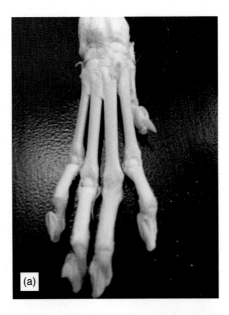

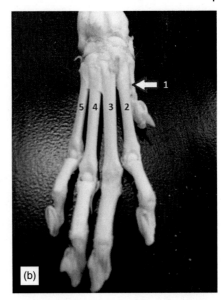

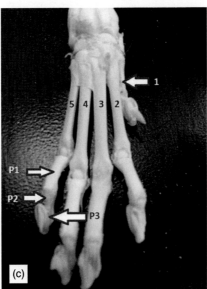

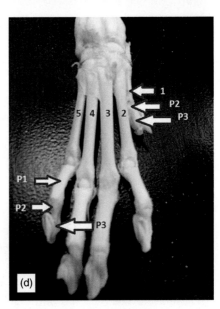

Figure 7.20 Live cat demonstrating grossly visible swelling associated with the left forepaw compared with the right. Source: Courtesy of Elizabeth Robbins, DVM.

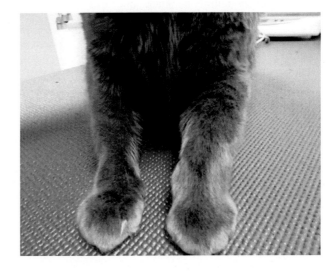

The orthopedic examination in the cat can be challenging, and student clinicians often become discouraged because unless there is an obvious fracture, abnormal physical examination findings are non-specific at best. For example, joint effusion is not pathognomonic. When it is identified at the carpus, it can result from trauma or degenerative joint disease; when it is identified at the shoulder, it can also result from a synovial cyst [39]. However, the better a clinician is able to localize the medical concern, the better equipped they will be when considering the most likely differential diagnoses and their approach to both the diagnostic work-up and the proposed treatment plans.

It is also important to replicate abnormal physical examination findings rather than to believe an isolated event. For example, a cat that might not prefer its feet to be touched might initially resist manipulation of the forepaw. It might be tempting to believe that cat is feeling pain and therefore localize the concern to that location, when in fact it might just be that the cat was simply startled the first time that manipulation was attempted.

The veterinarian should alert the owner that certain manipulations will be repeated, especially if there is a concern on the veterinarian's part that the manipulation may be painful, so that the owner knows there is a reason for the veterinarian continuing to induce pain.

7.4 The Appendicular Skeleton: The Hind Limb

Section 7.2.2 covered gait analysis relative to the whole patient. When considering gait analysis relative to the hind limbs, there are two classic gait abnormalities for the clinician to watch out for [40]:

- Unilateral hind limb lameness may cause the cat to have a hip hike: the hip of the affected leg elevates when bearing weight on the painful limb.
- Bilateral hind limb lameness may cause the cat to abbreviate its stride by taking short, choppy steps.

Broad categories of causes of forelimb lameness were reviewed in Section 7.3. The same categories could be responsible for lameness of the hind limbs.

Standing palpation follows gait analysis as an attempt to localize injury further and/or to appreciate normal structures, as in the case of performing a comprehensive wellness examination. Standing palpation assesses for [40]:

- Symmetry between the hind limbs in terms of bone contour: specifically, palpation concentrates on feeling for continuity of bone: are there open fractures?
- Symmetry between the hind limbs in terms of muscle mass: specifically, palpation concentrates on feeling

for the hamstrings, quadriceps, cranial tibial muscles, gastrocnemius, soleus, and the Achilles tendon [40].
- Symmetry between the hind limbs in terms of joints: specifically, palpation concentrates on joint diameter, the presence or absence of joint effusion, and the presence or absence of joint heat

As was discussed when considering palpation of the forelimbs, there is not one "right" way to palpate the hind limbs: the methodology of where to palpate and when is a matter of clinician preference. Some clinicians prefer to start distal and work their way up proximally, from the digits to the wings of the ilia [39]; others work preferentially in reverse. As mentioned, the author tends to perform standing palpation from proximal to distal because she finds that cats tend to resent manipulation of their feet and toes.

It matters less the order of the exam, and more that the clinician is systematic with the approach that makes the most sense so as to cover all of the following structures:

- the pelvic girdle, which includes the ilium, ischium, pubis, and acetabulum [50, 51];
- the femur, which comprises the thigh [50, 51];
- the tibia and fibula, which compose the lower leg [50, 51];
- the tarsus or ankle [50, 51];
- the metatarsals;
- the phalanges.

As with the forelimbs, each of the listed hind limb regions should be palpated superficially, followed by deep palpation and any associated range of motion manipulations through joints. It is common to begin this portion of the examination with the patient standing. However, by the time that range of motion manipulations are required, it is easiest to transition the patient into lateral recumbency. If one hind limb is known to be sensitive, then the author tends to examine that hind limb last [39].

When examining the pelvic girdle, the wings of the ilia and the ischiatic tuberosity are palpable [18, 50] (Figure 7.21).

Pelvic trauma is common in cats owing to their tendency to be involved in vehicular accidents [53, 58, 59]. When hit-by-car injuries are sustained, cats often experience femoral luxations or fractures [59]. In order for a cat to sustain the former type of traumatic injury, there has to have been a tear in the coxofemoral joint capsule and also in the teres ligament [53]. When femoral luxations occur in cats, 72% of the time they involve cranio-dorsal migration of the femur [53, 59]. Radiographs are confirmatory for this condition (Figure 7.22).

The astute clinician is able to diagnose cranio-dorsal coxofemoral luxation based upon abnormal physical examination findings alone. In a normal cat, the wings of the ilia, ischiatic tuberosities, and greater trochanters

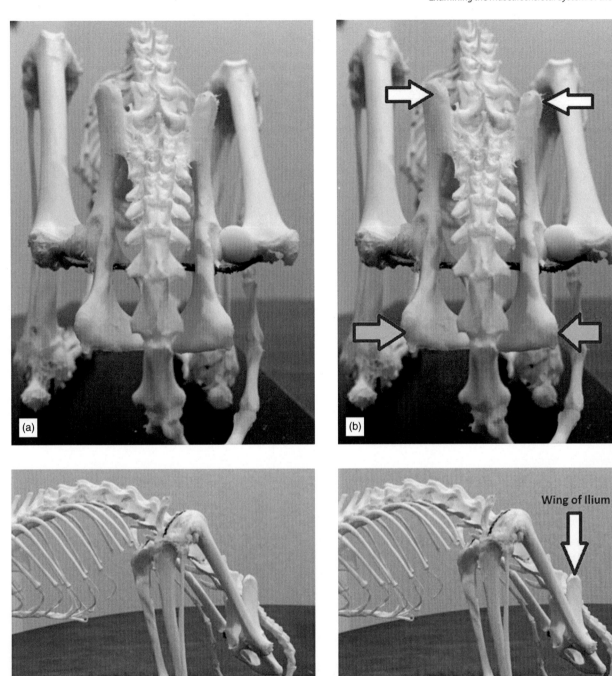

Figure 7.21 End-on, lateral, and aerial views of a plastic model of a cat skeleton, with the cat in a sphinx-like, crouched pose. (a) End-on view: the emphasis is on the pelvis, and (b) with the wings of the ilia identified by white arrows and the ischiatic tuberosities by pink arrows. (c) Lateral view: the emphasis is on the pelvis, and (d) with the wing of the left ilium identified by a white arrow and the left ischiatic tuberosity by a pink arrow. (*Continued*)

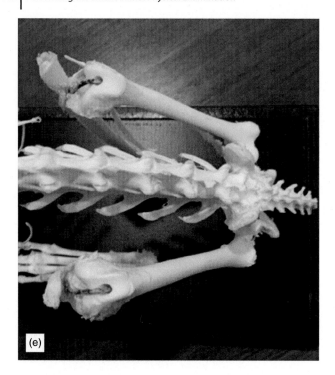
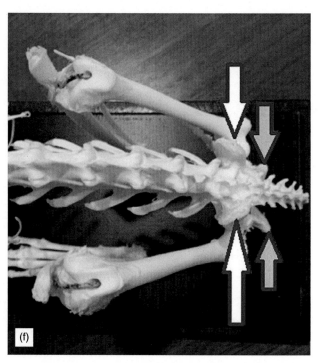

Figure 7.21 (*Continued*)
(e) Aerial view: the emphasis is on the pelvis, and (f) with the wings of the ilia identified by white arrows and the ischiatic tuberosities by pink arrows.

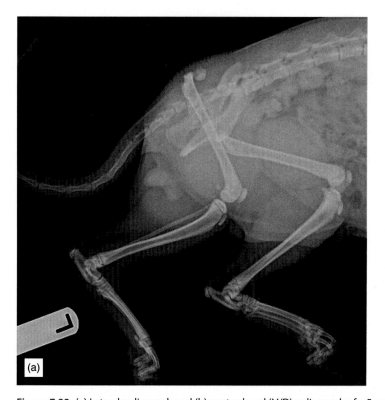
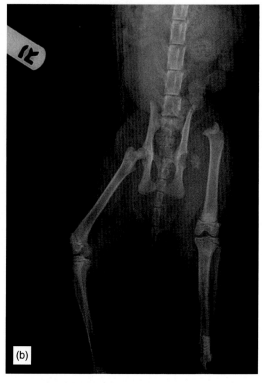

Figure 7.22 (a) Lateral radiograph and (b) ventrodorsal (V/D) radiograph of a 5-month-old intact male domestic short-haired kitten that had sustained a traumatic, oblique, closed fracture through the left femoral head and neck with cranio-dorsal displacement of the left femur relative to the coxofemoral joint.

Figure 7.23 (a) End-on view of a plastic model of a cat skeleton, with the cat in a sphinx-like, crouched pose. The emphasis is on the pelvis. The wings of the ilia are identified by white arrows, the ischiatic tuberosities by pink arrows, and the greater trochanters by blue arrows. (b) Note the imaginary triangle that is formed by the wings of the ilia (identified by white circles), the ischiatic tuberosities (pink circles), and the greater trochanters (blue circles).

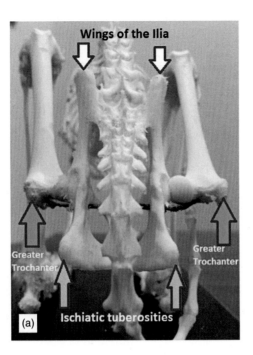
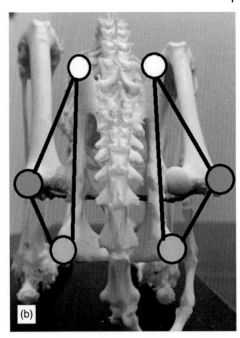

should form a triangle that is symmetrical on both the left and right sides (Figure 7.23). When there is a cranio-dorsal coxofemoral luxation, the greater trochanter on the affected side pathologically migrates in a cranio-dorsal direction, causing a disruption in this triangle [18] (Figure 7.24).

Another means by which to assess for cranio-dorsal coxofemoral luxation is for the clinician to place a thumb between the greater trochanter and the ischiatic tuberosity. Simultaneously, the clinician applies pressure to lift both hind limbs up gently and extend them caudally. Leg length is compared by assessing the location of the right and left calcanei. In cases involving cranio-dorsal coxofemoral luxation, the affected side will appear to have the shorter leg because the femur has been moved in a cranio-dorsal direction from its original seat within the acetabulum [18].

In addition to pelvic trauma, congenital pelvic deformities are possible. Although hip dysplasia has been classically linked to canine orthopedics, isolated cases of feline hip dysplasia were reported in the medical literature as early as the 1970s [60, 61]. The incidence is higher in purebreds especially Maine Coons, Himalayans, Siamese, Persians, the Abyssinian, and the Devon Rex [62, 63]. Radiographic prevalence ranges from 7 to 32% [62, 63].

Dysplastic hips are characterized as having a shallow acetabulum. Given that the feline acetabulum is already shallower than its canine counterpart, an even shallower acetabulum in a dysplastic hip results in inadequate coverage of the femoral head, if it is covered at all [38] (Figure 7.25).

As a result of hip dysplasia, cats may be reluctant to climb or descend stairs, and they may also exhibit varying degrees of lameness. As with many cases of orthopedic disease, owners may not pick up on subtle clinical signs.

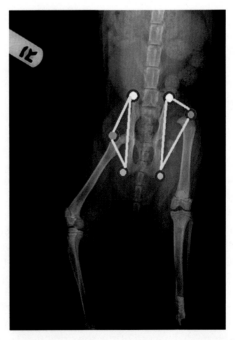

Figure 7.24 Compare this figure with Figure 7.23b. In this figure, note how the imaginary triangle that is formed by the wings of the ilia (identified by white circles), the ischiatic tuberosities (pink circles), and the greater trochanters (blue circles) is shifted owing to cranio-dorsal coxofemoral luxation of the left femur.

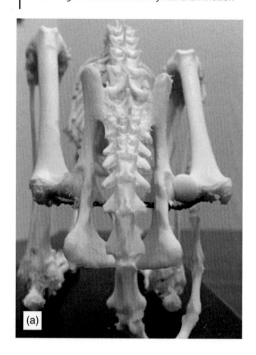

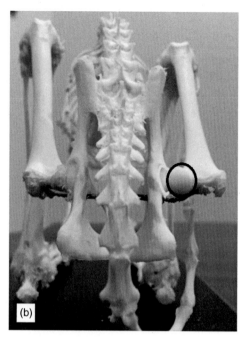

Figure 7.25 End-on-views of a plastic model of a cat skeleton, with the cat in a sphinx-like, crouched pose. The emphasis is on the pelvis, specifically on the coxofemoral joint. In (b), note how the right femoral head is not seated within the acetabulum. This is an example of right-sided hip dysplasia.

The patient may appear to be aclinical from the owner's perspective, yet the clinician may find abnormalities on the physical examination that raise the index of clinical suspicion. For example, they may pick up on hindquarter muscle atrophy due to disuse [53].

Radiographs are diagnostic for hip dysplasia: in dysplastic cats, they are confirmatory for the shallow acetabulum and femoral subluxation that is classic for the disease [38, 53]. However, radiographic signs do not correlate well with the severity of clinical disease. Mild changes on radiographs may be present in a cat that is clinical for advanced disease. By contrast, severe changes on radiographs may be found in a cat that presents with only subtle signs of disease [53].

The coxofemoral joint should be assessed for swelling, palpable heat that could indicate active inflammation, crepitus, pain, and tolerance of range of motion. Cats are not small dogs. Whereas dogs have 70–80° of flexion and 80–90° of extension at the hip, cats exhibit less hip flexion (30–60°) but significantly greater extension (100–165°) [53, 64].

The proximal femur is a key component of the coxofemoral joint. The femoral head, a hemispherical projection, sits within the pelvic acetabulum. Hyaline cartilage lines the articulating surface of the femoral head with the exception of the fovea capitis, a depression along the medial aspect of the proximal epiphysis. The fovea capitis is the site of attachment of the ligament of the head of the femur, which anchors the femur to the ventral acetabulum. The femoral neck supports the head and joins it to the proximal femoral epiphysis [50, 51, 65].

The proximal femur is exposed to large tensile and compressive forces during everyday activity, and the leaves of the trabeculae of the proximal femur are arranged to withstand these forces. Additional reinforcement is provided by the linea transversa, a ridge extending from the base of the femoral head to the greater trochanter. Together, the trabeculae and linea transversa counteract bending forces to stabilize the proximal femur and the coxofemoral joint [50, 51, 65, 66].

The greater trochanter further stabilizes the skeleton by serving as an attachment site for the middle gluteal, deep gluteal, and piriformis muscles. These muscles initiate hip extension, abduction, and medial rotation of the pelvic limb [50, 51, 65, 66].

The trochanteric fossa is a depression that is located medial to the greater trochanter and is the point of attachment for the internal and external obturator and gemelli muscles to achieve lateral rotation of the hip. Distal and caudomedial to the femoral neck is the lesser trochanter, where the iliopsoas muscle attaches to allow flexion of the hip [50, 51, 65, 66] (Figure 7.26).

As already mentioned, the greater trochanter is palpable on physical examination of the cat, in contrast to the remainder of the proximal femur, which is less easily accessed [18]. Yet proximal femoral fractures with and without greater trochanter involvement do occur and should be considered [67], especially in juvenile cats with unknown histories who present for clinical lameness. These fractures may be the result of trauma [67]. However, atraumatic fractures of the capital femoral epiphysis are on the rise in young, male cats

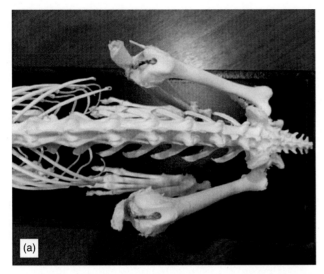 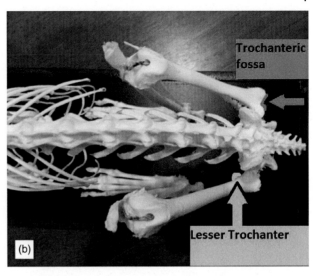

Figure 7.26 Aerial views of a plastic model of a cat skeleton, with the cat in a sphinx-like, crouched pose. The emphasis is on the femur. In (b), the trochanteric fossa is outlined in orange and the lesser trochanter in pink.

[67–72]. This condition is referred to as slipped capital femoral epiphysis (SCFE). The end result is displacement of the proximal femoral metaphysis from the capital femoral epiphysis through the growth plate [73]. Purebreds are overrepresented in case reports in the medical literature, including Siamese and Siamese mixes [70, 73], Maine Coons [68], British Blues [70, 74], Birmans [70], and Abyssinians [75]. Classically, there is no known history of trauma and the majority of the patients reported in the literature are described by their owners as having an "indoor only" lifestyle [72, 74].

When SCFE occurs, it is not always unilateral. In a 2001 study by Craig [73], five of 13 cats were bilaterally affected, compared with five of 26 in a 2002 study by McNicholas *et al.* [68]. Furthermore, of the 26 cats that were examined by McNicholas *et al.*, four that had initially presented with a unilateral fracture sustained a subsequent fracture in the contralateral femur. Thus, SCFE can be bilateral and affect both femoral heads and necks concurrently, or a fracture of the contralateral femur can occur separately from the first event.

Patients with SCFE typically exhibit varying degrees of acute, acute-on-chronic, or chronic lameness in the affected pelvic limb(s). More often, the owner reports apparent stiffness or weakness in the cat's hind end or the cat's decreased ability to jump [68, 70]. On physical examination, SCFE is not palpable. However, muscle atrophy at the hip and thigh of the affected limb(s) may be present and facilitate localization of disease [68]. Palpable crepitus over the hip joint as the hip is carried through its normal range of motion is commonly seen in cats with SCFE [68]. Hindlimb reflexes tend to be normal in cats with SCFE. However, proprioception of

the affected limb may be reduced [74]. A key feature of the orthopedic examination in cats with SCFE is pain on hip extension and occasionally pain on hip flexion [70, 76]. Palpation over the greater trochanter of the affected limb(s) may also elicit pain [76].

When SCFE is suspected, orthogonal radiographs of the pelvis and coxofemoral joints are important diagnostic tests. Radiographic findings that are characteristic of SCFE include loss of definition of the femoral neck with or without femoral neck sclerosis. It may be difficult to determine the borders of the femoral head, femoral neck, and the greater trochanter [74]. The femoral neck region often takes on an "apple core" appearance: it appears to be eroded due to bone destruction and/or resorption in the region of the proximal femoral metaphysis (Figure 7.27].

The femoral head may be grossly deformed or flattened. In some cases, complete femoral head separation is evident as an irregular radiolucent line across the femoral neck [70]. If a capital physeal fracture is apparent, there is typically minimal to no displacement. Chronic cases tend to demonstrate greater osteolysis [68, 77].

Returning to the main task at hand, performing an orthopedic examination of the feline hind limb, the body of the femur should be palpated for swelling, pain, and asymmetry between the left and right hind limbs. The medial and lateral epicondyles are palpable at the distal femur [50, 51].

The femoral trochlea, located at the cranial surface of the distal femur, between the medial and lateral epicondyles of the femur, is not palpable on physical examination (Figure 7.28). However, the patella or knee cap articulates with this smooth surface [50].

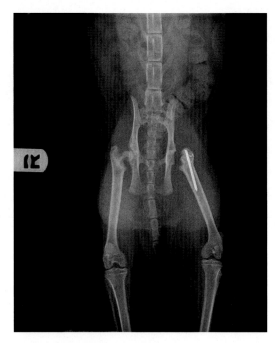

Figure 7.27 Ventrodorsal (V/D) radiograph of an 11-month-old intact male domestic short-haired kitten – the same kitten that in Figure 7.22, at 5 months of age, had sustained a traumatic, oblique, closed fracture through the left femoral head and neck with cranio-dorsal displacement of the left femur relative to the coxofemoral joint. The left femoral head and neck fracture had been surgically repaired. However, note the classic "apple core" appearance of the right femoral neck region. This patient was subsequently diagnosed with right femoral SCFE based upon histopathology.

The patella is palpable in cats [18] as an ossification within the tendon of insertion of the quadriceps femoris muscle, which extends the stifle [50]. To locate the patella, it may be easiest for the clinician first to identify the tibial crest, a prominence at the cranial aspect of the proximal tibia. Proximal to the tibial crest is the tibial tuberosity. The patellar tendon runs from the tibial tuberosity to the patella. Hence by tracking the patellar tendon proximally from the tibial tuberosity, the clinician should reach the patella (Figure 7.29).

The patella's ability to luxate should be tested on physical examination. Cats tend to have more laxity in their patellas than dogs, meaning that it is not uncommon for a normal cat to be able to luxate the patella with moderate force, provided that the patella immediately returns to its normal anatomical position once the force has abated [38, 53]. This would be considered a Grade 1 luxation in a dog, but can be normal in a cat.

When a cat has a so-called Grade 2 luxation, the patella is usually seated in its correct anatomical position. However, luxation is easily achieved. A Grade 3 luxation is characterized by a patella that is typically out of position, yet can be manually replaced to its normal anatomical location with ease. A Grade 4 luxation cannot be reduced: the patella is always seated out of position without the ability to replace it manually [38]. Patellar luxations in cats, like dogs, are considered congenital [38, 78], with apparent breed predispositions in the Devon Rex, Abyssinian, and domestic short-haired cats [78–85].

When patellar luxations occur, they are typically bilateral and medial [38, 53]. It is thought that they occur due to a developmentally shallower trochlear groove [53]. Over time, the increased motion of the patella in inappropriate locations causes erosion of articular cartilage on the trochlear ridge and predisposes the patient to osteoarthritis of the stifle joint. In moderate to severe cases, the affected patient may present with externally rotated stifles and a stiff, crouched gait [53].

In addition to localizing the patella and identifying whether or the not pathologic patellar luxation is present, the stifle or knee joint should be assessed

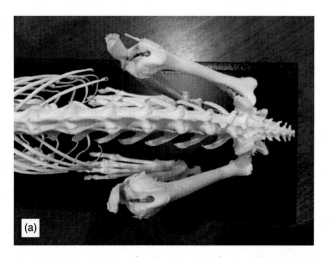

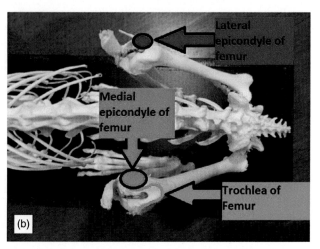

Figure 7.28 Aerial views of a plastic model of a cat skeleton, with the cat in a sphinx-like, crouched pose. The emphasis is on the femur. In (b) the femoral trochlea is outlined in blue, the medial femoral epicondyle is represented by an orange circle and the lateral femoral epicondyle by a purple circle.

Figure 7.29 Head-on views of the distal feline hind limb with focus on the cranial aspect of the tibia. In (b) the tibial crest is outlined as a blue triangle.

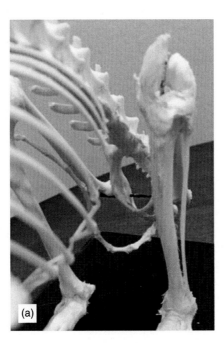

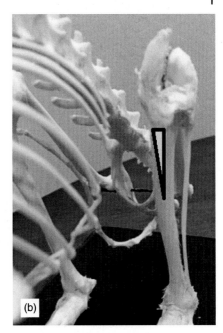

for swelling, palpable heat that could indicate active inflammation, crepitus, pain, and tolerance of range of motion. In the normal cat, the stifle joint can be maintained at 24° in flexion and 164° in extension as determined by goniometry [53].

The stifle joint is stabilized by several ligaments as it undergoes motion in the x-axis (flexion and extension) and y-axis (rotation): the medial and lateral collateral ligaments and the cranial and caudal cruciate ligaments [86]. The medial collateral ligament originates from the medial femoral epicondyle and the medial border of the tibia. It fuses with the joint capsule and attaches to the medial meniscus. Portions of this ligament selectively tighten throughout stifle flexion and extension to maintain the integrity of the joint [86, 87]. The lateral collateral ligament begins at the lateral femoral epicondyle and inserts on the head of the fibula. During flexion, this ligament is lax to allow for internal rotation of the stifle joint. By contrast, this ligament tightens during extension of the stifle [86, 87].

The cranial and caudal cruciate ligaments collectively prevent cranial translocation, movement of the tibia cranial to the femur, during weight bearing [87]. The caudomedial aspect of the lateral femoral condyle is the origin of the cranial cruciate ligament. From the condyle, the cranial cruciate ligament travels cranio-medially to insert on the cranial intercondyloid area of the tibia. Think of the cranial cruciate ligament as passing "like a hand in the pants pocket" [18]. Both its craniomedial and caudolateral bands remain taught through extension; however, the caudolateral band relaxes during flexion [86, 87]. The lateral surface of the medial femoral condyle is the origin of the caudal cruciate ligament.

From the condyle, the caudal cruciate ligament travels caudodistally to the popliteal notch of the tibia [86, 87].

The cranial and caudal cruciate ligaments cross each other as they course from origin to insertion; the cranial cruciate ligament is seated lateral to the caudal cruciate [87]. Rupture of the cranial cruciate ligament is more often seen clinically than tears of the caudal cruciate ligament, and classically both have been considered canine orthopedic diseases. However, cranial cruciate ligament rupture also occurs in cats. Historically, it was associated with traumatic injuries in cats such as high-rise syndrome, yet trauma is not always observed. More recent studies suggest that cranial cruciate ligament rupture in the cat may simply be the result of chronic ligament degeneration [38, 53, 88, 89].

When rupture of the cranial cruciate ligament occurs in the cat, the caudal cruciate ligament may follow suit. This causes pathologic hyperextension of the stifle, characterized by pronounced luxation of the tibia cranially. Additionally, the medial collateral ligament may be compromised [38]. Because cranial cruciate ligament injury destabilizes the stifle joint, the abnormal mobility of bone against bones leads to progressive wear and tear of the articular cartilage. The menisci tend to be damaged over time. When damage occurs, the lateral meniscus tends to be most often sacrificed [89]. In addition, the proximal patella, patellar groove, and mediodorsal tibia tend to develop radiographically diagnosed osteophytes [88].

Feline patients with cranial cruciate ligament injury are typically lame, with stifle effusion, and overt aversion to stifle manipulation by the attending clinician. There may or may not be a "click" when the stifle is put through its range of motion. When present, this "click" has historically been considered indicative of meniscal tearing. However, it is an inconsistent finding at best [53, 81].

When cranial cruciate ligament injury is suspected, it can be confirmed by the cranial drawer or tibial thrust tests [53, 90, 91]. The cranial drawer test is performed with the patient in lateral recumbency. If the patient's right stifle is suspected of cranial cruciate ligament injury, then the patient should be placed gently in left lateral recumbency so that the right hind limb is available for manipulation. In this example, the tip of the clinician's left index finger will be placed over the patella and his thumb will be placed over the femoral fabella. This serves to anchor the femur. The clinician then lays his right index finger over the tibial crest and plants his right thumb behind the head of the fibula. This stabilizes the proximal tibia. Holding the femur steady, the clinician then applies cranially directed force to the tibia with his right hand to attempt cranial translocation of the tibia. If this occurs, then the stifle has been pathologically hyperextended. The patient is said to be positive for cranial drawer, which confirms injury to the cranial cruciate ligament [18, 86] (Figure 7.30).

The tibial thrust test is also typically performed with the patient in lateral recumbency. The premise of this test is that when the tarsus is flexed while the stifle is extended, an intact cranial cruciate ligament should prevent hyperextension of the stifle. As before, if the patient's right stifle is suspected of cranial cruciate ligament injury, then the patient should be placed gently in left lateral recumbency so that the right hind limb is available for manipulation. The clinician gently lays his left index finger over patient's patella and tibial crest. He uses the placement of this forefinger to sense for abnormal cranial movement of the tibia as his right hand grasps the right metatarsal region and directs the tarsus into flexion. If cranial cruciate ligament injury is present, then forward motion of the tibia will be appreciated [18, 91] (Figure 7.31).

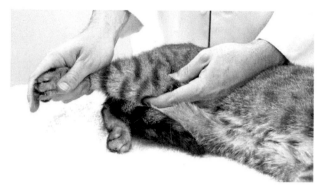

Figure 7.31 Testing for tibial thrust in this feline patient's right stifle. Source: Courtesy of the Media Resources Department at Midwestern University.

One should also assess for the stability of the medial and lateral collateral ligaments. To assess for medial collateral ligament stability, the patient is again placed in lateral recumbency with the limb of interest up and available for manipulation. The limb of interest is held in extension. The clinician grasps the limb's distal femur in one hand and the proximal tibia in the other. With the hand that is on the proximal tibia, the clinician attempts to abduct the tibia relative to the femur. If the medial collateral ligament is intact, the clinician should not feel displacement of the tibia [18].

To assess for lateral collateral ligament stability, the patient remains in lateral recumbency, with the "up" limb held in extension. The clinician grasps the limb's distal femur in one hand and the proximal tibia in the other. With the hand that is on the proximal tibia, the clinician attempts to adduct the tibia relative to the femur. If the lateral collateral ligament is intact, the clinician should not feel the lateral joint space open up [18].

Admittedly, these manipulations are easier to perform in a dog than a cat because dogs are more likely to tolerate them and because they tend to be larger, with more room for the clinician to insert his hands. Cats may also require sedation for the orthopedic examination to be comprehensive in a patient with suspected orthopedic disease.

When the orthopedic examination moves beyond the stifle joint to the crus, the clinician can consider the more cranially positioned tibia and the narrow fibula. The tibia is the primary weight-bearing bone of the crus; the function of the laterally located fibula is to serve as a site for muscle attachment [50]. The proximal tibia is flat to allow for articulation with the femur. The medial and lateral tibial condyles are separated from the medial and lateral femoral condyles only by the medial and lateral menisci, which are incomplete, biconcave discs [50]. Between the tibial condyles and caudally located is the popliteal notch. Recall that this is an attachment site for the caudal cruciate ligament [86, 87].

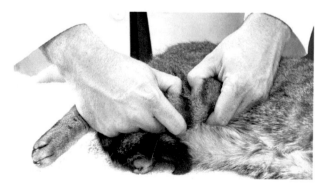

Figure 7.30 Testing for cranial drawer in this feline patient's right stifle. Source: Courtesy of the Media Resources Department at Midwestern University.

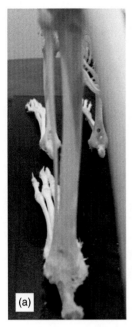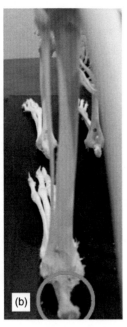

Figure 7.32 End-on views of the left crus and tarsus, with emphasis on the tuber calcanei, which is circled in blue in (b).

Distally, the tibia ends as the medial malleolus. Caudal to the medial malleolus are distinct notches and sulci that provide attachment sites for tarsal flexors [50].

Proximally, the head of the fibula articulates with the caudolateral aspect of the lateral tibial condyle. Distally, it ends as the lateral malleolus. Along the medial aspect of the lateral malleolus, there is an articulating surface that allows for the intimate connection involving the trochlea of the tibial tarsal bone or talus [50].

Although the tarsus is like the carpus in that they both consist of seven bones, there are three key differences.

First, both the tibia and fibula articulate only with the tibial tarsal bone, whereas the radius and ulna have a broader connection to the carpus. Second, the tarsus is three times longer than the carpus. Third, the tarsus contains an extremely varied set of tarsal bones based upon size and shape. The largest, longest bone of the tarsus is the calcaneus. Proximally, the calcaneus forms a prominent level, the tuber calcanei, upon which the calcaneal tendon inserts (Figure 7.32). Distally, it forms a stable joint with the tibial tarsal bone [50].

The clinician should assess the stability of the medial and lateral tarsal collateral ligaments, each of which is composed of two bands, a short and a long. To assess for instability of each band, the tarsus should be tested for displacement in flexion (damage to the short band will result in instability) and also the tarsus in extension (damage to the long band will result in instability).

The distal row of tarsal bones articulates with four metatarsal bones that are identified as being the second through fifth. The second metatarsal bone is the most medially located [50]. Each metatarsal bone bears three phalanges to form the second through fifth digits [50] (Figure 7.33).

Given the size of a cat's hind paw, it is very difficult to identify the individual tarsal bones through palpation alone, with the exception of the calcaneus. Therefore, the clinician's goal in examining the tarsus is less to identify individual bones and more to identify any abnormalities such as swelling, heat, crepitus, asymmetry between the left and right hind paw, and pain (Figure 7.34).

The clinician should also assess tarsal range of motion. In the normal cat, the tarsal joint can be maintained at 21° in flexion and 167° in extension as determined by goniometry [52].

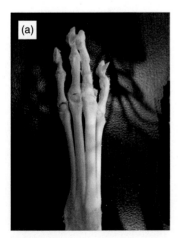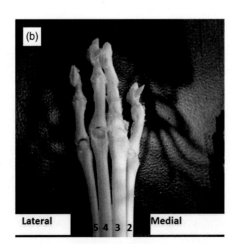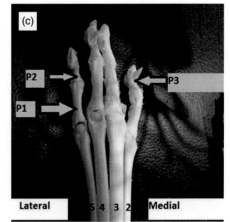

Figure 7.33 Aerial views of the left hind paw from a plastic model of the cat skeleton. In (b) the metatarsal bones are labeled 2–5, with the most medial metacarpal bone considered as 2 and the most lateral metacarpal bone as 5. In (c) the metatarsal bones are labeled 2–5 and the phalanges are labeled P1, P2, and P3, where P1 is the most proximal phalanx and P3 is the most distal.

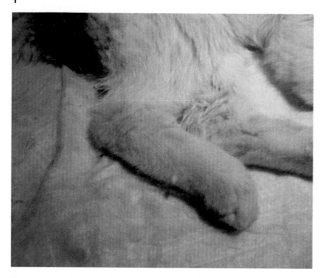

Figure 7.34 Live cat demonstrating grossly visible swelling associated with the right hind paw compared with the left. Source: Courtesy of Daniel Foy, MS, DVM, DACVIM, DACVECC.

The individual metatarsal bones can be palpated, as can the digits, taking care to manipulate them in such a way as to test for the ability to extend and retract the associated claws. However, the reality is that size is a huge limitation when it comes to examination of the hind paw, and fractures of tarsal, metatarsal bones, and phalanges can be missed when evaluated based on the physical examination alone [39]. Radiographs provide confirmation regarding the presence or absence of fractures and should be encouraged any time pain, swelling, or lameness is localized to the distal hind limb.

As already mentioned, the orthopedic examination can be challenging in the cat. However, the more student clinicians practice, the more likely they will be to pick up on subtle changes that can facilitate diagnostic, medical, and/or surgical management.

References

1 German, A.J. (2006) The growing problem of obesity in dogs and cats. *Journal of Nutrition*, **136** (7 Suppl.), 1940S–1946S.

2 German, A.J., Holden, S.L., Moxham, G.L. *et al.* (2006) A simple, reliable tool for owners to assess the body condition of their dog or cat. *Journal of Nutrition*, **136** (7 Suppl.), 2031S–2033S.

3 Bjornvad, C.R., Nielsen, D.H., Armstrong, P.J. *et al.* (2011) Evaluation of a nine-point body condition scoring system in physically inactive pet cats. *American Journal of Veterinary Research*, **72** (4), 433–437.

4 Laflamme, D. (1997) Development and validation of a body condition score system for cats: a clinical tool. *Feline Practice*, **25** (5–6), 13–18.

5 Michel, K.E., Anderson, W., Cupp, C., and Laflamme, D.P. (2011) Correlation of a feline muscle mass score with body composition determined by dual-energy X-ray absorptiometry. *British Journal of Nutrition*, **106** (Suppl. 1), S57–S59.

6 Freeman, L.M. (2012) Cachexia and sarcopenia: emerging syndromes of importance in dogs and cats. *Journal of Veterinary Internal Medicine*, **26** (1), 3–17.

7 Anker, S.D., Ponikowski, P., Varney, S. *et al.* (1997) Wasting as independent risk factor for mortality in chronic heart failure. *Lancet*, **349** (9058), 1050–1053.

8 Anker, S.D., Negassa, A., Coats, A.J. *et al.* (2003) Prognostic importance of weight loss in chronic heart failure and the effect of treatment with angiotensin-converting-enzyme inhibitors: an observational study. *Lancet*, **361** (9363), 1077–1083.

9 Freeman, L.M. and Roubenoff, R. (1994) The nutrition implications of cardiac cachexia. *Nutrition Reviews*, **52** (10), 340–347.

10 Baez, J.L., Michel, K.E., Sorenmo, K., and Shofer F.S. (2007) A prospective investigation of the prevalence and prognostic significance of weight loss and changes in body condition in feline cancer patients. *Journal of Feline Medicine and Surgery*, **9** (5), 411–417.

11 Scarlett, J.M. and Donoghue, S. (1998) Associations between body condition and disease in cats. *Journal of the American Veterinary Medical Association*, **212** (11), 1725–1731.

12 Doria-Rose, V.P. and Scarlett, J.M. (2000) Mortality rates and causes of death among emaciated cats. *Journal of the American Veterinary Medical Association*, **216** (3), 347–351.

13 Baldwin, K., Bartges, J., Buffington, T. *et al.* (2010) AAHA nutritional assessment guidelines for dogs and cats. *Journal of the American Animal Hospital Association*, **46** (4), 285–296.

14 Thayer, V. (2012) Deciphering the cat: the medical history and physical examination, in *The Cat: Clinical Medicine and Management* (ed. S.E. Little), Saunders Elsevier, St. Louis, pp. 26–39.

15 Bartges, J., Raditic, D., Kirk, C. *et al.* (2012) Nutritional management of diseases, in *The Cat: Clinical Medicine and Management* (ed. S.E. Little), Saunders Elsevier, St. Louis, pp. 255–288.

16 Little, S.E. (2012) Managing the senior cat, in *The Cat: Clinical Medicine and Management* (ed. S.E. Little), Saunders Elsevier, St. Louis, pp. 1166–1175.

17 Chandler, M. (2014) Nutrition for the surgical patient, in *Feline Soft Tissue and General Surgery* (eds. S.J. Langley-Hobbs, J.L. Demetriou, and J.F. Ladlow), Saunders Elsevier, St. Louis, pp. 55–58.

18 Hazewinkel, H.A.W., Meij, B.P., Theyse, L.F.H., and van Rijssen, B. (2009) Locomotor system, in *Medical*

History and Physical Examination in Companion Animals, 2nd edn. (eds. A. Rijnberk and F.J. van Sluijs), Saunders Elsevier, St. Louis, pp. 135–159.

19 Evans, H.E. (1993) Prenatal development, in *Miller's Anatomy of the Dog*, 3rd edn. (ed. H.E. Evans), Saunders Elsevier, Philadelphia.

20 Evans, H. (1958) Prenatal ossification in the dog. *Anatomical Record*, **130** (2), 406.

21 Dyce, K.M., Sack, W.O., and Wensing, C.J.G. (1996) Some basic facts and concepts, in *Textbook of Veterinary Anatomy*, 2nd edn. (eds. K.M. Dyce, W.O. Sack, and C.J.G. Wensing), Saunders, Philadelphia, pp. 1–31.

22 Stades, F.C., and Stokhof, A.A. (2009) Health certification, in *Medical History and Physical Examination in Companion Animals*, 2nd edn. (eds. A. Rijnberk and F.J. van Sluijs), Saunders Elsevier, St. Louis, pp. 245–246.

23 Kustritz, M.V.R. (2011) History and physical examination of the neonate, in *Small Animal Pediatrics: The First 12 Months of Life* (eds. M.E. Peterson and M.A. Kutzler), Saunders Elsevier, St. Louis, pp. 20–27.

24 Monfared, A.L. (2013) Anatomy of the Persian cat's skull and its clinical value during regional anesthesia. *Global Veterinaria*, **10** (5), 551–555.

25 Schlueter, C., Budras, K.D., Ludewig, E. *et al.* (2009) Brachycephalic feline noses: CT and anatomical study of the relationship between head conformation and the nasolacrimal drainage system. *Journal of Feline Medicine and Surgery*, **11** (11), 891–900.

26 Gunn-Moore, D. (2006) The cat with neck ventroflexion, in *Problem-Based Feline Medicine* (ed. J. Rand), Saunders Elsevier, Philadelphia, pp. 890–905.

27 Lantinga, E., Kooistra, H.S., and van Nes, J.J. (1998) Periodic muscle weakness and cervical ventroflexion caused by hypokalemia in a Burmese cat. *Tijdschrift voor Diergeneeskunde*, **123** (14–15), 435–437 (in Dutch).

28 Malik, R., Musca, F.J., Gunew, M.N. *et al.* (2015) Periodic hypokalaemic polymyopathy in Burmese and closely related cats: a review including the latest genetic data. *Journal of Feline Medicine and Surgery*, **17** (5), 417–426.

29 Dow, S.W., LeCouteur, R.A., Fettman, M.J., and Spurgeon, T.L. (1987) Potassium depletion in cats: hypokalemic polymyopathy. *Journal of the American Veterinary Medical Association*, **191** (12), 1563–1568.

30 Nemzek, J.A., Kruger, J.M., Walshaw, R., and Hauptman, J.G. (1994) Acute onset of hypokalemia and muscular weakness in four hyperthyroid cats. *Journal of the American Veterinary Medical Association*, **205** (1), 65–68.

31 Joseph, R.J., Carrillo, J.M., and Lennon, V.A. (1988) Myasthenia gravis in the cat. *Journal of Veterinary Internal Medicine*, **2** (2), 75–79.

32 Indrieri, R.J., Creighton, S.R., Lambert, E.H., and Lennon, V.A. (1983) Myasthenia gravis in two

cats. *Journal of the American Veterinary Medical Association*, **182** (1), 57–60.

33 Leon, A., Bain, S.A., and Levick, W.R. (1992) Hypokalaemic episodic polymyopathy in cats fed a vegetarian diet. *Australian Veterinary Journal*, **69** (10), 249–254.

34 van Nes, J.J., Meij, B.P., and van Ham, L. (2009) Nervous system, in *Medical History and Physical Examination in Companion Animals*, 2nd edn. (eds. A. Rijnberk and F.J. van Sluijs), Saunders Elsevier, St. Louis, pp. 160–174.

35 Lyons, L.A. (2015) DNA mutations of the cat: the good, the bad and the ugly. *Journal of Feline Medicine and Surgery*, **17** (3), 203–219.

36 Inoue, M., Hasegawa, A., and Sugiura, K. (2016) Morbidity pattern by age, sex and breed in insured cats in Japan (2008–2013). *Journal of Feline Medicine and Surgery*, **18** (12), 1013–1022.

37 Feldman, E.C. and Nelson, R.W. (2004) *Canine and Feline Endocrinology and Reproduction*, 3rd edn., Saunders, St. Louis.

38 Harasen, G.L.G. and Little, S.E. (2012) *Musculoskeletal diseases, in The Cat: Clinical Medicine and Management* (ed. S.E. Little), Saunders Elsevier, St. Louis, pp. 704–733.

39 Voss, K. and Steffen, F. (2009) Patient assessment, in *Feline Orthopedic Surgery and Musculoskeletal Disease* (eds. P.M. Montavon, K. Voss, and S.J. Langley-Hobbs), Saunders Elsevier, St. Louis, pp. 3–20.

40 Kerwin, S. (2012) Orthopedic examination in the cat: clinical tips for ruling in/out common musculoskeletal disease. *Journal of Feline Medicine and Surgery*, **14** (1), 6–12.

41 Leonard, C.A. and Tillson, M. (2001) Feline lameness. *Veterinary Clinics of North America: Small Animal Practice*, **31** (1), 143–163, vii.

42 Arnoczky, S.P. and Tarvin, G.B. (1981) Physical examination of the musculoskeletal system. *Veterinary Clinics of North America: Small Animal Practice*, **11** (3), 575–593.

43 Piermattei, D.L., Flo, G.L., and DeCamp C.E. (2006) *Brinker, Piermattei and Flo's Handbook of Small Animal Orthopedics and Fracture Repair*, 4th edn., Saunders, Philadelphia.

44 Breur, G.J., McDonough, S.P., and Todhunter, R.J. (2011) The musculoskeletal system, in *Small Animal Pediatrics: The First 12 Months of Life* (eds. M.E. Peterson and M.A. Kutzler), Saunders Elsevier, St. Louis, pp. 443–460.

45 Barone, G. (2012) Neurology, in *The Cat: Clinical Medicine and Management* (ed. S.E. Little), Saunders Elsevier, St. Louis, pp. 734–767.

46 Baral, R.M. (2012) Diseases of the intestines, in *The Cat: Clinical Medicine and Management* (ed. S.E. Little), Saunders Elsevier, St. Louis, pp. 466–495.

47 Hardie, E.M., Roe, S.C., and Martin, F.R. (2002) Radiographic evidence of degenerative joint disease in geriatric cats: 100 cases (1994–1997). *Journal of the American Veterinary Medical Association*, **220** (5), 628–632.

48 Clarke, S.P., Mellor, D., Clements, D.N. *et al.* (2005) Prevalence of radiographic signs of degenerative joint disease in a hospital population of cats. *Veterinary Record*, **157** (25), 793–799.

49 Lund, E.M., Armstrong, P.J., Kirk, C.A. *et al.* (1999) Health status and population characteristics of dogs and cats examined at private veterinary practices in the United States. *Journal of the American Veterinary Medical Association*, **214** (9), 1336–1341.

50 Evans, H.E. (1993) The skeleton, in *Miller's Anatomy of the Dog*, 3rd edn. (ed. H.E. Evans), Saunders Elsevier, Philadelphia, pp. 122–218.

51 Gilbert, S.G. (1989) *Pictorial Anatomy of the Cat*, University of Washington Press, Seattle.

52 Jaeger, G.H., Marcellin-Little, D.J., Depuy, V., and Lascelles, B.D. (2007) Validity of goniometric joint measurements in cats. *American Journal of Veterinary Research*, **68** (8), 822–826.

53 Grierson, J. (2012) Hips, elbows and stifles: common joint diseases in the cat. *Journal of Feline Medicine and Surgery*, **14** (1), 23–30.

54 Lascelles, B.D. (2010) Feline degenerative joint disease. *Veterinary Surgery*, **39** (1), 2–13.

55 Hardie, E.M. (1997) Management of osteoarthritis in cats. *Veterinary Clinics of North America: Small Animal Practice*, **27** (4), 945–953.

56 Valastro, C., Di Bello, A., and Crovace, A. (2005) Congenital elbow subluxation in a cat. *Veterinary Radiology and Ultrasound*, **46** (1), 63–64.

57 Rossi, F., Vignoli, M., Terragni, R. *et al.* (2003) Bilateral elbow malformation in a cat caused by radio-ulnar synostosis. *Veterinary Radiology and Ultrasound*, **44** (3), 283–286.

58 Meeson, R. and Corr, S. (2011) Management of pelvic trauma: neurological damage, urinary tract disruption and pelvic fractures. *Journal of Feline Medicine and Surgery*, **13** (5), 347–361.

59 Basher, A.W.P., Walter, M.C., and Newton, C.D. (1986) Coxofemoral luxation in the dog and cat. *Veterinary Surgery*, **15** (5), 356–362.

60 Kolde, D. (1974) Pectineus tenectomy for treatment of hip dysplasia in a domestic cat. *Journal of the American Animal Hospital Association*, **10**, 564–565.

61 Hayes, H., Wilson, G., and Burt, J. (1999) Feline hip dysplasia. *Journal of the American Animal Hospital Association*, **15**, 447–448.

62 Langenbach, A., Giger, U., Green, P. *et al.* (1998) Relationship between degenerative joint disease and hip joint laxity by use of distraction index and Norberg angle measurement in a group of cats. *Journal of the American Veterinary Medical Association*, **213** (10), 1439–1443.

63 Keller, G.G., Reed, A.L., Lattimer, J.C., and Corley, E.A. (1999) Hip dysplasia: a feline population study. *Veterinary Radiology and Ultrasound*, **40** (5), 460–464.

64 Chandler, J.C. and Beale, B.S. (2002) Feline orthopedics. *Clinical Techniques in Small Animal Practice*, **17** (4), 190–203.

65 Guiot, L.P., Demianiuk, R.M., and Dejardin, L.M. (2012) Fractures of the femur, in *Veterinary Surgery: Small Animal*, vol. 1 (eds. K.M. Tobias and S.A. Johnston), Saunders Elsevier, St. Louis, pp. 865–905.

66 Sebastiani, A.M. and Fishbeck, D.W. (1998) *Mammalian Anatomy: The Cat*, Morton Publishing, Englewood, CO.

67 Phillips, I.R. (1979) A survey of bone fractures in the dog and cat. *Journal of Small Animal Practice*, **20** (11), 661–674.

68 McNicholas, W.T., Jr., Wilkens, B.E., Blevins, W.E. *et al.* (2002) Spontaneous femoral capital physeal fractures in adult cats: 26 cases (1996–2001). *Journal of the American Veterinary Medical Association*, **221** (12), 1731–1736.

69 Lafuente, P. (2011) Young, male neutered, obese, lame? Non-traumatic fractures of the femoral head and neck. *Journal of Feline Medicine and Surgery*, **13** (7), 498–507.

70 Queen, J., Bennett, D., Carmichael, S. *et al.* (1998) Femoral neck metaphyseal osteopathy in the cat. *Veterinary Record*, **142** (7), 159–162.

71 Forrest, L.J., O'Brien, R.T., and Manlet, P.A. (1999) Feline capital physeal dysplasia syndrome. *Veterinary Radiology and Ultrasound*, **40**, 672.

72 Burke, J. (2003) Physeal dysplasia with slipped capital femoral epiphysis in a cat. *Canadian Veterinary Journal/Revue Vétérinaire Canadienne*, **44** (3), 238–239.

73 Craig, L.E. (2001) Physeal dysplasia with slipped capital femoral epiphysis in 13 cats. *Veterinary Pathology*, **38** (1), 92–97.

74 Ridge, P.A. (2006) What is your diagnosis? Destructive bony lesions of the proximal femoral metaphysis. *Journal of Small Animal Practice*, **47** (5), 291–293.

75 Fischer, H.R., Norton, J., Kobluk, C.N. *et al.* (2004) Surgical reduction and stabilization for repair of femoral capital physeal fractures in cats: 13 cases (1998–2002). *Journal of the American Veterinary Medical Association*, **224** (9), 1478–1482.

76 Isola, M., Baroni, E., and Zotti, A. (2005) Radiographic features of two cases of feline proximal femoral dysplasia. *Journal of Small Animal Practice*, **46** (12), 597–599.

77 Chandler, E.A., Hilbery, A.D.R., and Gaskell, C.J. (2004) *Feline Medicine and Therapeutics*, 3rd edn., Iowa State Press, Ames, IA.

78 Flecknell, P. and Gruffydd-Jones, T. (1979) Congenital luxation of the patellae in the cat. *Feline Practice*, **9**, 18–20.

79 L'Eplattenier, H. and Montavon, P. (2002) Patellar luxation in dogs and cats: pathogenesis and diagnosis. *Compendium: Continuing Education for the Practicing Veterinarian*, **24** (3), 234–240.

80 Loughlin, C., Kerwin, S., Hosgood, G. *et al.* (2006) Clinical signs and results of treatment in cats with patellar luxation: 42 cases (1992–2002). *Journal of the American Veterinary Medical Association*, **228** (9), 1370–1375.

81 Scott, H. and McLaughlin, R. (2007) *Feline Orthopedics*, Manson Publishing, London.

82 Smith, G.K., Langenbach, A., Green, P.A. *et al.* (1999) Evaluation of the association between medial patellar luxation and hip dysplasia in cats. *Journal of the American Veterinary Medical Association*, **215** (1), 40–45.

83 Engvall, E. and Bushnell, N. (1990) Patellar luxation in Abyssinian cats. *Feline Practice*, **18** (4), 20–22.

84 Houlton, J.E.F. and Meynink, S.E. (1989) Medial patellar luxation in the cat. *Journal of Small Animal Practice*, **30** (6), 349–352.

85 Johnson, M.E. (1986) Feline patellar luxation – a retrospective case-study. *Journal of the American Animal Hospital Association*, **22** (6), 835–838.

86 Palmer, R. (2005) *Diagnosing Cranial Cruciate Ligament Pathology*, http://veterinarymedicine. dvm360.com/diagnosing-cranial-cruciate-ligament-pathology (accessed 2 May 2016).

87 Evans, H.E. (1993) Arthrology, in *Miller's Anatomy of the Dog*, 3rd edn. (ed. H.E. Evans), Saunders Elsevier, Philadelphia, pp. 219–257.

88 Voss, K., Langley-Hobbs, S.J., and Montavon, P.M. (2009) Stifle joint, in *Feline Orthopedic Surgery and Musculoskeletal Disease* (eds. P.M. Montavon, K. Voss, and S.J. Langley-Hobbs), Saunders Elsevier, St. Louis, pp. 475–490.

89 Harasen, G.L. (2005) Feline cranial cruciate rupture: 17 cases and a review of the literature. *Veterinary and Comparative Orthopaedics and Traumatology*, **18** (4), 254–257.

90 Thomson, M. (2006) The cat with lameness, in *Problem-Based Feline Medicine* (ed. J. Rand), Saunders Elsevier, Philadelphia, pp. 976–991.

91 Henderson, R.A. and Milton, J.L. (1978) Tibial compression mechanism – diagnostic aid in stifle injuries. *Journal of the American Animal Hospital Association*, **14** (4), 474–479.

8

Evaluating the Nervous System of the Cat

8.1 Assessing Behavior and Mental Status

Neurologic dysfunction is not always restricted to loco-motion and gait. At its most subtle, neurologic dysfunc-tion can involve abnormal behavior that is sporadic or owner reported based on observations witnessed within the home environment [1, 2].

Owners may report dysphonia, a state of altered vocalizations, with or without apparent confusion [1, 2]. Owners may witness their cat staring into space or head-pressing into walls [2]. Owners may describe exag-gerated responses, mania, or reduced responsiveness of the cat to its surroundings.

Historical data can be especially telling [3, 4] with regard to progression of underlying disease, and the client should be questioned into terms of

- description of the behavior;
- onset;
- duration;
- frequency;
- time of day;
- apparent connection to other activities.

Owners should be encouraged to provide audiovisual recordings as able, especially when the observed behav-iors are infrequent and unlikely to be present on physical examination.

After taking a thorough history, the clinician should make initial observations regarding the patient and its interactions within the examination room prior to physi-cally examining it. Although the clinician may not wit-ness some or all of the behaviors that were described by the client, he or she may identify additional findings to augment or clarify the client's concerns [5].

The clinician should first consider whether the patient is conscious [2, 5]. A conscious patient is said to be awake and aware of its surroundings [1, 4]. Note that the patient's response to the environment may vary, yet it may still be considered conscious. For instance, three very different patients may be hypervigilant, attentive, and quietly aware, yet all three states are compatible with consciousness (Figure 8.1).

It is important to recognize that an alert cat does not necessarily have to be interactive, as is evident in Fig-ure 8.1c. To decide whether or not a cat is alert, the clinician should determine if it is responding appropri-ately to environmental stimuli. For instance, it would be abnormal for an anxious adult cat in a high-stress environment such as an examination room to sleep.

Consciousness is not all-or-nothing [1, 2, 4]: there is a sliding scale to qualify reductions in consciousness. In order of increasing severity, patients may be described as follows [2, 5]:

- depressed;
- obtunded;
- stuporous;
- comatose.

A depressed patient is aware of, yet less responsive towards its surroundings. Some clinicians might describe the patient's behavior as being lethargic. The patient tends to be less active (Figure 8.2). The classic example of a neurologically normal, yet depressed patient is one that is febrile. Depression can also be due to non-infec-tious diseases, such as a lesion within the central nervous system [4].

A cat that is attempting to hide may or may not be depressed. It is important to remember that a hiding cat may simply be scared. When there is any question regarding the motivation underlying the "escape from sight" behavior, the clinician should look for non-verbal clues [6] (see Section 1.9 for details). In particular, the astute clinician should note pupil size and shape: dilated, rounded pupils tend to convey increased sympathetic tone. Ear carriage, the presence or absence of piloerec-tion, and tail posture may also help to differentiate a fearful cat from one that is depressed.

An obtunded patient is mentally dull with a markedly decreased response to external stimuli. When a patient is stuporous, responses are limited to noxious stimuli.

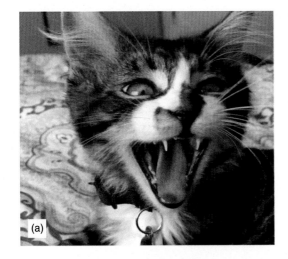

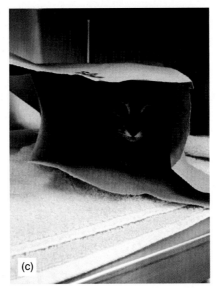

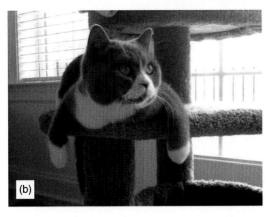

Figure 8.1 (a) Hypervigilant patient that is overstimulated in the clinic environment to the point of reacting with a hiss and spit. Source: Courtesy of Hilary Lazarus. (b) Attentive, alert patient in its home environment. Source: Courtesy of Richard and Jill Englar. (c) Quietly aware, yet conscious patient, trying to retreat from view.

This is a patient that can be roused, but it takes effort on the clinician's part to do so. Once a patient is comatose, it loses the ability to respond even to noxious stimuli. Nothing provokes a response. The patient acts as if deeply under general anesthesia: not awake and unresponsive to its surroundings [1–4].

Stuporous and comatose patients are relatively easy to discern. It can be more challenging to differentiate depression from obtundation, especially because there is an element of subjectivity as to where one category blurs into the next. Clinicians may need to rely on creative strategies designed to stimulate a reaction in the patient: for instance, clapping one's hands may provoke the patient to raise its head and point its ears in the direction of the sound. A depressed patient may react slowly, but surely. An obtunded patient may be even slower to react, only to promptly resume its original state when the clapping has ceased [1].

Consciousness matters to the clinician because any alternation from the norm can be indicative of diffuse or focal central nervous system disease. When both cerebral hemispheres are involved or when the brainstem's ascending reticular activating system (ARAS) is impacted, the patient's state of consciousness may be reduced [2, 4].

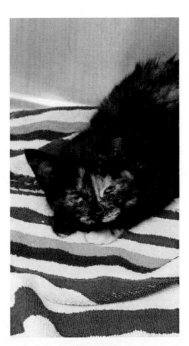

Figure 8.2 This patient is depressed secondary to an upper respiratory infection. The patient's eyes are dull and the eyelids are droopy. The fur along the topline over the lumbosacral spine is unkempt. This patient has not been grooming well. This patient appears to be unwell.

8.2 Assessing Posture

Posture should be taken into consideration relative to the age of the patient. At birth, kittens are able to lift their head; however, they are unable to maintain themselves in an upright posture until roughly 2 weeks of age [7, 8] (Figure 8.3).

Flexor tone predominates for the first few days of life, creating the classic comma shape that is characteristic of newborns. This allows newborns to be flaccid and portable when scruffed by their mother [9, 10] (Figure 8.4).

Extensor dominance eventually overtakes flexor tone in kittens at variable ages, sometime between a few days and a few weeks of life, until eventually the musculature develops a coordinated approach rather than all-or-none [11].

By 1 month of age, the kitten's posture should mirror an adult's: the head and neck are held upright, with right- and left-sided symmetry, and the trunk should be held evenly without a unilateral tilt. When standing, the

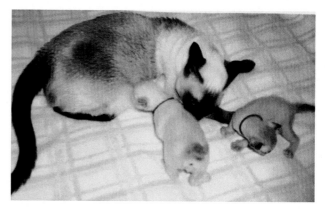

Figure 8.4 Note the predominant flexor tone, which is especially pronounced in the kitten on the right.

weight distribution between limbs should be roughly equal [1, 4] (Figure 8.5).

Asymmetry in head and neck carriage may be subtle, but clinically important. The astute clinician should identify and note the presence of a head tilt, the direction of the head tilt, and whether or not there is concurrent facial asymmetry (Figure 8.6).

If there is a head tilt, care must be taken to clarify that it is truly of neurologic origin rather than the by-product of severe external ear canal disease. In the author's experience, a handful of cats have presented with head tilts secondary to marked unilateral bacterial or mixed

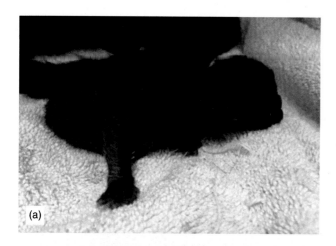

(a)

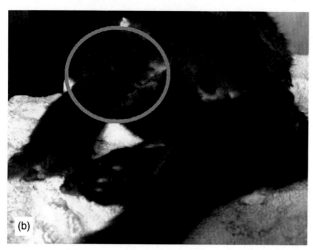

(b)

Figure 8.3 (a) This 2-hour-old kitten is able to raise its head. (b) By being able to raise its head, this 2-hour-old kitten is able to nurse.

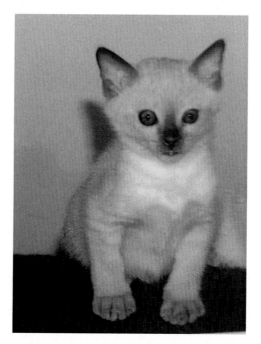

Figure 8.5 Note the age-appropriate posture in this 6-week-old kitten. There is symmetry between the ears and eyes. There is no head tilt.

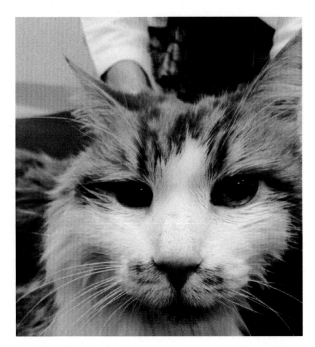

Figure 8.6 Note the asymmetry when comparing the palpebral fissure of the right and left eyelids. Although it is difficult to appreciate in this image, this patient had concurrent anisocoria and a diagnosis of cryptococcosis. Source: Courtesy of Andrew Weisenfeld, DVM.

otitis externa. Therefore, any cat presenting with a head tilt should be subjected to a thorough otoscopic examination with cytologic evaluation of any exudate.

In patients that present with a head tilt, it is important to consider if there is concurrent ataxia or nystagmus that may be suggestive of underlying vestibular disease. In classic vestibular disease, the head tilt is ipsilateral to the lesion. However, if vestibular disease is bilateral, the head tilt may be extinguished [12]. In patients with both a head tilt and circling behavior, vestibular disease is less likely and thalamic and cerebral diseases are prioritized [4, 12].

Abnormalities in neck posture may be due to underlying musculoskeletal disease or neurologic dysfunction. See Section 7.2.1 to review muscular weakness as a cause of neck ventroflexion [13–20]. Additional causes for posture abnormalities of the cervical region include congenital malformations and acquired orthopedic disease. For instance, abnormal shaping of the vertebral column can lead to [1]

- scoliosis, a sideways deviation in the spinal column;
- kyphosis, a dorsal deviation in the spinal column;
- lordosis, a ventral deviation in the spinal column.

When neck posture abnormalities are due to neurologic dysfunction, the neck is often twisted rather than simply deviated in a state referred to as torticollis [4].

Patients may have a normal head and neck posture yet position one or more limbs in space abnormally. In these cases, a more thorough investigation of the affected limb is required by means of palpation and postural reflexes to assist with lesion localization [3]. Abnormal postures are not isolated to weight-bearing, standing patients. Patients that are recumbent are also subject to changes in posture that are easily recognized and, when present, denote serious neurologic dysfunction [4, 5]:

- Extension of all limbs in recumbency, with or without opisthotonus (head and neck dorsiflexion) is called decerebrate rigidity. It signifies the presence of a brain stem lesion.
- Thoracic limb extension with hip flexion and opisthotonus is characteristic of acute cerebellar injury and is referred to as decerebellate rigidity.
- Thoracic limb extension with bilateral pelvic limb paralysis is characteristic of thoracolumbar spinal segment injury and is referred to as the Schiff–Sherrington posture.

8.3 Assessing Coordination and Gait

In order for a patient to stand, it must have a functional, intact musculoskeletal system that is capable of bearing weight and also proprioceptive function to provide feedback as to where its body is relative to the surrounding space. For the same patient to initiate and maintain movement, there must be integration of and communication between the peripheral and central nervous systems. Muscles and tendons possess receptors capable of detecting stretch as from locomotion. These messages are then conveyed to higher centers via ascending spinal tracts in order for the brain stem and cerebellum to coordinate movement. Unlike in primates, cats rely less on the cerebrum to contribute to gait [2]. Nonetheless, a lesion in any of the steps along this signaling process may adversely impact gait [4].

As discussed in Chapter 7, gait analysis in cats is challenging at best. Even the most tolerant cat on physical examination may balk at being asked to walk and trot on command. More typically, cats prefer to stay hunched or frozen rather than ambulating within the examination room. As a result, the same challenges that the orthopedic examination presents in cats hold true for the neurologic examination: the clinician's assessment of gait may be limited to owner-provided audiovisual recordings that demonstrate the cat's mobility within its natural home environment [21–23].

Even when a feline patient is ambulatory in the examination room, experience is the veterinary student's best teacher. It takes time to be able to discriminate accurately and repeatedly between subtleties in gait abnormalities.

Becoming a gait expert is therefore well beyond the scope of this text. What veterinary students should instead focus on, initially, is evaluating the strength, coordination, and symmetry of the gait. These are challenging enough to master [3].

A normal gait should be smooth, strong, and even. Forelimb stride should be roughly equivalent to hind limb stride. Foot placement should be solid, without hesitation, and crisp, meaning that each foot strikes the ground and comes up off the ground without the dorsal surface of the paw knuckling [4].

Subtle gait changes are most easily detected when the patient makes tight turns or sudden movements [3, 4]; however, this is far less easy to reproduce in cats than dogs, which can be guided in their movement by leashes.

When gait changes are noted, the clinician should record which one or more limbs are affected because so doing assists with lesion localization. Paresis is said to occur when there is voluntary movement that is hindered because of underlying weakness. This term may be adjusted to describe the location of apparent weakness as follows [3, 5]:

- Tetraparesis implies that all four limbs are affected.
- Hemiparesis implies that one side of the body is affected.
- Paraparesis implies that both pelvic limbs are affected.
- Monoparesis implies that only one limb is affected.

The clinician should designate which side of the body is affected when the condition is unilateral. For example, the clinician should specify that a patient has right-sided hemiparesis or monoparesis of the left forelimb.

When weakness is present, it may or may not be linked to exertion. For example, in cases of myasthenia gravis, weakness intensifies as movement continues: the patient starts out strong and then loses momentum. This should be documented in the medical record as it facilitates diagnosis [3].

Paresis may also be classified based upon the origin of the underlying problem. In order to generate a gait, the patient must have functional interaction between the upper motor neuron (UMN) system within the central nervous system and the lower motor neuron (LMN) system as the connection piece between the central nervous system and the innervated muscles. UMN paresis results from an inability to generate a gait at the level of the central nervous system. LMN paresis results from difficulty supporting weight. A patient with UMN paresis will demonstrate a delay in the swing phase of the gait whereas a patient with LMN paresis will demonstrate abbreviated strides and/or collapse the limb when weight is applied [2].

Paralysis, on the other hand, describes a situation in which there is complete loss of voluntary movement [3, 5]:

- Tetraparalysis implies that all four limbs are affected.
- Hemiparalysis implies that one side of the body is affected.
- Paraparalysis implies that both pelvic limbs are affected.
- Monoparalysis implies that only one limb is affected.

As was the case in conditions involving paresis, the clinician is encouraged to designate which side of the body is affected when paralysis is unilateral. For example, the clinician should specify that a patient has right-sided hemiparalysis or monoparalysis of the left forelimb.

In addition to the presence and strength of voluntary movement, the quality of the gait should be assessed. The clinician should ask if the gait appears to be coordinated. Gait incoordination that is not attributable to weakness is referred to as ataxia [2, 4]. There are three main categories of ataxia [4, 5]: cerebellar ataxia, vestibular ataxia, and proprioceptive or sensory ataxia.

Cerebellar ataxia stems from underlying cerebellar disease that results in an abnormal rate, range, or force of movement. A classic example of cerebellar ataxia is the "toy soldier" gait, where the patient has a very stilted, high-stepping, over-reaching gait, each step of which may also demonstrate exaggerated flexion [3].

Vestibular ataxia reflects a true lack of balance. This may be due to peripheral vestibular disease, as in medical conditions that involve the tympanic bulla, or central vestibular disease, as occurs when lesions arise at the cerebello-ponto-medullary angle [12]. When there is unilateral vestibular disease, the patient will lean, drift, or fall toward one side. This may be overt or subtle. The patient may simply try to lean against the examination room wall as it walks to "hold itself up." A head tilt may or may not be present [4, 12]. When vestibular disease is bilateral, the patient tends to be reluctant to move and classically presents with wide, wild side-to-side swaying of the head and neck [4, 12].

Proprioceptive or sensory ataxia occurs when there is a lesion in the peripheral nerve, dorsal root, spinal cord, or brain stem. This adversely affects the patient's ability to sense where its limbs are positioned in space. As a result, the patient appears to be clumsy and exceptionally uncoordinated. Clients may say that their cat appears to be intoxicated. Cats with this type of ataxia will typically try to stand with a wide base to attempt stability. They also often "knuckle," meaning that they scuff or even stand upon the dorsal aspect of one or more feet. There may also be concurrent paresis because motor pathways often overlap with proprioceptive pathways [4, 12].

8.4 Assessing Postural Reactions

Because gait can be such a challenge to evaluate in cats for the aforementioned reasons, it is important for the clinician to follow up on gait analysis with an assessment of postural reactions. Postural reactions provide supplemental data with regard to whether the cat knows where its head and neck, body, and feet are relative to each other in space. In order for the cat to have a spatial sense of its own anatomy relative to its environment, all components of the nervous system (both the central nervous system and the peripheral nervous system) must be intact and functionally communicating with one another. When there is dysfunction in one or more parts of the pathway, there will be deficits in one or more postural responses. Deficits in postural reactions may be more apparent to the veterinary student than the subtleties of gait analysis [2, 4].

The most common postural reactions that are assessed in cats or are at least attempted are the following [1–5]:

- proprioceptive positioning;
- placing response;
- hopping;
- hemi-walking;
- wheel-barrowing.

Proprioceptive positioning is sometimes referred to as position sense [3] or the knuckling-over reflex [1]. This test requires the clinician to evaluate each foot. With the patient standing and supported, the clinician methodically grasps each paw, one at a time, and positions it such that the dorsal surface comes into contact with the ground [1, 3–5, 24]:

- The front paws are most easily accessed from their respective side. For example, the left front paw is most accessible from the left side whereas the right front paw is most accessible from the right.
- The hind paws are most easily accessed when the veterinarian stands behind the patient with the patient facing away from the veterinarian.

Supporting the patient throughout the examination is essential. A patient may have normal proprioception but "fail" this test because of weakness. Supporting the patient eliminates the risk that weakness will yield inaccurate test results.

A patient with normal proprioception will "recognize" that the dorsum of the paw is not an appropriate anatomic position to maintain and will quickly right its paw so that the palmar or plantar aspect makes contact with the floor instead, as is the normal posture of a standing cat [3, 5]. A patient with normal proprioception may even anticipate the clinician's attempt to place its paw in a way that does not feel right anatomically. The patient may even refuse to allow the paw to be misplaced on the floor [1, 3, 5]. By contrast, a patient that has one or more lesions along the reflex arc will not attempt to right the wrong, and will remain standing as is, trying to bear weight abnormally on the dorsal surface of the affected paw [3, 5].

Ideally, each paw should be tested at least twice to be certain that the results are repeatable. The clinician should note whether the patient corrects or fails to correct each paw placement, and should be cognizant of the relative time it takes to right each foot. If one or more feet are sluggish compared with the others, the astute clinician should make a note of this in the medical record, as this may assist with lesion localization.

Assessment of this reflex is technically easy and should be well tolerated by the veterinary patient in that it does not induce pain or discomfort. However, it can be challenging to reproduce conclusive results repeatedly in cats because they tend not to like having their feet touched. Cats may refuse this examination altogether: they may refuse to stand, they may hunch, or they may curl themselves up into a frozen ball [1, 2]. For cats that are intolerant of this component of the neurologic examination, tactile and visual placement tests or hopping may be more fruitful [1, 2].

The tactile placement test is performed with the patient held by the clinician, facing forwards, in front of a horizontal surface such as an examination room table. The clinician covers the cat's eyes so that it cannot see what is directly in front of it. With the cat's visual field obstructed, the clinician then moves the cat toward the horizontal surface so that the dorsal aspects of the cat's distal forelimbs come into contact with the table's edge. As soon as the cat contacts the table edge, it should respond by placing its paws on the table. Both forelimbs can be tested simultaneously, although occasionally a normal patient will not respond on the side that is being held. In this case, the patient should be retested while holding the opposite side. The test is also less reliable when used to assess the hind limbs [1, 4, 5, 25]. A patient that has proprioceptive deficits in the forelimbs is unlikely to replace its paws [1].

The visual placement test is performed much as described for the tactile placement test with one exception: the patient's visual field is unobstructed. As the cat is advanced toward the horizontal surface, it typically flexes its forelimbs well in advance of contacting the table's edge, then extends both forelimbs to bear weight on the table's surface [1, 3, 5].

If the cat remains uncooperative, proprioception can be assessed by placing a sheet of paper under one foot of the standing cat. The clinician can then slowly slide the paper away from being directly under the cat's body. A cat with a normal proprioceptive response will pull its foot back to a normal standing posture whereas a cat with an abnormal response will fall over in the direction in which the paper is moving [1].

Whereas both the tactile and visual placement tests are primarily associated with the forelimbs, the hopping test can be used to evaluate reliably both forelimb and hind limb function in terms of the limb's ability to support weight and to recognize its position in space. The patient is lifted off the ground and supported with the exception of the limb being tested. That limb is then brought into contact with the floor, bearing the patient's weight as the limb is moved laterally. Because this sideways motion displaces the center of gravity of the patient, the patient "falls" toward the newly established center of gravity, causing a "hopping" motion in the normal patient [1, 3–5, 25]. Each limb should be tested and contralateral sides should be compared. This test has the potential to detect subtle weakness and asymmetry. However, the test's usefulness depends upon the patient. Not all cats tolerate hopping; many refuse to hop and will do anything to avoid giving the clinician the response that they are looking for, including laying down.

Hemi-hopping, otherwise referred to as hemi-walking, is a variation of the hopping test: it tests ipsilateral limbs concurrently. To test the patient's left forelimb and left hind limb, its right forelimb and right hind limb are lifted off the ground as it is pushed to the left. By contrast, the test the patient's right forelimb and right hind limb, its left forelimb and left hind limb are lifted off the ground as it is pushed to the right [3–5, 12, 25].

Wheel-barrowing is yet another variation of the hopping test: it tests forelimbs or hind limbs concurrently [1, 3–5]:

- To test both forelimbs, the patient is supported under the abdomen. Without the hind limbs coming into contact with the ground, the patient is encouraged to move forward. In a normal patient, the forelimbs will alternate movements.
- To test both hind limbs, the patient is supported under each axillary region with its thoracic end raised so that the forelimbs do not come into contact with the ground. With the patient standing, in effect, upright on both hind limbs, it is encouraged to move backwards.

Abnormal patients will either stumble because they lose their foot placement or they will scuff the dorsal surface of their paws on the ground [3].

8.5 Assessing for Other Abnormal Movements

Involuntary movements tend to be of less clinical significance in veterinary patients than in human patients; however, these can be self-reported by the client or documented clinically. These so-called dyskinesias often have blurred definitions in the veterinary literature and may be difficult to describe because of perceived overlap between them [1, 4]. The three most commonly identified dyskinesias are

1) tremors;
2) tics;
3) myoclonus.

Tremors are defined as rhythmic trembling of one or more body parts that involve antagonistic muscle groups. They may be focal or generalized. They may be triggered by metabolic disturbances such as hypocalcemia or they may be clinical signs of toxicosis as from mycotoxins or metaldehyde. When they are associated with goal-oriented movement, as when a cat lowers its head into its food bowl, they are further categorized as intention tremors [4].

When tremors occur because of developmental pathology, they typically reflect an underlying cerebellar disorder. Cerebellar hypoplasia is one of the most commonly recognized congenital and developmental disorders in cats [7, 26–29]. Cerebellar hypoplasia of kittens is most notably associated with the in utero infection of pregnant queens with the feline panleukopenia virus. Kittens may also be infected immediately postnatally with the same virus or iatrogenically infected in utero when an immunologically naïve queen is vaccinated with a modified live FVRCP vaccine [7, 26–32].

The feline panleukopenia virus exerts a cytopathic effect on rapidly dividing cells. These include the cells of the cerebellum. As a result, the cerebellum of affected kittens is hypoplastic [7, 26–29]. Not every kitten in a litter has to be affected [27]. However, those who are tend to develop clinical signs between 2 and 4 weeks of age [7, 27]. These clinical signs will either remain static throughout life or may improve [7, 27]. Improvement is thought to be due to patient compensation as the cat learns how best to navigate its environment [26].

The tremor that characterizes cerebellar hypoplasia is typically generalized and exaggerated with a slow frequency of 2–6 times per second [26]. The tremor tends to intensify with goal-oriented movement [26] to the extent that kittens may fall over as they attempt to eat, drink, or use the litterbox. Cats with cerebellar hypoplasia may also present with ataxia due to cerebellar dysfunction [26]. Despite their involuntary incoordination, cats with cerebellar hypoplasia are highly functional and can lead high-quality lives. If examined at rest, they appear in all other ways to be "normal" cats (Figure 8.7) – they simply require a safe living environment where they are protected from harm should they tumble [25].

In contrast to a tremor, a tic is a contraction of one or more muscle groups. When they occur in veterinary patients, tics often involve the facial muscles. Tics and tremors are both frequently observed in feline patients with permethrin toxicosis [33].

Figure 8.7 (a) At rest, one would never know that this patient is afflicted with cerebellar hypoplasia. (b) Despite being afflicted with cerebellar hypoplasia, this patient is still able to ambulate and explore its environment. Source (a), (b): Courtesy of Juliane Daggett, MBS.

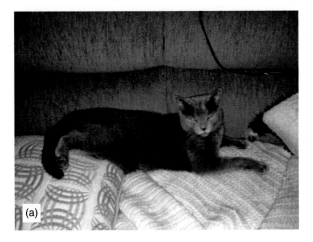 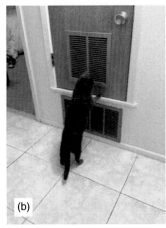

Myoclonus is an exaggerated or violent tic, with an extremely intense, albeit brief, muscle contraction that results in a very pronounced jerking of the affected body part. Myoclonus is less commonly seen in feline patients and is more commonly seen in dogs with encephalitis as from canine distemper virus [4].

8.6 Evaluating the Spinal Reflexes

A reflex is an automatic, spontaneous response to a stimulus. It is hard-wired into the body: the patient does not have to think about it in order for it to occur [2, 34]. Spinal cord reflexes were discovered when patients that had undergone experimental spinal cord transection still retained certain stereotypic functions despite segments of the spinal cord being permanently severed from connections to the brain [34].

At its most basic, a spinal reflex occurs when a peripheral receptor receives a stimulus. The receptor transmits the message to a sensory neuron that synapses with interneurons within an integration center – in this case, the spinal cord. The outcome is a "reply" sent via interneurons to a part of the body that can do something in response to the initial stimulus. The resultant action is effected by the motor neuron [34].

Spinal reflexes are considered to be normal only when all components of this "communication" are functional. There must be an intact pathway. If there is not, it is up to the clinician to determine which part of the pathway is "broken." When there is a "break" in the pathway, the quality of one or more reflexes may be impacted and observed on neurologic examination [3].

Abnormal reflexes may be described as [1, 4, 5]

- exaggerated;
- weak;
- absent.

Recognizing the quality of the reflex compared with what is expected in a normal patient may help to assist with the localization of a neurologic lesion.

Another way to facilitate lesion localization is to break the spinal cord into various segments [2, 5]:

- C1–C5;
- C6–T2;
- T3–L3;
- L4–L6;
- L7–S3.

The segments are grouped in such a way that each cluster has a characteristic mix of neurologic signs [2, 4, 5]:

- C1–C5 lesions cause so-called upper motor neuron (UMN) signs in all four limbs. UMN signs are characterized by loss of muscle inhibition, which causes an increase in muscle tone and exaggerated reflexes.
- C6–T2 lesions cause mixed signs: the thoracic limbs demonstrate lower motor neuron (LMN) signs of decreased muscle tone and decreased to absent reflexes. In contrast, the pelvic limbs demonstrate UMN signs.
- T3–L3 lesions cause no abnormalities in the thoracic limbs; however, they cause UMN signs in the pelvic limbs.
- L4–L6 lesions cause no abnormalities in the thoracic limbs; however, they cause LMN signs in the pelvic limbs.
- L7–S3 lesions also cause LMN signs to the tail and perineum.

Different nerves are associated with each spinal segment cluster. The astute clinician can make use of spinal reflexes to test different spinal cord segments in order to assess the integrity of their associated nerves [2, 4, 5].

It is important to note, however, that not all reflexes are equally reliable. Some are much more difficult to elicit than others. Some are also very user dependent – so much so that unless the clinician makes use of them daily, they cannot be sure that the result is accurate. The two most reliable spinal reflexes that can be performed in the cat are [2]:

1) the patellar reflex;
2) the withdrawal or flexor reflex.

Both of these reflexes are present in the neonatal kitten; however, they may be difficult to appreciate [7].

There is not one right way to perform these reflexes. Depending upon where and by whom the clinician was trained, patient positioning may vary. It becomes less important that the cat is positioned in dorsal recumbency, as suggested by Garosi [2] and de Lahunta and Glass [25], or in lateral recumbency, as suggested by Thomas and Dewey [5]. Of greater significance is the repeatability of the results obtained when eliciting each reflex. Repeatability is more likely when both the clinician and patient are comfortable, and when the clinician has had extensive practice with eliciting each reflex in order to make an accurate determination as to its quality.

For both the patellar reflex and the withdrawal reflex, the author prefers that the cat be placed in lateral recumbency. The patellar reflex evaluates whether or not the femoral nerve and the associated L4–L6 segments of the spinal cord are intact. With the patient restrained in lateral recumbency, the clinician uses one hand to support the limb that is "up" by seating this hand under the medial thigh. The stifle of the "up" limb is positioned so that it is partially flexed. The clinician then uses the other hand to swing the plexor, a reflex hammer, firmly and smoothly to make contact with the patellar ligament. The stifle should respond by automatically extending [2, 4, 5, 25].

If the patellar reflex is weak or absent, then a lesion is likely to be present within the femoral nerve itself or within the L4–L6 spinal segments. However, severe stifle disease can also result in the same weak or absent patellar reflex, reminding the clinician that the patient must be evaluated as a whole rather than taking into consideration only the results of the neurologic examination, which are not intended to stand alone. Accurate lesion localization requires the clinician to integrate all diagnostic findings to create a clinical picture that best fits a given patient [2].

If the patellar reflex is exaggerated and there are no concurrent abnormalities in gait and postural reactions, the patient is likely to be overexcited or tense, without true neurologic disease. However, an exaggerated patellar reflex in combination with other gait and postural deficits is likely suggestive of an UMN lesion cranial to L4 [2]. The patellar reflex may also appear to be exaggerated if the flexor muscles of the stifle, those that typically counteract stifle extension that is elicited in the reflex arc, have decreased tone as from a lesion within the sciatic nerve or spinal cord segments caudal to L6 [2].

The withdrawal reflex assesses the integrity of different nerves and different spinal segments depending on whether it is performed on a thoracic or a hind limb. When performed on the thoracic limb, the withdrawal reflex evaluates the C6–T2 spinal cord segments as well as the musculocutaneous, axillary, median, ulnar, and radial nerves. When performed in the hind limb, the withdrawal reflex evaluates the L7–S1 segments and the sciatic nerve [2, 4, 5, 25].

With the patient restrained in lateral recumbency, the clinician pinches interdigital skin or a nail bed on each limb, one limb at a time, with the limb being tested held in extension. When the thoracic limb is tested, the patient should automatically respond by flexing the shoulder, elbow, and carpus to pull the limb away from the clinician. When the pelvic limb is tested, the patient should automatically respond by flexing the hip, stifle, and hock to pull the limb away from the clinician. The contralateral limb should be unaffected, meaning that if the right hind limb is evaluated for the withdrawal reflex, the left hind limb should not respond. If the contralateral limb extends when the opposite limb is being tested for the withdrawal reflex, an abnormal crossed-extensor reflex is present and requires further investigation [2, 4, 5, 25]. The only exception is in a newborn kitten up to 17 days of age, during which time a crossed extensor reflex can be considered normal [7, 8].

A third spinal reflex that should be performed in the neurologic examination of every patient, feline or canine, is the perineal or anal reflex. This was briefly described in Section 6.5.8 when reviewing key points of the rectal examination. The perineal reflex is a means by which to assess anal tone. To determine if there is appropriate tone, the clinician touches the anal rim with a gloved forefinger. An anus with normal tone will "wink" as the anal sphincters close. Decreased or absent tone is suggestive of a lesion in the S1–S3 segments or dysfunctional anal innervation from branches of the pudendal nerve [5]. In addition, the perineal reflex also results in flexion of the tail. Failure of the patient to tail-tuck suggests that there may be a lesion within the caudal spinal cord segments [5]. In a neonatal kitten up to 3 weeks of age, stimulation of the perineal region also triggers elimination [7].

A fourth spinal reflex that may be performed is the panniculus or cutaneous trunci reflex. The clinician uses a hemostat to gently pinch the skin lateral to the spine, beginning in the lumbosacral region and moving cranially, one vertebra at a time. Both the patient's left and right lateral sides should be tested. When performed in the normal patient, the panniculus reflex results in contraction of the cutaneous trunci muscles. This contraction will be evident as a twitch over the thoracolumbar region due to the integrity of the lateral thoracic nerve and C8–T1 spinal segments [4, 5]. If contraction of the cutaneous trunci muscles is not evident at a discrete cut-off point, then a lesion is likely to be present anywhere from one to four segments cranially [5].

Additional spinal reflexes may be tested in the cat, but are beyond the scope of this text given that their reliability and reproducibility in the feline patient are questionable and highly user dependent. In the thoracic limb, these include [2, 4, 5, 25]:

- the extensor carpi radialis or triceps reflex, which assesses the integrity of the radial nerve in the thoracic limb and C7–T1 spinal cord segments;
- the biceps reflex, which evaluates the spinal cord segments C6–C8 and also the musculocutaneous nerve.

In the pelvic limb, the author does not routinely test for the gastrocnemius reflex. This evaluates the sciatic nerve and primarily L7–S1 segments; however, this reflex is difficult to elicit in a normal patient, let alone one with neurologic dysfunction [5].

8.7 Assessing the Cranial Nerves

After evaluating the gait and postural reactions, the clinician typically assesses the cranial nerves [25]. The cranial nerves consist of 12 pairs that originate from the brain itself. Their functions to different regions of the body (primarily the head, neck, and trunk) vary. Some are heavily involved in the perception of special senses – vision, olfaction, audition, and taste – whereas others contribute to sensation, muscle contraction, and glandular or organ function. They are numbered in order from where they arise within the brain, from cranial to caudal, as cranial nerve I through XII [5]:

- CN I: the olfactory nerve;
- CN II: the optic nerve;
- CN III: the oculomotor nerve;
- CN IV: the trochlear nerve;
- CN V: the trigeminal nerve;
- CN VI: the abducent nerve;
- CN VII: the facial nerve;
- CN VIII: the vestibulocochlear nerve;
- CN IX: the glossopharyngeal nerve;
- CN X: the vagus nerve;
- CN XI: the accessory nerve;
- CN XII: the hypoglossal nerve.

Of the 12 pairs of cranial nerves, not all are routinely tested during a routine physical examination. For example, there is no clinical reason that makes it necessary to test each patient's ability to differentiate subtly between different scents. Although it has been established that cats tend to find certain scents aversive – particularly citrus, aloe, pine, eucalyptus, and alcohol

[35, 36] – it would be challenging to assess objectively whether a given patient is capable of detecting each and every odor.

Similarly, the cochlear portion of CN VIII is not routinely tested in the wellness examination. Unlike human patients, who can articulate a concern about the loss of hearing, veterinary patients rely upon their owners to sense their deficit. Even then, when loss of hearing is suspected, it is clinically rare to pursue diagnostic confirmation because hearing loss in cats is not typically medically or surgically managed.

If the clinician and client wish, they could pursue electrodiagnostic testing such as brainstem auditory evoked response (BAER), as was discussed briefly in Section 3.3. [37–41]. More often than using BAER, clients and clinicians diagnose deafness presumptively based upon client-relayed history in combination with physical examination findings such as the tendency for white-coated cats with blue eyes to be deaf. This combination of coat and eye color is genetically linked to apoptosis of the inner ear's hair cells, resulting in hearing impairment shortly after birth [42–49].

Other than CN I and CN VIII, most of the other cranial nerves are tested either in sequence, within the context of a comprehensive neurologic examination, or in isolation, as they relate to other body systems that are tested throughout the wellness examination.

8.7.1 Reviewing the Ocular Reflexes Associated with the Cranial Nerves

CN II is one of several components in the visual pathway that convey the special sense of vision to a patient. For a patient to be visual, the cat must have a functional eye, retina, CN II, optic tract, and occipital cortex. To assess a patient's vision, the clinician may observe whether or not it visually tracks an object such as a cotton ball that is dropped from a height, as from a hand to the ground. This rudimentary test is effective at differentiating visual from avisual patients if the patient is alert, aware, and observant. However, it cannot establish the fineness of the patient's vision: the clarity and crispness of the patient's sight [3, 5].

Another rudimentary test of the patient's vision is to create an obstacle course or maze within the examination room or treatment area. The maze need not be extravagant – it may consist of a series of cardboard boxes or open cage doors. The purpose of the maze is to test an ambulatory patient's ability to navigate through the obstacles by observing them and changing course accordingly [3].

Pupil size is dependent upon a balance between sympathetic and parasympathetic pathways. The former is in many ways tied to the attitude and emotional status of the patient: stress as triggered by "fight or flight"

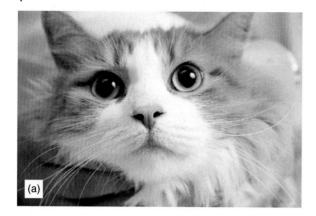

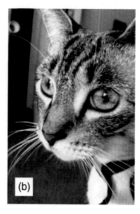

Figure 8.8 (a) Stressed feline patient with bilaterally dilated pupils due to sympathetic stimulation. Source: Courtesy of the Media Resources Department at Midwestern University. (b) Patient with miotic pupils due to abundant ambient lighting. Source: Courtesy of Samantha Rudolph.

tends to dilate both pupils due to abundant sympathetic stimulation (Figure 8.8a). By contrast, parasympathetic pathways facilitate pupillary response to the amount of ambient light: strong light tends to induce pupillary constriction or miosis (Figure 8.8b), whereas low ambient lighting causes pupillary dilation or mydriasis. CN III has a parasympathetic component that is responsible for facilitating miosis [2].

Together, CN II and CN III must be functional in order to elicit a positive pupillary light reflex (PLR). Recall from Section 3.2.8 that there are two variations of PLRs: direct and consensual. To perform a direct PLR, a bright light is shone into the eye that is being evaluated. If CN II and CN III are intact, then CN III will modulate entry of the light into the eye by constricting the pupil. A normal pupil should constrict in response to the light. In addition, the pupil of the contralateral eye should also constrict. This is referred to as the consensual PLR [1, 3, 5, 25]. PLRs are present in kittens as early as 5–14 days after birth [7].

Note that the patient's degree of mydriasis may complicate the clinician's ability to test for PLRs. The clinic setting is often stressful for feline patients, many of which present with bilaterally symmetrical, dilated pupils. When such dilation is pronounced, a normal cat does not always constrict its pupils in response to weak light sources such as a penlight. A stronger light source is often required to obtain PLRs in stressed feline patients [50].

Recall that, as discussed in Section 3.2.8, positive PLRs do not guarantee that the patient is visual. Normal PLRs will be present in a patient that is cortically blind. This explains why multiple tests are required in order for lesion localization to be accurate [37, 50].

If the patient is visual yet lacks one or both PLRs and/or exhibits pupillary asymmetries, then there is a lesion either in CN III or in the sympathetic innervation of the eye [3]. Horner's syndrome is an example of the latter and is characterized by miosis of the affected eye [51]. In addition, there is concurrent enophthalmos, ptosis (upper eyelid droopiness), and a pronounced nictitating membrane [51].

Nasopharyngeal polyps, in particular those involving the middle ear, commonly result in Horner's syndrome [52]. Recall from Section 5.4.1 that nasopharyngeal polyps occur primarily in young cats. These cats typically present with stertor due to upper airway obstruction during the inspiratory part of the respiratory cycle. An oropharyngeal examination under sedation may assist with the diagnosis; however, advanced imaging such as a CT scan may be indicated to evaluate the upper airway sinuses to rule out turbinate destruction and/or mass effect [53].

A transient Horner's syndrome is also possible to see in the postoperative period following a ventral bulla osteotomy due to inadvertent disruption of the sympathetic nerve fibers that pass through the tympanic bulla [52] (Figure 8.9).

In addition to the PLR, one additional ocular reflex tests the integrity of CN II. Recall the menace response, as reviewed in Section 3.2.8. The menace response tests CN II and CN VII. The clinician makes a threatening gesture toward each eye. A patient with a positive menace response must first see the threat and then blink as a protective function. It is important that the clinician takes care not to touch the eyelids themselves in the process or to create excessive air currents, because although the outcome may be the same (the patient blinks), it will be due to touch as a stimulus rather than vision [37, 50]. Kittens develop a menace response in both eyes during the first 4 weeks of life [7], although it may take until 2–3 months of age for it to become consistent [3].

One additional ocular reflex should be reviewed at this time. Recall the palpebral reflex, as discussed in Section 3.2.8. The palpebral reflex tests CN V and CN VII. The clinician touches the medial canthus of each eyelid. A neurologically normal cat with this reflex intact will blink due to tactile stimulation. In order to do so, the cat must first sense the clinician's contact via CN V and then blink via CN VII [37, 50]. Kittens develop the palpebral reflex within the first 3 days of life [7].

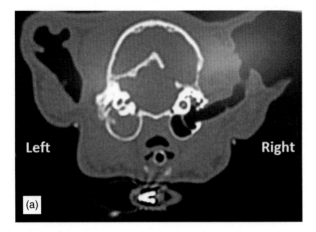

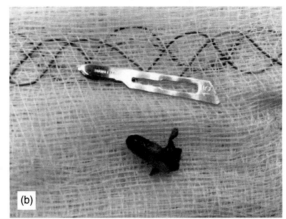

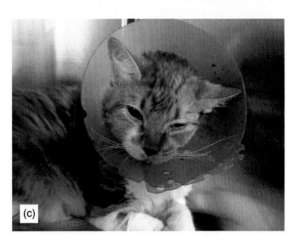

Figure 8.9 (a) Transverse CT scan demonstrating appreciable fluid in the left tympanic bulla. (b) Nasopharyngeal polyp after surgical extraction. (c) Post-operative ptosis and pronounced nictitating membrane OS in a feline patient that underwent ventral bulla osteotomy.

8.7.2 Reviewing the Cranial Nerves Associated with Ocular Movement

Coordinated movement of the eyes is facilitated by CN III, IV, and VI [3, 5, 25], which innervate the extraocular muscles. Strabismus results when there is dysfunction in one or more of the extraocular muscles. The resulting misalignment between the eyes prevents them from directing their gaze at the same point in space at the same time. As a result, binocular vision and depth perception may be compromised [54–57].

Whereas in human medicine the presence of strabismus typically indicates dysfunction within the extraocular eye muscles themselves [55, 56], strabismus in veterinary medicine typically stems from underlying neuropathy. The direction of the strabismus confers which cranial nerve is impacted:

- Ventrolateral strabismus involves CN III.
- Rotatory strabismus involves CN IV.
- Medial strabismus involves CN VI.

Strabismus can occur in one or both eyes and is common in Siamese cats [37, 58–60]. See Figure 3.16 for an example of a feline patient with strabismus.

8.7.3 Reviewing the Cranial Nerves Associated with Tactile Sensation

The role of CN V in the sensory portion of the palpebral reflex via its ophthalmic branch has already been reviewed. In this reflex, CN V is responsible for sensing tactile stimulation at the level of the medial canthus.

The ophthalmic branch of CN V can also be assessed when the clinician touches a saline-moistened cotton-tipped applicator to the cornea. This so-called corneal reflex requires the ophthalmic branch of CN V to recognize tactile stimulation, which then alerts CN VI to retract the globe [5].

CN V is also responsible for detecting tactile sensation in other regions of the face. For instance, facial sensation can be assessed by taking the tips of a hemostat or cotton-tipped applicator and touching the nasal septum. A patient with an intact maxillary branch of CN V will pull away from the stimulus. A patient that does not attempt to escape the stimulus likely has a lesion in the maxillary branch of CN V [5].

The maxillary branch of CN V can also be assessed when the upper lip adjacent to the maxillary canine tooth is pinched. The author makes use of this technique much less commonly in the cat because in her opinion it is more aversive than the aforementioned technique and is more likely to result in fractious behavior on the part of the patient [5]. For similar reasons, the author does not tend to test the mandibular branch of CN V: the lower lip adjacent to the mandibular canine tooth is pinched and the patient is expected to withdraw its head [5].

8.7.4 Reviewing the Cranial Nerves Associated with Muscle Movement Other Than Ocular

CN V, VII, and XI innervate select muscle groups within the body. When these muscles exhibit changes in form or function, their associated cranial nerves may be implicated [5]:

- The muscles of mastication are innervated by CN V. Dysfunction within CN V may lead to atrophy of the temporalis or masseter muscles or a weak or "dropped" jaw.
- The positions of the eyelids and lip folds are innervated by CN VII. If ptosis is present or if lip folds are droopy, dysfunction of CN VII may be considered.
- The trapezius muscle, which straddles the dorsal shoulder and upper back, is innervated by CN XI. Dysfunction of this nerve will lead to atrophy of this muscle. However, this atrophy may be so subtle that it is rarely, if ever, appreciated in the affected patient.

8.7.5 Reviewing the Cranial Nerves Associated with Digestion

CN IX, X, and XII assist with digestion. When these digestive functions are observed to be dysfunctional by either the client or clinician on physical examination, their associated cranial nerves may be implicated [5]:

- CN IX and X help to coordinate the swallowing reflex. Patients with deficits in one or both of these nerves may have a client-reported history of dysphagia or regurgitation. In the dog, a finger is often advanced into the caudal pharyngeal region to elicit a gag in order to confirm that both nerves are functional. However, this is not typically done in the cat for safety reasons.
- The tongue is innervated by CN XII. A patient with a deficit in this nerve may have difficulty lapping up water or prehending food. The patient may also have "tongue droop," meaning that the tongue involuntarily hangs out of the mouth. The author does not typically grab the tongue with gauze in a feline patient as she might be so inclined in a canine patient to assess tongue strength; however, if she did and found the tongue to be weak, she would consider dysfunction within CN XII to be a possibility.

8.7.6 Reviewing the Cranial Nerves Associated with Maintaining Posture

The vestibular portion of CN VIII helps the body to maintain itself in equilibrium. The patient is able to sense changes in head position without losing balance. The patient is also able to keep images focused on the retina when the head is turning by moving the eyes in the opposite the direction to the head due to coordination between the eyes and the vestibular apparatus [5]. A patient with a dysfunctional vestibular portion of CN VIII may exhibit a head tilt, abnormal (rather than physiologic) nystagmus, or ataxia with a broad-based stance.

8.8 Assessing Nociception

Nociception refers to the patient's perception of pain as an aversive experience that can result from either an actual or an anticipated stimulus [61–64]. Perception of pain is unique to the individual [64]. Pain perception may be influenced by the patient's age, health status, and past experiences [62]. Pain may be acute or chronic; it may also be additive [64]. Furthermore, pain is not just the immediate sensation, but also the after-effects: how pain alters the patient's emotional status becomes equally important [63–65].

Veterinary patients present a challenge to clinicians because they cannot articulate in words recognizable in the human language what it is that they are experiencing. Human patients can identify and convey the timeline of pain (onset, duration, progression), the intensity of the pain, and the pain's characteristics (stabbing, burning, throbbing, tingling, etc.) Veterinary patients rely upon owners and the veterinary team to pick up on behavioral or other observational cues that may be suggestive that pain exists [63, 64].

The burden is therefore on the clinician to anticipate, recognize, intervene, manage, and reevaluate pain not just during surgical procedures or hospital stays, but at each and every visit [64, 65]. This has been referred to in the medical literature as the PLATTER approach [65]:

- **PL**an;
- **A**nticipate;
- **T**rea**T**;
- **E**valuate;
- **R**eturn.

This acronym serves as an important reminder that to manage pain effectively, the clinician must invest in a patient-tailored plan that is revised as needed rather than falling back upon the old-school, cookie-cutter approach to pharmacologic therapy. Drugs may still represent one appropriate arm of therapy. However, effective pain management may also need to take into consideration proper nursing care, gentle handling, behavioral therapy, exercise, nutrition and weight management, range of motion exercises, and other physiotherapy, therapeutic laser, and other complementary modalities [62].

Pain used to be considered an afterthought, but is now considered to be as important to every patient as obtaining the temperature, pulse, and respiratory rate. Some practices have automatically inserted it into the medical record as the fourth vital sign [64, 65].

Several pain scales have been devised for use in veterinary patients [63]. Early scoring systems that have been clinically employed include the Numerical Rating Scale (NRS), the Visual Analogue Scale (VAS), and the Simple Descriptive Scale (SDS) as a means to assess pain on an individual patient basis [64, 66, 67]. When using these scales, subjectivity is a concern: inter-observer variability has been observed, which is thought to limit the scales' reliability [64].

Subsequent pain scoring systems have been developed for use as clinical decision-making tools that combine numerical pain ratings with composite behavioral observations [64]. These highlight the importance of recognizing that a patient's behavior can be indicative of the presence, persistence, and intensity of pain [62, 63, 68]. For example, the Melbourne Pain Scale incorporates an assessment of canine posture, activity, mental status, vocalization, and response to palpation [68, 69]. Colorado State University Veterinary Teaching Hospital designed and implemented a similar composite scale for both cats and dogs [70, 71].

When considering pain recognition in cats, pupil size, heart rate, and respiratory rate are inconsistent. Behavior is still considered to be the superior indicator [64, 72]. Understanding the patient's "normal" behavior – that is, what is considered to be the norm for the individual cat by those who best understand the patient, the client – is critical to the identification of new behaviors, particularly those that are consistently out of character. For example, a cat that is consistently people-friendly within the clinic environment should be flagged as a potential concern if that cat suddenly disengages, hides itself from observers, and/or resorts to defensive aggression. Similarly, the cat that is always fastidious about grooming yet suddenly presents in the clinic with a soiled or otherwise unkempt, matted coat should flag the clinician's attention that something pathologic, including pain, could be a contributing factor [64].

Additional behavior changes that may reflect underlying pain in cats include changes in activity; changes in appetite; excessive grooming, for instance, of surgical sites; the guarding of surgical sites as from a tense abdomen post-ovariohysterectomy; and changes in elimination habits such as abandoning the litter box and resorting to house soiling [64].

Posture can be a significant behavioral cue. A feline patient that is curled up, sleeping, in a normal position is less likely to be in pain than a cat that is hunched up under itself, particularly if the tucked up cat is attempting to disappear from sight. This cat may be experiencing psychologic pain as from stress or true physical pain, particularly if this patient is observed to be hunched in the postoperative period. Additional postural cues that may be indicative of pain in cats are a head held low, or a patient that is constantly shifting weight from one limb to another [64].

Facial expressions can be telling when it comes to recognizing pain or the potential for pain in the clinic setting. Cats that exhibit a furrowed brow or squinted eyes are more likely to be in pain than those displaying a slow blink, which is more characteristic of cats that are relaxed in social settings [64].

The utility of composite scales is that they are technically easy to use and encourage the veterinary team to rely heavily on observation – not just once, but at repeated intervals – emphasizing again the importance of continuity of care. Few scales have been assessed for validity and reliability. At this point, it likely matters less which scale is used in a clinical setting and more that pain is being considered in each and every veterinary patient, not just those undergoing surgery [64].

Composite scales also paint a more complete picture of patient well-being by evaluating multiple criteria rather than just one. The clinician is more likely to identify areas where the patient deviates from its norm because more aspects of the patient are observed and recorded.

For example, let us consider three separate patients with three different locations of physical pain that can be induced by various maneuvers in the physical examination:

- A cat with structural brain disease demonstrates a pain response when the clinician applies firm and constant pressure on the skull just above the zygomatic arch.
- A cat with neck pain resists movement of the neck in the direction that elicits pain.
- A cat with a lumbosacral lesion reacts painfully when firm, downward pressure is applied to the sacrum.

Despite the fact that pain is present in all three cats, the pain response between them is likely to vary. Not all cats may react in the same way, and not all cats may experience the same intensity of pain. If all three cats in the scenario outlined were painful, yet only one criterion was observed, one or more cats may be wrongly labeled as non-painful.

By using composite scales to observe more variables, the definition of what constitutes pain is broadened. This allows the astute clinician to recognize that pain is expressed in multiple forms that may include, but are not limited to:

- The patient attempting to escape.
- The patient's attention being drawn to the area that was touched. A patient that was looking away from the clinician may suddenly turn its head in the clinician's direction.
- The patient vocalizing (growling, hissing, yowling).
- The patient attempting to physically harm the clinician.

Moreover, the repeated use of composite scales in the same patient over time helps to improve the veterinary team's understanding of how each patient responds to external and internal stimuli, and how medical intervention in response to the perceived pain has impacted the extent of the painful response that the patient is displaying.

In addition to making use of composite scales, it is important that clinicians test the intactness of pain pathways, from a neurologic perspective, to assess whether aversive stimuli are making it through the spinal cord as signals to the brain, where they are consciously perceived. A failure to perceive pain is informative and may help the clinician to localize the lesion by identifying where the signal is successfully received in the patient versus where it is not.

When clinicians test the integrity of pain pathways, they are interested in two different types of pain [1, 5]:

1) superficial pain;
2) deep pain.

Superficial pain originates in the skin. To test a patient's perception of superficial pain, the clinician uses a hemostat to grasp a skin fold at the site of interest. The clinician waits for the patient to settle, then gradually increases the "squeeze" of the hemostat to pinch the skin. Pinching ceases as soon as the patient provides an appropriate response [1, 5]:

- The patient may twitch the skin.
- The patient may react vocally.
- The patient may try to bite.
- The patient may try to escape.

All of these responses are indicative that the noxious event was felt.

In contrast to superficial pain, deep pain refers to what its name implies: it arises deep to the skin and its pathways are less likely to be damaged than those at the body's surface. Accordingly, deep pain is only tested when the patient fails to respond to the clinician's attempts to elicit a superficial pain test [1, 5].

To assess a patient's ability to perceive deep pain, the clinician begins by pinching the toes or the tail with his fingers. If this elicits no response, the clinician graduates from using fingertips to a hemostat. As with the superficial pain test, the clinician gradually increases the "squeeze" of the hemostat to pinch with incrementally greater force to elicit a response. A limb withdrawal is not enough: this merely tells the clinician that the reflex is intact. The clinician is looking for the patient to react by turning its head in the direction of the stimulus, vocalizing, or attempting to bite [1, 5]. The absence of deep pain, as from severe spinal cord compression or other lesions, is suggestive of severe damage at the level of the spinal cord and carries a guarded prognosis for recovery.

References

1 van Nes, J.J., Meij, B.P., and van Ham, L. (2009) Nervous system, in *Medical History and Physical Examination in Companion Animals* (eds. A. Rijnberk and F.J. vanSluijs), Saunders Elsevier, St. Louis, pp. 160–174.

2 Garosi, L. (2009) Neurological examination of the cat. How to get started. *Journal of Feline Medicine and Surgery*, **11** (5), 340–348.

3 Averill, D.R., Jr. (1981) The neurologic examination. *Veterinary Clinics of North America: Small Animal Practice*, **11** (3), 511–521.

4 Thomas, W.B. (2000) Initial assessment of patients with neurologic dysfunction. *Veterinary Clinics of North America: Small Animal Practice*, **30** (1), 1–24, v.

5 Thomas, W.B. and Dewey, C.W. (2008) Performing the neurologic examination, in *A Practical Guide to Canine and Feline Neurology*, 2nd edn. (ed. C.W. Dewey), Wiley-Blackwell, Ames, IA, pp. 53–74.

6 Overall, K.L. (1997) *Clinical Behavioral Medicine for Small Animals*, Mosby, St. Louis.

7 Lavely, J.A. (2006) Pediatric neurology of the dog and cat. *Veterinary Clinics of North America: Small Animal Practice*, **36** (3), 475–501, v.

8 Hoskins, J.D. (1990) Clinical evaluation of the kitten – from birth to eight weeks of age. *Compendium: Continuing Education for the Practicing Veterinarian*, **12** (9), 1215–1225.

9 Kustritz, M.V.R. (2011) History and physical examination of the neonate, in *Small Animal Pediatrics: The First 12 Months of Life* (eds. M.E. Peterson and M.A. Kutzler), Saunders Elsevier, St. Louis, pp. 20–27.

10 Hoskins, J.D. and Partington, B.P. (2001) Physical examination and diagnostic imaging procedures, in *Veterinary Pediatrics: Dogs and Cats from Birth to Six Months*, 3rd edn. (ed. J.D. Hoskins), Saunders Elsevier, Philadelphia, pp. 6–7.

11 Beaver, B.V. (1980) Neuromuscular development of *Felis catus. Laboratory Animals*, **14** (3), 197–198.

12 Parent, J.M. (2006) The cat with a head tilt, vestibular ataxia, or nystagmus, in *Problem-Based Feline Medicine* (ed. J. Rand), Saunders Elsevier, Philadelphia, pp. 835–851.

13 Gunn-Moore, D. (2006) The cat with neck ventroflexion, in *Problem-Based Feline Medicine* (ed. J. Rand), Saunders Elsevier, Philadelphia, pp. 890–905.

14 Lantinga, E., Kooistra, H.S., and van Nes, J.J. (1998) Periodic muscle weakness and cervical ventroflexion caused by hypokalemia in a Burmese cat. *Tijdschrift voor Diergeneeskunde*, **123** (14–15), 435–437 (in Dutch).

15 Malik, R., Musca, F.J., Gunew, M.N. *et al.* (2015) Periodic hypokalaemic polymyopathy in Burmese and closely related cats: a review including the latest genetic data. *Journal of Feline Medicine and Surgery*, **17** (5), 417–426.

16 Dow, S.W., LeCouteur, R.A., Fettman, M.J., and Spurgeon, T.L. (1987) Potassium depletion in cats: hypokalemic polymyopathy. *Journal of the American Veterinary Medical Association*, **191** (12), 1563–1568.

17 Nemzek, J.A., Kruger, J.M., Walshaw, R., and Hauptman, J.G. (1994) Acute onset of hypokalemia and muscular weakness in four hyperthyroid cats. *Journal of the American Veterinary Medical Association*, **205** (1), 65–68.

18 Joseph, R.J., Carrillo, J.M., and Lennon, V.A. (1988) Myasthenia gravis in the cat. *Journal of Veterinary Internal Medicine*, **2** (2), 75–79.

19 Indrieri, R.J., Creighton, S.R., Lambert, E.H., and Lennon, V.A. (1983) Myasthenia gravis in two cats. *Journal of the American Veterinary Medical Association*, **182** (1), 57–60.

20 Leon, A., Bain, S.A., and Levick, W.R. (1992) Hypokalaemic episodic polymyopathy in cats fed a vegetarian diet. *Australian Veterinary Journal*, **69** (10), 249–254.

21 Voss, K. and Steffen, F. (2009) Patient assessment, in *Feline Orthopedic Surgery and Musculoskeletal Disease* (eds. P.M. Montavon, K. Voss, and S.J. Langley-Hobbs), Saunders Elsevier, St. Louis, pp. 3–20.

22 Kerwin, S. (2012) Orthopedic examination in the cat: clinical tips for ruling in/out common musculoskeletal disease. *Journal of Feline Medicine and Surgery*, **14** (1), 6–12.

23 Leonard, C.A. and Tillson, M. (2001) Feline lameness. *Veterinary Clinics of North America: Small Animal Practice*, **31** (1), 143–163, vii.

24 Chrisman, C.L. (2006) The neurologic examination. *Clinician's Brief, January*, 11–16.

25 de Lahunta, A. and Glass, E. (2009) The neurologic examination, in *Veterinary Neuroanatomy and Clinical Neurology*, 4th edn. (eds. A. deLahunta, E. Glass, and M. Kent), Saunders Elsevier, St. Louis, pp. 487–501.

26 Bagley, R.S. (2006) The cat with tremor or twitching, in *Problem-Based Feline Medicine* (ed. J. Rand), Saunders Elsevier, Philadelphia, pp. 852–869.

27 Hoskins, J.D. and Shelton, G.D. (2001) The nervous and neuromuscular systems, in *Veterinary Pediatrics: Dogs and Cats from Birth to Six Months*, 3rd edn. (ed. J.D. Hoskins), Saunders, Philadelphia, pp. 425–462.

28 Blythe LL. (2011) The neurologic system, in *Small Animal Pediatrics: The First 12 Months of Life* (eds. M.E. Peterson and M.A. Kutzler), Saunders Elsevier, St. Louis, pp. 418–435.

29 Barone, G. (2012) Neurology, in *The Cat: Clinical Medicine and Management* (ed. S.E. Little), Saunders Elsevier, St. Louis, pp. 734–767.

30 Willoughby, K. and Kelly, D.F. (2002) Hereditary cerebellar degeneration in three full sibling kittens. *Veterinary Record*, **151** (10), 295–298.

31 Johnson, R.H., Margolis, G., and Kilham, L. (1967) Identity of feline ataxia virus with feline panleucopenia virus. *Nature*, **214** (5084), 175–177.

32 Kilham, L. and Margolis, G. (1966) Viral etiology of spontaneous ataxia of cats. *American Journal of Pathology*, **48** (6), 991–1011.

33 Richardson, J.A. and Little, S.E. (2012) Toxicology, in *The Cat: Clinical Medicine and Management* (ed. S.E. Little), Saunders Elsevier, St. Louis, p. 919.

34 Jennings, D.P. and Bailey, J.G. (2004) Spinal control of posture and movement, in *Dukes' Physiology of Domestic Animals*, 12th edn. (ed. W.O. Reece), Comstock, Ithaca, NY, pp. 892–903.

35 Herron, M.E. and Shreyer, T. (2014) The pet-friendly veterinary practice: a guide for practitioners. *Veterinary Clinics of North America: Small Animal Practice*, **44** (3), 451–481.

36 Rodan, I., Sundahl, E., Carney, H. *et al.* (2011) AAFP and ISFM feline-friendly handling guidelines. *Journal of Feline Medicine and Surgery*, **13** (5), 364–375.

37 Rijnberk, A. and vanSluijs, F.S. (eds.) (2009) *Medical History and Physical Examination in Companion Animals*, Saunders Elsevier, St. Louis.

38 Bach, J.P., Lupke, M., and Wefstaedt, P. (2013) Deafness in the dog and cat: aetiology, diagnostics and treatment. *Tierarztliche Praxis. Ausgabe K, Kleintiere/ Heimtiere*, **41** (6), 421–427; quiz, 8 (in German).

39 Sims, M.H. (1988) Electrodiagnostic evaluation of auditory function. *Veterinary Clinics of North America: Small Animal Practice*, **18** (4), 913–944.

40 Dijkshoorn, N.A. and van der Wel, T. (1997) Screening for deafness in companion animals. *Tijdschrift voor Diergeneeskunde*, **122** (6), 168–169 (in Dutch).

41 Cook, L.B. (2004) Neurologic evaluation of the ear. *Veterinary Clinics of North America: Small Animal Practice*, **34** (2), 425–435, vi.

42 Stokking, L.B. and Campbell, K.C. (2004) Disorders of pigmentation, in *Small Animal Dermatology Secrets* (ed. K.C. Campbell), Hanley & Belfus, Philadelphia, pp. 352–255.

43 Cat Fanciers' Association (2004) *Cat Colors FAQ: Cat Color Genetics*, http://www.fanciers.com/other-faqs/color-genetics.html (accessed 12 April 2016).

44 Cvejic, D., Steinberg, T.A., Kent, M.S., and Fischer, A. (2009) Unilateral and bilateral congenital sensorineural deafness in client-owned pure-breed white cats. *Journal of Veterinary Internal Medicine*, **23** (2), 392–395.

45 Strain, G.M. (1999) Congenital deafness and its recognition. *Veterinary Clinics of North America: Small Animal Practice*, **29** (4), 895–907, vi.

46 Luttgen, P.J. (1994) Deafness in the dog and cat. *Veterinary Clinics of North America: Small Animal Practice*, **24** (5), 981–989.

47 Strain, G.M. (2007) Deafness in blue-eyed white cats: the uphill road to solving polygenic disorders. *Veterinary Journal*, **173** (3), 471–472.

48 Geigy, C.A., Heid, S., Steffen, F. *et al.* (2007) Does a pleiotropic gene explain deafness and blue irises in white cats? *Veterinary Journal*, **173** (3), 548–553.

49 Bergsma, D.R. and Brown, K.S. (1971) White fur, blue eyes, and deafness in the domestic cat. *Journal of Heredity*, **62** (3), 171–185.

50 deLahunta, A., Glass, E., and Kent, M. (eds.) (2009) *Veterinary Neuroanatomy and Clinical Neurology*, 4th edn., Saunders Elsevier, St. Louis.

51 Bagley, R.S. (2006) The cat with anisocoria or abnormally dilated or constricted pupils, in *Problem-Based Feline Medicine* (ed. J. Rand), Saunders Elsevier, Philadelphia, pp. 870–889.

52 Baines, S.J. (2014) Pharynx, in *Feline Soft Tissue and General Surgery* (eds. S.J. Langley-Hobbs, J.L. Demetriou, and J.F. Ladlow), Saunders Elsevier, St. Louis, pp. 617–634.

53 Quimby, J. and Lappin, M.R. (2012) The upper respiratory tract, in *The Cat: Clinical Medicine and Management* (ed. S.E. Little), Saunders Elsevier, St. Louis, pp. 846–861.

54 Maggs, D.J., Miller, P.E., and Ofri, R. (2013) *Slatter's Fundamentals of Veterinary Ophthalmology*, 5th edn., Saunders Elsevier, St. Louis.

55 Gunton, K.B., Wasserman, B.N., and DeBenedictis, C. (2015) Strabismus. *Primary Care*, **42** (3), 393–407.

56 Campos, E.C. (2008) Why do the eyes cross? A review and discussion of the nature and origin of essential infantile esotropia, microstrabismus, accommodative esotropia, and acute comitant esotropia. *Journal of AAPOS*, **12** (4), 326–331.

57 Ketring, K.L. and Glaze, M.B. (2012) *Atlas of Feline Ophthalmology*, 2nd edn., Wiley-Blackwell, Ames, IA.

58 Rengstorff, R.H. (1976) Strabismus measurements in the Siamese cat. *American Journal of Optometry and Physiological Optics*, **53** (10), 643–646.

59 Blake, R. and Crawford, M.L. (1974) Development of strabismus in Siamese cats. *Brain Research*, **77** (3), 492–496.

60 Hyde, J.E. (1962) Cross-eyedness: a study in Siamese cats. *American Journal of Ophthalmology*, **53**, 70–75.

61 de Lahunta, A. and Glass, E. (2009) General sensory systems: general proprioception and general somatic afferent, in *Veterinary Neuroanatomy and Clinical Neurology*, 4th edn. (eds. A. deLahunta, E. Glass, and M. Kent), Saunders Elsevier, St. Louis, pp. 221–242.

62 Epstein, M., Rodan, I., Griffenhagen, G. *et al.* (2015) 2015 AAHA/AAFP Pain Management Guidelines for Dogs and Cats. *Journal of the American Animal Hospital Association*, **51** (2), 67–84.

63 Balakrishnan, A. and Benasutti, E. (2012) Pain assessment in dogs and cats. *Today's Veterinary Practice, March/April*, 68–74.

64 Mathews, K., Kronen, P.W., Lascelles, D. *et al.* (2014) Guidelines for recognition, assessment and treatment of pain: WSAVA Global Pain Council members and co-authors of this document. *Journal of Small Animal Practice*, **55** (6), E10–E68.

65 AAHA/AAFP Pain Management Guidelines Task Force Members, Hellyer, P., Rodan, I. *et al.* (2007) AAHA/AAFP Pain Management Guidelines for Dogs and Cats. *Journal of Feline Medicine and Surgery*, **9** (6), 466–480.

66 Holton, L.L., Scott, E.M., Nolan, A.M. *et al.* (1998) Comparison of three methods used for assessment of pain in dogs. *Journal of the American Veterinary Medical Association*, **212** (1), 61–66.

67 Hudson, J.T., Slater, M.R., Taylor, L. *et al.* (2004) Assessing repeatability and validity of a visual analogue scale questionnaire for use in assessing pain and lameness in dogs. *American Journal of Veterinary Research*, **65** (12), 1634–1643.

68 Hansen, B.D. (2003) Assessment of pain in dogs: veterinary clinical studies. *ILAR Journal*, **44** (3), 197–205.

69 Firth, A.M. and Haldane, S.L. (1999) Development of a scale to evaluate postoperative pain in dogs. *Journal of the American Veterinary Medical Association*, **214** (5), 651–659.

70 Hellyer, P.W., Uhrig, S.R., and Robinson, S.G. (2006) *Feline Pain*, http://csu-cvmbs.colostate.edu/Documents/anesthesia-pain-management-pain-score-feline.pdf (accessed 30 May 2016).

71 Hellyer, P.W., Uhrig, S.R., and Robinson, S.G. (2006) *Canine Pain*, http://csu-cvmbs.colostate.edu/Documents/anesthesia-pain-management-pain-score-canine.pdf (accessed 30 May 2016).

72 Brondani, J.T., Luna, S.P., and Padovani, C.R. (2011) Refinement and initial validation of a multidimensional composite scale for use in assessing acute postoperative pain in cats. *American Journal of Veterinary Research*, **72** (2), 174–183.

Part Two

Performing the Canine Physical Examination

9

Setting the Stage: Canine-Friendly Practice and Low-Stress Handling

9.1 Challenges Faced in Canine Practice

The human–animal bond has evolved over time such that companion animals reside in the majority of households within the Western Hemisphere and are more often than not considered to be members of the immediate family [1–3]. This strong relationship between humans and their non-human counterparts has resulted in appreciable documented physical, physiological, social, and psychological benefits [1, 4, 5]. Yet when the bond is broken, companion animal-owning clients are often at a loss as to whom to turn to, leaving the patient at increased risk of relinquishment, abandonment, or euthanasia [1, 6–13].

Behavior problems are one of the primary reasons for relinquishment of canine and feline patients to shelters [7, 8, 10–12, 14, 15]. Behavior problems are also a frequently cited reason why patients that are adopted from shelters may be returned [8, 10, 16]. Particularly damaging to the human-animal bond are behavioral concerns regarding canine aggression toward people and inter-dog aggression [14, 17]. According to a nationwide survey by Salman *et al.* in 1998, roughly 10% of cases of canine relinquishment involve aggression [10]. Of these, nearly 70% of the implicated dogs have bitten one or more people [10]. When behaviors are considered incompatible with the maintenance of the human–animal bond, euthanasia is often considered. A study by Patronek and Dodman in 1999 estimated that 224,000 cats and dogs were destroyed annually as a result of underlying behavioral concerns [18].

The euthanasia of otherwise medically healthy patients on account of behavior likely represents a combination of unrealistic owner expectations for the companion pet and a failure of the veterinary clinic to intervene appropriately and to proactively recognize and manage behavioral concerns [11, 12, 19]. The veterinary team shares responsibility for failing these patients because of the established interconnection between mental and physical health [6, 20]. The burden is on the veterinarian to incorporate a holistic approach to wellness that includes open discussion regarding various aspects of preventive medicine, including behavior [6, 21]. Yet many veterinarians discount behavior as being less significant in the list of topics for discussion in wellness visits. In 2004, when Greenfield *et al.* asked small animal clinicians to rank important skillsets or knowledge bases in which new graduates should be proficient, a working knowledge of animal behavior did not even factor into the top 10 [22].

Many veterinarians feel ill-equipped to address behavioral concerns [6, 18]. As a result, only one-fourth of veterinarians on average routinely ask clients whether or not an underlying behavioral concern exists [6, 11, 12, 18]. Clients report that they typically experience even less discussion with regard to behavior within the examination room: a 1997 nationwide survey by the AVMA indicated that behavior counseling did not account for even 1% of veterinary services during a routine wellness visit [23]. As a result, clients have not classically relied upon the veterinary team for advice regarding inappropriate behavior. In fact, up to 93% of cat-owners acknowledged seeking out non-veterinary advice for the management of house soiling, and roughly one-fourth did not even contact the veterinarian about the issue at all [24]. Those in the latter group admitted to having reservations about whether the veterinarian would know how to intervene effectively [24].

Yet behavior issues are not going away, and companion animals will continue to present for behavioral concerns that could limit their lives if the veterinary team fails to acknowledge and address them [6]. Behavioral issues may also have an underlying medical basis: they may be the first observable indicator that a patient's health is compromised [6]. The veterinarian must be held accountable for leading this discussion so that they can anticipate the development of behavior issues before they occur. This means that each and every patient should receive a behavioral assessment at each and every visit [15]. This assessment should be incorporated into the patient's permanent medical record, allowing the veterinary team to recognize trends [15].

Although a significant proportion of companion animals that are relinquished to shelters on account of behavior are adults [25], behavior issues are rarely isolated events [8] and often have their origin early in life. Fear and distrust at a young age frequently carry over into adulthood: fearful puppies at 8 weeks of age are at an increased risk of being persistently fearful at 18 months [26, 27].

The astute veterinarian must therefore be able and willing to recognize signs of discomfort in veterinary patients [15]. These signs should be discussed with the client on a case-by-case basis to establish whether the deviation from normal behavior is expected or unexpected, contextual or generalized [15]. This allows for a two-sided conversation between the veterinary team and the client, the aim of which is problem-solving before the human–animal bond is fractured.

Not only does an open door of communication regarding animal behavior improve patient outcomes by delaying or reducing risk of relinquishment, it also improves recognition of behavior concerns by the veterinary team in such a way that improves their safety. The veterinary profession is not without occupational risks, and animal-related injuries in veterinary practice are commonplace [28–30]. In a 2009 Canadian survey of 809 veterinarians, 64% reported one or more scratches, 63% reported one or more bite wounds, and 20% reported one or more post-wound infections [28]. Companion animal veterinarians are also 4.4 times more likely to be bitten than their equine counterparts [28]. From a safety perspective alone, it is critical that the veterinary team recommit itself to behavior assessment, particularly a working knowledge of body posture [15].

At the same time, there is a growing body of literature to suggest that forced restraint and punitive training are counter-productive [15]. It used to be that a rough, physical approach to handling was the norm, and that it did not matter how many technicians it took to pin down a dog for a nail trim provided that the job got done. The old-school philosophy was less about patient welfare and more about efficiency [31]. It has since been established that such measures only perpetuate, if not intensify, fear-based aggression and that more appropriate, humane measures are indicated to manage each patient successfully based upon its individual needs [31].

9.2 The Concept of Low-Stress Handling

Just as feline-friendly practice was developed in order that the veterinary profession adapt to cats' physical, physiological, and psychological needs rather than the other way round, the concept of low-stress handling was pioneered by such animal advocates as Dr. Sophia Yin [32]. The phrase erroneously implies that it pertains solely to the physical restraint of patients within the clinic setting. However, low-stress handling involves much more than patient restraint. It encompasses a philosophy of leadership without force, built upon understanding what motivates a patient and using positive reinforcement to promote acceptable behaviors both in and outside the examination room. The cornerstone of low-stress handling is a working knowledge of animal behavior: understanding how to read patients' non-verbal cues and how accordingly to react appropriately to create a safer, calmer environment for all involved.

Whereas cats are by nature solitary [33–35], dogs within their natural environment tend to be social and sociable [36]. Dogs tend to live in extended family groups to raise altricial young that require 18–36 months to reach social maturity. Even well into adulthood, canine patients tend to display infantile behavior patterns such as begging and passive submission. Relationships between pack members tend to be hierarchal, with day-to-day disputes resolved more often than not by deferential behavior. Dogs, like cats, prefer to avoid conflict management through combat when possible [36].

Because humans may identify several parallels between their social system and that of canids, it is tempting to anthropomorphize. Yet canine signals are strictly canine signals and need to be interpreted as such. Often what clients may consider to be friendly behavior directed at their dog is viewed differently from the canine perspective. For example, certain gestures that are strictly human, such as embraces, may be perceived as threatening by a dog [36].

Low-stress handling therefore aims to reinterpret the world of the veterinary clinic as seen through the eyes of the canine patient. As such, low-stress handling must begin as soon as the patient enters the clinic. Dogs may be social creatures; however, the clinic environment is considered to be unfamiliar territory full of new and potentially terrifying sights, sounds, and senses. Just as the majority of feline patients benefit from being minimally exposed to conspecifics and other species [37], so, too, do dogs. A canine-friendly practice should have a designated dog-only waiting room or at least one that is spatially segregated (Figure 9.1).

When at all possible, the practice should structure its appointment schedule so as to minimize wait times. When unforeseen circumstances extend the wait, canine patients should be directed into dog-only examination rooms as soon as possible.

While en route to the examination room, most clinics expect that canine patients will consent to walking up onto a low profile, electronic floor scale. These scales can be a source of stress because their metal surfaces are highly reflective and they may also feel cold and slippery to the patient. See Section 1.5 regarding the use of non-slip mats to place over the scale's surface to afford greater security in foot placement.

Scales may also create stress due to location. For example, scales are often tucked into corners where they

Figure 9.1 (a) Dog-designated and (b) cat-designated waiting room, as identified by the outline of the dog or cat stenciled into the floor design.

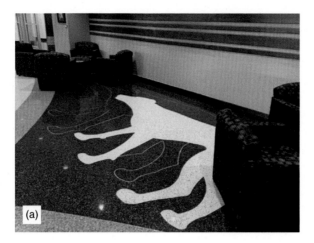
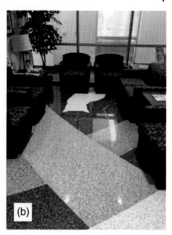

are less obtrusive and out of view; however, this placement may feel threatening to a dog that is already fearful because in a sense it further backs the dog into a corner (Figure 9.2a). A preferred approach may be to abandon the floor scale altogether and instead opt for a digital platform scale: the patient is able to be weighed on the examination room table (Figure 9.2b).

If the examination rooms have windows facing the interior of the corridor, blinds may be installed to reduce visual stimuli (see Figure 1.4).

As was the case with cat-only examination rooms, the exterior of dog-designated examination rooms may be fitted with a sliding card to denote when the rooms are occupied. This prevents unknowing staff from entering an occupied room with closed blinds and inadvertently allowing the patient to escape into the hospital corridor (see Figure 1.5).

When canine patients are required to be admitted into the hospital, one or more dog-designated wards should be available to decrease inter-species exposure. The author has the privilege of working in a facility with two separate dog-designated wards, into which dogs are admitted based upon size (Figure 9.3). This allows smaller dogs to be confined to a room with smaller dogs, and larger dogs with larger dogs, so as to lessen tension and undue stress based upon vast differences in size.

As was the case with feline patients, canine cages should not face each other (Figure 9.4). When they do, dogs see other dogs, which may be a significant source of stress.

See Sections 1.3 and 1.4 to review how light and sound in the practice setting may be aversive. Although cats' hearing exceeds dogs' in terms of range – dogs hear up to 15,000–60,000 cycles per second compared with

Figure 9.2 (a) Low-profile floor scale, backed into a corner. Although many canine patients will not balk at being asked to walk onto this scale, the position of the scale in a corner may intensify fear in a patient that is scared. (b) Digital platform scale, incorporated into the design of the examination room table. This allows patients to be weighed when they are standing on the examination room table, rather than requiring them to walk onto a floor scale that may be an added stressor.

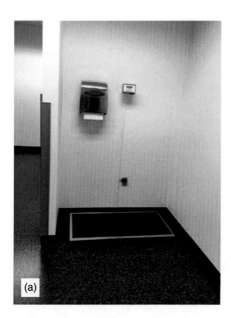
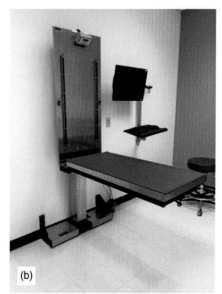

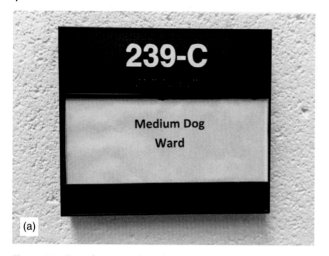 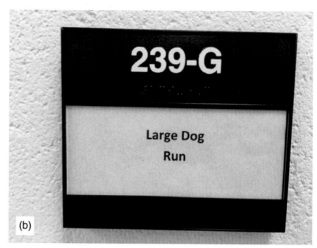

Figure 9.3 Dog-designated wards designed to house (a) small- to medium-sized dogs and (b) large-breed dogs.

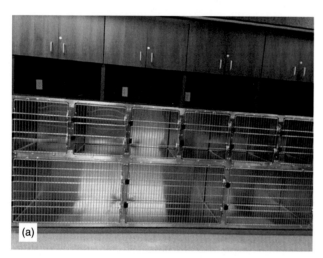 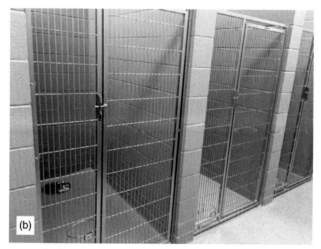

Figure 9.4 (a) Stackable cages that house small- to medium-sized dogs. Note that these are stackable, without the ability of housed patients to see other housed patients. (b) Side-by-side kennel runs that house large-breed dogs. Note that these kennels do not allow patients to see other patients because they do not face one another.

20,000–100,000 in cats – dogs still exceed the hearing capabilities of people [36]. Accordingly, the veterinary team should be conscientious when it comes to noise, recognizing that it may be a noxious stimulus for veterinary patients.

9.3 White Coat Syndrome

White coat syndrome is stress-induced activation of the sympathetic nervous system in response to veterinary paraphernalia, in particular the white coat, causing transient hypertension [38–41]. White coat syndrome has been reported in both dogs and cats [42, 43]. The impact of stress-induced hypertension [44–48] is not necessarily minor [49]. Human patients who have experienced white coat syndrome are at risk of developing target organ damage, particularly in

the cardiovascular system, kidneys, and eyes [44, 45, 50–52]. In canine patients, the kidneys are most affected [53]. Renal damage from persistent hypertension may result in the development of proteinuria with the urinalysis testing positive for microalbuminuria [52–54]. Of all canine breeds, racing Greyhounds appear to be most at risk of target organ damage due to unchecked, sustained hypertension. This is because from a cardiovascular perspective, racing Greyhounds are "built" differently from other canine breeds. The cardiovascular traits that make racing Greyhounds distinct include the following:

- more viscous blood [55];
- a higher than normal baseline hematocrit [55];
- increased left ventricular mass and volume [56, 57];
- higher than normal baseline systolic blood pressure [55, 58].

Although these cardiovascular traits collectively adapt Greyhounds to racing, they concurrently predispose the dogs to target organ damage because their resting blood pressure when measured in the clinic setting is routinely 10–20 mmHg higher than that of other canine species [53]. In other words, their systolic blood pressure is already nearer to levels at which target organ damage is anticipated, so there is less leeway in a Greyhound experiencing white coat syndrome for blood pressure to rise without adverse effect [49]. When Greyhounds become hypertensive, the majority demonstrate abnormal findings on urinalysis subsequent to exposure to the stressor: 84% of hypertensive Greyhounds develop microalbuminuria [59].

White coat syndrome is a real phenomenon, hence prevention is much preferred to treatment. Prevention should begin early in life before negative associations in veterinary patients with regard to the clinic environment are learned and reinforced. Just as clinicians immunize against infectious diseases, so the veterinary team should consider the importance of immunizing against fear. One way to do so is by hosting in-clinic socialization classes. These are intended to promote the clinic experience and interactions with the veterinary team as positive and interactive rather than aversive and domineering. Positive reinforcement, verbal praise, and both toy and treat rewards collectively inspire a relaxed environment in which the patient can feel safe and unstressed [60].

In addition to interacting with staff, puppies should be encouraged to explore examination rooms under supervision and in so doing become exposed to commonplace veterinary paraphernalia. Allowing pets access to see and touch this equipment on their own, voluntarily, without being forced to submit to invasive procedures sets the stage for patients to feel in control and therefore less afraid. In particular, puppies should be exposed to stethoscopes and white coats before problem visits arise. The idea is that veterinary equipment should become so commonplace and benign that they no longer incite fear or distrust. Instead, they become a non-event [60].

For this to occur, patients need to be encouraged to explore at their own rate rather than "flooding" them with every piece of veterinary equipment at once. Flooding is the process of exposing a patient to an all-or-nothing stimulus that has historically provoked a negative response in the patient with the hope of ultimately extinguishing the patient's reaction. For example, if a human patient had a phobia of elevators and flooding were employed in an attempt to lessen the fear, the patient would be forced into an elevator for extended periods of time until they no longer feared the elevator [61].

Similarly, if a canine patient were afraid of the doorbell, flooding would include playing an audio recording of the doorbell ringing over and over again, at maximum volume, without pause, until the patient's adverse reaction to it reduced in intensity [61, 62].

Flooding has the potential to be exceedingly stressful. Because it has the potential to exacerbate fear, thereby creating a perpetually fearful dog, its use is no longer advised by many veterinary behaviorists. In its place, desensitization is preferred. Desensitization incorporates gradual exposure to the adverse stimulus to build confidence sequentially and, in so doing, lessen fear [61].

Desensitization may occur in the clinic; however, owing to time constraints it is often much more successfully initiated and followed through at home, within a safe and familiar environment. For example, patients may be desensitized against white coats or other medical attire such as scrubs by having them on hand at home, where the patient may be gradually exposed. Patients may then sniff at the objects voluntarily and/or paw at them, when left out. If the patient exhibits avoidance behavior, the owner may encourage its involvement with the object that incites distrust by using a trail of treats to coax the patient to approach. Initially, this method requires a potentially extensive time commitment on the part of the client; however, the initial investment is likely to pay off in subsequent veterinary visits because the patient has already experienced the unfamiliar object in its own environment on its own terms, and has learned to associate the object's use with positive rewards [60].

This is why veterinarians frequently emphasize how important it is for the client to acclimate new puppies to as many aspects of the veterinary examination as possible, as early in life as able. For instance, it is not uncommon for the author to ask owners of new puppies to stroke the feet, touch between the toes, lift the lips, and lift the pinnae. Because fear and distrust at a young age are likely to carry over into adulthood, anything that the veterinary–client partnership can do now to reduce fear is a step in the right direction [26, 27].

Note that despite the best efforts of both the clinician and the owner, white coat syndrome is not always preventable [60]. Patients that have been poorly socialized or that have experienced trauma may never be fully at ease within a clinic setting [60]. Furthermore, heritability plays a role, and certain patients are genetically predisposed to nervousness. These individuals are pre-wired to respond fearfully to novel stimuli. As a result, their innate fear may be a challenge to overcome – all the more reason for the veterinary team to assess each patient behaviorally, taking into account genetic history, when available through selective breeding, patient temperament, and patient reactivity. Only by proactively anticipating stressors for patients can the veterinary team fully embrace the concept of low-stress handling to advance patient welfare.

9.4 The Role of Scent

Of domestic species, dogs are equipped with the best olfactory capabilities. This acuity has been attributed to the amount of surface area devoted to olfaction: 7000 mm^2 in dogs compared with 500 mm^2 in people. Additionally, dogs have 2.8×10^8 olfactory cells, compared with 2.0×10^7 in humans [36].

Hence canine olfactory acuity is exquisitely sensitive. Even if a scent is diluted out to 1% of the strength that is detectable by people, scent recognition in the dog is possible [63]. This sensory perception is what makes it possible for dogs to detect fingerprints on glass 6 weeks after they were created [64] and to differentiate identical twins based upon olfaction alone [65]. A study involving police dogs demonstrated a 93.3% success rate in identifying individuals by scent [66]. In addition, the dogs could identify accurately the region of the body from where the scent originated [66].

Because scent recognition is strong in the dog, it is not surprising that pheromones play a significant role in canine communication [36]. Depending upon the individual dog and the intent behind its message, scent marking may include feces, anal sac secretions, urine, vaginal secretions, secretions from the merocrine sweat glands of the paw pads, and secretions from the sebaceous glands of interdigital skin [67].

Fecal marking is more common in males than females [68], but anal sac secretions coat every bowel movement of every dog with a unique identifier [36, 69]. In addition, anal sac secretions may be released when dogs are excited or anxious [36]. It is not uncommon for fearful dogs to express their anal glands at the veterinary clinic. This fishy, semi-rancid odor is unmistakably detectable by human members of the veterinary team in addition to any other dog in the vicinity.

Urine marking occurs more frequently than fecal marking, especially in free-ranging males [36]. Its purpose may be sexual, as a means to advertise sexual status or receptivity. However, more commonly, its context is social, providing information about the specific individual, its social group, and its social status [36, 70]. Around 50% of male dogs mark with urine by 13 months of age [71, 72], and by 24 months of age, 94% of all dogs, male and female, urine mark [72].

Scratching may or may not accompany urine and fecal marking. However, paw pad and interdigital secretions also carry identifiers and intra-species messages.

Vaginal secretions of receptive, intact females are more important than urine marking when it comes to attracting males [36].

Clearly, the canine nose is fine-tuned to detect a number of scents from a number of different regions of the body, all of which may carry messages of varying intent.

Working dogs make their living by employing their noses. Their function is reliant upon olfaction and their ability to discriminate between scents. It is for this reason that owners of tracking and/or field trial dogs prefer that the veterinary team avoid the administration of intra-nasal vaccinations whenever possible: these may cause the patient to display clinical signs that, although transient, may reduce olfactory acuity for up to 6 weeks [36].

Because dogs are so acutely aware of each other and the environment through their sense of smell, they may perceive the kennel or clinic settings as barrages of olfactory messages that may be distracting, if not petrifying. Such fear can result in escape or avoidance behaviors, excessive vocalization, ptyalism, over-grooming, destructiveness, and/or aggressive tendencies, all of which represent inappropriate coping mechanisms [36, 73].

Just as veterinarians have attempted to alleviate fear-based behaviors in cats through the use of pheromones, it was hypothesized that the same effect could be replicated in dogs given their olfactory acuity [74]. Because feline facial pheromone is not part of the canine olfactory language, another compound had to be considered: that compound was dog appeasing pheromone (DAP).

DAP is naturally produced by the bitch 3 days post-parturition by the intermammary sebaceous glands [75]. This is thought to convey a sense of security to the pups before and after nursing [76]. The idea that this pheromone could be synthesized in the laboratory and used to address fear and separation anxiety in the adult dog was favorably received by the veterinary profession. Synthetic analogues of DAP have since been commercialized in both spray and diffuser forms. There is also a collar-infused version that is worn by the patient. All versions have been studied in a variety of settings, to target a variety of behavioral concerns. DAP has been evaluated in the kennel [73, 74], clinic [77], socialization class [78], and automobile [79], and within the home environment [80, 81]. The use of DAP to combat various noise-related phobias such as fireworks [82–85] and thunder [76] has also been explored. DAP has not been proven to reduce house soiling during the night effectively in newly adopted dogs [86].

Whether or not DAP is effective in all settings and for all fears remains to be determined. A systematic review of the literature by Frank *et al.* concluded that evidence for the efficacy of DAP is lacking [87]. However, the use of DAP is not harmful: it either is or is not effective. Therefore, DAP may be employed by the veterinary team or its use may be encouraged among owners as one means of behavioral modification that may result in stress reduction.

9.5 The Role of Advance Preparation

As was the case in feline veterinary medicine, the first canine veterinary visit sets the tone for both the current and subsequent visits. It is critical that the veterinary team plan ahead and anticipate the patient's needs. Examination rooms should be equipped with easily laundered toys and highly palatable treats. If a patient is known to be reserved or timid, but food motivated, the client may be instructed to fast the patient so that treats are more likely to be accepted from the veterinary team. This will help to make the visit a more pleasurable experience for the client and patient alike [31].

9.6 Examination Room Etiquette: Setting the Tone for Initial Veterinary Interactions with the Dog

As was discussed in Section 1.8, the veterinary profession has historically prioritized efficiency. Companion animals have not always been handled with consideration as to their welfare. The welfare of the veterinary team typically came first [31]. Unfortunately, what was safe and efficient for veterinary professionals was not always in the best interest of the patient. "Problem dogs," much like cats, were handled with "brudacaine," not recognizing that this only perpetuated fear, avoidance behaviors, and/or the development of fear-based aggression.

The philosophy underlying low-stress handling of dogs favors patient-centered, relationship-based care. The welfare of each individual patient is considered, and the veterinary team strives to transition into the physical examination rather than diving in head-first, without allowing the patient to acclimate [32].

Once the client and patient have settled into the examination room, the client may be encouraged to release the patient's leash, provided that it is not known to be offensively aggressive. This gives the dog the opportunity to explore the environment while the veterinary team takes a medical history from the client. During history taking, the clinician can take note of the patient's body posture, respiration, and emotional state.

When given the freedom of being off-leash, some patients will walk over to the clinician, sniff shoes, or even nudge their muzzles against the clinician's side. In a sense, they are giving the veterinary team a once-over and trying to feel out whether or not the clinician is "okay" to approach.

Other patients refuse to leave their owner's side. Still others remain hidden in the far corner of the examination room or tucked as far as possible underneath examination room benches or client legs. For these patients, it is best not to approach them in a threatening manner. The veterinary team would do well to avoid towering over the patient. When it is time to approach the patient, the clinician should lower his body to its level [88].

With the owner's permission, the veterinary team may benefit from tossing treats to the patient so that it forms a positive association with the staff. The patient should be greeted cheerfully, in a "happy" voice. If the patient responds with a tail wag, then the clinician may offer a treat directly to the patient in the palm of the hand [88].

As the dog acclimates to the examination room, the clinician should also avoid direct stares. Direct stares can be perceived as threats, especially to a dog in an unfamiliar environment. Instead, the clinician should avert his gaze initially to allow the dog to adjust to his presence [88].

The clinician should be aware of his body language at all times and avoid rapid hand movements, especially those that involve reaching a hand out quickly in front of the dog's face [88]. Instead, move slowly and calmly. Just as is said routinely in feline medicine, you must "go slow to go fast" [33].

If a patient remains tucked up underneath an examination room chair or remains cowered in the corner, it is important to avoid dragging it from its hideaway if at all possible. This is the equivalent in feline medicine of "dumping" cats out of their carriers onto the examination room table. The action of physically forcing a patient out of hiding removes its sense of control over the situation and may in turn provoke defensive aggression.

9.7 Recognizing Body Language

Just as the veterinary team must be aware of its body language and its potential effects on the patient, it is critical for them to read the patient's non-verbal signals prior to approaching and handling the patient [31].

Visually, dogs communicate with each other and with other species through body posture, coat, tail position, eyes, ears, and mouth. These signals are used to communicate immediate messages over short distances. By contrast, olfaction is typically relied upon to convey long-lasting messages and vocalizations function to communicate over long distances [36].

Although there are breed differences with regard to postural communication [36], there are shared commonalities that the veterinary team should be able to recognize with certainty.

A dog, especially a juvenile, that stands with a lowered front end and an elevated hind end, with rump up, paws out, and tail wagging is signaling a "play bow." This is a dog that wants to play (Figure 9.5).

An alert but relaxed dog may be standing, seated, or lying down. This is a dog that, regardless of stance, is interested and engaged in its surroundings without becoming antagonistically reactive or fearful. The fur is not piloerected as from arousal. The tail is either wagging or relaxed rather than tucked (Figure 9.6).

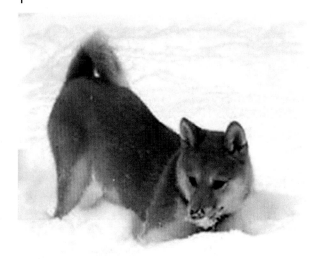

Fearful dogs display obvious postural changes to communicate their unease with the current situation or environment. A dog that is afraid shifts its weight backwards so that there is a whole-body lean away from the object or individual that is inducing the fear (Figure 9.7a). As fear intensifies, the patient continues to tuck its head and neck until they are parallel with the dorsum; its ventral abdomen contacts the ground; the tail tucks underneath of the caudal abdomen; and the dog attempts to withdraw from its surroundings (Figure 9.7b) [36, 88].

More subtle signs of fear in the dog are yawning, licking the lips, and/or sweating profusely through the paw pads [88]. A timid or uncertain patient may also display its sclera prominently (Figure 9.8).

Figure 9.5 Shiba Inu demonstrating a "play bow." Source: Courtesy of Alan Fink Fine Art.

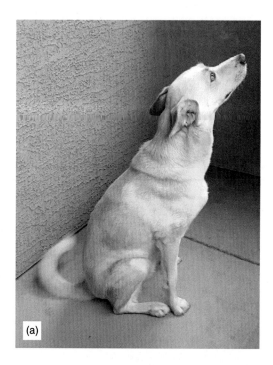

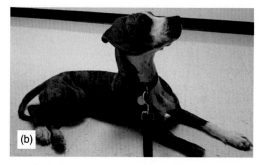

Figure 9.6 (a) Seated, alert, and relaxed patient that is focused and awaiting instructions from its owner. Source: Courtesy of Sarah Ciamello. (b) Alert, yet relaxed patient in a clinic setting, lying down while retaining focus on the veterinary team. Source: Courtesy of Analucia P. Aliaga.

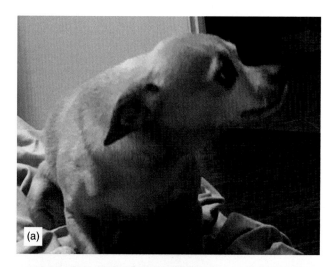

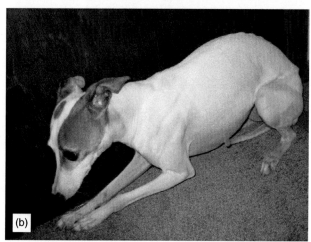

Figure 9.7 (a) A fearful Chihuahua. Note that it is beginning to lean back away from that which induced fear, and that its head and neck are slightly lowered. Source: Courtesy of Lydia T. McDaniel. (b) An intensely fearful canine patient. Note that the head and neck are parallel with the dog's dorsum and the tail is tucked. The patient's ventral abdomen is contacting the floor, and the patient is as pressed up against the wall as is possible. The patient is also averting its gaze. Source: Courtesy of Danna Kedrowski.

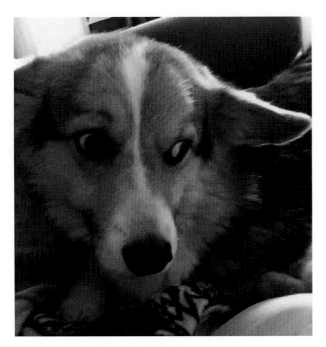

Figure 9.8 Patient demonstrating uncertainty by means of bilaterally prominent sclera. Note also the classic "airplane ear" carriage that is suggestive of the patient's lack of confidence. Source: Courtesy of Cora R. Zenko.

may be present in fearful patients in addition to those that are antagonistic. It is thought that fearful dogs with piloerection tend to have bimodal distribution of the affected fur, over the shoulders and at the hips, whereas antagonistic dogs often have piloerect fur along the entire dorsum [36].

Dogs that expose their ventral abdomen with all four limbs flexed and tail tucked are conveying submission (Figure 9.11a). These patients may urinate or exhibit ptyalism to demonstrate fear or uncertainty. This behavior is both neotenic and instinctual: puppies routinely exhibit their behavior toward the adult members of their pack. An adult dog will "ask" the pup to display deference through submissive posture by pinning the pup by its neck [36].

Note that not all patients that expose their abdomen are fearful. Some dogs are simply relaxed and their exposure of the ventral abdomen conveys trust: they are unconcerned about allowing access to a vulnerable region of the body (Figure 9.11b).

The novice clinician may initially consider it difficult to differentiate exposure of the ventral abdomen due to fear from that which is due to comfort and security. In these situations, the clinician should combine his assessment

By contrast, assertive and potentially antagonistic dogs lean forward or into their forequarters (Figure 9.9) [36]. Assertively antagonistic dogs may also have a broad-based stance in the hindquarters to allow for rapid changes in direction should the patient decide to pivot [36].

Dogs that are reactive to their environment may also display piloerection (Figure 9.10). Note that piloerection

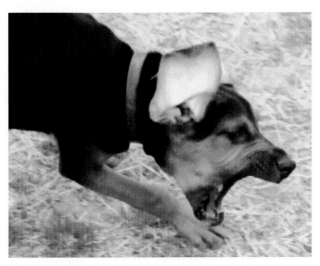

Figure 9.9 Assertively antagonistic patient demonstrating a forward poise toward the object or individual of interest. Source: Courtesy of Lauren A. Beren.

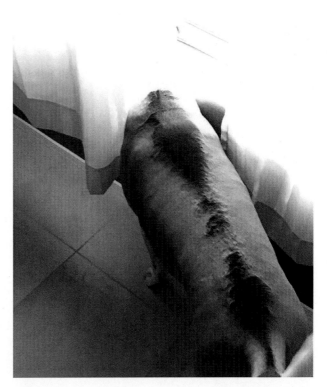

Figure 9.10 Aroused dog that is looking out of the window, with piloerection of the fur. Its head is hidden behind the curtain. Note the bimodal distribution of piloerect fur. Source: Courtesy of Kiefer Hazard.

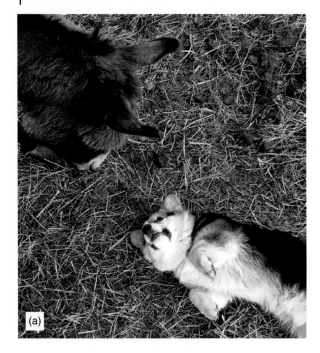

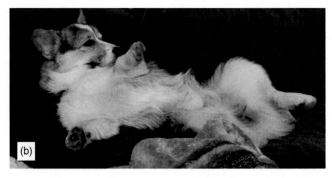

Figure 9.11 (a) Patient exposing ventral abdomen. (b) The same patient as in (a), in his home environment, relaxed and comfortable enough to expose his ventral abdomen. Source (a), (b): Courtesy of Cora R. Zenko.

of the patient's postural communication with additional visual cues such as the eyes, ears, mouth, and tail.

Eye contact or the lack thereof may be assessed by the astute clinician to assist with the behavioral assessment of each and every canine patient. Fearful patients tend to avert their gaze (Figure 9.12a). They may even redirect their gaze with frequency to various parts of the examination room. If the intensity of the fear becomes overwhelming, they may also narrow their palpebral fissures so as to keep the eyes mostly closed [36, 88]. By contrast, a relaxed, confident, or aggressive patient will provide direct eye contact [36] (Figure 9.12b).

Pupil size also accurately reflects the dog's underlying emotional state, provided that ambient lighting is adequate and is not a contributing factor. A fearful dog exhibits mydriasis due to activation of the body's sympathetic "fight or flight" response (Figure 9.13a). Contrast that with the pupils of a non-adrenalized canine patient (Figure 9.13b).

Note that whether or not a dog's pupils are dilated, they tend to take on a rounded appearance compared with the cat, which has more elliptical or slit-like pupils when they are miotic.

A dog also communicates visually through ear carriage, although ear carriage in the dog may also be highly dependent upon the breed. As a broad generalization, alert dogs typically have symmetrical ear carriage, with both ears erect and directed toward a shared stimulus (Figure 9.14a). Dogs that are uncertain or are exhibiting heightened awareness of their surroundings tend to have asymmetric ears, meaning that one or both ears are swiveled with the inner pinnae directed sideways (Figure 9.14b). Symmetrically flatted ears, pinned down against the top of the head, denote defensiveness: the patient is on guard and may feel forced to strike out aggressively as a means of self-defense (Figure 9.14c) [36].

Some dog breeds do not typically have erect ears [36]. For example, it can be normal in Border Collies for the ears to lay flat against the head in a neutral position (Figure 9.15a). This flattened appearance to the ears conveys a very different message to that reflected in Figure 9.14c. The Border Collie depicted in Figure 9.15a is not warning anyone: it is simply aware of its environment and is neutral toward it. Note that Border Collies' ears are likely to change position from a neutral to a semi-erect position when their interest in their surroundings is piqued (Figure 9.15b).

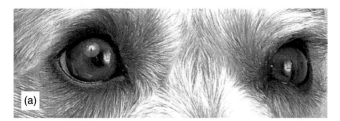

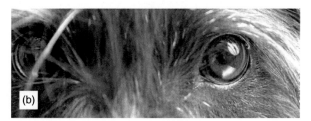

Figure 9.12 (a) Note the averted gaze in this timid patient. (b) Note the direct stare in this confident patient. Source (a), (b): Courtesy of the Media Resources Department at Midwestern University.

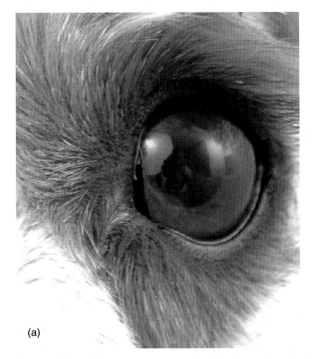

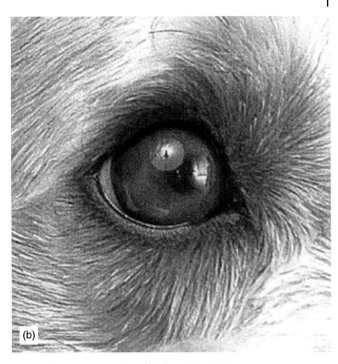

Figure 9.13 (a) Bilateral mydriasis in a timid canine patient. (b) Normal pupil size in a non-adrenalized canine patient. Source (a), (b): Courtesy of the Media Resources Department at Midwestern University.

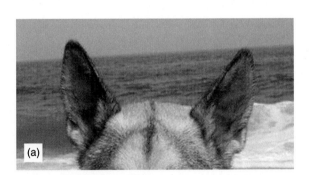

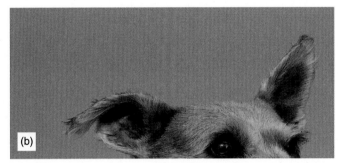

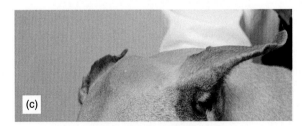

Figure 9.14 (a) This dog's upright ears suggest that it is paying attention. In loving memory of Rachel Beard, DVM. (b) The patient's ears do not match. This dog may be unsure, confused, or trying to cue in to what is happening to the right of him without breaking his gaze. (c) The patient's ears are pinned back. This is a "red flag" to practitioners that the patient is feeling threatened. Source (a)–(c): Courtesy of the Media Resources Department at Midwestern University.

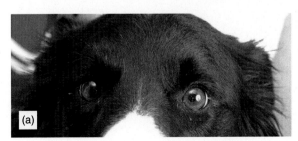

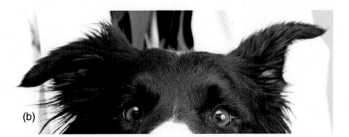

Figure 9.15 (a) Normal neutral ear position and (b) alert ear positioning in a Border Collie. Source (a), (b): Courtesy of the Media Resources Department at Midwestern University.

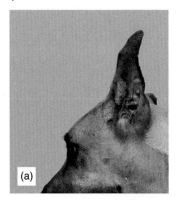

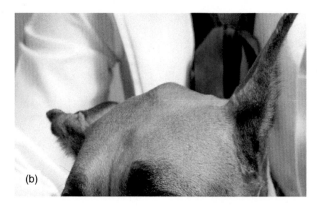

Figure 9.16 Normal appearance of cropped ears as seen (a) from the side and (b) from the front in a Great Dane. Source (a), (b): Courtesy of the Media Resources Department at Midwestern University.

Some breeds, such as Great Danes, have cropped ears, which gives them a characteristically unusual conformation from the front and from the side (Figure 9.16).

In addition to using their eyes and ears to communicate, dogs may also incorporate their oral cavity, specifically their teeth. Dogs that are confident and assertive tend to square their jawline and expose their most rostral teeth, the canines and incisors (Figure 9.17a). By contrast, dogs that are described as being fearfully aggressive are conflicted as to whether to attack or not. They would prefer to deflect the antagonistic encounter, but will attack if sufficiently threatened. These dogs tend to expose their caudal teeth as well as their rostral teeth (Figure 9.17b). In addition, their ventral neck is exposed and their field of vision is partially obstructed by a raised head that leans slightly backwards [36].

Tail carriage is yet another means by which dogs visually communicate although, like the ears, tail carriage in the dog may also be highly dependent upon the breed.

As a broad generalization, a wagging tail communicates that the dog is in a good frame of mind. It is willing and eager to interact. By contrast, a tucked tail signals lack of confidence and uncertainty compared with a tail held in a neutral position (Figure 9.18) [36].

As is the case with ears, certain breeds have unusual, yet distinct tail carriage that ought to be recognized as normal by the veterinary team. For example, the Shiba Inu breed of dogs always has a tail that is fixed in a curled position atop the rump (Figure 9.19). In these dogs, it is difficult to assess temperament based upon tail position alone and the clinician must take cues from other features.

Collectively, body posture, coat, eyes, ears, mouth, and tail carriage paint a picture of how each canine patient is perceiving the environment and help the clinician to determine how the patient is likely to react [36]. Being able to recognize aggressive tendencies through body language is critical. Once these have been identified, the

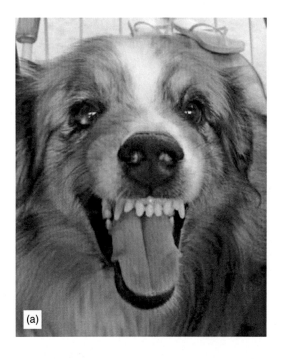

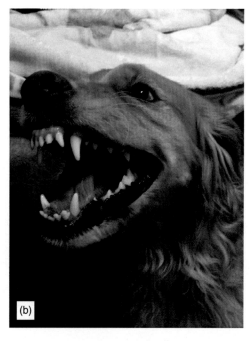

Figure 9.17 (a) Confident, assertive dog. Note how the dog is baring its most rostral teeth and the lips are curled in a snarl. Source: Courtesy of Stephani Ruppert. (b) This canine patient is conflicted. Note the fully exposed oral cavity, including the molars, the exposed neck, and the slightly raised head with a subtle backwards lean. Source: Courtesy of Kaylee and Christiana Otterson, Midwestern University CVM 2019.

Figure 9.18 (a) This patient's tucked tail denotes a lack of confidence and comfort with the current situation. (b) Note the neutral position in this canine patient that is alert, yet relaxed. Source (a), (b): Courtesy of the Media Resources Department at Midwestern University.

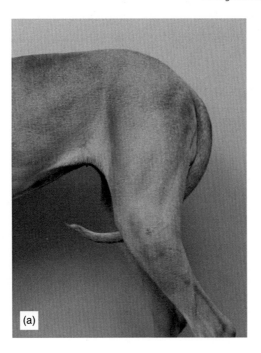
(a)

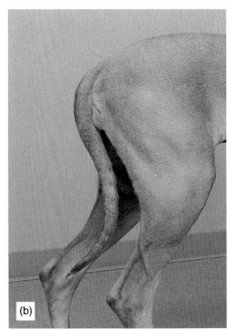
(b)

clinician can adjust their approach to the patient. The goal is to prevent the tendencies from escalating into full-out aggression that worsens with each subsequent visit [31].

Because it is time consuming and frustrating to manage these patients in a clinic setting where time constraints are likely, it is tempting to respond to these fearful patients without patience and with excessive force. It is equally tempting to label these patients as "difficult" or, simply put, "bad dogs." However, it is important to understand that in a clinical setting, the primary reason underlying a patient's aggressive tendencies is fear. Unless the veterinary team takes measures now to address this fear, it will only intensify, making subsequent visits much more challenging [31].

Reasonable attempts should be made in every situation to lessen fear through a soft, gentle voice, the offering of treats, the altering of the clinician's own body language so as not to convey direct threats, and the provision of time to allow the patient ample opportunity to acclimate [31].

9.8 Creative Approaches to Challenging Interactions with Canine Patients

When canine patients continue to threaten the safety of the veterinary team despite multiple attempts at low-stress handling, additional tools are necessary to make patient handling possible. Sometimes all that is necessary is some creative thinking on the part of the veterinary team: some dogs perform better in the absence of their owners. Others preferentially tolerate physical examinations when they are positioned on the examiner's lap as opposed to the examination room table [31].

Some dogs may benefit from periodic breaks in the examination so as to prevent over-stimulation that escalates into aggression [31]. Others may benefit from staging the appointment so as to end on a positive note. For example, if it was a struggle to get the patient vaccinated, but the patient ultimately conceded with positive

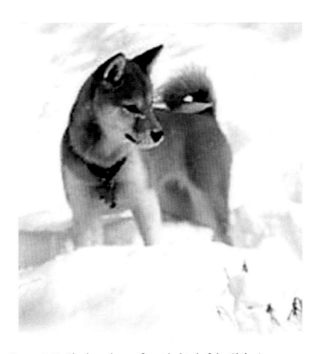

Figure 9.19 The breed-specific curled tail of the Shiba Inu. Source: Courtesy of Alan Fink Fine Art.

reinforcement, then there is little sense proceeding with a toe nail trim. Better to end with success than to push the limits of a patient's tolerance. The nail trim can be attempted at the next visit.

Staging appointments requires an open discussion between the clinician and the client regarding which procedures should be prioritized. The procedure that is the priority for both members of the medical care team will be performed first. Other procedures are performed sequentially, as needed, at subsequent visits so as to limit the amount of stress that a patient encounters on any given day.

On occasion, it may be necessary to reschedule the examination in the event that a patient is truly intractable. "Brudacaine" is not the answer; a different set of circumstances on a different day is [31]. The patient may benefit from prescribed anxiolytics to be given prior to the next appointment [31].

The patient may need to be rescheduled for a specific time of day [31]. For instance, in the author's experience, patients that tend to get over-stimulated often perform better when scheduled for the first appointment of the day, before the clinic is inundated with olfactory cues from other stressed patients. The patient may benefit from avoiding the waiting room altogether and entering the clinic through a different entranceway. Alternatively, the patient may be more tractable if examined in a different location, for example, in the treatment area or the supply room. The author has even on rare occasions examined a patient in the parking lot! In this circumstance, the change in venue markedly improved the outcome and the patient tolerated a comprehensive physical examination with the owner present [31].

It may also be appropriate for a clinician to recommend that the client try an at-home veterinarian for patients that are exceptionally fearful in the clinic setting. It is important that the client knows why this recommendation is being made and that the clinician truly has the welfare of the patient in mind. Maintaining an open, honest dialogue with the clients about these challenging patients is critical so that misunderstandings do not occur. Both the clinician and the client can usually come to an agreement regarding any decision that clearly puts the patient's needs first.

9.9 Other Canine Handling Tools

Despite the veterinary team's best attempts to get by without commercially available products for safer handling of fractious patients, they cannot afford to become injured or to allow the client to become injured. These patients may require "toweling" or muzzling to protect staff, client, and patient alike [31]. "Toweling" is similar to the "kitty burrito" approach that was discussed in Section 1.10. However, rather than covering the entire dog as is done with the cat in a "kitty burrito," the towel is used to restrain dogs by creating a barrier between the its head and neck and the clinician.

The author prefers to use "toweling" in small- to medium-sized dogs, especially brachycephalic breeds, that are resistant to being handled and/or are attempting to bite. A bath towel, rather than a hand towel, is rolled to resemble a pool noodle. Each end of the rolled towel is held in the restrainer's ipsilateral hand. That is, the left side of the rolled towel is held in the restrainer's left hand and the right side of the rolled towel is held in the restrainer's right hand. The restrainer's hands are held just enough apart so that the rolled towel hangs in a "U" shape. With the dog in a standing position, the towel is held so that the dog's head slides between the "U" of the towel. The ends of the towel are then twisted. Now the dog cannot pull out.

There are also times when the use of a muzzle is indicated to prevent physical harm to the veterinary team. As was the case with cat muzzles, there are also several different canine options. Most veterinary practices are equipped with the classic nylon or leather muzzle. These come in a variety of sizes and function to keep the patient's mouth tightly closed (Figure 9.20) [31].

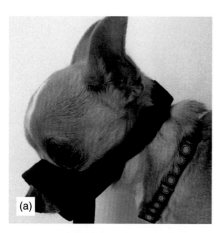
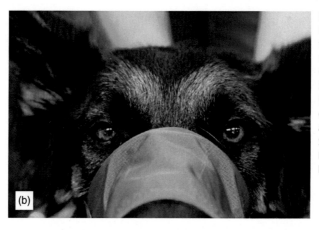

Figure 9.20 (a) Chihuahua fitted with a nylon muzzle. Source: Courtesy of Jule Schweighoefer. (b) Large-sized dog fitted with a nylon muzzle. Source: Courtesy of Elizabeth Robbins, DVM.

The potential concern with the aforementioned muzzles is that they do not provide for the patient's ability to pant. The way in which they keep the mouth tightly closed inhibits panting, and the majority of patients that are fearful have increased ventilation. Preventing a patient from panting may in fact intensify its stress. From an anthropomorphic standpoint, the patient may feel that it is not able to take in sufficient air and may struggle further in an attempt to rectify the situation [31].

Basket muzzles are preferred to nylon or leather because they do not prohibit panting. They also allow the patient to drink naturally, and are safe if left on a kenneled patient, for example if the patient is in-between examinations or diagnostic procedures. They come in different varieties to fit the various muzzle shapes and sizes of different breeds (Figure 9.21). [31]

As is evident in Figure 9.21, basket muzzles may be purchased by clients to use in the home environment for two purposes: one, so that clients of clinic-aggressive dogs can acclimate patients to wear a muzzle prior to a veterinary visit [31], and second, so that clients of dog-aggressive dogs can still enjoy outdoor time with their pets.

As an alternative approach to muzzling and in the event that a site distal to the dog's face and head needs to be examined, an Elizabethan collar may be placed on the canine patient to prevent it from reaching the clinician with its mouth (see Figure 1.29, which demonstrates the use of an Elizabethan collar in a feline patient). Note that the Elizabethan collar must be longer than anticipated to make sure that it extends well beyond the muzzle.

A fearful patient may also benefit from wearing a body wrap such as a Thundershirt, which applies pressure to the torso to simulate swaddling (Figure 9.22). It is believed that anxiety is diminished when evenly applied pressure is provided over the body's core [89–91].

In addition to body wraps, there are face wraps such as Calming Caps that function to reduce visual stimuli

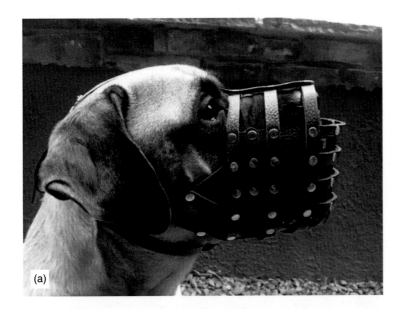

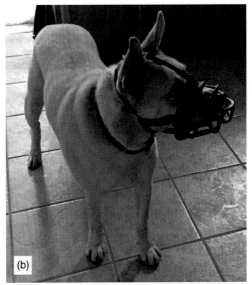

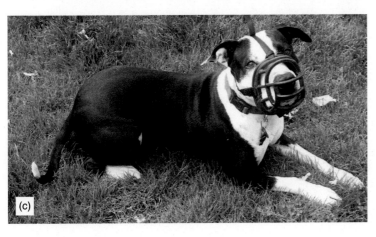

Figure 9.21 (a) Giant-breed dog fitted with a basket muzzle, viewed from the side. Source: Courtesy of Miranda Frolich. (b) Large-breed dog fitted with a basket muzzle. Source: Courtesy of Kyley Olson. (c) Alternative type of basket muzzle. Source: Courtesy of Danielle N. Cucuzella.

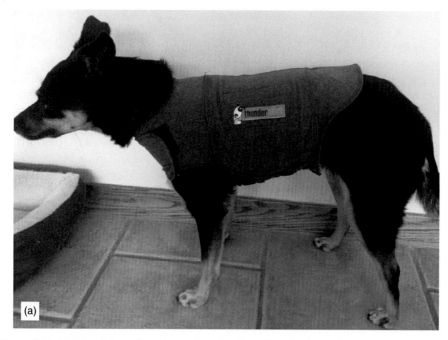
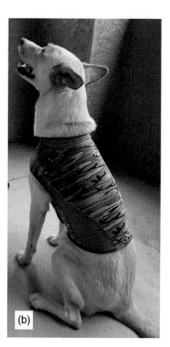

Figure 9.22 (a) Lateral view of a canine patient donning a Thundershirt. Source: Courtesy of Jule Schweighoefer. (b) Alternative view of a canine patient wearing a body wrap. Source: Courtesy of Sarah Ciamello.

(Figure 9.23). Because the patient's vision is filtered through fabric, the dog is less likely to be overstimulated via its visual field. The utility of this cap is in any procedure that is likely to cause visual stimulation such as nail trims and blood draws [31].

As was discussed in Chapter 1, there are times when chemical restraint is appropriate to minimize patient stress and to improve safety for the veterinary team. Intramuscular injections that are reversible are preferred because they are fast-acting, are easy to administer in a fractious patient, and their duration can be terminated when the physical examination or the diagnostic procedure is completed. As is the case any time medications are prescribed and administered, sedation

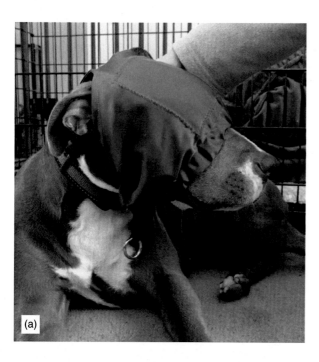
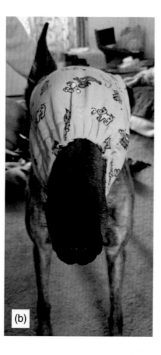

Figure 9.23 (a) Lateral view of a canine patient donning a Calming Cap. (b) Canine patient wearing a Calming Cap, viewed from the front. Source (a), (b): Courtesy of Leni Kaplan, MS, DVM.

protocols should be tailored to the individual based upon age, health status, underlying disease processes, and the duration for which sedation is required. All of these can be difficult to predict in a patient that has never before been examined and is intolerant of handling. However, it is the responsibility of the attending clinician to weigh risks versus benefits. These should be effectively communicated to the client in order to assist them with decision-making, a significant component of relationship-centered care [31, 92].

References

1 Coe, J.B., Young, I., Lambert, K. *et al.* (2014) A scoping review of published research on the relinquishment of companion animals. *Journal of Applied Animal Welfare Science: JAAWS*, **17** (3), 253–273.

2 Case, L. (2008) Perspectives on domestication: the history of our relationship with man's best friend. *Journal of Animal Science*, **86** (11), 3245–3251.

3 Hines, L.M. (2003) Historical perspectives on the human–animal bond. *American Behavioral Scientist*, **47** (1), 7–15.

4 Barker, S.B. and Wolen, A.R. (2008) The benefits of human–companion animal interaction: a review. *Journal of Veterinary Medical Education*, **35** (4), 487–495.

5 Wells, D.L. (2009) The effects of animals on human health and well-being. *Journal of Social Issues*, **65** (3), 523–543.

6 Seibert, L.M. and Landsberg, G.M. (2008) Diagnosis and management of patients presenting with behavior problems. *Veterinary Clinics of North America: Small Animal Practice*, **38** (5), 937–950, v.

7 Houpt, K.A., Honig, S.U., and Reisner, I.R. (1996) Breaking the human–companion animal bond. *Journal of the American Veterinary Medical Association*, **208** (10), 1653–1659.

8 Horwitz, D.F. (2008) Managing pets with behavior problems: realistic expectations. *Veterinary Clinics of North America: Small Animal Practice*, **38** (5), 1005–1021, vi.

9 Scarlett, J.M., Salman, M.D., New, J.G., Jr., and Kass, P.H. (1999) Reasons for relinquishment of companion animals in U.S. animal shelters: selected health and personal issues. *Journal of Applied Animal Welfare Science: JAAWS*, **2** (1), 41–57.

10 Salman, M.D., New, J.G., Jr., Scarlett, J.M. *et al.* (1998) Human and animal factors related to relinquishment of dogs and cats in 12 selected animal shelters in the United States. *Journal of Applied Animal Welfare Science: JAAWS*, **1** (3), 207–226.

11 Patronek, G.J., Glickman, L.T., Beck, A.M. *et al.* (1996) Risk factors for relinquishment of dogs to an animal shelter. *Journal of the American Veterinary Medical Association*, **209** (3), 572–581.

12 Patronek, G.J., Glickman, L.T., Beck, A.M. *et al.* (1996) Risk factors for relinquishment of cats to an animal shelter. *Journal of the American Veterinary Medical Association*, **209** (3), 582–588.

13 Miller, D.D., Staats, S.R., Partlo, C., and Rada, K. (1996) Factors associated with the decision to surrender a pet to an animal shelter. *Journal of the American Veterinary Medical Association*, **209** (4), 738–742.

14 Seksel, K. (2008) Preventing behavior problems in puppies and kittens. *Veterinary Clinics of North America: Small Animal Practice*, **38** (5), 971–982, v–vi.

15 Hammerle, M., Horst, C., Levine, E. *et al.* (2015) 2015 AAHA Canine and Feline Behavior Management Guidelines. *Journal of the American Animal Hospital Association*, **51** (4), 205–221.

16 Wells, D.L. and Hepper, P.G. (2000) Prevalence of behaviour problems reported by owners of dogs purchased from an animal rescue shelter. *Applied Animal Behaviour Science*, **69** (1), 55–65.

17 Ledger, R.A. and Baxter, M.R. (1997) The development of a validated test to assess the temperament of dogs in a rescue shelter, in *Proceedings of the First International Conference on Veterinary Behavioural Medicine, 1997*, Birmingham, UK (eds. D.S. Mills, S.E. Heath, and L.J. Harrington), Universities Federation for Animal Welfare, Wheathampstead, pp. 87–92.

18 Patronek, G.J. and Dodman, N.H. (1999) Attitudes, procedures, and delivery of behavior services by veterinarians in small animal practice. *Journal of the American Veterinary Medical Association*, **215** (11), 1606–1611.

19 Landsberg, G.M., Shaw, J., and Donaldson, J. (2008) Handling behavior problems in the practice setting. *Veterinary Clinics of North America: Small Animal Practice*, **38** (5), 951–969, v.

20 McMillan, F.D. (2005) Stress, distress, and emotion: distinctions and implications for mental well-being, in *Mental Health and Well-Being in Animals* (ed. F.D. McMillan), Blackwell, Ames, IA, pp. 93–111.

21 McMillan, F.D. and Rollin, B.E. (2001) The presence of mind: on reunifying the animal mind and body. *Journal of the American Veterinary Medical Association*, **218** (11), 1723–1727.

22 Greenfield, C.L., Johnson, A.L., and Schaeffer, D.J. (2004) Frequency of use of various procedures, skills, and areas of knowledge among veterinarians in private small animal exclusive or predominant practice and proficiency expected of new veterinary school graduates. *Journal of the American Veterinary Medical Association*, **224** (11), 1780–1787.

23 Gehrke, B.C. (1997) The 1997 AVMA survey of US pet-owning households regarding services and

products purchased and expenditures during their pet's most recent veterinary medical visit. *Journal of the American Veterinary Medical Association,* **211** (6), 706–708.

24 Bergman, L., Hart, B.L., Bain, M., and Cliff, K. (2002) Evaluation of urine marking by cats as a model for understanding veterinary diagnostic and treatment approaches and client attitudes. *Journal of the American Veterinary Medical Association,* **221** (9), 1282–1286.

25 Scarlett, J.M., Salman, M.D., New, J.G., and Kass, P.H. (2002) The role of veterinary practitioners in reducing dog and cat relinquishments and euthanasias. *Journal of the American Veterinary Medical Association,* **220** (3), 306–311.

26 Godbout, M., Palestrini, C., Beauchamp, G., and Frank, D. (2007) Puppy behavior at the veterinary clinic: a pilot study. *Journal of Veterinary Behavior,* **2** (4), 126–135.

27 Godbout, M. and Frank, D. (2011) Persistence of puppy behaviors and signs of anxiety during adulthood. *Journal of Veterinary Behavior,* **6** (1), 126–135.

28 Epp, T. and Waldner, C. (2012) Occupational health hazards in veterinary medicine: zoonoses and other biological hazards. *Canadian Veterinary Journal/ Revue Vétérinaire Canadienne,* **53** (2), 144–150.

29 Jeyaretnam, J. and Jones, H. (2000) Physical, chemical and biological hazards in veterinary practice. *Australian Veterinary Journal,* **78** (11), 751–758.

30 Epp, T. and Waldner, C. (2012) Occupational health hazards in veterinary medicine: physical, psychological, and chemical hazards. *Canadian Veterinary Journal/Revue Vétérinaire Canadienne,* **53** (2), 151–157.

31 Moffat, K. (2008) Addressing canine and feline aggression in the veterinary clinic. *Veterinary Clinics of North America: Small Animal Practice,* **38** (5), 983–1003, vi.

32 Yin, S. (2016) *Low Stress Handling,* CattleDog Publishing, Davis, CA, https://drsophiayin.com/low-stress-handling/ (accessed 31 May 2016).

33 Rodan, I., Sundahl, E., Carney, H. *et al.* (2011) AAFP and ISFM feline-friendly handling guidelines. *Journal of Feline Medicine and Surgery,* **13** (5), 364–375.

34 Rodan, I., Sundahl, E., Carney, H. *et al.* (2011) Feline focus: AAFP and ISFM feline-friendly handling guidelines. *Compendium: Continuing Education for the Practicing Veterinarian,* **33** (12), E3.

35 Bowen, J. and Heath, S. (2005) *An Overview of Feline Social Behaviour and Communication: Behaviour Problems in Small Animals: Practice Advice for the Veterinary Team,* Saunders, Philadelphia.

36 Overall, K.L. (1997) Normal canine behavior, in *Clinical Behavioral Medicine for Small Animals* (ed. K.L. Overall), Mosby, St. Louis, pp. 10–44.

37 Scherk, M. (2013) *The cat-friendly practice, in BSAVA Manual of Feline Practice: A Foundation Manual* (eds. A. Harvey and S. Tasker), British Small Animal Veterinary Association, Gloucester.

38 Verdecchia, P., Schillaci, G., Borgioni, C. *et al.* (1995) White coat hypertension and white coat effect – similarities and differences. *American Journal of Hypertension,* **8** (8), 790–798.

39 Ogedegbe, G. (2008) White-coat effect: unraveling its mechanisms. *American Journal of Hypertension,* **21** (2), 135.

40 Cardillo, C., Defelice, F., Campia, U., and Folli, G. (1993) Psychophysiological reactivity and cardiac end-organ changes in white coat hypertension. *Hypertension,* **21** (6), 836–844.

41 Palmer, B.M., Lynch, J.M., Snyder, S.M., and Moore, R.L. (2001) Renal hypertension prevents run training modification of cardiomyocyte diastolic Ca^{2+} regulation in male rats. *Journal of Applied Physiology,* **90** (6), 2063–2069.

42 Marino, C.L., Cober, R.E., Iazbik, M.C., and Couto, C.G. (2011) White-coat effect on systemic blood pressure in retired racing greyhounds. *Journal of Veterinary Internal Medicine,* **25** (4), 861–865.

43 Belew, A.M., Barlett, T., and Brown, S.A. (1999) Evaluation of the white-coat effect in cats. *Journal of Veterinary Internal Medicine,* **13** (2), 134–142.

44 Verdecchia, P., Schillaci, G., Borgioni, C. *et al.* (1995) White coat hypertension and white coat effect. Similarities and differences. *American Journal of Hypertension,* **8** (8), 790–798.

45 Ogedegbe, G. (2008) White-coat effect: unraveling its mechanisms. *American Journal of Hypertension,* **21** (2), 135.

46 Belew, A.M., Barlett, T., and Brown, S.A. (1999) Evaluation of the white-coat effect in cats. *Journal of Veterinary Internal Medicine,* **13** (2), 134–142.

47 Zimmerman, R.S. and Frohlich, E.D. (1990) Stress and hypertension. *Journal of Hypertension Supplement,* **8** (4), S103–S107.

48 Verdecchia, P., Porcellati, C., Schillaci, G. *et al.* Ambulatory blood pressure. *An independent predictor of prognosis in essential hypertension. Hypertension,* **24** (6), 793–801.

49 Marino, C.L., Cober, R.E., Iazbik, M.C., and Couto, C.G. (2011) White-coat effect on systemic blood pressure in retired racing Greyhounds. *Journal of Veterinary Internal Medicine,* **25** (4), 861–865.

50 Cardillo, C., De Felice, F., Campia, U., and Folli, G. (1993) Psychophysiological reactivity and cardiac end-organ changes in white coat hypertension. *Hypertension,* **21** (6 Pt. 1), 836–844.

51 Palmer, B.F. (2001) Impaired renal autoregulation: implications for the genesis of hypertension and hypertension-induced renal injury. *American Journal of the Medical Sciences,* **321** (6), 388–400.

52 Palmer, B.F. (2001) Renal dysfunction complicating the treatment of hypertension. *New England Journal of Medicine,* **347** (16), 1256–1261.

53 Brown, S., Atkins, C., Bagley, R. *et al.* (2007) Guidelines for the identification, evaluation, and management of systemic hypertension in dogs and cats. *Journal of Veterinary Internal Medicine,* **21** (3), 542–558.

54 Lees, G.E., Brown, S.A., Elliott, J. *et al.* (2005) American College of Veterinary Internal Medicine. Assessment and management of proteinuria in dogs and cats: 2004 ACVIM Forum Consensus Statement (small animal). *Journal of Veterinary Internal Medicine*, **19** (3), 377–385.

55 Bodey, A.R. and Rampling, M.W. (1999) Comparison of haemorrheological parameters and blood pressure in various breeds of dog. *Journal of Small Animal Practice*, **40** (1), 3–6.

56 Schneider, H.P., Truex, R.C., and Knowles J.O. (1964) Comparative observations of the hearts of mongrel and greyhound dogs. *Anatomical Record*, **149**, 173–179.

57 Pape, L.A., Price, J.M., Alpert, J.S., and Rippe, J.M. (1986) Hemodynamics and left ventricular function: a comparison between adult racing greyhounds and greyhounds completely untrained from birth. *Basic Research in Cardiology*, **81** (4), 417–424.

58 Cox, R.H., Peterson, L.H., and Detweiler, D.K. (1976) Comparison of arterial hemodynamics in the mongrel dog and the racing greyhound. *American Journal of Physiology*, **230** (1), 211–218.

59 Surman, S.E. (2010) *The Relationship Between Systemic Hypertension, Proteinuria, and Renal Histopathology in Clinically Healthy Retired Racing Greyhounds*, Graduate School of Ohio State University, Columbus, OH.

60 Cromwell-Davis, S.L. (2007) White coat syndrome: prevention and treatment. *Compendium: Continuing Education for the Practicing Veterinarian*, **29** (3), 163–165.

61 Overall, K.L. (1997) Treatment of behavioral problems, in *Clinical Behavioral Medicine for Small Animals* (ed. K.L. Overall), Mosby, St. Louis, pp. 274–292.

62 Levis, D.J. (1980) Implementing the technique of implosive therapy, in *Handbook of Behavioral Interventions: A Clinical Guide* (eds. A.J. Goldstein and E.B. Foa), John Wiley & Sons, Inc., New York, 1980, pp. 92–151.

63 Moulton, D.G. (1960) Studies in olfactory acuity. 4. Relative detectability of n-aliphatic acids by the dog. *Animal Behaviour*, **8**, 117–128.

64 King, J.E., Markee, J.E., and Becker, R.F. (1964) Studies on olfactory discrimination in dogs. 3. Ability to detect human odour trace. *Animal Behaviour*, **12** (2–3), 311.

65 Kalmus, H. (1955) The discrimination by the nose of the dog of the individual human odours and in particular the odours of twins. *British Journal of Animal Behaviour*, **3**, 25–31.

66 Toner, B.S. and Miller, D.I., Jr. (1993) Olfactory discrimination of individual human odors using experienced tracking police and work dogs. *Animal Behavior Consultants Newsletter*, **10** (4), 2–4.

67 Bradshaw, J.W.S. and Brown, S.L. (1990) Behavioral adaptations of dogs to domestication, in *Pets, Benefits, and Practice* (ed. I.H. Berger), British Veterinary Association Publications, London, pp. 18–24.

68 Sprague, R.H. and Anisko, J.J. (1973) Elimination patterns in the laboratory beagle. *Behaviour*, **47** (3), 257–267.

69 Fox, M.W. and Bekoff, M. (1975) The behaviour of dogs, in *The Behaviour of Domestic Animals*, 3rd edn. (ed. E.S.E. Hafez), Williams & Wilkins, Baltimore, pp. 370–409.

70 Scott, J.P. and Fuller, J.L. (1965) *Genetics and the Social Behavior of the Dog*, University of Chicago Press, Chicago.

71 Borchelt, P.L. (1984) Behavior development of the puppy in the home environment, in *Nutrition and Behavior of Dogs and Cats* (ed. R.S. Anderson), Pergamon Press, New York, pp. 165–174.

72 Borchelt, P.L. (1984) Development of behaviour in the dog during maturity, in *Nutrition and Behavior of Dogs and Cats* (ed. R.S. Anderson), Pergamon Press, New York, pp. 189–197.

73 Tod, E., Brander, D., and Waran, N. (2005) Efficacy of dog appeasing pheromone in reducing stress and fear related behaviour in shelter dogs. *Applied Animal Behaviour Science*, **93** (3–4), 295–308.

74 Grigg, E.K. and Piehler, M. (2015) Influence of dog appeasing pheromone (DAP) on dogs housed in a long-term kennelling facility. *Veterinary Record Open*, **2** (1), e000098.

75 Pageat, P. and Gaultier, E. (2003) Current research in canine and feline pheromones. *Veterinary Clinics of North America: Small Animal Practice*, **33** (2), 187–211.

76 Landsberg, G.M., Beck, A., Lopez, A. *et al.* (2015) Dog-appeasing pheromone collars reduce sound-induced fear and anxiety in beagle dogs: a placebo-controlled study. *Veterinary Record*, **177** (10), 260.

77 Mills, D.S., Ramos, D., Estelles, M.G., and Hargrave, C. (2006) A triple blind placebo-controlled investigation into the assessment of the effect of dog appeasing pheromone (DAP) on anxiety related behaviour of problem dogs in the veterinary clinic. *Applied Animal Behaviour Science*, **98** (1–2), 114–126.

78 Denenberg, S. and Landsberg, G.M. (2008) Effects of dog-appeasing pheromones on anxiety and fear in puppies during training and on long-term socialization. *Journal of the American Veterinary Medicine Association*, **233** (12), 1874–1882.

79 Estelles, M.G. and Mills, D.S. (2006) Signs of travel-related problems in dogs and their response to treatment with dog-appeasing pheromone. *Veterinary Record*, **159** (5), 143.

80 Gaultier, E., Bonnafous, L., Vienet-Legue, D. *et al.* (2008) Efficacy of dog-appeasing pheromone in reducing stress associated with social isolation in newly adopted puppies. *Veterinary Record*, **163** (3), 73–80.

81 Gaultier, E., Bonnafous, L., Vienet-Lague, D. *et al.* (2009) Efficacy of dog-appeasing pheromone in reducing behaviours associated with fear of unfamiliar people and new surroundings in newly adopted puppies. *Veterinary Record*, **164** (23), 708–714.

82 Sheppard, G. and Mills, D.S. (2003) Evaluation of dog-appeasing pheromone as a potential treatment for dogs fearful of fireworks. *Veterinary Record*, **152** (14), 432–436.

83 Mills, D.S., Estelles, M.G., Coleshaw, P.H., and Shorthouse, C. (2003) Retrospective analysis of the treatment of firework fears in dogs. *Veterinary Record*, **153** (18), 561–562.

84 Levine, E.D. and Mills, D.S. (2008) Long-term follow-up of the efficacy of a behavioural treatment programme for dogs with firework fears. *Veterinary Record*, **162** (20), 657–659.

85 Levine, E.D., Ramos, D., and Mills, D.S. (2007) A prospective study of two self-help CD based desensitization and counter-conditioning programmes with the use of dog appeasing pheromone for the treatment of firework fears in dogs (*Canis familiaris*). *Applied Animal Behaviour Science*, **105** (4), 311–329.

86 Taylor, K. and Mills, D.S. (2007) A placebo-controlled study to investigate the effect of dog appeasing pheromone and other environmental and management factors on the reports of disturbance and house soiling during the night in recently adopted puppies (*Canis familiaris*). *Applied Animal Behaviour Science*, **105** (4), 358–368.

87 Frank, D., Beauchamp, G., and Palestrini, C. (2010) Systematic review of the use of pheromones for treatment of undesirable behavior in cats and dogs. *Journal of the American Veterinary Medical Association*, **236** (12), 1308–1316.

88 Yin, S. (2007) Simple handling techniques for dogs. *Compendium: Continuing Education for the Practicing Veterinarian*, **29** (6), 352–358.

89 Grandin, T. (1992) Calming effects of deep touch pressure in patients with autistic disorder, college students, and animals. *Journal of Child and Adolescent Psychopharmacology*, **2** (1), 63–72.

90 Grandin, T. (1989) Voluntary acceptance of restraint by sheep. *Applied Animal Behaviour Science*, **23** (3), 257–261.

91 Cottam, N., Dodman, N.H., and Ha, J.C. (2013) The effectiveness of the Anxiety Wrap in the treatment of canine thunderstorm phobia: an open-label trial. *Journal of Veterinary Behavior*, **8** (3), 154–161.

92 Herron, M.E. and Shreyer, T. (2014) The pet-friendly veterinary practice: a guide for practitioners. *Veterinary Clinics of North America: Small Animal Practice*, **44** (3), 451.

10

Assessing the Big Picture: the Body, the Coat, and the Skin of the Dog

10.1 Forms of Identification

In the United States alone, over two million owned dogs go missing annually [1]. During any given 5-year period, that number represents 14% of owned dogs nationally [1]. The recovery rate of lost owned dogs is reasonably high at 93% [2], which is attributed to the fact that dog-owners are more likely to frequent animal shelters to look for their missing companion than are cat-owners, and an estimated 89% of owners have provided their dogs with some form of identification [1].

Visible forms of identification such as collars with tags that provide client contact information are most efficient when it comes to reunification: finders of lost dogs can read the tag and contact the owner without delay [2–4] (Figure 10.1).

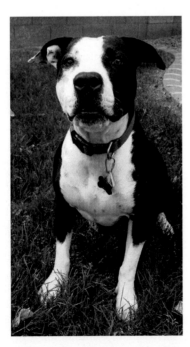

Figure 10.1 Canine patient outfitted with visual identification: a collar with tags that provide client contact information. Source: Courtesy of Danielle N. Cucuzella.

Owners are more likely to use collars with identification tags when they are provided as a courtesy by the veterinary clinic: compliance with collar wearing by dogs increased from 14% to 84% over 8 weeks following the receipt of a courtesy collar [5]. The downside to collar use is that a collar can be removed intentionally, altered, or lost. If this is the only form of identification for the patient, then the dog's likelihood of being returned to its owner is significantly diminished in the absence of a second identifier.

In addition to collars with identification tags, permanent forms of patient identification such as tattoos or microchips are preferred [2]. Microchips are rice-sized electronic forms of patient identification that are typically implanted into the subcutaneous tissue between the shoulder blades (Figure 10.2a and b). Microchips often come with an identifying tag for the collar as an additional reminder to finders of lost dogs that the dog is microchipped (Figure 10.2c). This increases the likelihood that a finder of a lost dog will take it to a veterinary clinic as opposed to a shelter, to be scanned [4]. Scanning a patient is necessary to reveal the unique identifying number of each microchip (Figure 10.2d). This unique identifier is registered to the pet-owner, whose contact information can be accessed from a central database.

The use of microchips has been proven to increase the rate of owner recovery of dogs in shelters from 22% to 52% [6]. Accordingly, the veterinary team should take care to incorporate discussions about patient identification into wellness and new patient examinations. Even better, scanning for microchips should be integrated into the physical examination to ensure that previously placed chips are still functional, and as a reminder to owners to update contact information [2].

Clinics may also want to consider registering contact information for the patient as a courtesy to the client to make sure that registration is complete [2]. A study by Lord *et al.* found that only 58.1% of microchipped lost dogs and cats that ended up at shelters had in fact been registered [6]. Of those registered, many were linked to out-of-date contact information,

Performing the Small Animal Physical Examination, First Edition. Ryane E. Englar.
© 2017 John Wiley & Sons, Inc. Published 2017 by John Wiley & Sons, Inc.

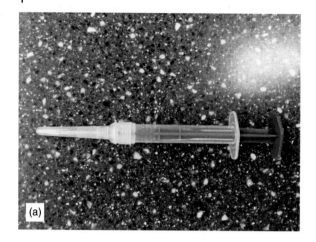

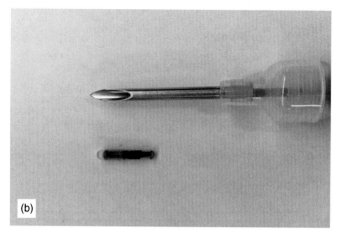

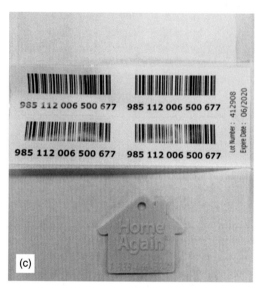

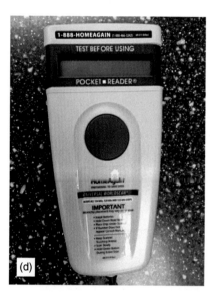

Figure 10.2 (a) Needle and syringe used to administer a microchip to a patient. The needle has been capped. (b) Microchip and needle for size comparison. Note that the microchip is approximately the size of a grain of rice. (c) Identifying tag that comes with the microchip to signify to finders of lost dogs that the patient in question is both owned and microchipped. (d) Example of a so-called universal microchip scanner.

with incorrect listings for telephone numbers or residential addresses [6]. At best, this leads to unnecessary delays in reunions between clients and lost dogs. In worst-case scenarios, reunions fail to occur: they are thwarted by missing links in client contact information.

Microchips are considered to be safe and efficacious, with few reports of microchip failure, microchip migration, implantation reactions (hematomas), and injection site tumors [7–9]. As a result, dogs and cats have been required to be microchipped in Australia since 1999 [9]. Whether the United States follows suit and requires compulsory microchipping remains to be seen. However, the use of microchips within the United States has certainly been advocated.

10.2 Body Condition Scoring

Just as it is the responsibility of the veterinary team to recommend patient identification, the burden falls upon the veterinary profession to provide nutritional recommendations as part of each patient's individualized wellness plan. Nutritional recommendations include a comprehensive review of the patient's diet, the diet's nutrient profile, feeding management, and environmental factors such as husbandry, the use of treats in training, whether or not the patient has to compete for resources in multi-pet households, and the presence or absence of environmental stimulation [10].

A major component of nutritional screening for every patient includes an assessment of the patient's body condition score (BCS). A contributing factor to BCS is the patient's body weight [10]. Weight can be a challenging physical examination parameter to regulate because it is so multifactorial [11–18]. Some factors, such as signalment and lifestyle, are beyond the clinician's control [19]. Sedentary lifestyles are commonplace within the companion animal population; in these cases, patients tend to mirror the activity levels of the people who live under the same roof [15, 20–22]. The veterinary team may recommend an increase in activity level; however, ultimately it is up to the members of the patient's family to buy in and follow through.

Pre-existing, underlying endocrine disease and medically necessitated pharmacologic interventions may further compound the issue [19]. For example, a patient that requires prolonged steroid therapy is likely to exhibit the adverse effect of polyphagia, which in turn promotes weight gain [19].

As a result of the factors outlined above, weight gain is increasing in frequency in the companion animal population [12]. Some clinicians have even considered it to be a shared epidemic between human and pet populations, particularly within the Western hemisphere [23–26].

Increased body weight raises concerns about canine welfare [12]. Increased body weight adversely impacts the musculoskeletal and endocrine systems by predisposing dogs to lameness and diabetes mellitus [11, 15, 19, 27, 28]. Specifically, overweight and obese dogs are predisposed to degenerative orthopedic diseases, such as osteoarthritis, and also the development of insulin resistance [29–31]. Dogs that are overweight are also at increased risk of asymptomatic bacteriuria, which may promote ascending urinary tract infections or urolithiasis [25]. In addition, abdominal obesity increases the risk of cardiovascular disease in dogs [32].

Lifespan is reduced in overweight dogs by 2 years on average [30, 33]. This may be due to an increased risk of developing cancer if overweight or obese dogs model their human counterparts when it comes to cancer biology: obesity in people has been linked to higher risks for developing colorectal carcinoma [34], postmenopausal breast adenocarcinoma [35], esophageal–gastric adenocarcinoma [36, 37], and hepatocellular carcinoma [38].

A dog is considered to be overweight when its body weight is 10% or more above that which is considered optimal based upon its breed and frame, and a dog is considered to be obese when its body weight is 15% or more above optimal [39]. Depending upon the country surveyed, anywhere from 10 to 40% of the owned canine population is obese [40–44]. The percentage of overweight dogs is even higher. In France, 38.8% of dogs were

considered overweight when assessed by the veterinary team compared with 41% in Australia and 52% in the United Kingdom [40, 45–47].

Compared with assessment of body weight by trained eyes among members of the veterinary team, clients tend to underestimate. For example, of the 41% of Australian dogs that veterinary professionals flagged as being overweight, only 25% were considered overweight by their owners [40, 46].

Although clients seem to be able to identify correctly silhouettes of generic canine body shapes as being ideal or under- or overweight, they do not always seem willing or able to label their own pet as weighing more than is ideal [40, 48, 49]. For example, a study by White *et al.* identified distinct discrepancies between veterinary and client perceptions about canine weight: 39% of clients felt that the veterinarian was incorrect in assessing that their dog was overweight [11]. Although 79% of those surveyed by White *et al.* confirmed that the client had discussed weight with the veterinary team, there was great variability as to whether or not the client supported the veterinary team's assessment [11].

However, being overweight is not the only concern that is relevant to the welfare of veterinary patients. Being underweight carries its own risks and it, too, may be associated with increased morbidity and mortality [50]. In addition, when weight loss is linked to an underlying disease process, it may color owners' perceptions of quality of life and may contribute to premature decision-making regarding euthanasia [50, 51].

Therefore, it is critical that the veterinary team discuss nutrition and weight status openly with clients in order to acknowledge, clarify, and address weight concerns. Body weight should be documented at each visit and trends in body weight over time should be analyzed so that the veterinary team may intervene as needed [10, 52].

However, the use of body weight alone can be challenging because it does not take into account anticipated differences in body weight based upon breed or the individual's build and body composition. One solution in human medicine is to calculate the body mass index (BMI) in addition to recording body weight. The BMI measures weight relative to height to tailor nutritional recommendations to the individual based upon build and stature.

Human medicine is also able to use portable bioimpedance monitors to establish the percentage of body composition that is body fat; however, these non-invasive devices are inaccurate in obese dogs [53].

Body composition in humans and dogs can be obtained with accuracy despite obesity using dual-energy X-ray absorptiometry (DEXA). Unfortunately, this is more of an academic procedure rather than a clinical reality in veterinary medicine owing to the cost of obtaining and maintaining such equipment [54, 55]. Preliminary work with morphometric measurements has led to the development of equations that are able to predict body fat as a percentage of body composition [55–57]; however, these are not yet routinely used in the clinical setting.

A more commonly used method in veterinary medicine is to assess for body condition score (BCS) using either a five- or nine-point scale [58, 59]. Both scales assess BCS along a sliding scale, in which the extremes of one and nine reflect emaciation and morbid obesity, respectively. When used to assess patients with <45% body fat, these scales have been validated [55, 59]. They may be used to approximate the percentage of body fat in dogs, and calculate energy requirements for dogs based upon their respective body condition scores. Unfortunately, as the percentage of body fat in veterinary patients exceeds 45%, both the five- and nine-point scales fall short of accurately predicting body fat as determined in the laboratory by DEXA [55]. This is of concern given the upward trends in pet obesity worldwide [13, 27, 46].

It may be that veterinary medicine of the future may need to increase reliance on morphometric methods for greater accuracy in patients that are morbidly obese while at the same time taking into account the effect of breed on body composition [55]. For example, chondrodystrophic dogs and dogs with prominent, muscular heads such as Staffordshire Terriers may require additional measurements to predict body composition more accurately [55]. Furthermore, different breeds have different norms in terms of ideal body fat. Young Papillons and young Labradors, for example, have more body fat than young Great Danes [56]. As they age, Great Danes lay down additional body fat whereas Papillons and Labradors do not [56].

Until veterinary medicine comes to a consensus on how best to address body composition in the obese patient, BCS is the best approach, understanding that it is not without its limitations.

The author prefers to reference the Purina nine-point system of body condition scoring (Figure 10.3). Much like the five-point system, the Purina nine-point system determines BCS by assessing visible and palpable landmarks, taking into account both lateral and aerial views of the patient.

Because BCS as determined by this method relies upon the clinician putting their hand on the patient, BCS cannot always be accurately discerned through observation alone. The visual assessment of a patient, as through photographs, is adequate as an initial screening tool; however, its accuracy hinges on observer experience. Less experienced observers are more likely to vary in accuracy [60].

The author has provided photographs of canine BCS in an attempt to provide guidelines for the visual learner. These photographs are not a replacement for a live patient for a hands-on examination. They are, simply put, a starting point.

The importance of palpation can be highlighted when evaluating dogs with extensive coat coverage. Breeds with medium to thick, plush coats are at risk of being over-scored because the heaviness of the fur dwarfs otherwise typically visible characteristics. For this reason, the clinician must come to rely even more upon their palpation skills, especially with regard to the ribcage, lumbar vertebrae, waist line, and wings of the ilia (Figure 10.4).

As mentioned, BCS is not without its limitations. At best, it is a subjective measurement, unlike weight, hence it may vary between observers who are evaluating the same patient [61]. However, it provides a starting point to initiate a conversation with the client about the patient's current plane of nutrition.

According to the Purina nine-point system for assessing BCS for dogs (Figure 10.3), dogs are underweight if they score a BCS of 1, 2, or 3:

- A dog that is classified as a BCS of 1 is emaciated as from neglect or end-stage protein-losing enteropathy. If short-haired, these dogs have visually prominent ribs, lumbar vertebrae, and pelvic bones that are evident without palpation. There is no palpable body fat and muscle mass is overwhelmingly poor. The waist line is exaggerated. The patient takes on a skeletal appearance (Figure 10.5).
- A dog that is classified as a BCS of 2 is considered to be moderately underweight, with easily visible ribs, lumbar vertebrae, and pelvic bones; however, compared to dogs with a BCS of 1, dogs with a BCS of 2 have adequate muscle mass. The abdominal tuck remains pronounced, and there is still no palpable fat (Figure 10.6).
- A dog that is classified as a BCS of 3 is considered to be mildly underweight. The ribs may or may not be visible, but they are easy to palpate without overlying fat. The pelvic bones, such as the wings of the ilia, are prominent, and the tips of the spinous processes of the lumbar vertebrae are visible. Overall, there is minimal body fat. The waist line is obvious.

The author considers dogs with a BCS of 4 to be a "lean normal" or what she refers to as an "athletic build." The "lean normal" patient has easily palpable, but not visible, ribs with minimal fat coverage, and a prominent abdominal tuck (Figure 10.7).

According to the Purina nine-point system, dogs are considered ideal if they score a BCS of 5. These patients are well proportioned and they have a visible waist and palpable ribs without an excess of fat coverage (Figure 10.8).

The author considers dogs with a BCS of 6 to be slightly overweight. There is a slight excess of fat covering otherwise palpable ribs. One can discern the waist, but it is not prominent (Figure 10.9).

Body Condition System

1. Ribs, lumbar vertebrae, pelvic bones and all bony prominences evident from a distance. No discernible body fat. Obvious loss of muscle mass.

2. Ribs, lumbar vertebrae pelvic bones easily visible. No palpable fat. Some evidence of other bony prominence. Minimal loss of muscle mass.

3. Ribs easily palpated and may be visible with no palpable fat. Tops of lumbar vertebrae visible; pelvic bones becoming prominent. Obvious waist and abdominal tuck.

4. Ribs easily palpable, with minimal fat covering. Waist easily noted, viewed from above. Abdominal tuck evident.

5. Ribs palpable, without excess fat covering. Waist observed behind ribs when viewed from above. Abdomen tucked up when viewed from side.

6. Ribs palpable with slight excess fat covering; waist is discernible viewed from above but is not prominent; abdominal tuck apparent.

7. Ribs palpable with difficulty; heavy fat cover. Noticeable fat deposits over lumbar area and base of tail. Waist absent. No abdominal tuck may be present.

8. Ribs not palpable under very heavy fat cover, or palpable only with significant pressure. Heavy fat deposits over lumbar area and base of tail. Waist absent. No abdominal tuck. Obvious abdominal distention may be present.

9. Massive fat deposits over thorax, spine and base of tail. Waist and abdominal tuck absent. Fat deposits on neck and limbs. Obvious abdominal distention.

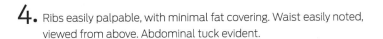
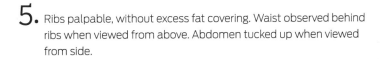
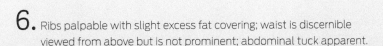
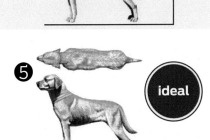
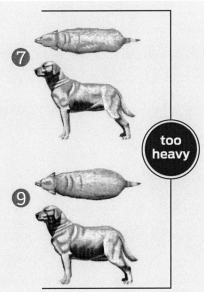

Figure 10.3 Assessing canine BCS using the Purina nine-point system. Source: Courtesy of Nestlé Purina PetCare.

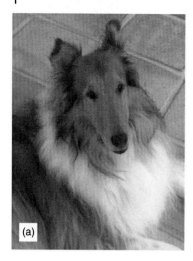
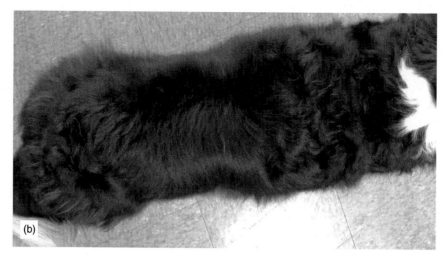

Figure 10.4 (a) Note the challenges that a heavy coat presents when BCS is determined using visible landmarks alone. This patient may be over-scored unless it is palpated, given that visual landmarks are difficult to appreciate under this plush coat. Source: Courtesy of Rozalyn Donner. (b) Note the challenges that a medium coat presents when determining BCS using visible landmarks alone. The aerial view is misleading: without palpation to supplement the clinician's physical examination findings, the patient may be over-scored. Source: Courtesy of the Media Resources Department at Midwestern University.

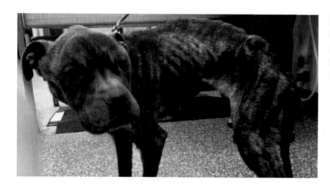

Figure 10.5 This canine patient has a BCS of 1. Note the prominent, easy-to-appreciate skeletal structures such as the rib cage, the dorsal spinous processes of the vertebral column, and the ilia. This patient was overtly malnourished from neglect. Source: Courtesy of Karen Burks, DVM.

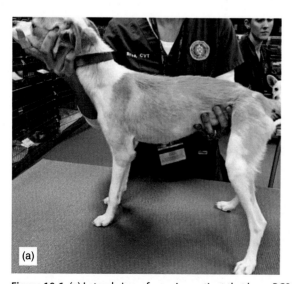
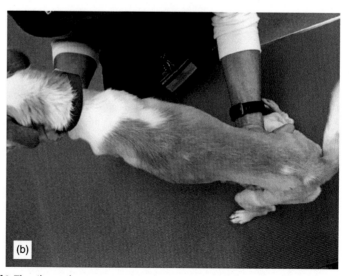

Figure 10.6 (a) Lateral view of a canine patient that has a BCS of 2. The ribs are less easy to appreciate compared with Figure 10.5, but they are very easy to palpate owing to lack of overlying fat coverage. (b) Aerial view of the same canine patient with a BCS of 2. Note the bony prominences and the prominent abdominal tuck.

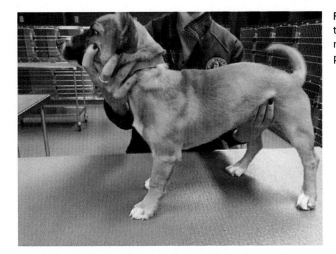

Figure 10.7 Lateral view of a canine patient that has a BCS of 4. Note that the ribs are not visible, although they are easy to palpate, with minimal fat coverage. There is a prominent waist, especially if this patient were viewed from above.

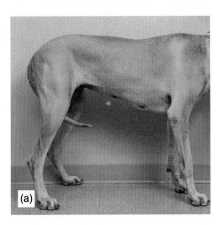

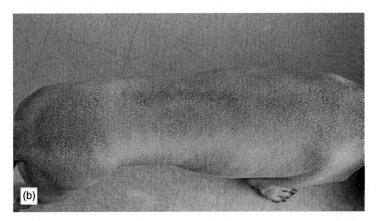

Figure 10.8 A patient with a BCS of 5. (a) In this lateral view, the patient's abdominal tuck is apparent. (b) In this aerial view, the patient's waist is easy to appreciate. Source (a), (b): Courtesy of the Media Resources Department at Midwestern University.

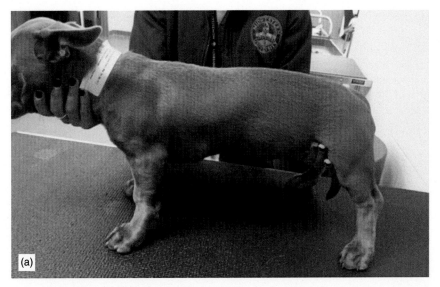

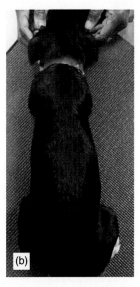

Figure 10.9 A patient with a BCS of 6. (a) In this lateral view, it is difficult to appreciate the patient's waist line as easily as in Figure 10.8a. Palpation is needed to appreciate also that the ribs are palpable, but have slightly more fat covering than would be considered normal. (b) In this aerial view, it is difficult to appreciate the patient's waist line or ribs. Palpation is needed to appreciate that the ribs are palpable, but have slightly more fat covering than would be considered normal.

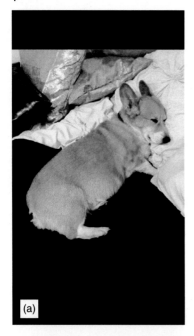

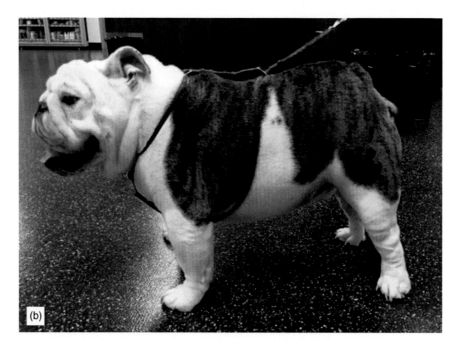

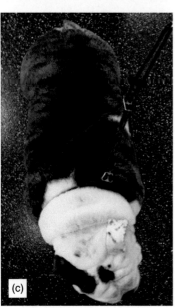

Figure 10.10 Patients with a BCS of 7. (a) Note the loss of abdominal tuck. Source: Courtesy of Rayeanne Solano. (b) This English Bulldog is beginning to display visible deposits of fat in the lumbar region and is also losing its abdominal tuck. (c) Aerial view of the same English Bulldog as in (b). Note that it is equally difficult to appreciate the patient's waist when viewed from above.

According to the Purina nine-point system, dogs are overweight if they score a BCS of 7, 8, or 9:

- A dog that is classified as a BCS of 7 is considered to be mildly overweight (Figure 10.10). It is possible, but challenging, to feel the ribcage owing to heavy fat coverage, and fat deposits may be starting to accumulate over the lumbar region and tail base. The waist is absent, as is the abdominal tuck.
- A dog that is classified as a BCS of 8 is considered to be moderately overweight (Figure 10.11). It is not possible to feel the ribcage owing to heavy fat coverage, and there is no waist line. Fat deposits are easily seen

and palpable in the lumbar region bilaterally and also at the tail base. There may also be visible rounding of the ventral abdomen due to fat deposition.
- A dog that is classified as a BCS of 9 is considered to be morbidly obese (Figure 10.12). Fat deposits are extensive: in addition to prominent lumbar "love handles," fat is present over the neck, thorax, spine, tail, and limbs.

BCS tends to be underutilized by the veterinary team [61], yet it should be used at each visit as a screening tool [62] to assist with clinician recognition of trends.

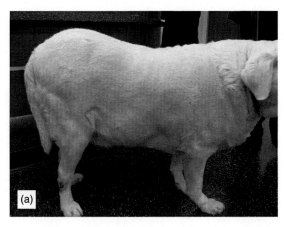
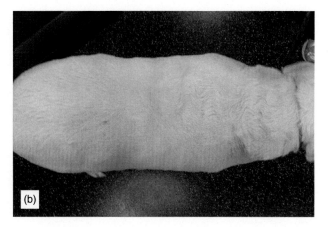

Figure 10.11 A patient with a BCS of 8. (a) Note the loss of abdominal tuck in this lateral view and also the prominent fat deposits over the caudal rump and ventral abdomen. (b) Aerial view of same patient. Note the prominent fat deposits over the shoulder blades.

When assessing BCS, keep in mind that not all dogs are "built" the same in terms of size, shape, build, stature, and body composition. As mentioned, there are breed-specific differences in body composition [56] and also individual variability. Some dogs will score a BCS of 7 for their entire life: they always have been and always will be, simply put, "big dogs." Other dogs will score a BCS of 3 for their entire life: they always have been and always will be, simply put, "skinny."

More important than noting consistency is to note trends. Changes in body size or shape may occur prior to the development of overt clinical signs that owners may recognize. The "big dog" that was always a BCS of 7 and is now a 4 on physical examination, without any identifiable changes in diet or feeding routine at home, should be flagged as needing a more extensive work-up.

It is the responsibility of the veterinary team to engage the client in a discussion about the risks associated with being under- or overweight. As already

noted, many owners do not recognize weight as a medical concern. Accordingly, the burden is on the veterinary team to address the topic of weight management, and to work with the client to convince them of its importance [23].

10.3 Assessing Hydration

In addition to BCS, the hydration status of a patient is one of many indicators of whole-body wellness. See Section 2.3 for an extensive discussion regarding the importance of clinical history taking in the assessment of hydration. Recall that the physical examination augments the history to paint a complete clinical picture of the patient. In order to characterize hydration status for each patient, the veterinary professional should examine skin turgor, mucous membrane moistness, eye position within the orbits, heart rate, peripheral pulse quality, capillary refill time, and whether or not there is jugular distension [62]. Canine cardiovascular findings are described in Chapter 13.

This section emphasizes skin turgor, which evaluates the skin's elasticity. It can be assessed by grasping a generous fold of skin at the nape of the neck or between the shoulder blades. This skin fold is classically lifted up, pinched between the examiner's thumb and index fingers or twisted to one side by the examiner's flick of the wrist. Some refer to this process as intentionally "tenting the skin" (Figure 10.13).

The skin fold is then released and the savvy practitioner observes that one of two outcomes is possible:

- In a euhydrated patient, there is appreciable skin elasticity. The fold of skin returns to its normal position almost instantaneously. In other words, there is not a persistent "skin tent."

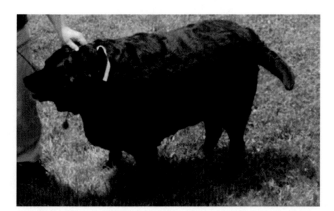

Figure 10.12 Lateral view of a morbidly obese patient with BCS of 9. Note the abundance of fat deposits, particularly at the neck, cranioventral chest, and topline.

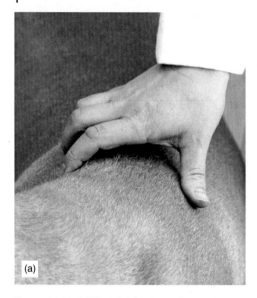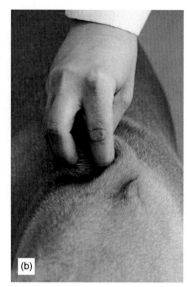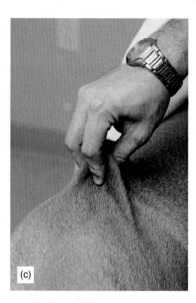

Figure 10.13 (a) The clinician is getting ready to grasp a skin fold between the shoulder blades to assess hydration. (b) The clinician is twisting the patient's skin to assess hydration. (c) The clinician is tenting the patient's skin to assess hydration. Source (a)–(c): Courtesy of the Media Resources Department at Midwestern University.

- As the patient dehydrates, there is a progressive loss of skin elasticity that leads to slow-to-bounce-back skin. The skin is said to be "sluggish" – it does not seem motivated to return to its normal position. As dehydration progresses, the skin fold does not return at all but remains "tented."

See Section 2.3 to review the limitations of skin tenting, how to corroborate a presumptive diagnosis of dehydration based upon physical examination findings with relevant clinicopathologic data, and how to estimate the percentage dehydration in any given patient.

10.4 Breed Designation

If this is the patient's first visit to the practice, it behooves the clinician to take a moment to recognize distinguishing features that may be unique to the patient's breed. These breed-specific identifiers are important to note in any medical record and may assist with patient identification.

Dog owners frequently self-identify the patient's breed, and they may or may not be accurate in their assessment. For example, in the author's experience, a number of pit bull terriers that are presented to the clinic are misrepresented as alternative breeds or breed-mixes – most notably as Labradors, Boxers, or Labrador–Boxer crosses.

The emergence of breed-specific legislation [63–66] with its resultant breed-specific restrictions and/or

bans may have contributed to the overt mislabeling of breeds by some individuals to circumvent the law. This legislation is most typically written against Pit Bull Terriers, but depending upon the municipality, may include Staffordshire Bull Terriers, American Staffordshire Terriers, or any other dog with a Pit Bull-like appearance [63].

The concern with regard to Pit Bull Terriers and Pit Bull-like breeds is that the injuries they cause are thought to be associated with extensive morbidity and mortality [67–70]. Dog bite injuries remain a serious concern in public health, involving approximately 1.5% of the human population of the United States annually [70–73]. Because dog bites are largely considered preventable [67, 73–75], breed-specific legislation was designed to be protective and proactive. Whether or not it is effective remains controversial [76–79].

Unfortunately, there is a concurrent demand for shelters to re-home immense numbers of companion animals annually [80]. In the United Kingdom alone during 2010, shelter intake of dogs reached 89,571, split between 536 rescue organizations [81]. The American Society for the Prevention of Cruelty to Animals (ASPCA) estimates that 7.6 million companion animals enter an estimated 13,600 community animal shelters nationwide [82]. Many of these unwanted or homeless dogs include Pit Bull Terriers or Pit Bull-like breeds [80]. These breeds tend to have longer shelter stays [86] or are euthanized at accelerated rates within shelters [84–86]. Accordingly, 41% of shelter workers in regions affected by breed-specific legislation admitted to intentionally mislabeling dogs of restricted breeds to increase their chance for adoption [80]. Shelter workers may also rely upon physical characteristics and traits as a primary means by which shelter dogs are assigned to a breed [80], yet even first- and second-generation crosses of two purebred dogs of differing breeds exhibit immense diversity in terms of physical appearance [87].

Breed labels, regardless of their accuracy, impact length of stay in shelters and adoptability [83]. Breed labels also impact client perceptions as to how the dog is expected to behave. For example, the Border Collie is perceived by the general pet-owning population to be highly intelligent and therefore trainable, whereas the Pit Bull Terrier faces stereotypes of being less approachable and more difficult to train [83].

Understanding client perception as it relates to breed is an important consideration for any clinician: eliciting the client's perspective regarding breed paves the way for an open dialogue between the clinician and the client that allows for shared mutual understanding between expectations and reality.

10.5 Inspecting the Coat: First Impressions

One of the most important integumentary characteristics for the clinician to recognize and record is coat length and whether or not the patient belongs to a "furless" breed. A handful of "furless" breeds of dog have been reported since Darwin referred to one as the "Turkish naked dog with defective teeth" [88]. Other rarities include the African Sand Dog and the Egyptian Dog. By comparison, the best known breeds include the Chinese Crested dog and the Mexican Hairless dog. None of these are truly 100% devoid of hair; they all have sparse truncal coverage with more hair than elsewhere

concentrated on the dorsum of the head and at the tip of the tail [88].

An autosomal dominant monogenic gene is responsible for conferring the phenotypic characteristics of the Mexican Hairless dog with regard to its coat coverage or the lack thereof [89]. Mexican Hairless dogs are also known to have abnormal sebaceous glands [88] and an epidermis that is heavily concentrated with melanocytes [90]. Not surprisingly, their skin is delicate and at increased risk of damage from ultraviolet (UV) irradiation [90–92]. Along their topline and also along the limbs and prepuce, comedones are commonplace as plugged follicles otherwise referred to as "blackheads" [93].

Hairlessness in the Chinese Crested dog is also inherited as an autosomal semi-dominant trait. Heterozygotes share the classic phenotype that characterizes the breed, although there is some variation in the extent to which a patient is truly hairless [94, 95]. Heterozygous Chinese Crested dogs exhibit true hypotrichosis. Nearly one-third of all follicles are dysplastic and, as is the case with the Mexican Hairless dogs, comedones are common. It is important when reviewing the physical examination with the clients of these dogs that the clinician note these as normal findings for the breed.

If the patient has a coat, it should be described in terms of texture, especially if it is unique. The majority of dogs have straight coats. However, the Labradoodle may have a coat that is naturally straight, wavy, or curled (Figure 10.14a). Similarly, the Miniature Poodle may also have a coat with curls (Figure 10.14b).

If the patient has a coat, it should also be evaluated in terms of length and thickness relative to what is considered the norm for the breed standard (Figure 10.15). Coat length may seem obvious as a visible characteristic and may therefore be easy to overlook. However, it is important to recognize, record, and review with

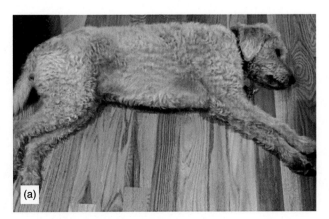
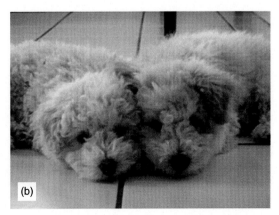

Figure 10.14 (a) Example of a curly-coated Labradoodle. Source: Courtesy of Ambika Vaid. (b) Example of a curly-coated Miniature Poodle. Source: Courtesy of Christine Chen.

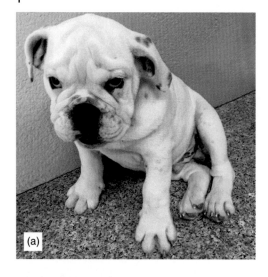

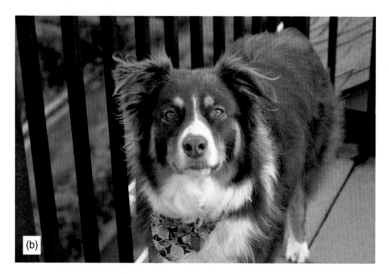

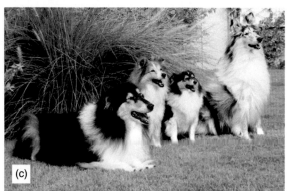

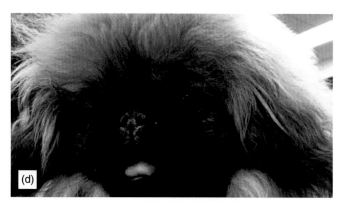

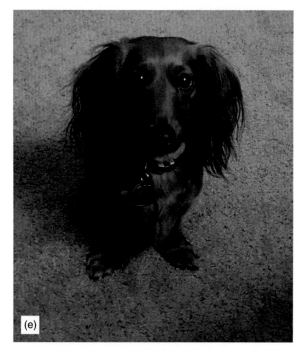

Figure 10.15 (a) Example of a typical English Bulldog coat, which is classically short. Source: Courtesy of Shirley Yang, DVM. (b) Example of a typical Australian Shepherd coat, which is classically medium in length. Source: Courtesy of Stephanie Harris. (c) Several examples of the classic Collie coat. Source: Courtesy of B. Santos. (d) Example of a typical Pekingese coat. (e) Example of the coat of a typical long-haired miniature Dachshund. Source: Courtesy of Marissa Haglund, Midwestern University CVM 2019.

the client because the coat at its current length may require routine upkeep to maintain it in good health. Owners may look to veterinarians for information as to proper care and coat maintenance, and some owners may elect to alter the coat length accordingly to prevent matting and other complications associated with coats of certain lengths.

In addition to coat length, coat odor is an important consideration. Every patient has its own unique smell from apocrine and sebaceous gland secretions and by-products of resident bacterial populations. However, there are times when the veterinarian will be overtaken by an odor that is clearly abnormal. When this occurs, closer inspection is warranted. Sometimes the odor is a "red herring" – it may be a by-product of the environment in which the patient has been living, for example, the smell of smoke on the coat of a dog that lives with a smoker. However, when the smell is acrid, do not overlook it: it is a clue to look deeper. Skin lesions, metabolic disease, or both may be to blame.

10.6 Identifying Coat Colors and Coat Patterns

Coat colors and coat patterns, which refer to combinations of colors, are additional patient-specific characteristics that should be documented within the medical record any time the veterinary team is meeting a patient for the first time.

There are several dog coat patterns that the clinician should recognize:

- solid;
- bicolor;
- tricolor;
- merle;
- harlequin;
- brindle;
- brindlequin;
- sable;
- agouti;
- color-point;
- speckled or ticked;
- fawn.

Solid dogs are characterized as having coats with only one color. Black, brown, blue, red, gold, cream, and white are typical base colors for canine coats [96] (Figure 10.16).

Just as white-coated cats with blue eyes tend to be deaf owing to hereditary apoptosis of the hair cells in the inner ear [97–104], so pigment-associated deafness exists in dogs and has been identified in over 90 breeds [105–112]. Most notably, pigment-associated deafness

has been reported in the Dalmatian, Jack Russell Terrier, English Setter, English Cocker Spaniel, Whippet, and Border Collie [112]. It is associated with recessive alleles, specifically those associated with the piebald and merle genes [105]. Both genes suppress melanocytes [105]. This causes white or diluted pigmentation of the skin and hair and potentially blue irises [105]. When the stria vascularis of the cochlear duct is also impacted, deafness results [105].

Clients of dogs that are presumed to be congenitally deaf may report that their dog does not respond to verbal cues. A sleeping puppy, for example, may not come when called. It may not even seem to be aware when the client returns home and walks through the front door.

As a supplement to this clinical history, the patient may be selected to undergo electrodiagnostic testing such as brain-stem auditory-evoked response (BAER) [113–117]. BAER is more frequently performed in dogs than in cats to provide a definitive diagnosis. Breeders may ask to have this test performed at as early as 5–6 weeks of age, when the cochlear cells will have had time to develop and/or degenerate. The goal in obtaining a diagnosis is twofold: (1) for the direct benefit of the patient so that the household is cognizant of the need to communicate via hand signals and other cues, and (2) to remove the patient from the breeding pool because this type of congenital deafness is hereditary [105].

Several colors have multiple names depending upon the breed of dog [96]:

- The breed-specific terminology for the color brown may be "liver" or "chocolate," as in chocolate Labradors.
- The breed-specific terminology for the color red may be "orange," "red–gold," "ruby," or "cinnamon," as in cinnamon Chow Chows.
- The breed-specific terminology for the color gold may be "apricot," "wheaten," "tawny," "straw," "honey," "blonde," or "lemon," as in lemon-colored Beagles.

Some color names are highly breed specific. For example, deadgrass is a color that is referenced most typically in Chesapeake Bay Retrievers (Figure 10.17). The color deadgrass can vary from a solid tan to straw to a very light cream that is almost white in appearance [118].

Bicolor dogs are characterized as having coats with two colors. Black and white, also known as the "tuxedo" color combination, and blue ("gray") and white are classic examples of this coat pattern. As is the case with tuxedo cats, tuxedo dogs can be primarily black or primarily white (Figure 10.18). Tuxedo dogs may also be short, medium, or long-haired [96].

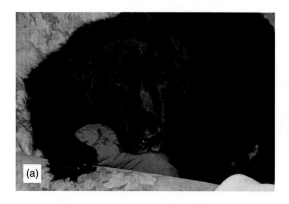

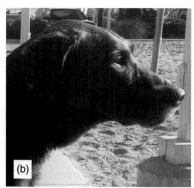

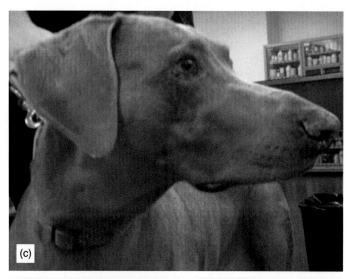

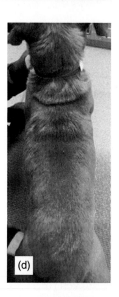

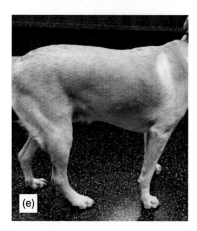

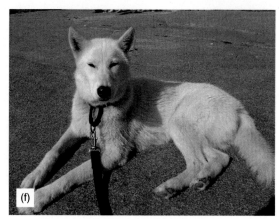

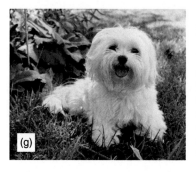

Figure 10.16 (a) Example of a solid black coat in a Newfoundland dog. (b) Example of a solid brown coat in a dog. Source: Courtesy of Jess Darmofal. (c) Example of a solid blue coat in a Weimaraner. Source: Courtesy of Elizabeth Robbins, DVM. (d) Example of a solid red coat in a dog. (e) Example of a solid gold coat in a Labrador Retriever dog. (f) Example of a solid cream coat in a husky. Source: Courtesy of Garrett Rowley, 2018 DVM. (g) Example of a solid white coat in a Maltese. Source: Courtesy of Richard Vallejos.

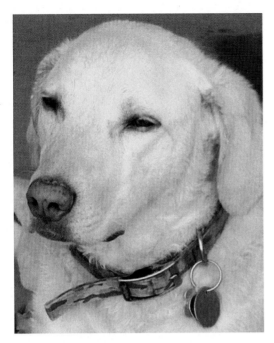

Figure 10.17 Example of a deadgrass coat in a Chesapeake Bay Retriever. Source: Courtesy of Jess Darmofal.

Tricolor dogs are characterized as having coats with three colors, typically black, brown, or blue on the dog's upper parts, with a white ventrum, and tan highlights (Figure 10.19) [96].

The merle coat pattern resembles a marbled coat. It is commonly seen in Australian Shepherds. When a merle pattern is present in a Dachshund, the dog is sometimes referred to as being dappled [96]. Blue merle refers to a marbling of the blue coat color; liver merle refers to a marbling of the brown coat color (Figure 10.20). As mentioned, the merle gene is associated with a higher inci-

dence of deafness and blue-colored irises [105] (Figure 10.21).

In addition, the merle coat pattern is linked with microphthalmia, congenitally under-sized eyes [119–122]. When microphthalmia alone is present, the patient typically has vision. However, when combined with multiple ocular anomalies (MOA), the clinical picture for the patient is consistent with merle ocular dysgenesis (MOD), which may be blinding. In addition to microphthalmia, these patients may also present with corneal, iridal, pupillary, scleral, and retinal defects. Microcornea, iris coloboma, anisocoria, lens luxation, retinal dysplasia, and retinal detachment have been documented [120].

Because the merle gene creates marbling of color throughout the coat, it can also create marbling of the skin, nose, and paw-pads (Figure 10.22). The mottled skin is easiest to appreciate along the ventrum and medial thighs where there is typically less coat coverage [123].

Note that mottled skin pigmentation is not limited to dogs with the merle gene, and may also occur in other breeds of dogs that do not carry the merle gene (Figure 10.23).

The harlequin coat pattern is a modification of the merle gene. It is specific to Great Danes. Rather than a marbling of the coat, the harlequin gene confers discrete color patches (Figure 10.24). For instance, a harlequin Great Dane may be described as white with black and/or gray patches much like a piebald horse or cow [96, 124].

The brindle coat pattern is a striped pattern. In its classic form it may be referred to as the "tiger striped" pattern. The stripes are a mixture of black with brown, tan, or gold (Figure 10.25). The brindle coat pattern is common in Boxers, Bulldogs, and Great Danes [96, 125, 126].

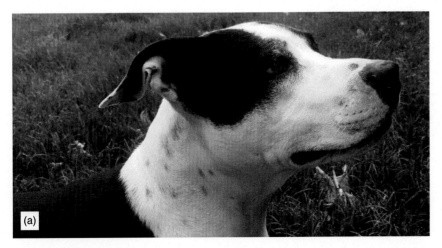
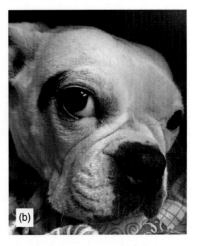

Figure 10.18 (a) Example of a tuxedo coat pattern in a dog. Source: Courtesy of Danielle N. Cucuzella. (b) Alternative example of a tuxedo coat pattern in a dog. Note how this dog is primarily white with just a trace of black. Source: Courtesy of Rozalyn Donner.

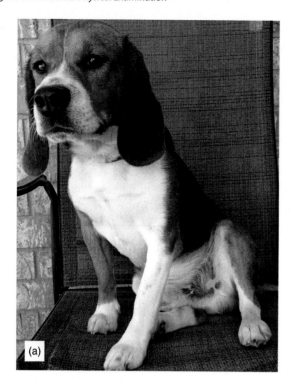

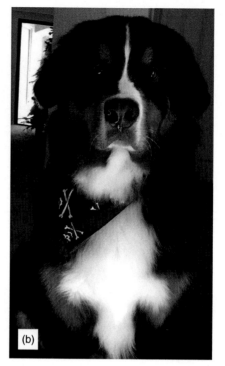

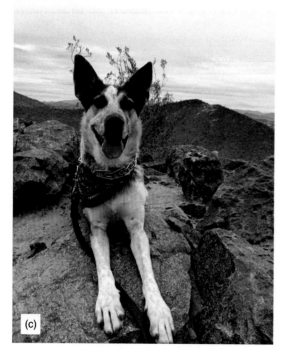

Figure 10.19 (a) Example of a tricolor Beagle. Source: Courtesy of Jordanne M. Diaz. (b) Example of a tricolor Bernese Mountain Dog. Source: Courtesy of Kim Wallitsch. (c) Alternative example of a tricolor dog. Source: Courtesy of Samantha Rudolph.

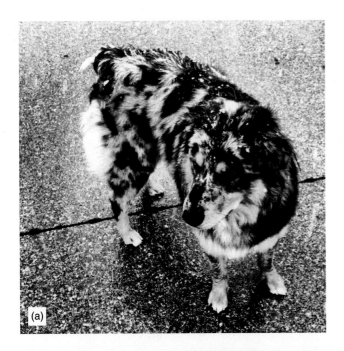

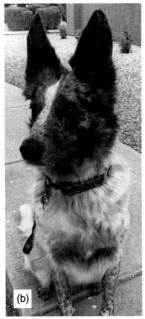

Figure 10.20 (a) Example of a blue merle Sheltie dog. Source: Courtesy of Lauren A. Beren. (b) Alternative example of a blue merle dog. Source: Courtesy of Brittany L. Lasak. (c) Example of a red merle Australian Shepherd. Source: Courtesy of Amanda Rappaport. (d) Alternative example of a red merle mixed-breed dog. Source: Courtesy of Arielle Hatcher.

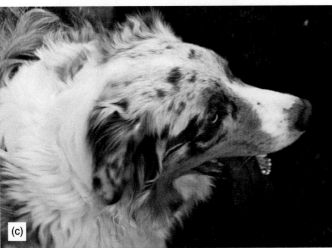

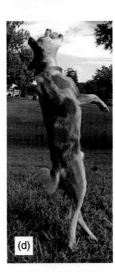

Figure 10.21 Note the blue iris in this dog with a merle coat pattern. These commonly go hand-in-hand. Source: Courtesy of Heather Gould.

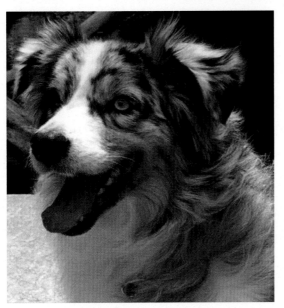

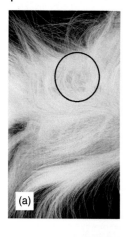

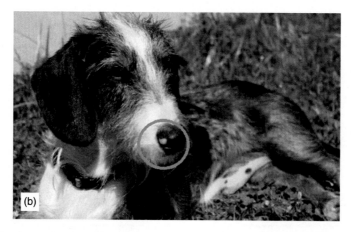

Figure 10.22 (a) Note the subtle skin mottling that is evident underneath the ventral abdominal fur in this canine patient with a merle coat pattern. (b) Note the mottled pigment on the nose of this dapple Dachshund. Source: Courtesy of R. Lewis, LVT.

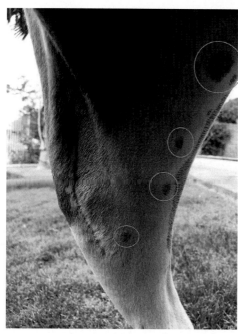

Figure 10.23 This patient lacks the merle gene but happens to have mottled skin pigmentation along the medial thigh. Source: Courtesy of Kiefer Hazard.

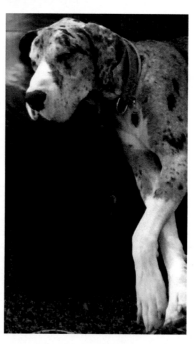

Figure 10.24 An example of a harlequin Great Dane. Source: Courtesy of Daniel J. Fletcher, PhD, DVM, DACVECC.

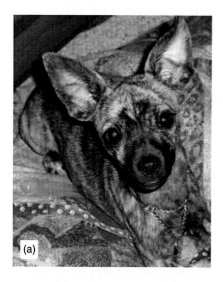

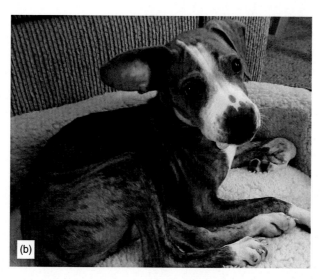

Figure 10.25 (a) Example of a brindle dog. Source: Courtesy of Kaitlen Betchel. (b) Alternative example of a brindle dog that happens also to have a white stripe down the bridge of its muzzle. Source: Courtesy of Analucia P. Aliaga.

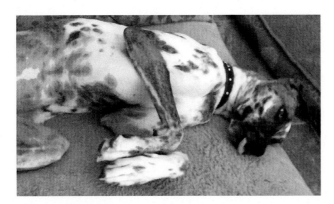

Figure 10.26 Example of a brindlequin Great Dane. Source: Courtesy of Rozalyn Donner.

A brindlequin is a coat pattern that is specific to Great Danes. It is a blend of the harlequin pattern in which the splotches of color are brindle (Figure 10.26) [127].

A sable pattern refers to hairs that are tipped black. This pattern is classically found in German Shepherds (Figure 10.27) [96].

The agouti pattern refers to hairs that are banded (Figure 10.28). This pattern is typically seen in Keeshonds [96].

Point coloration is a common coat pattern in the Rottweiler and Doberman. The coat is solid black with the exception of tan "points" or splotches above the eyes, on the facial cheeks, on the neck just below the head, on the chest, on the lower legs, and on the medial aspects of the legs. Sometimes this color pattern is simply referred to as "black and tan" rather than as "point coloration" (Figure 10.29).

The speckled or ticked coat pattern is typically seen in Australian Cattle Dogs (Figure 10.30). The ticking of the fur is created by the presence of agouti hairs. These are banded, with several different colors along their length. The second colored fur is typically darker and, when "stamped" against the lighter background fur, creates distinct contrast. For example, in the Australian cattle dog, the ticking of the hairs with a black base creates a moth-eaten blue–gray appearance [96].

The fawn coat pattern is typically seen in pugs and puggles (Figure 10.31). Fawn refers to a tannish yellow or cream base coat color with a dark facial mask [96].

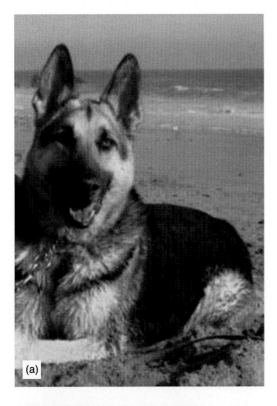

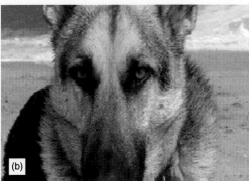

Figure 10.27 (a) Sable coat pattern in a German Shepherd and (b) close-up of the sable coat pattern. In loving memory of Rachel Beard, DVM.

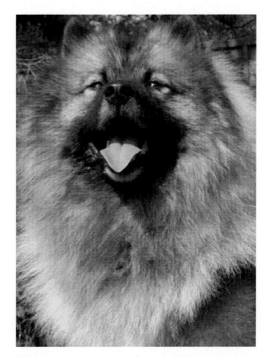

Figure 10.28 Example of the agouti coat pattern that is seen in Keeshonds.

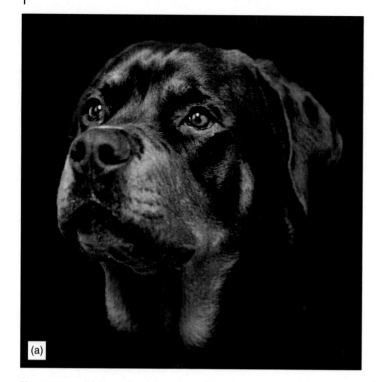

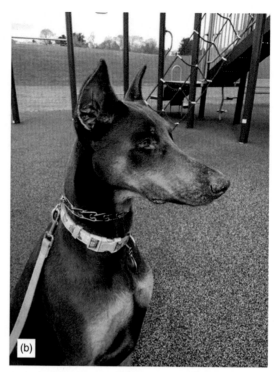

Figure 10.29 (a) Example of the color point coloration pattern that is seen in the Rottweiler. Source: Courtesy of Zabzoo Services. (b) Example of the color point coloration pattern that is seen in the Doberman. Source: Courtesy of Courtney Keller.

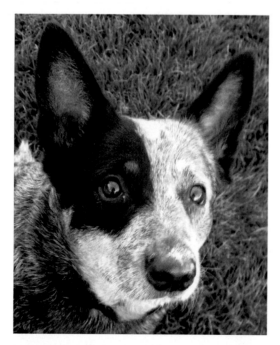

Figure 10.30 The ticked pattern of an Australian Cattle Dog. Source: Courtesy of Kayla M. Kerstetter.

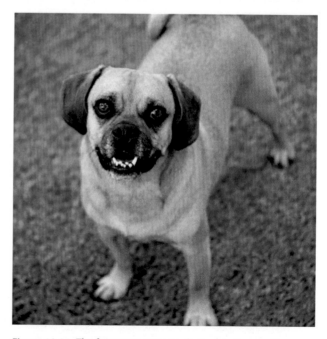

Figure 10.31 The fawn coat pattern of a Puggle. Source: Courtesy of Shelby Newton.

10.7 Assessing Coat Quality

Coat quality should be assessed and documented. In particular, the clinician should note whether the coat is well groomed or unkempt, shiny or dull (Figure 10.32). Recent changes in coat quality should raise a red flag.

In addition, the clinician should assess coat quality in terms of fullness: is there hypotrichosis or alopecia? If either is present, then the following questions ought to be considered:

- Is the hypotrichosis or alopecia focal or diffuse?
- Is the hypotrichosis or alopecia progressing?
- Is the hypotrichosis or alopecia bilaterally symmetrical?
- Is the hypotrichosis or alopecia associated with particular coat color(s)?

Color dilution alopecia is an uncommon, inherited skin disease that has been reported in increasing numbers in Doberman Pinschers, Dachshunds, Miniature Pinschers, Schnauzers, Yorkshire Terriers, Italian Greyhounds, Whippets, Shetland Sheepdogs, and Chihuahuas. Coats of affected patients are aesthetically normal at birth; however, between 6 months and 2 years of age, they progressively thin out over the dorsum of the trunk, but only in regions where there are color-diluted hairs. In particular, fawn hairs are affected because fawn is a dilution of red or brown, and blue hairs are affected because blue is a dilution of black. The head, tail, and limbs are typically, but not always, spared (Figure 10.33) [128–130].

Histologically, dogs with color dilution alopecia have defects in pigment production and storage, follicle structure, and keratinization [130]. As a result, what hairs remain in the color-diluted regions are sparse and of poor quality [129]. The shafts fracture easily, and the underlying skin tends to be both scaly and prone to secondary pyoderma [129].

Black hair follicular dysplasia is the primary differential for color dilution alopecia. From a histological approach, the two conditions are identical. The only difference is that in the former condition, only black hairs are affected and tan areas are spared [129–133].

Another form of non-pathological focal alopecia is breed-related canine pattern baldness, reported primarily in Dachshunds, but also in Doberman Pinschers, Chihuahuas, Boston Terriers, Boxers, and Whippets. Affected patients typically develop hypotrichosis in early adulthood that then progresses to alopecia. The alopecia is symmetrical and most commonly affects the lateral aspects of the pinnae and also the post-auricular regions (Figure 10.34). However, it may also impact the cranioventral neck, chest, and ventrum [134].

Greyhounds have a similar condition that is characterized by focal alopecia of the caudolateral thighs that may or may not extend cranially up the ventrum. Like canine pattern baldness in Dachshunds, this so-called idiopathic bald thigh syndrome of Greyhounds causes early-adulthood onset of hair thinning that progresses to hair loss. This is purely cosmetic and does not require treatment [135].

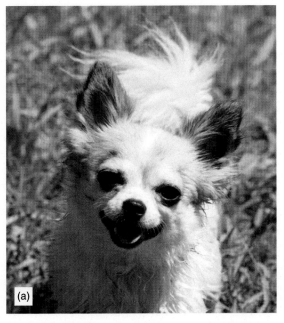
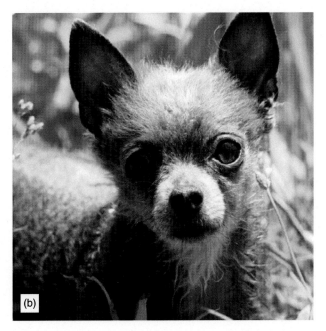

Figure 10.32 (a) Example of a well-groomed, shiny, healthy coat. (b) Example of a poor-quality, brittle, dry coat with an abnormal, almost woolly texture to the fur. Source (a), (b): Courtesy of Cheri Erwin.

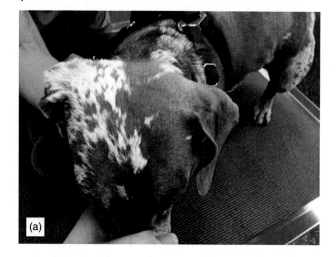

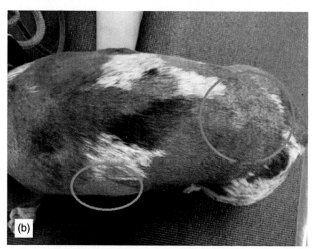

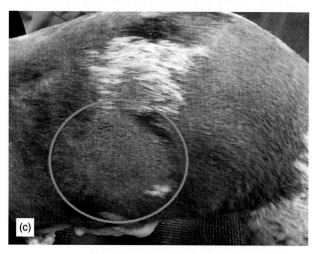

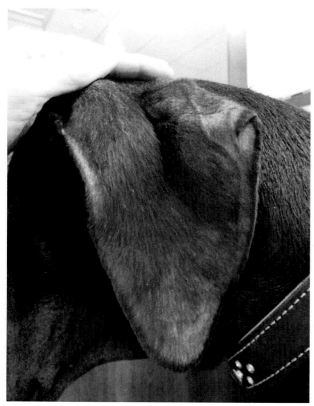

Figure 10.34 Presumptive canine pattern baldness in a Doberman Pinscher affecting the lateral aspect of both pinnae. Only the right pinna is shown here. Source: Courtesy of Elizabeth Robbins, DVM.

Figure 10.33 (a) Example of a canine patient with color dilution alopecia. Note that the head has been spared. (b) Example of a canine patient with color dilution alopecia associated with blue regions of the coat. Note that in the circled regions, both along the dorsum and at the caudal rump, fur coverage is becoming sparse. (c) Example of a canine patient with color dilution alopecia associated with blue regions of the coat. Note that in the circled region along the dorsum, fur coverage is sparse.

More often than not, focal areas of alopecia are the result of underlying pathology. The list of differential diagnoses for focal alopecia is extensive, as are the innumerable locations where focal alopecia can present itself. However, broad categories include bacterial [136], fungal [137], and parasitic skin disorders [138]. When alopecia has a truncal distribution, it tends to be associated with endocrinopathies [139, 140]. In addition, focal alopecia may be congenital [141] or caused by traumatic injuries, including vaccinations [142, 143], and self-induced fur-mowing [144, 145] as discussed in Section 2.6 (Figures 10.35).

When dogs exhibit "fur-mowing," their compulsive licking tends to be concentrated focally on a distal limb. Over time, this leads to the development of focal alopecia with secondary changes to the surrounding skin. The skin typically becomes firm, proliferative, and ulcerative. The lesion may weep. Even when the patient is prevented from licking, these lesions notoriously take a significant time to resolve spontaneously, given that they often have developed chronic changes in addition to secondary bacterial infections that may run deep to the skin. Such a lesion is typically referred to as a lick granuloma, which is the result of acral lick dermatitis. The most common

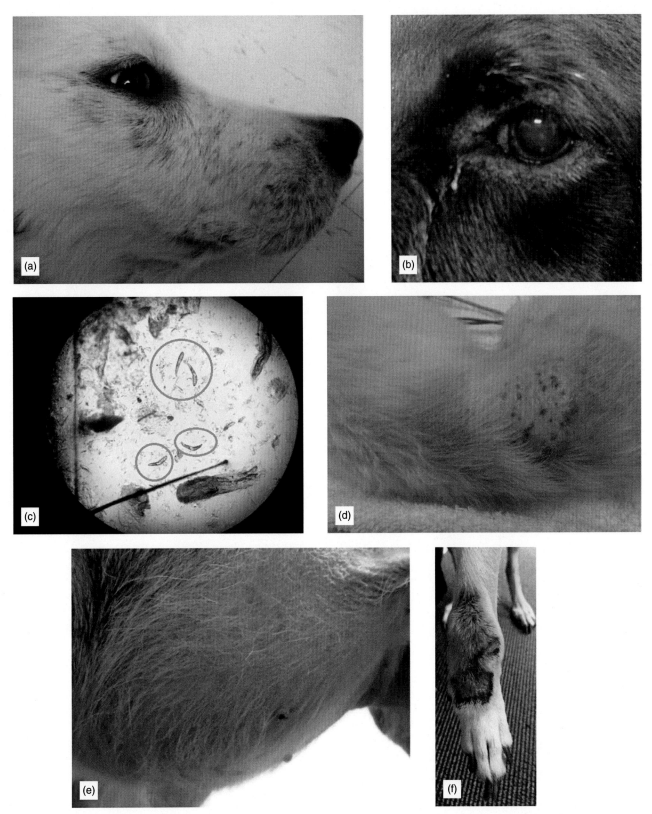

Figure 10.35 (a) Example of a juvenile canine patient with a patchy, moth-eaten facial hypotrichosis secondary to focal demodicosis. Source: Courtesy of Samantha Thurman, DVM. (b) Example of an adult canine patient with focal peri-ocular alopecia secondary to generalized demodicosis. Source: Courtesy of Elizabeth Robbins, DVM. (c) Light microscope view of Demodex canis. (d) Maltese in left lateral recumbency with right lateral flank visible. Note the extensive flank-associated alopecia that developed several weeks after the rabies vaccination was administered. This region of alopecia was biopsied and the pathologist reported post-vaccinal rabies panniculitis – ischemic dermatopathy. Source: Courtesy of Samantha Thurman, DVM. (e) Hypotrichosis associated with the caudoventral abdomen. This was bilaterally symmetrical. The patient also had a concurrent pot-bellied appearance that raised the clinician's suspicion that an endocrinopathy might be present. Source: Courtesy of Patricia Bennett, DVM. (f) Alopecia associated with a traumatic wound at the left distal antebrachium. Source: Courtesy of Samantha Thurman, DVM. (*Continued*)

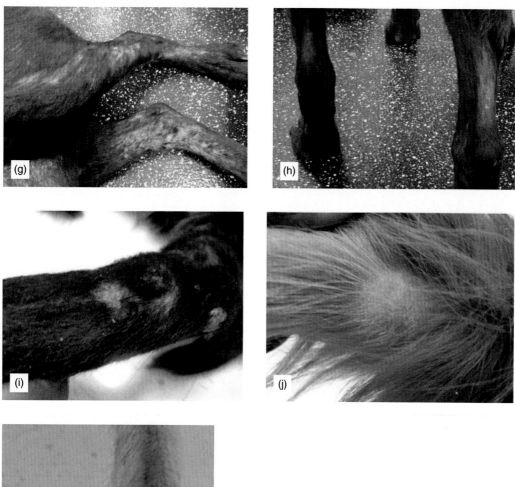

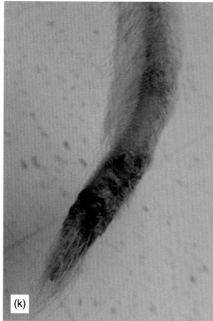

Figure 10.35 (*Continued*)
(g) Example of an adult canine patient with patchy, moth-eaten alopecia at the thighs and distal hind limbs secondary to generalized demodicosis. Source: Courtesy of Elizabeth Robbins, DVM. (h) Hypotrichosis of the caudal distal hind limbs. Source: Courtesy of Elizabeth Robbins, DVM.
(i) Hypotrichosis of the left plantar tarsus and metatarsus. Source: Courtesy of Patricia Bennett, DVM. (j) Alopecia of the tail base. Source: Courtesy of Patricia Bennett, DVM.
(k) Alopecia of the distal tail. Source: Courtesy of Patricia Bennett, DVM.

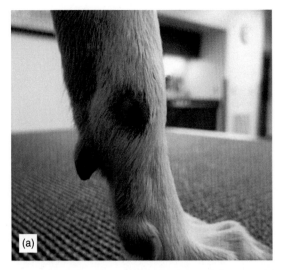
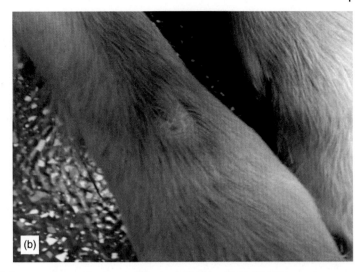

Figure 10.36 (a) Lick granuloma at the medial aspect of the left tarsus. Source: Courtesy of Elizabeth Robbins, DVM. (b) Lick granuloma at the cranial aspect of the right antebrachium. Source: Courtesy of Patricia Bennett, DVM.

locations for lick granulomas are the dorsal carpus, metacarpus, tarsus, and metatarsus (Figure 10.36) [146].

10.8 Inspecting the Skin

The clinician should part the fur to inspect the surface of the skin and to evaluate it for the present of ectoparasites (Figure 10.37).

The clinician should also evaluate the integrity of the skin. This refers to whether or not the skin is abraded and, if so, to what extent. Disrupted skin integrity is often the result of external trauma; however, it may also be self-induced, as was mentioned with reference to acral lick dermatitis (Figure 10.38).

A thorough assessment of the skin should also take into account any changes in pigmentation. Some changes in pigmentation, such as nasal depigmentation,

are idiopathic, yet strictly cosmetic. Nasal depigmentation is common in dogs, especially yellow Labrador Retrievers, Golden Retrievers, Alaskan Malamutes, and Siberian Huskies. Sometimes it is referred to as Dudley nose. Affected patients have a pigmented nose at birth; however, as they age, the nose lightens (Figure 10.39). This lightening may be seasonal, it may resolve spontaneously, or it may be a change that is permanent. The nose itself is not abraded; only the pigment is affected [147].

On the other hand, changes to nasal pigment with concurrent skin lesions may reflect underlying pathology such as pigmentary changes following wound healing from traumatic injury (Figure 10.40), solar dermatitis, or autoimmune diseases such as pemphigus foliaceus [148].

While evaluating for pigmentary changes of the integumentary system, the clinician should also screen for any

Figure 10.37 (a) Parting fur in a black dog to evaluate the surface of the skin. (b) Parting fur in a white dog to evaluate the surface of the skin. Source: Courtesy of Patricia Bennett, DVM.

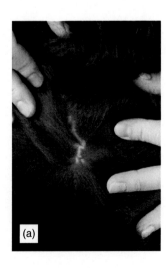
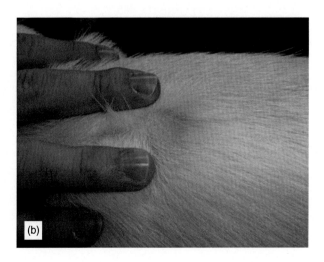

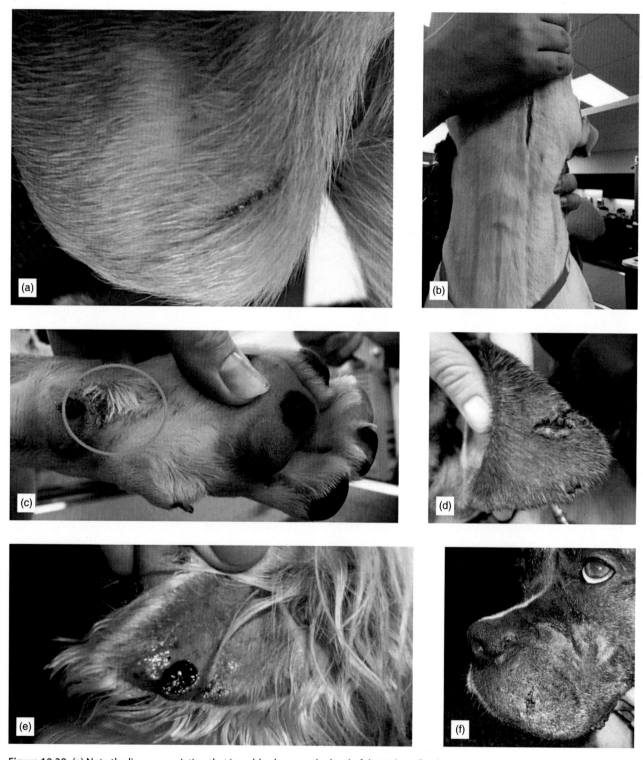

Figure 10.38 (a) Note the linear excoriation that is scabbed over at the level of the right stifle. (b) Note the linear excoriation at the ventral neck secondary to rough play at doggie day care. (c) Note the abrasive injury distal to the carpal paw pad, circled in blue. (d) Wound on the ventral left pinna. Source: Courtesy of Elizabeth Robbins, DVM. (e) Open wound on the ventral right pinna. Source: Courtesy of Elizabeth Robbins, DVM. (f) Facial wounds. Source: Courtesy of Patricia Bennett, DVM. (*Continued*)

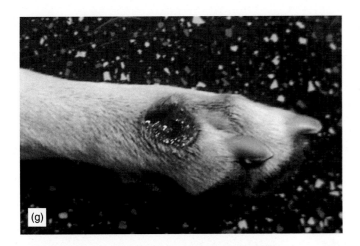

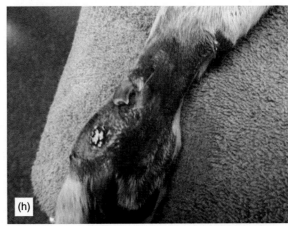

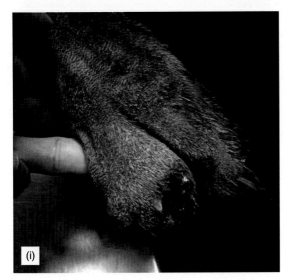

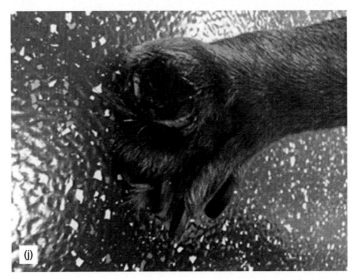

Figure 10.38 (*Continued*)
(g) Open wound at the medial left metatarsus. Source: Courtesy of Elizabeth Robbins, DVM. (h) Extensive lack of skin integrity at the palmar aspect of the right antebrachium caused by a pressure sore secondary to splint placement. Source: Courtesy of Patricia Bennett, DVM. (i) Eroded digit secondary to digital squamous cell carcinoma that was confirmed after digital amputation with histopathology. Source: Courtesy of Amanda Maltese, DVM. (j) Eroded digit. Source: Courtesy of Samantha Thurman, DVM.

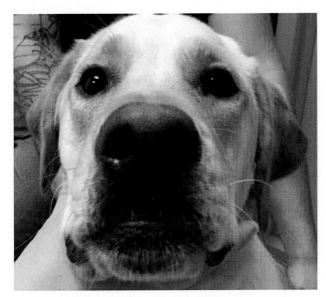

Figure 10.39 Note the onset of nasal depigmentation in this yellow Labrador Retriever.

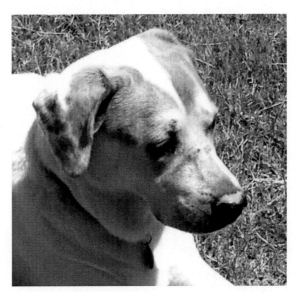

Figure 10.40 Change in nasal pigment following a traumatic injury to the dorsal aspect of the nasal planum. Source: Courtesy of Juliane Daggett, MBS.

areas of active bruising as this may reflect either an injury to the underlying soft tissues or coagulopathy [149–151] (Figure 10.41).

In addition to bruising, the clinician should note if the skin is icteric (Figure 10.42a). Icterus refers to the yellowish discoloration of the body that is the result of excessive bilirubin. Icterus may be present due to increased hemolysis [152–154], liver disease [155, 156], or biliary tract obstruction [157, 158]. As the underlying disease progresses, icterus may develop in additional regions of the body rather than remaining isolated to the skin. For instance, the patient may present with icteric sclera and/or icteric mucous membranes (Figure 10.42b and c).

10.9 Primary Skin Lesions

The skin should be evaluated for any of the following primary skin lesions during every comprehensive physical examination [113, 159]:

- Papule: a small elevation of the skin, typically less than 0.25 cm (Figure 10.43).

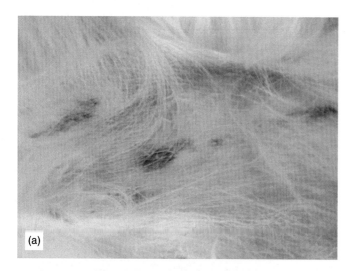

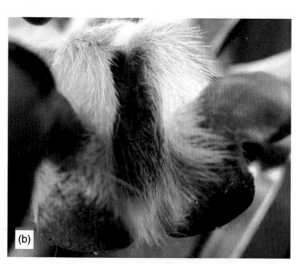

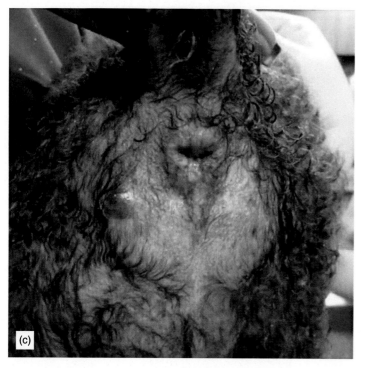

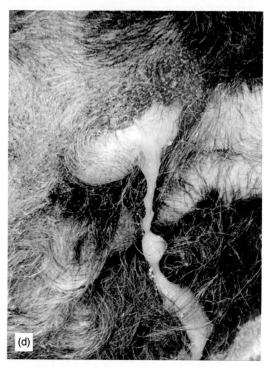

Figure 10.41 (a) Bruising along the ventral abdominal wall. Source: Courtesy of Elizabeth Robbins, DVM. (b) Bruising of the interdigital space secondary to a phalangeal fracture. Source: Courtesy of Patricia Bennett, DVM. (c) Perineal bruising secondary to anal gland impaction. Source: Courtesy of Patricia Bennett, DVM. (d) Peri-anal bruising secondary to anal gland abscess that has ruptured in this canine patient. Source: Courtesy of Shannon Carey, DVM.

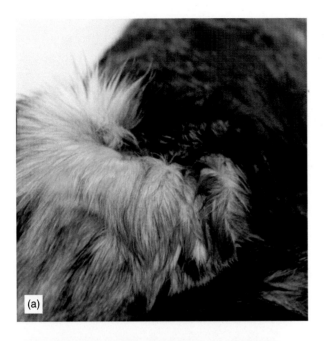

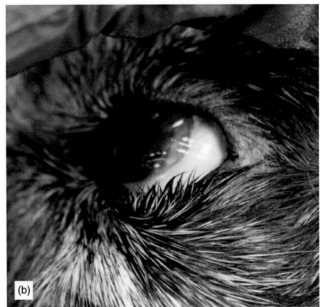

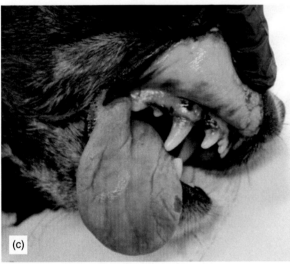

Figure 10.42 (a) Note how the skin diffusely has icteric undertones in this canine patient. (b) Note the icteric sclera in this canine patient. (c) Note the extensive icterus of this patient's mucous membranes and tongue. Source (a)–(c): Courtesy of Ali Brower, DVM, DACVP.

- Nodule: a large papule, typically up to 1 cm in diameter (Figure 10.44).
- Tumor: a large nodule, typically greater than 1 cm (Figure 10.45).
- Pustule: a pus-filled papule, colloquially referred to as a "pimple" (Figure 10.46).
- Vesicle: an elevation that is fluid filled but devoid of purulent material.
- Bulla: a large vesicle, typically greater than 0.5 cm.
- Wheal: a focal allergic reaction.
- Plaque: an elevation with a flat rather than rounded top.

When lesions are identified and recorded in the medical record, the veterinarian should be as descriptive as possible and should take care to document the following:

- the number of lesions;
- the size of the lesions;
- the location of the lesions;
- the configuration of the lesions;
- the progression of the lesions, either as reported by the history or as observed if this is a recheck examination.

A "skin map" may be used to keep track of lesions as they develop, progress, and/or resolve.

When recording the size of the lesions, be accurate. Always measure with calipers rather than "guesstimating." The use of calipers is increasingly recommended in human healthcare to improve accuracy at time of diagnosis and also to chart response to treatment more accurately [160] (Figure 10.45j).

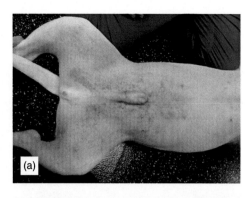

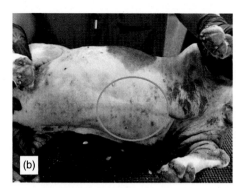

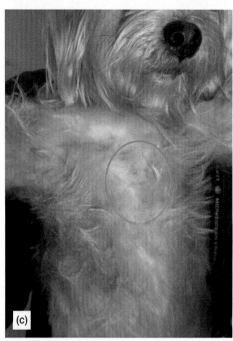

Figure 10.43 (a) Papular rash in the inguinal region. There are hundreds of papules that comprise this rash that was thought to be caused by contact dermatitis. Source: Courtesy of Elizabeth Robbins, DVM. (b) Papular rash along ventrum. Focus on the area circled in blue. This patient also has concurrent hyperpigmentation and lichenification; however, the area of interest is the circled region, in which papules are evident. (c) Papular rash at the cranioventral chest.

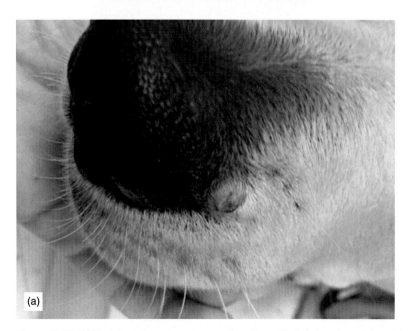

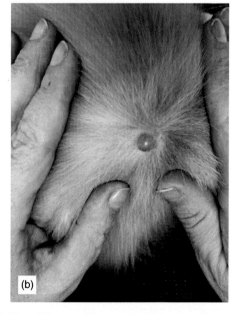

Figure 10.44 (a) Nodule at the mucocutaneous junction at the left dorsolateral rim of the bridge of the nose. Presumptive histiocytoma in a 6-month-old dog that resolved spontaneously over the course of 3 months. (b) Cystic nodule at the dorsal aspect of the head. (Continued)

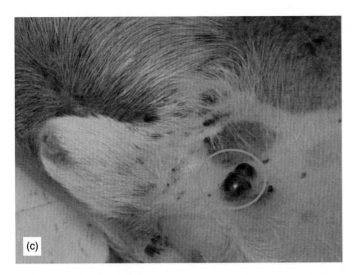

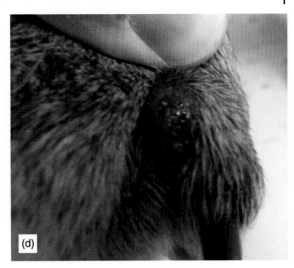

Figure 10.44 (*Continued*)
(c) Melanotic nodules in the inguinal region. (d) Nodule located in the interdigital space of this canine patient. Source: Courtesy of Patricia Bennett, DVM.

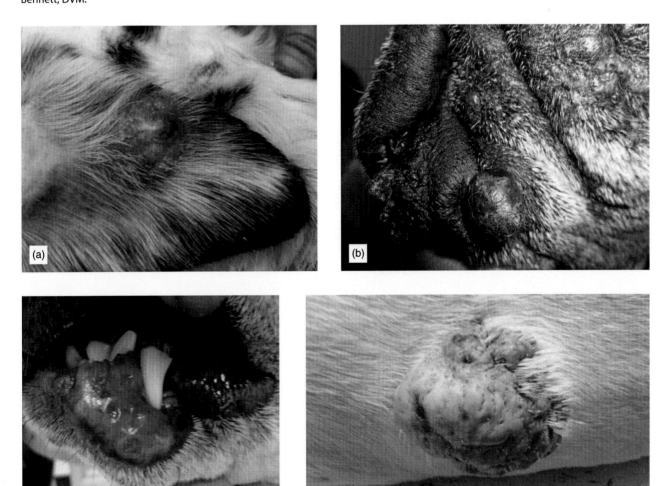

Figure 10.45 (a) Tumor along the ventral aspect of the left pinna. Source: Courtesy of Patricia Bennett, DVM. (b) Tumor associated with the right lower lip fold in a Pug. Source: Courtesy of Elizabeth Robbins, DVM. (c) Extensive tumor associated with the inner aspect of the lower left lip, buccal to the left mandibular canine tooth. This tumor is characterized as having an ulcerative surface thought to be attributed to occlusive trauma. Source: Courtesy of Patricia Bennett, DVM. (d) Cauliflower-like tumor located along the dorsum in a dog. (*Continued*)

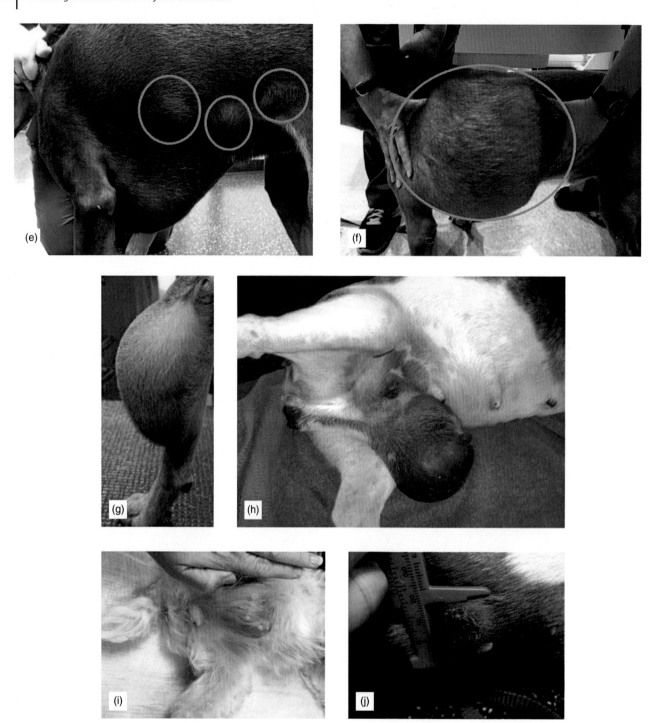

Figure 10.45 (*Continued*)
(e) Several subcutaneous tumors along the ventrolateral body wall in a Doberman Pinscher. These are presumptive lipomas. (f) Extensive tumor arising from the cranial surface of this patient's antebrachium, causing appreciable distortion in the limb's silhouette. Source: Courtesy of Patricia Bennett, DVM. (g) Extensive left axillary and thoracic wall mass. Source: Courtesy of Samantha Thurman, DVM. (h) Tumor associated with the right caudal mammary chain. Source: Courtesy of Patricia Bennett, DVM. (i) Extensive tumor associated with the caudo-ventral abdomen, incorporating the left caudal mammary chain. Source: Courtesy of Samantha Thurman, DVM. (j) Using calipers to quantify tumor size. Source: Courtesy of Samantha Thurman, DVM.

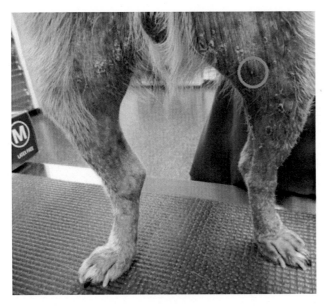

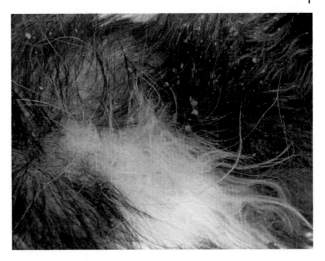

Figure 10.47 Excessive scale. Source: Courtesy of Patricia Bennett, DVM.

Figure 10.46 Extensive papulopustular rash within the inguinal region of this patient and extending down the caudo-medial aspect of both thighs. Note the isolated pustule circled in blue. Source: Courtesy of Elizabeth Robbins, DVM.

10.10 Secondary Skin Lesions

Secondary skin lesions should also be identified if present on physical examination and include the following [113, 159]:

- Scale: loose flakes of skin, colloquially referred to as "dandruff" (Figure 10.47).
- Collarette: what is left after a pustule ruptures (Figure 10.48).

- Crust: dried exudate and keratin that form over the skin's surface (Figure 10.49).
- Scab: dried fibrin and platelet plug that caps the surface of a wound, under which a new layer of skin begins to form (Figure 10.50).
- Comedone: a plug of oil and dead skin cells at the surface of a pore (a "blackhead").
- Lichenification: abnormally thick, leathery skin that typically signifies chronic skin irritation, inflammation, and/or infection (Figure 10.51).
- Hyperpigmentation: dark gray to black discoloration of the skin that typically signifies chronic skin irritation, inflammation, and/or infection (Figure 10.52).

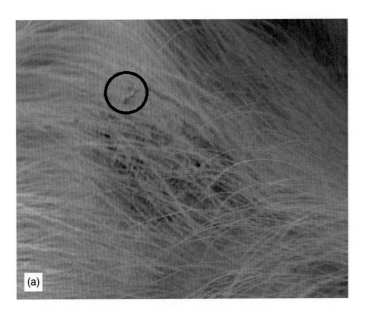

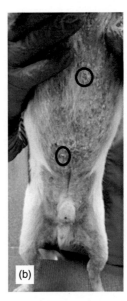

Figure 10.48 (a) Collarette located along the ventrum of a patient, circled in black. Source: Courtesy of Patricia Bennett, DVM. (b) Extensive lesions along the ventrum. Two collarettes are circled in black; however, there are several more that can be identified. Source: Courtesy of Elizabeth Robbins, DVM.

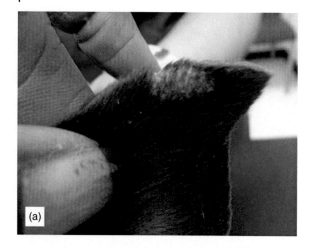

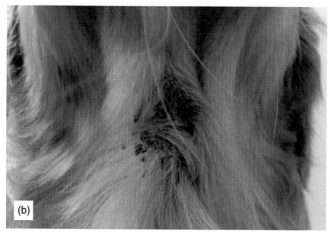

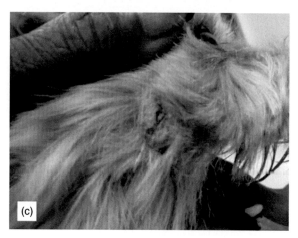

Figure 10.49 Crusting at (a) the tip of a pinna, (b) the ventral neck and (c) the right cheek. The patient is looking toward the right and its mouth is open to support it panting. Source (a)–(c): Courtesy of Patricia Bennett, DVM.

Figure 10.50 Example of several scabs. Source: Courtesy of Patricia Bennett, DVM.

10.11 Miscellaneous Skin Lesions

Some changes in the skin are related to pressure points. A common example is the development of an elbow callus characterized by hardened, thickened skin (Figure 10.53). Although these lesions may occur as a natural response to pressure, most notably in large to giant breed dogs, calluses may also develop in dogs that are persistently recumbent [161].

Recumbent dogs are also at risk of developing pressure sores, as are dogs with improperly fitted or poorly padded bandages (Figure 10.54). Whereas a callus is protective, a pressure sore is not. Pressure sores are most likely to develop over the bony prominences of the limbs such as the lateral humeral epicondyle, greater femoral trochanter, and tuber calcanei. In addition, pressure sores may occur at the level of the pelvis, most notably at the tuber coxae and ischiatic tuberosities. These may be superficial or they may delve beyond the subcutaneous tissue and reach bone [161].

Another lesion of interest that tends to form over bony prominences is the elbow hygroma (Figure 10.55). This thick-walled, bursa-like structure occurs at the lateral aspect of the olecranon. When it occurs, its presentation is typically bilateral and the patient appears to be pain-

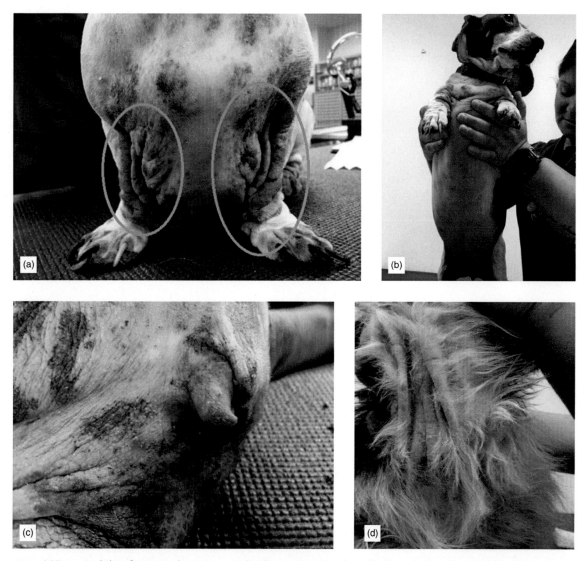

Figure 10.51 (a) Extensive lichenification at the cranioventral axillary regions. Note how the skin is thickened and elephant-like. (b) Same patient as in (a), approximately 1 month into systemic antibiotic therapy. Note how much "softer" the skin appears. (c) Example of peri-vulvar and perineal lichenification. (d) Example of ventral neck lichenification due to *Malassezia* dermatitis. Source: Courtesy of Patricia Bennett, DVM.

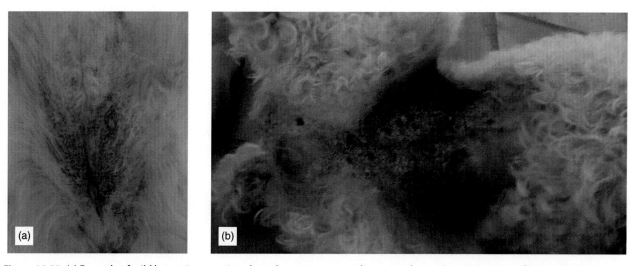

Figure 10.52 (a) Example of mild hyperpigmentation along the ventrum secondary to pyoderma. Source: Courtesy of Samantha Thurman, DVM. (b) Severe hyperpigmentation along the caudo-ventral abdomen. Source: Courtesy of Angie Mexas, DVM, DACVIM. (*Continued*)

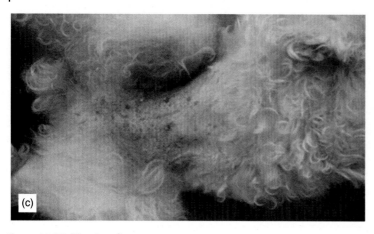
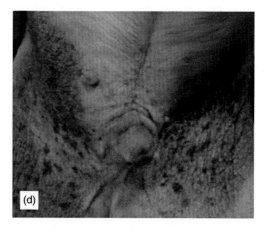

Figure 10.52 (*Continued*)
(c) Same patient as in (b) with lessening hyperpigmentation attributed to treatment for atopy. Source: Courtesy of Angie Mexas, DVM, DACVIM. (d) Concurrent hyperpigmentation and lichenification in the inguinal region of a male dog. Source: Courtesy of Elizabeth Robbins, DVM.

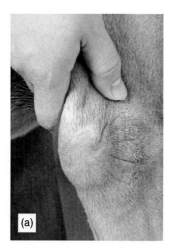
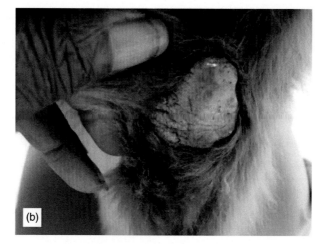

Figure 10.53 (a) Elbow callus in an otherwise healthy young adult Great Dane. This patient had bilateral elbow calluses. Only the right side is pictured here. Source: Courtesy of the Media Resources Department at Midwestern University. (b) More prominent elbow callus in an otherwise healthy adult dog. This patient also had bilateral elbow calluses. Only the right side is pictured here. Source: Courtesy of Patricia Bennett, DVM.

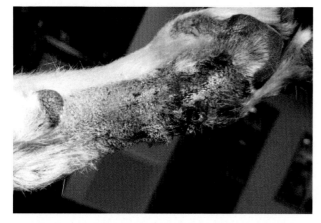
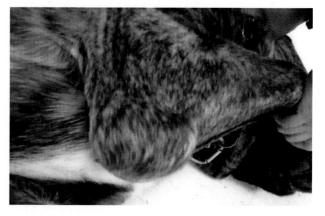

Figure 10.54 Palmar aspect of the distal right forelimb. Note the extensive pressure sore secondary to an improperly fitted splint. Source: Courtesy of Patricia Bennett, DVM.

Figure 10.55 Right-sided elbow hygroma. Source: Courtesy of Patricia Bennett, DVM.

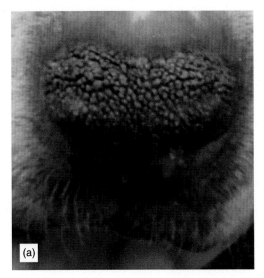

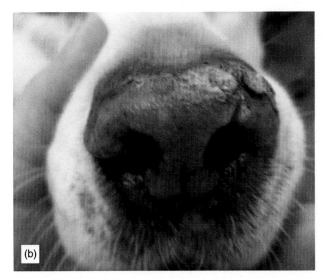

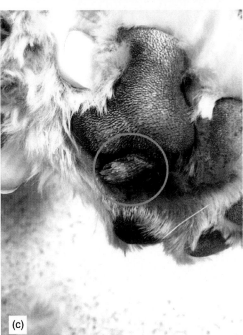

Figure 10.56 (a) Frond-like projections on the nose, (b) crusting of the dorsalmost nasal planum, and (c) frond-like projection on the footpad, all attributed to idiopathic nasodigital hyperkeratosis. Source (c): Courtesy of Kate Anderson, DVM.

free. Young, large to giant breed dogs are most at risk because they have yet to form a protective callus over the bony prominence. As a result of repeated trauma, such as the dog flopping onto the ground to lay down as part of its daily routine, the patient develops this pocket of fluid surrounded by a fibrous capsule. Surgical excision is difficult owing to the location. Medical management is more often pursued and aimed at eliminating elbow trauma from the patient's day-to-day experience, such as by improving padding of surfaces on which they lay [161, 162].

10.12 Hyperkeratosis

Hyperkeratosis refers to the thickening of the outermost layer of the epidermis, the stratum corneum, usually due to excessive keratin. For reasons that are not yet understood, nasodigital hyperkeratosis is common as canine patients age. This may result in overt crusting of the nasal planum and/or the development of frond-like projections on the nose (Figure 10.56a and b). When the footpads are affected, horny growths may develop (Figure 10.56c). These may become painful if their location is such that they exert constant pressure against adjacent footpads [163].

Note that these patients are otherwise clinically healthy, compared with patients who develop hyperkeratosis secondary to infectious disease such as canine distemper virus or autoimmune diseases such as pemphigus foliaceus [163].

Idiopathic nasodigital hyperkeratosis may also mirror hereditary nasal parakeratosis of Labrador Retrievers, a familial condition that is more typically associated with

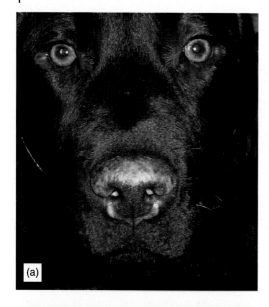

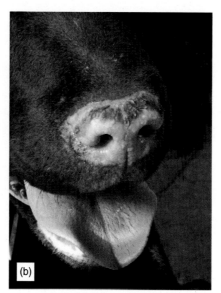

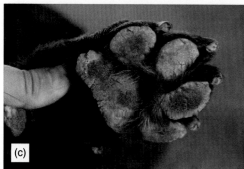

Figure 10.57 (a) Early depigmentation of the nose, attributed to hereditary nasal parakeratosis of Labrador retrievers. (b) Progressive nasal depigmentation with the accumulation of frond-like projections on dorsal rim of the nasal planum, attributed to hereditary nasal parakeratosis of Labrador Retrievers. (c) Hyperkeratosis of the foot pads, attributed to hereditary nasal parakeratosis of Labrador Retrievers. Source (a)–(c): Courtesy of Jackie Kucskar, DVM.

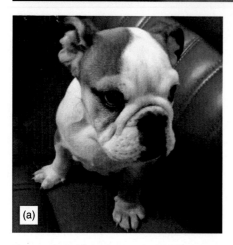

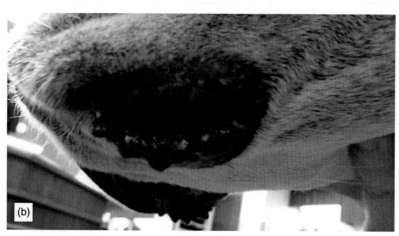

Figure 10.58 (a) Extensive nasal folds in an English Bulldog puppy. Source: Courtesy of Shirley Yang, DVM. (b) Cheilitis due to a moist erosive dermatitis associated with the lower lip fold. Source: Courtesy of Patricia Bennett, DVM.

the nasal planum, but may also involve the footpads (Figure 10.57). This condition is uncommon and is thought to be inherited through an autosomal recessive gene. Affected individuals develop hyperkeratotic lesions as early as 6 months of age. These lesions may worsen over time, plateau, or come and go. Spontaneous cures are rare; however, like idiopathic nasodigital hyperkeratosis, these patients are not in pain and are able to maintain a good quality of life [164].

10.13 Skin Folds

Certain breeds have integumentary systems with impressive surface areas due to prominent skin folds. These skin folds may be associated with the following [165]:

- the face, as in nasal or lip folds (Figure 10.58);
- the trunk and/or the legs, as demonstrated by Chinese Shar Peis and Basset Hounds;

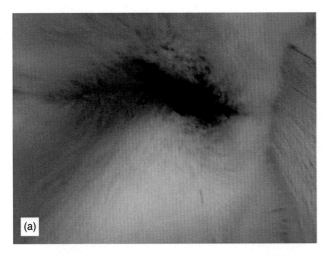
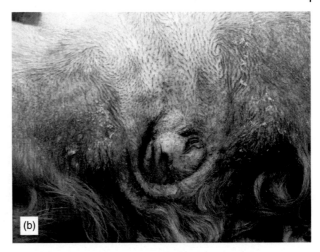

Figure 10.59 (a) This dog's vulva is so recessed that it is difficult even to visualize. All that can be seen is appreciable peri-vulvar discoloration. Source: Courtesy of Patricia Bennett, DVM. (b) Moderately recessed vulva with a prominent dorsal peri-vulvar skin fold. Source: Courtesy of Samantha Thurman, DVM.

- the vulva, as seen in obese females or in those with recessed vulvas (Figure 10.59);
- the base of the tail, as in brachycephalic breeds such as the English Bulldog.

These excessive skin folds increase the likelihood that the patient may develop a secondary bacterial skin infection. Excess moisture, as from the patient licking between the folds, creates an ideal environment for bacteria and/or yeast to flourish, and because these areas are not open to air dry, owner involvement to maintain good hygiene such as by using cleansing wipes may be necessary to guard proactively against infection [165].

10.14 Nails and Paw Pads

The head, neck, and torso are relatively easy to remember when evaluating the skin. Paws and claws, however, are often forgotten. It is important to examine both in order to evaluate for abrasions and other evidence of "wear and tear." Because the nails may be considered extensions of the skin, they should be included in every comprehensive physical examination. In particular, they should be evaluated in terms of their quality: are they worn evenly, broken, or overgrown? (Figure 10.60).

Figure 10.60 (a) Examining the nails. A cursory examination reveals that these nails appear to be evenly worn. Source: Courtesy of the Media Resources Department at Midwestern University. (b) These nails are also evenly worn. Source: Courtesy of the Media Resources Department at Midwestern University. (c) Note the fractured nail. These nails are not evenly worn. Source: Courtesy of the Media Resources Department at Midwestern University. (d) The nail associated with the third digit of the left hind paw has entirely broken off. Source: Courtesy of Patricia Bennett, DVM. (*Continued*)

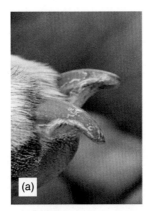
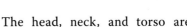
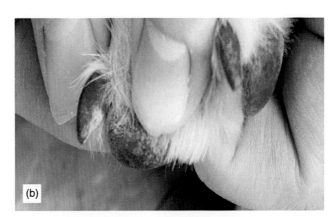
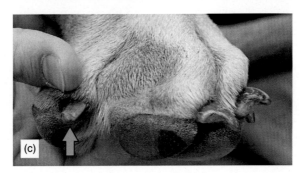
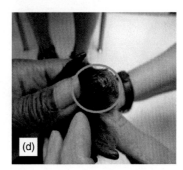

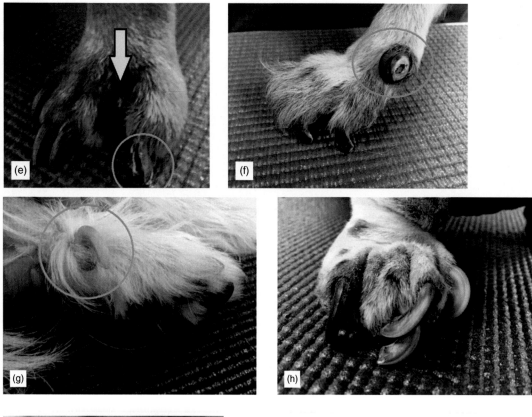

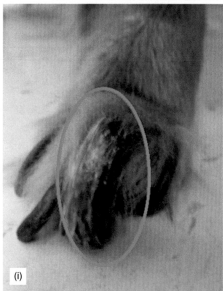

Figure 10.60 (*Continued*)
(e) Note the split nail encircled in blue as well as the apparently infected, moist interdigital space identified by the light blue arrow. Source: Courtesy of Patricia Bennett, DVM. (f) Note the exceptionally long dewclaw associated with the right forepaw. (g) This patient has a rear dewclaw associated with the left hind paw. Note how overgrown it is. (h) All of this patient's nails are overgrown. They are evenly, albeit poorly worn. (i) These nails are all overgrown. However, note the discrepancy in thickness between the nails. The nail that is circled in blue is exceptionally thick compared with the rest.

In addition to examining the nails, the interdigital spaces should be evaluated for lesions and for brown discoloration of the fur that might suggest excessive licking or over-grooming (Figure 10.61).

The clinician should also evaluate the paw pads. Normal "wear and tear" is to be expected, and the extent to which this is present may depend upon both the dog and the environment. However, there should not be cracks, fissures, or other erosions (Figure 10.62).

Lastly, concerning the integumentary system and the feet, the clinician should evaluate the skin between the digital and carpal or tarsal paw pads, noting any abnormalities (Figure 10.63).

10.15 Skin Incisions

If the patient has been operated on, the clinician should take care to evaluate the skin incision to assess patient progress with regard to healing (Figure 10.64). Palpable heat and

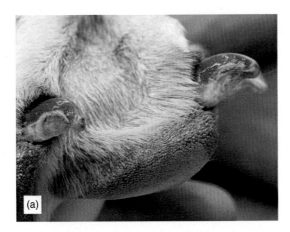

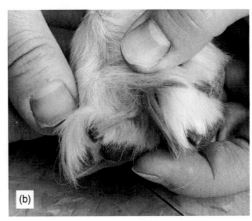

Figure 10.61 (a) The interdigital space depicted in this patient is normal. There are no excoriations, abrasions, or ulcerations. The skin is pink rather than red. The skin is dry as opposed to moist. (b) The interdigital fur is discolored brown. This patient has been licking excessively between the toes. This may be suggestive of underlying irritation, inflammation, or even infection. Source (a), (b): Courtesy of the Media Resources Department at Midwestern University.

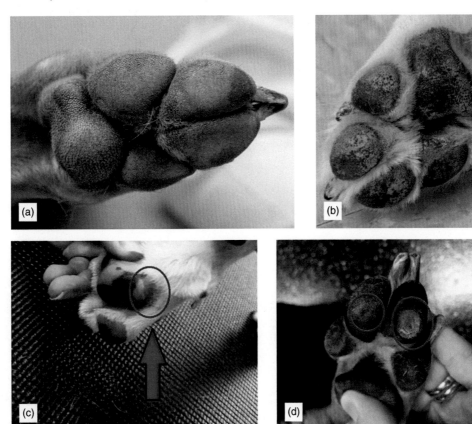

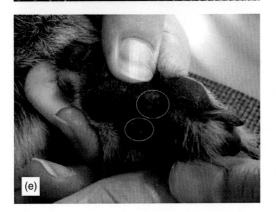

Figure 10.62 (a) Normal paw pads in a canine patient. Source: Courtesy of the Media Resources Department at Midwestern University. (b) An alternative example of normal paw pads in a canine patient. Note that some patients, such as this one, have a mottled appearance to the paw pads. This can be normal. Source: Courtesy of the Media Resources Department at Midwestern University (c) Note the abrasion at the medial aspect of the carpal pad. (d) Note the abrasions encircled in red at the digital pads along the plantar aspect of this hind paw. Source: Courtesy of Samantha Thurman, DVM. (e) Note how the surface of the paw pads has been eroded.

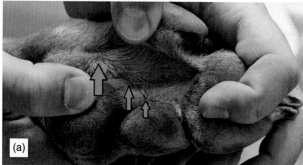

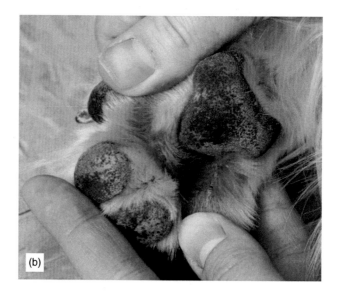

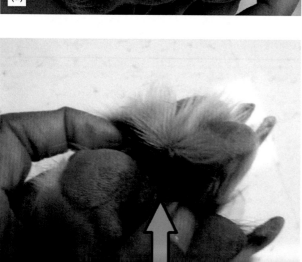

Figure 10.63 (a) Note the mild, focal areas of erythema. Source: Courtesy of the Media Resources Department at Midwestern University. (b) Note the brown discoloration of the fur that is due to excessive licking in this pruritic patient. Source: Courtesy of the Media Resources Department at Midwestern University. (c) Note the marked erythema. Source: Courtesy of Patricia Bennett, DVM.

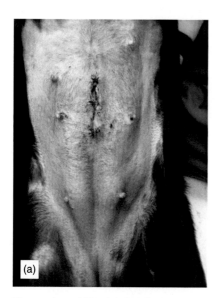

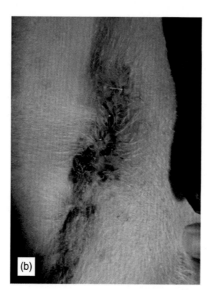

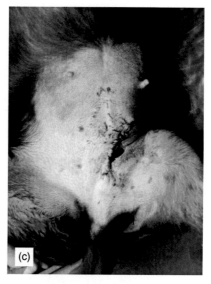

Figure 10.64 (a) Evaluating the surgery site following ovariohysterectomy. (b) Surgical dehiscence with yellow–green purulent discharge from the surgery site. Source: Courtesy of Patricia Bennett, DVM. (c) Another example of surgical dehiscence. Source: Courtesy of Andrew Weisenfeld, DVM.

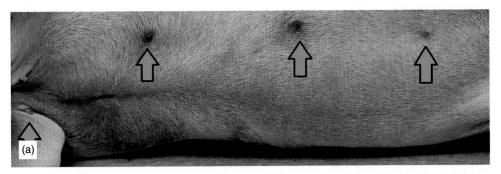
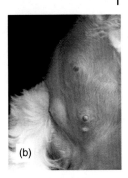

Figure 10.65 (a) View of the ventral mid-to-caudal abdomen demonstrating the position and spacing of four sets of mammary glands in a canine patient that has never experienced gestation. The cranial most set of glands is not captured in this photograph. Source: Courtesy of the Media Resources Department at Midwestern University. (b) View of the ventral mid-to-caudal abdomen demonstrating the prominence of the mammary chain in a pregnant bitch 7 days prior to whelping. Source: Courtesy of Nechama Bloom.

visible redness may be suggestive of inflammation, which is considered to be normal in the immediate post-operative period. The clinician should identify whether or not the redness persists and/or progresses, and note the development of any papulopustular rash that may be suggestive of a developing surgical site infection. The clinician should also evaluate the stability of the suture line: is there appropriate skin-to-skin apposition or is there surgical dehiscence? In the event of surgical dehiscence, any drainage should be noted in terms of amount, color, and consistency.

10.16 Mammary Glands

Dogs typically have five sets of mammary glands, so 10 glands in total. Glands will not be developed in males or in spayed females that have never had a litter (Figure 10.65). However, it is still important to palpate over each gland in both sexes because mammary masses do occur and can be aggressive.

It is also important to evaluate each nipple for peri-areolar dermatitis (see Figure 2.50). This can be a clinically important sign of autoimmune disease in dogs. Additionally, in the lactating bitch, the veterinarian should assess each mammary gland for asymmetry, swelling, redness, discharge, or heat on palpation. The presence of one or more of these findings may indicate mastitis. If the patient is tolerant, the clinician may also take care to express each gland to make sure that the patient is producing milk and to evaluate the milk's consistency [113, 166].

References

1 Weiss, E., Slater, M., and Lord, L. (2012) Frequency of lost dogs and cats in the United States and the methods used to locate them. *Animals*, **2** (2), 301–315.

2 Dingman, P.A., Levy, J.K., Rockey, L.E., and Crandall, M.M. (2014) Use of visual and permanent identification for pets by veterinary clinics. *Veterinary Journal*, **201** (1), 46–50.

3 Lord, L.K., Wittum, T.E., Ferketich, A.K. *et al.* (2007) Search and identification methods that owners use to find a lost dog. *Journal of the American Veterinary Medical Association*, **230** (2), 211–216.

4 Lord, L.K., Wittum, T.E., Ferketich, A.K. *et al.* (2007) Search methods that people use to find owners of lost pets. *Journal of the American Veterinary Medical Association*, **230** (12), 1835–1840.

5 Weiss, E., Slater, M.R., and Lord, L.K. (2011) Retention of provided identification for dogs and cats seen in veterinary clinics and adopted from shelters in Oklahoma City, OK, USA. *Preventive Veterinary Medicine*, **101** (3–4), 265–229.

6 Lord, L.K., Ingwersen, W., Gray, J.L., and Wintz, D.J. (2009) Characterization of animals with microchips entering animal shelters. *Journal of the American Veterinary Medical Association*, **235** (2), 160–167.

7 Veterinary Medicines Directorate (2014) VMD launches adverse events monitoring scheme for microchips. *Veterinary Record*, **174** (17), 419.

8 Laurence, C. (2010) Microchipping update. *Journal of Small Animal Practice*, **51** (3, Suppl.), 4–7.

9 Gyles, C. (2013) Checking for microchips. *Canadian Veterinary Journal/Revue Vétérinaire Canadienne*, **54** (2), 111–112.

10 Baldwin, K., Bartges, J., Buffington, T. *et al.* (2010) AAHA nutritional assessment guidelines for dogs and cats. *Journal of the American Animal Hospital Association*, **46** (4), 285–296.

11 White, G.A., Hobson-West, P., Cobb, K. *et al.* (2011) Canine obesity: is there a difference between veterinarian and owner perception? *Journal of Small Animal Practice*, **52** (12), 622–626.

12 Yam, P.S., Butowski, C.F., Chitty, J.L. *et al.* (2016) Impact of canine overweight and obesity on health-related quality of life. *Preventive Veterinary Medicine*, **127**, 64–69.

13 Courcier, E.A., Thomson, R.M., Mellor, D.J., and Yam, P.S. (2010) An epidemiological study of environmental factors associated with canine obesity. *Journal of Small Animal Practice*, **51** (7), 362–367.

14 Degeling, C., Burton, L., snd McCormack, G.R. (2012) An investigation of the association between socio-demographic factors, dog-exercise requirements, and the amount of walking dogs receive. *Canadian Journal of Veterinary Research/Revue Canadienne de Recherche Vétérinaire*, **76** (3), 235–240.

15 German, A.J. (2006) The growing problem of obesity in dogs and cats. *Journal of Nutrition*, **136** (7 Suppl.), 1940S–1946S.

16 Gossellin, J., Wren, J.A., and Sunderland, S.J. (2007) Canine obesity: an overview. *Journal of Veterinary Pharmacology and Therapeutics*, **30** (Suppl. 1), 1–10.

17 Laflamme, D.P. (2006) Understanding and managing obesity in dogs and cats. *Veterinary Clinics of North America: Small Animal Practice*, **36** (6), 1283–1295, vii.

18 Bland, I.M., Guthrie-Jones, A., Taylor, R.D., and Hill, J. (2009) Dog obesity: owner attitudes and behaviour. *Preventive Veterinary Medicine*, **92** (4), 333–340.

19 German, A.J. (2010) Obesity in companion animals. *Companion Animal Practice*, **32**, 42–50.

20 Shoveller, A.K., DiGennaro, J., Lanman, C., and Spangler, D. (2014) Trained vs untrained evaluator assessment of body condition score as a predictor of percent body fat in adult cats. *Journal of Feline Medicine and Surgery*, **16** (12), 957–965.

21 Michel, K. and Scherk, M. (2012) From problem to success: feline weight loss programs that work. *Journal of Feline Medicine and Surgery*, **14** (5), 327–336.

22 Lund, E., Armstrong, P.J., Kirk, C. *et al.* (2005) Prevalence and risk factors for obesity in adult cats from private US veterinary practices. *International Journal of Applied Research in Veterinary Medicine*, **3**, 88–96.

23 Sandoe, P., Palmer, C., Corr, S. *et al.* (2014) Canine and feline obesity: a One Health perspective. *Veterinary Record*, **175** (24), 610–616.

24 Day, M.J. (2010) One Health: the small animal dimension. *Veterinary Record*, **167** (22), 847–849.

25 Wynn, S.G., Witzel, A.L., Bartges, J.W. *et al.* (2016) Prevalence of asymptomatic urinary tract infections in morbidly obese dogs. *PeerJ*, **4**, e1711.

26 Nijland, M.L., Stam, F., and Seidell, J.C. (2010) Overweight in dogs, but not in cats, is related to overweight in their owners. *Public Health Nutrition*, **13** (1), 102–106.

27 Lund, E.M., Armstrong, P.J., Kirk, C.A., and Klausner, J.S. (2006) Prevalence and risk factors for obesity in adult dogs from private U.S. veterinary practices. *International Journal of Applied Research in Veterinary Medicine*, 4, 177–186.

28 Markwell, P.J., Vanerk, W., Parkin, G.D. *et al.* Obesity in the dog. *Journal of Small Animal Practice*, **31** (10), 533–537.

29 Weeth, L.P., Fascetti, A.J., Kass, P.H. *et al.* Prevalence of obese dogs in a population of dogs with cancer. *American Journal of Veterinary Research*, **68** (4), 389–398.

30 Kealy, R.D., Lawler, D.F., Ballam, J.M. *et al.* (2002) Effects of diet restriction on life span and age-related changes in dogs. *Journal of the American Veterinary Medical Association*, **220**, 1315–1320.

31 Mattheeuws, D., Rottiers, R., Kaneko, J.J., and Vermeulen, A. (1984) Diabetes mellitus in dogs: relationship of obesity to glucose tolerance and insulin response. *American Journal of Veterinary Research*, **45** (1), 98–103.

32 Thengchaisri, N., Theerapun, W., Kaewmokul, S., and Sastravaha, A. (2014) Abdominal obesity is associated with heart disease in dogs. *BMC Veterinary Research*, **10**, 131.

33 Lawler, D.F., Larson, B.T., Ballam, J.M. *et al.* (2008) Diet restriction and ageing in the dog: major observations over two decades. *British Journal of Nutrition*, **99** (4), 793–805.

34 Wei, E.K., Giovannucci, E., Wu, K. *et al.* (2004) Comparison of risk factors for colon and rectal cancer. *International Journal of Cancer*, **108** (3), 433–442.

35 van den Brandt, P.A., Spiegelman, D., Yaun, S.S. *et al.* (2000) Pooled analysis of prospective cohort studies on height, weight, and breast cancer risk. *American Journal of Epidemiology*, **152** (6), 514–527.

36 Crew, K.D. and Neugut, A.I. (2004) Epidemiology of upper gastrointestinal malignancies. *Seminars in Oncology*, **31** (4), 450–464.

37 Forman, D. (2004) Review article: oesophago-gastric adenocarcinoma – an epidemiological perspective. *Alimentary Pharmacology & Therapeutics*, **20** (Suppl. 5), 55–60; discussion, 1–2.

38 Wang, X.J., Yuan, S.L., Lu, Q. *et al.* (2004) Potential involvement of leptin in carcinogenesis of hepatocellular carcinoma. *World Journal of Gastroenterology*, **10** (17), 2478–2481.

39 Laflamme, D.P. (2001) Challenges with weight-reduction studies. *Compendium: Continuing Education for the Practicing Veterinarian*, **23**, 45–50.

40 Robertson, I.D. (2003) The association of exercise, diet and other factors with owner-perceived obesity in privately owned dogs from metropolitan Perth, WA. *Preventive Veterinary Medicine*, **58** (1–2), 75–83.

41 Anderson, R.S. (1973) Obesity in the dog and cat. *Veterinary Annual*, **1441**, 182–186.

42 Crane, S.W. (1991) Occurrence and management of obesity in companion animals. *Journal of Small Animal Practice*, **32** (6), 275–282.

43 Sloth, C. (1992) Practical management of obesity in dogs and cats. *Journal of Small Animal Practice*, **33** (4), 178–182.

44 Wolfsheimer, K.J. (1994) Obesity in dogs. *Compendium: Continuing Education for the Practicing Veterinarian*, **16** (8), 981.

45 Colliard, L., Ancel, J., Benet, J.J. *et al.* (2006) Risk factors for obesity in dogs in France. *Journal of Nutrition*, **136** (7), 1951s–1954s.

46 McGreevy, P.D., Thomson, P.C., Pride, C. *et al.* (2005) Prevalence of obesity in dogs examined by Australian veterinary practices and the risk factors involved. *Veterinary Record*, **156** (22), 695.

47 Holmes, K.L., Morris, P.J., Abdulla, Z. *et al.* (2007) Risk factors associated with excess body weight in dogs in the U.K. *Journal of Animal Physiology and Animal Nutrition*, **91**, 166–167.

48 Scarlett, J.M., Donoghue, S., Saidla, J., and Wills, J. (1994) Overweight cats: prevalence and risk factors. *International Journal of Obesity and Related Metabolic Disorders*, **18** (Suppl. 1), S22–S28.

49 Courcier, E.A., Mellor, D.J., Thomson, R.M., and Yam, P.S. (2011) A cross sectional study of the prevalence and risk factors for owner misperception of canine body shape in first opinion practice in Glasgow. *Preventive Veterinary Medicine*, **102** (1), 66–74.

50 Freeman, L.M. (2012) Cachexia and sarcopenia: emerging syndromes of importance in dogs and cats. *Journal of Veterinary Internal Medicine*, **26** (1), 3–17.

51 Mallery, K.F., Freeman, L.M., Harpster, N.K., and Rush, J.E. (1999) Factors contributing to the decision for euthanasia of dogs with congestive heart failure. *Journal of the American Veterinary Medical Association*, **214** (8), 1201.

52 Freeman, L., Becvarova, I., Cave, N. *et al.* (2011) WSAVA nutritional assessment guidelines. *Compendium: Continuing Education for the Practicing Veterinarian*, **33** (8), E1–E9.

53 German, A.J., Holden, S.L., Morris, P.J., and Biourge, V. (2010) Comparison of a bioimpedance monitor with dual-energy X-ray absorptiometry for noninvasive estimation of percentage body fat in dogs. *American Journal of Veterinary Research*, **71** (4), 393–398.

54 Lauten, S.D., Cox, N.R., Brawner, W.R., Jr., and Baker, H.J. (2001) Use of dual energy X-ray absorptiometry for noninvasive body composition measurements in clinically normal dogs. *American Journal of Veterinary Research.*, **62** (8), 1295–1301.

55 Witzel, A.L., Kirk, C.A., Henry, G.A. *et al.* (2014) Use of a novel morphometric method and body fat index system for estimation of body composition in overweight and obese dogs. *Journal of the American Veterinary Medical Association*, **244** (11), 1279–1284.

56 Jeusette, I., Greco, D., Aquino, F. *et al.* (2010) Effect of breed on body composition and comparison between various methods to estimate body composition in dogs. *Research in Veterinary Science*, **88** (2), 227–232.

57 Mawby, D.I., Bartges, J.W., d'Avignon, A. *et al.* (2004) Comparison of various methods for estimating body fat in dogs. *Journal of the American Animal Hospital Association*, **40** (2), 109–114.

58 Laflamme, D. (1997) Development and validation of a body condition score system for dogs. *Canine Practice*, **22** (4), 10–15.

59 Toll, P.W., Yamka, R.M., Schoenherr, W.D. *et al.* (2010) Obesity, in *Small Animal Clinical Nutrition* (eds. M. S. Hand, C.D.Thatcher, R.L.Remillard *et al.*), Mark Morris Institute, Topeka, KS, pp. 501–542.

60 Gant, P., Holden, S.L., Biourge, V., and German, A.J. (2016) Can you estimate body composition in dogs from photographs? *BMC Veterinary Research*, **12**, 18.

61 Burkholder, W.J. (2000) Use of body condition scores in clinical assessment of the provision of optimal nutrition. *Journal of the American Veterinary Medical Association*, **217** (5), 650–654.

62 DiBartola, S.P. and Bateman, S. (2006) Introduction to fluid therapy, in *Fluid, Electrolyte, and Acid–Base Disorders in Small Animal Practice*, 3rd edn. (ed. S.P. DiBartola), Saunders Elsevier, St. Louis, pp. 325–344.

63 Raghavan, M., Martens, P.J., Chateau, D., and Burchill, C. (2013) Effectiveness of breed-specific legislation in decreasing the incidence of dog-bite injury hospitalisations in people in the Canadian province of Manitoba. *Injury Prevention*, **19** (3), 177–183.

64 Ledger, R.A., Orihel, J.S., Clarke, N. *et al.* (2005) Breed specific legislation: considerations for evaluating its effectiveness and recommandations for alternatives. *Canadian Veterinary Journal/Revue Vétérinaire Canadienne*, **46** (8), 735–743.

65 Beaver, B.V., Baker, M.D., Gloster, R.C. *et al.* (2001) A community approach to dog bite prevention. *Journal of the American Veterinary Medical Association*, **218** (11), 1732–1749.

66 Burstein, D. (2004) Breed specific legislation: unfair prejudice and ineffective policy. *Animal Law*, **10**, 313–361.

67 Overall, K.L. and Love, M. (2001) Dog bites to humans – demography, epidemiology, injury, and risk. *Journal of the American Veterinary Medical Association*, **218** (12), 1923–1934.

68 Hess, G. (1996) Pro canine breed-specific legislation. *Canadian Veterinary Journal/Revue Vétérinaire Canadienne*, **37** (12), 712.

69 Shuler, C.M., DeBess, E.E., Lapidus, J.A., and Hedberg, K. (2008) Canine and human factors related to dog bite injuries. *Journal of the American Veterinary Medical Association*, **232** (4), 542–546.

70 Bini, J.K., Cohn, S.M., Acosta, S.M. *et al.* (2011) Mortality, mauling, and maiming by vicious dogs. *Annals of Surgery*, **253** (4), 791–797.

71 Voelker, R. (1997) Dog bites recognized as public health problem. *JAMA*, **277** (4), 278, 280.

72 Weiss, H.B., Friedman, D.I., and Coben, J.H. (1998) Incidence of dog bite injuries treated in emergency departments. *JAMA*, **279** (1), 51–53.

73 Gilchrist, J., Sacks, J.J., White, D., and Kresnow, M.J. (2008) Dog bites: still a problem? *Injury Prevention*, **14** (5), 296–301.

74 Presutti, R.J. (2001) Prevention and treatment of dog bites. *American Family Physician*, **63** (8), 1567–1572.

75 Ozanne-Smith, J., Ashby, K., and Stathakis, V.Z. (2001) Dog bite and injury prevention – analysis, critical review, and research agenda. *Injury Prevention*, **7** (4), 321–326.

76 Rosado, B., Garcia-Belenguer, S., Leon, M., and Palacio, J. (2007) Spanish dangerous animals act: effect on the epidemiology of dog bites. *Journal of Veterinary Behavior*, **2** (5), 166–174.

77 Cornelissen, J.M.R. and Hopster, H. (2010) Dog bites in The Netherlands: a study of victims, injuries, circumstances and aggressors to support evaluation of breed specific legislation. *Veterinary Journal*, **186** (3), 292–298.

78 Klaassen, B., Buckley, J.R., and Esmail, A. (1996) Does the dangerous dogs act protect against animal attacks: a prospective study of mammalian bites in the accident and emergency department. *Injury*, **27** (2), 89–91.

79 De Keuster, T., Lamoureux, J., and Kahn, A. (2006) Epidemiology of dog bites: a Belgian experience of canine behaviour and public health concerns. *Veterinary Journal*, **172** (3), 482–487.

80 Hoffman, C.L., Harrison, N., Wolff, L., and Westgarth, C. (2014) Is that dog a pit bull? A cross-country comparison of perceptions of shelter workers regarding breed identification. *Journal of Applied Animal Welfare Science*, **17** (4), 322–339.

81 Stavisky, J., Brennan, M.L., Downes, M., and Dean, R. (2010) Demographics and economic burden of un-owned cats and dogs in the UK: results of a 2010 census. *BMC Veterinary Research*, **8** (1), 163.

82 American Society for the Prevention of Cruelty to Animals (2016) *Pet Statistics*, http://www.aspca.org/animal-homelessness/shelter-intake-and-surrender/pet-statistics (accessed 10 January 2017).

83 Gunter, L.M., Barber, R.T., and Wynne, C.D. (2016) What's in a name? Effect of breed perceptions and labeling on attractiveness, adoptions and length of stay for pit-bull-type dogs. *PLoS One*, **11** (3), e0146857.

84 Clevenger, J. and Kass, P.H. (2003) Determinants of adoption and euthanasia of shelter dogs spayed or neutered in the University of California Veterinary Student Surgery Program compared to other shelter dogs. *Journal of Veterinary Medical Education*, **30** (4), 372–378.

85 Lepper, M., Kass, P.H., and Hart, L.A. (2002) Prediction of adoption versus euthanasia among dogs and cats in a California animal shelter. *Journal of Applied Animal Welfare Science*, **5** (1), 29–42.

86 Lord, L.K., Wittum, T.E., Ferketich, A.K. *et al.* (2006) Demographic trends for animal care and control agencies in Ohio from 1996 to 2004. *Journal of the American Veterinary Medical Association*, **229** (1), 48–54.

87 Scott, J.P. and Fuller, J.L. (1965) *Genetics and the Social Behavior of the Dog*, University of Chicago Press, Chicago.

88 Goto, N., Imamura, K., Miura, Y. *et al.* (1987) The Mexican hairless dog, its morphology and inheritance. *Jikken Dobutsu/Experimental Animals*, **36** (1), 87–90.

89 Kimura, T., Ohshima, S., and Doi, K. (1993) The inheritance and breeding results of hairless descendants of Mexican hairless dogs. *Laboratory Animals*, **27** (1), 55–58.

90 Kimura, T., Kuroki, K., and Doi, K. (1998) Dermatotoxicity of agricultural chemicals in the dorsal skin of hairless dogs. *Toxicologic Pathology*, **26** (3), 442–447.

91 Kimura, T. and Doi, K. (1994) Responses of the skin over the dorsum to sunlight in hairless descendants of Mexican hairless dogs. *American Journal of Veterinary Research*, **55** (2), 199–203.

92 Kimura, T. and Doi, K. (1995) Dorsal skin reactions to sunlight and artificial ultraviolet light in hairless descendants of Mexican hairless dogs. *Experimental Animals*, **45**, 293–299.

93 Kimura, T. and Doi, K. (1996) Spontaneous comedones on the skin of hairless descendants of Mexican hairless dogs. *Experimental Animals*, **45** (4), 377–384.

94 Wiener, D., Gurtner, C., Panakova, L. *et al.* (2013) Clinical and histological characterization of hair coat and glandular tissue of Chinese crested dogs. *Veterinary Dermatology*, **24**, 274-e62.

95 Robinson, R. (1985) Chinese crested dog. *Journal of Heredity*, 76, 217–218.

96 Wikipedia (2016) *Coat (Dog)*, https://en.wikipedia.org/wiki/Coat_(dog) (accessed 10 January 2017).

97 Stokking, L.B. and Campbell, K.C. (2004) Disorders of pigmentation, in *Small Animal Dermatology Secrets* (ed. K.C. Campbell), Hanley & Belfus, Philadelphia, pp. 352–355.

98 Cat Fanciers Association (2016) *Cat Colors FAQ: Cat Color Genetics*, http://www.fanciers.com/other-faqs/color-genetics.html (accessed 12 April 2016).

99 Cvejic, D., Steinberg, T.A., Kent, M.S., and Fischer, A. (2009) Unilateral and bilateral congenital sensorineural deafness in client-owned pure-breed white cats. *Journal of Veterinary Internal Medicine*, **23** (2), 392–395.

100 Strain, G.M. (1999) Congenital deafness and its recognition. *Veterinary Clinics of North America: Small Animal Practice*, **29** (4), 895–907, vi.

101 Luttgen, P.J. (1994) Deafness in the dog and cat. *Veterinary Clinics of North America: Small Animal Practice*, **24** (5), 981–989.

102 Strain, G.M. (2007) Deafness in blue-eyed white cats: the uphill road to solving polygenic disorders. *Veterinary Journal*, **173** (3), 471–472.

103 Geigy, C.A., Heid, S., and Steffen, F. *et al.* (2007) Does a pleiotropic gene explain deafness and blue irises in white cats? *Veterinary Journal*, **173** (3), 548–553.

104 Bergsma, D.R. and Brown, K.S. (1971) White fur, blue eyes, and deafness in the domestic cat. *Journal of Heredity*, **62** (3), 171–185.

105 Strain, G.M. (2012) Canine deafness. *Veterinary Clinics of North America: Small Animal Practice*, **42** (6), 1209–1224.

106 Strain, G.M., Kearney, M.T., Gignac, I.J. *et al.* (1992) Brainstem auditory evoked potential assessment of

congenital deafness in Dalmatians: associations with phenotypic markers. *Journal of Veterinary Internal Medicine*, **6**, 175–182.

107 Strain, G.M. (2004) Deafness prevalence and pigmentation and gender associations in dog breeds at risk. *Veterinary Journal*, **167**, 23–32.

108 Platt, S., Freeman, J., di Stefani, A. *et al.* (2006) Prevalence of unilateral and bilateral deafness in Border Collies and association with phenotype. *Journal of Veterinary Internal Medicine*, **20** (6), 1355–1362.

109 Strain, G.M., Clark, L.A., Wahl, J.M. *et al.* (2009) Prevalence of deafness in dogs heterozygous or homozygous for the merle allele. *Journal of Veterinary Internal Medicine*, **23** (2), 282–286.

110 Sommerlad, S., McRae, A.F., McDonald, B. *et al.* (2010) Congenital sensorineural deafness in Australian stumpy-tail cattle dogs is an autosomal recessive trait that maps to CFA10. *PLoS One*, **5** (10), e13364.

111 De Risio, L., Lewis, T., Freeman, J. *et al.* (2011) Prevalence, heritability and genetic correlations of congenital sensorineural deafness and pigmentation phenotypes in the Border Collie. *Veterinary Journal*, **188** (3), 286–290.

112 Comito, B., Knowles, K.E., and Strain, G.M. (2012) Congenital deafness in Jack Russell terriers: prevalence and association with phenotype. *Veterinary Journal*, **193** (2), 404–407.

113 Rijnberk, A. and vanSluijs, F.S. (eds.) (2009) *Medical History and Physical Examination in Companion Animals*, 2nd edn., Saunders Elsevier, St. Louis.

114 Bach, J.P., Lupke, M., and Wefstaedt, P. (2013) Deafness in the dog and cat: aetiology, diagnostics and treatment. *Tierarztliche Praxis, Ausgabe K, Kleintiere/ Heimtiere*, 41 (6), 421–427; quiz, 8 (in German).

115 Sims, M.H. (1988) Electrodiagnostic evaluation of auditory function. *Veterinary Clinics of North America: Small Animal Practice*, **18** (4), 913–944.

116 Dijkshoorn, N.A. and van der Wel, T. (1997) Screening for deafness in companion animals. *Tijdschrift voor Diergeneeskunde*, **122** (6), 168–169 (in Dutch).

117 Cook, L.B. (2004) Neurologic evaluation of the ear. *Veterinary Clinics of North America: Small Animal Practice*, **34** (2), 425–435, vi.

118 American Chesapeake Club (2014) *Color in the Chesapeake Bay Retriever*, http://www.amchessieclub.org/standard/discussion.html (accessed 10 January 2017).

119 Hédan, B., Corre, S., Hitte, C. *et al.* (2006) Coat colour in dogs: identification of the *Merle* locus in the Australian shepherd breed. *BMC Veterinary Research*, **2**, 9.

120 Bauer, B.S., Sandmeyer, L.S., and Grahn, B.H. (2015) Diagnostic ophthalmology. Microphthalmos and multiple ocular anomalies (MOA) OU consistent with merle ocular dysgenesis (MOD). *Canadian Veterinary Journal/Revue Vétérinaire Canadienne*, **56** (7), 767–768.

121 Gelatt, K.N., Powell, N.G., and Huston, K. (1981) Inheritance of microphthalmia with coloboma in the Australian shepherd dog. *American Journal of Veterinary Research*, **42** (10), 1686–1690.

122 Dausch, D., Wegner, W., Michaelis, W., and Reetz, I. (1978) Eye changes in the merle syndrome in the dog. *Albrecht von Graefes Archiv für klinische und experimentelle Ophthalmologie*, **206** (2), 135–150 (in German).

123 Wikipedia (2016) *Merle (Dog Coat)*, https://en.wikipedia.org/wiki/Merle_(dog_coat) (accessed 6 June 2016).

124 Sponenberg, D.P. (1985) Inheritance of the harlequin color in Great Dane dogs. *Journal of Heredity*, **76** (3), 224–225.

125 Wikipedia (2016) *Brindle*, https://en.wikipedia.org/wiki/Brindle (accessed 6 June 2016).

126 Kerns, J.A., Cargill, E.J., Clark, L.A. *et al.* (2007) Linkage and segregation analysis of black and brindle coat color in domestic dogs. *Genetics*, **176** (3), 1679–1689.

127 Wikipedia (2016) *Brindlequin*, https://en.wikipedia.org/wiki/Brindlequin (accessed 6 June 2016).

128 Medleau, L. and Hnilica, K A. (2006) Color dilution alopecia (color mutant alopecia), in *Small Animal Dermatology: A Color Atlas and Therapeutic Guide*, 2nd edn. (eds. L. Medleau and K.A. Hnilica), Saunders Elsevier, St. Louis, pp. 253–254.

129 Kim, J.H., Kang, K.I., Sohn, H.J. *et al.* (2005) Color-dilution alopecia in dogs. *Journal of Veterinary Science*, **6** (3), 259–261.

130 Perego, R., Proverbio, D., Roccabianca, P., and Spada, E. (2009) Color dilution alopecia in a blue Doberman pinscher crossbreed. *Canadian Veterinary Journal/Revue Vétérinaire Canadienne*, **50** (5), 511–514.

131 Munday, J.S., French, A.F., and McKerchar, G.R. (2009) Black-hair follicular dysplasia in a New Zealand Huntaway dog. *New Zealand Veterinary Journal*, **57** (3), 170–172.

132 von Bomhard, W., Mauldin, E.A., Schmutz, S.M. *et al.* (2006) Black hair follicular dysplasia in Large Munsterlander dogs: clinical, histological and ultrastructural features. *Veterinary Dermatology*, **17** (3), 182–188.

133 Knottenbelt, C.M. and Knottenbelt, M.K. (1996) Black hair follicular dysplasia in a tricolour Jack Russell terrier. *Veterinary Record*, **138** (19), 475–476.

134 Medleau, L. and Hnilica, K.A. (2006) *Canine pattern baldness, in Small Animal Dermatology: A Color Atlas and Therapeutic Guide*, 2nd edn. (eds. L. Medleau and K.A. Hnilica), Saunders Elsevier, St. Louis, p. 256.

135 Medleau, L. and Hnilica, K.A. (2006) Idiopathic bald thigh syndrome of greyhounds, in *Small Animal Dermatology: A Color Atlas and Therapeutic Guide*, 2nd edn. (eds. L. Medleau and K.A. Hnilica), Saunders Elsevier, St. Louis, p. 257.

136 Pin, D., Carlotti, D.N., Jasmin, P. *et al.* (2006) Prospective study of bacterial overgrowth syndrome in eight dogs. *Veterinary Record*, **158** (13), 437–441.

137 Outerbridge, C.A. (2006) Mycologic disorders of the skin. *Clinical Techniques in Small Animal Practice*, **21** (3), 128–134.

138 Mueller, R.S. (2012) An update on the therapy of canine demodicosis. *Compendium: Continuing Education for the Practicing Veterinarian*, **34** (4), E1–E4.

139 Zur, G. and White, S.D. (2011) Hyperadrenocorticism in 10 dogs with skin lesions as the only presenting clinical signs. *Journal of the American Animal Hospital Association*, 47 (6), 419–427.

140 Frank, L.A. (2006) Comparative dermatology – canine endocrine dermatoses. *Clinics in Dermatology*, **24** (4), 317–325.

141 Chastain, C.B. and Swayne, D.E. (1985) Congenital hypotrichosis in male Basset Hound littermates. *Journal of the American Veterinary Medical Association*, **187** (8), 845–846.

142 Wilcock, B.P. and Yager, J.A. (1986) Focal cutaneous vasculitis and alopecia at sites of rabies vaccination in dogs. *Journal of the American Veterinary Medical Association*, **188** (10), 1174–1177.

143 Bensignor, E. (1999) What is your diagnosis? Post-rabies-vaccination alopecia. *Journal of Small Animal Practice*, **40** (4), 151, 189.

144 Virga, V. (2003) Behavioral dermatology. *Veterinary Clinics of North America: Small Animal Practice*, **33** (2), 231–251, v–vi.

145 Woods-Kettelberger, A., Kongsamut, S., Smith, C.P. *et al.* (1997) Animal models with potential applications for screening compounds for the treatment of obsessive–compulsive disorder. *Expert Opinion on Investigational Drugs*, **6** (10), 1369–1381.

146 Medleau, L. and Hnilica, K.A. (2006) Acral lick dermatitis (lick granuloma, acral pruritic nodule), in *Small Animal Dermatology: A Color Atlas and Therapeutic Guide*, 2nd edn. (eds. L. Medleau and K.A. Hnilica), Saunders Elsevier, St. Louis, pp. 328–330.

147 Medleau, L. and Hnilica, K.A. (2006) Nasal depigmentation, in *Small Animal Dermatology: A Color Atlas and Therapeutic Guide*, 2nd edn. (eds. L. Medleau and K.A. Hnilica), Saunders Elsevier, St. Louis, p. 290.

148 Medleau, L. and Hnilica, K.A. (eds.) (2006) *Small Animal Dermatology: A Color Atlas and Therapeutic Guide*, 2nd edn., Saunders Elsevier, St. Louis.

149 Lobetti, R.G. and Dippenaar, T. (2000) Von Willebrand's disease in the German shepherd dog. *Journal of the South African Veterinary Association*, **71** (2), 118–121.

150 Stokol, T., Parry, B.W., and Mansell, P.D. (1995) Von Willebrand's disease in Scottish Terriers in Australia. *Australian Veterinary Journal*, **72** (11), 404–407.

151 Parry, B.W., Howard, M.A., Mansell, P.D., and Holloway, S.A. (1988) Haemophilia A in German shepherd dogs. *Australian Veterinary Journal*, **65** (9), 276–279.

152 Blundell, R. and Adam, F. (2013) Haemolytic anaemia and acute pancreatitis associated with zinc toxicosis in a dog. *Veterinary Record*, **172** (1), 17.

153 Piek, C.J. (2011) Canine idiopathic immune-mediated haemolytic anaemia: a review with recommendations for future research. *Veterinary Quarterly*, **31** (3), 129–141.

154 Mills, J.N., Day, M.J., Shaw, S.E., and Penhale, W.J. (1985) Autoimmune haemolytic anaemia in dogs. *Australian Veterinary Journal*, **62** (4), 121–123.

155 Rissi, D.R. and Brown, C.A. (2014) Diagnostic features in 10 naturally occurring cases of acute fatal canine leptospirosis. *Journal of Veterinary Diagnostic Investigation*, **26** (6), 799–804.

156 Wouters, A.T., Casagrande, R.A., Wouters, F. *et al.* (2013) An outbreak of aflatoxin poisoning in dogs associated with aflatoxin B1-contaminated maize products. *Journal of Veterinary Diagnostic Investigation*, **25** (2), 282–287.

157 Smalle, T.M., Cahalane, A.K., and Koster, L.S. (2015) Gallbladder mucocoele: a review. *Journal of the South African Veterinary Association*, **86** (1), 1318.

158 Kirpensteijn, J., Fingland, R.B., Ulrich, T. *et al.* (1993) Cholelithiasis in dogs: 29 cases (1980–1990). *Journal of the American Veterinary Medical Association*, **202** (7), 1137–1142.

159 Miller, W.H., Griffin, C.E., Campbell, K.L. *et al.* (2013) *Muller & Kirk's Small Animal Dermatology*, 7th edn. Saunders Elsevier, St. Louis.

160 Wasson, J., Amonoo-Kuofi, K., Scrivens, J., and Pfleiderer, A. (2012) Caliper measurement to improve clinical assessment of palpable neck lumps. *Annals of the Royal College of Surgeons of England*, **94** (4), 256–260.

161 Fossum, T.W., Duprey, L.P., and O'Connor, D. (2007) Surgery of the integumentary system, in *Small Animal Surgery*, 3rd edn. (eds. T.W. Fossum, L.P. Duprey, and D.O'Connor), Elsevier, Boston, pp. 159–259.

162 Johnston, D.E. (1975) Hygroma of the elbow in dogs. *Journal of the American Veterinary Medical Association*, **167** (3), 213–219.

163 Medleau, L. and Hnilica, K.A. (2006) Idiopathic nasodigital hyperkeratosis, in *Small Animal Dermatology: A Color Atlas and Therapeutic Guide*, 2nd edn. (eds. L. Medleau and K.A. Hnilica), Saunders Elsevier, St. Louis, pp. 316–318.

164 Medleau, L. and Hnilica, K.A. (2006) Hereditary nasal parakeratosis of Labrador retrievers, in *Small Animal Dermatology: A Color Atlas and Therapeutic Guide*, 2nd edn. (eds. L. Medleau and K.A. Hnilica), Saunders Elsevier, St. Louis, p. 319.

165 Medleau, L. and Hnilica, K.A. (2006) Skin fold dermatitis, in *Small Animal Dermatology: A Color Atlas and Therapeutic Guide*, 2nd edn. (eds. L. Medleau and K.A. Hnilica), Saunders Elsevier, St. Louis, pp. 26–28.

166 Johnston, S.D. and Hayden, D.W. (1980) Non-neoplastic disorders of the mammary glands, in *Current Veterinary Therapy*, vol. VII (ed. R.W. Kirk), Saunders, Philadelphia, pp. 1224–1226.

11

Examining the Head of the Dog

11.1 Skull Shape: Function Versus Cosmesis

Anatomically, the skull is both the scaffold upon which the face is built and the protector of the central nervous system. Despite the universality of these roles, skull shapes vary immensely between species and breeds [1, 2].

In nature, structure evolved to maximize efficiency: skull shape was primarily functional. For example, the common ancestor of the domestic dog, the gray wolf (*Canis lupus*) [3, 4], developed and retained a dolichocephalic skull shape to support predation. There is a confirmed relationship between the size of the skull, the size of the eyes, and the visual field [3]. The long and narrow head of the gray wolf, in addition to its long and narrow muzzle, is positively correlated with eyes of increased diameter and also increased total number of retinal ganglion cells [3, 5]. Furthermore, nose length is a determinant of retinal ganglion topography: where retinal cells concentrate is largely dependent upon skull shape [3]. The dolichocephalic skull as seen in the wolf has been linked to a horizontally aligned visual streak of retinal ganglion cells as opposed to a strongly concentrated area centralis in brachycephalic breeds [3]. This visual streak in the gray wolf, combined with orbits that are seated less forward facing [4], confers the ability to scan the periphery, a predatory advantage that facilitates the pursuit of prey [1]. Without an area centralis, the wolf is less adept at seeing directly in front of its face; however, what is lost in terms of central visual acuity is gained in peripheral sight such that the wolf is a tremendously skilled hunter [1, 6].

Based on archeological records, the domestication of the dog took place between 15,000 and 36,000 years ago [4, 7]. These progenitors of the modern-day dog were adopted by the human race to fulfill a niche that was purely functional: to be their master's hunters, herders, or protectors [1, 4, 8, 9]. For example, two dolichocephalic breeds, the Afghans and Salukis, were selectively bred for the purpose of hunting small prey. Their craniofacial configuration enhanced their abilities as hunters, much like it did for their ancestor, the gray wolf, by improving their peripheral vision [3, 4, 10]. They could more easily scan the horizon for prey [3, 4, 10].

Likewise, other favorable traits were selected for that promoted the function for which the dog was acquired. For example, breeding became selective to reproduce pointers that point and setters that set [9]. Because hunting behaviors are heritable [11–13], selective breeding for function effectively established lineages that met the needs of those who owned them.

As domestication progressed, other structural and anatomic changes took root. The dog underwent encephalization: like other domesticated species, its brain-to-body size ratio increased [4]. Yet portions of the brain that had been committed to fight-or-flight, such as the limbic system, which was essential for survival in wolves, were markedly reduced in the dog [14–16]. Compared with the wolf, the modern day dog's brain is decreased in size by roughly 30% [14, 16]. As brain morphology changed, it is likely that changes in skull shape followed suit [4], as was the case in silver foxes that were domesticated in Russia over a 40-year period [16, 17]. In addition to skull shape, juvenile physical characteristics and behavioral traits of the wolf were retained [15, 18–20].

With the emergence of the Kennel Club in the United Kingdom in 1873 [4, 21], dogs began to exit the workforce and enter the arena as participants in dog shows designed to showcase the morphological and increasingly aesthetic aspects of each individual breed standard [1]. In many cases, appearance was prioritized over function when selecting for conformation to produce what society valued to be the most desirable phenotype [9].

Currently, there are over 400 dog breeds worldwide [4, 22], most of which bear little to no resemblance to the gray wolf, despite sharing 98.8% of their mitochondrial DNA sequence [4, 23, 24]. Morphology varies immensely between dog breeds [4]. In particular, many breeds are defined and recognized by their skull shape [4]. For example, the classic downward-pointing muzzle of bull terriers and the dome-shaped Chihuahua are unmistakable (Figure 11.1).

Whereas the wolf has a uniform skull length of 30 cm, dog breeds exhibit immense variability [3]. Although puppies are relatively uniform in terms of muzzle size at birth, breeds with dolichocephalic skulls experience appreciable postnatal growth of their snouts [14]. This

Performing the Small Animal Physical Examination, First Edition. Ryane E. Englar.
© 2017 John Wiley & Sons, Inc. Published 2017 by John Wiley & Sons, Inc.

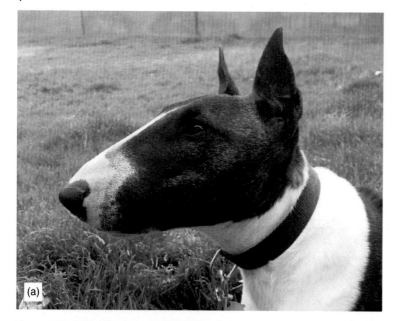
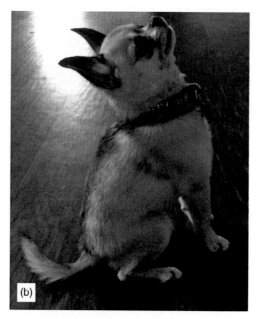

Figure 11.1 (a) Profile view of a Bull Terrier, demonstrating the classic, breed-specific appearance of its head and muzzle. Source: Courtesy of Danielle N. Cucuzella. (b) Profile view of a Chihuahua, demonstrating the classic, breed-specific, dome-shaped appearance of its calvarium. Source: Courtesy of Kaitlen Betchel.

growth continues until adulthood, at which point the length of each dog's skull is breed-dependent and ranges from 7 to 28 cm [3].

The cephalic index (CI) also contributes to diversity between breeds as the ratio of the width of the skull to its length [6]. The CI for the gray wolf is 51–52 [25], whereas domesticated dog breeds have a CI ranging from 42 to 98.54 [6, 25]. The higher the CI, the wider is the skull

compared with its length, hence the emergence of the brachycephalic breeds. Compared with those with dolichocephalic skulls, brachycephalic breeds have broad, short skulls that give their muzzle a "pushed in" appearance [4, 26–28] (Figure 11.2).

In addition, brachycephalic breeds tend to have shallow orbits that are spaced further apart than would be the case in a dolicocephalic dog [4]. These features are

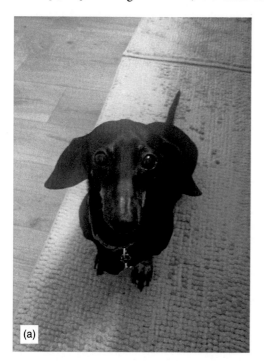
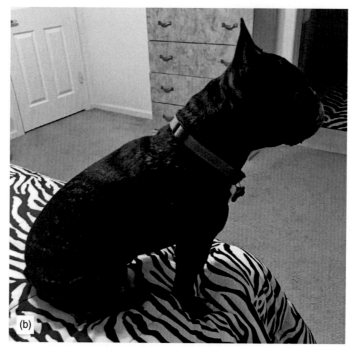

Figure 11.2 (a) Profile view of a Dachshund as an example of a dolichocephalic breed. Source: Courtesy of Meghan Teixeira. (b) Profile view of a French Bulldog as an example of a brachycephalic breed. Source: Courtesy of Cailin McElhenny.

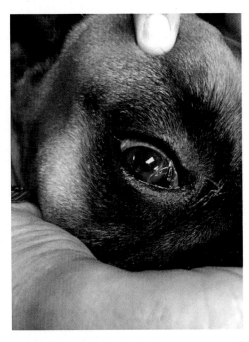

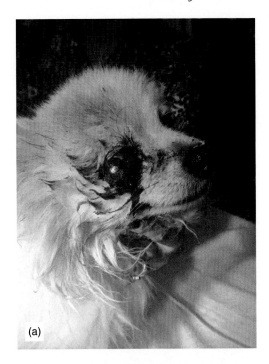

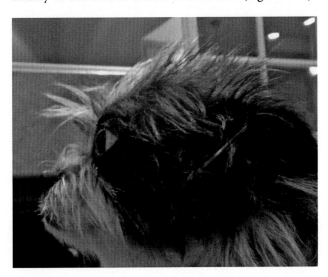

Figure 11.3 This patient is fluorescein positive, meaning that there is a corneal ulcer OD in the region of stain uptake. Source: Courtesy of Samantha Thurman, DVM.

preferred in the general dog-owning population [29], perhaps because the wide-eyed appearance of brachycephalic breeds provides the perception that they are more engaged with their owners [1]. Unfortunately, this desirable phenotype from an aesthetic perspective is medically unsound. Brachycephalic breeds are 20 times more likely to develop one or more corneal ulcers than breeds without brachycephalic skulls (Figure 11.3) [30]. Of brachycephalic breeds, the pug is most at risk [30].

Brachycephalic breeds are also more likely to have over-sized palpebral fissures and protruding eyes secondary to the shallow nature of the orbits (Figure 11.4).

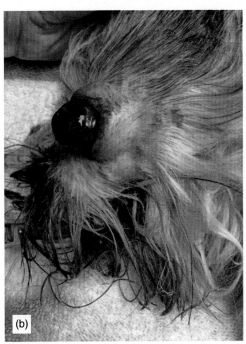

Figure 11.5 (a) Proptosis in a small-breed dog. Source: Courtesy of Andrew Weisenfeld, DVM. (b) Side view of a dog with proptosis. Source: Courtesy of Amanda Maltese, DVM.

This combination may make it difficult to close the eyelids fully. As a result, tear film is inadequately spread and the cornea is likely to experience exposure keratitis [30]. The brachycephalic patient may also be more at risk of proptosis (Figure 11.5).

Additionally, because the skin overlying the muzzle is reduced in length in proportion to the facial skeleton in brachycephalic breeds, the skin is forced into nasal folds

Figure 11.4 This patient has a "bug-eyed" appearance, meaning that its eyes are very pronounced. Source: Courtesy of David May.

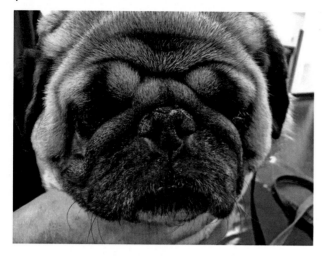

Figure 11.6 Head-on view of a Pug with extensive nasal folds.

(Figure 11.6), the hairs of which may then come into contact with one or both corneas. This so-called nasal fold trichiasis is painful and in some cases may require surgical intervention to eliminate the inappropriate contact [30].

Furthermore, to accommodate space limitations within the shortened braincase, brachycephalic breeds have altered cerebral positioning by shifting the olfactory bulb rostrally and having a more ventrally rotated cerebral axis [25]. These changes may affect information processing in brachycephalic breeds: the way in which they perceive external stimuli may differ from that in breeds with other skull shapes due to altered brain morphology [6].

The mesaticephalic or mesocephalic skull shape represents a mid-point between the dolichocephalic and brachiocephalic builds. In the mesocephalic breed of dog, such as a Weimaraner, Labrador Retriever, and Puggle, the skull width and length are roughly equal (Figure 11.7).

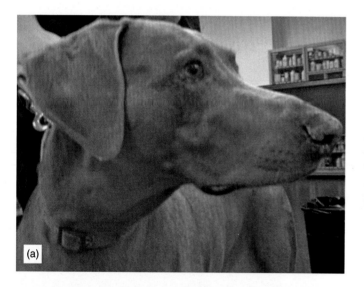

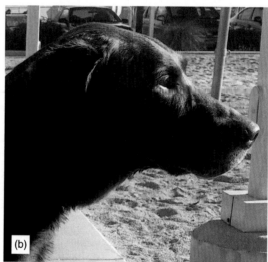

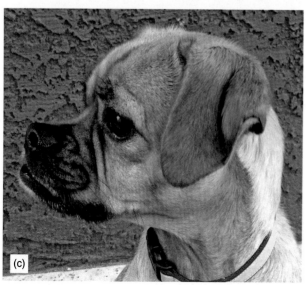

Figure 11.7 (a) Profile view of a Weimaraner as an example of a mesocephalic breed. Source: Courtesy of Elizabeth Robbins, DVM. (b) Profile view of a Labrador Retriever as an example of a mesocephalic breed. Source: Courtesy of Jess Darmofal. (c) Profile view of a Puggle as an example of a mesocephalic breed. Source: Courtesy of Kara N. Jones.

The degree of a dog's trainability is thought to vary by breed [31–34]. The mesocephalic breeds are perceived by the general public to be more trainable [35].

Some have criticized the dolichocephalic/mesocephalic/brachycephalic classification system for skull size and shape as being too simplistic [22, 36]. CI is preferred because it represents a continuum rather than a category [25, 37], but even CI has its limitations. For example, the Papillon and Pug are morphologically distinct based upon the shape of the calvarium; however, when these breeds are classified by CI, they are lumped into the same category [36].

It is therefore less important that the clinician knows the CI for every patient and more important to be aware of risk factors for disease that are based upon the patient's skull shape. In this way, the clinician is able to anticipate the level of care that such a patient may require. This then needs to be articulated to the client so that breeders and dog owners are made aware of the care necessary to maintain good quality of life. For example, the clinician needs to educate owners of brachycephalic breeds that aforementioned health concerns are probable based upon morphological characteristics alone.

11.2 Facial symmetry

Once skull shape has been identified and recorded, the veterinarian should assess for facial symmetry. Facial symmetry can be a challenge if the patient is crouched or tucking the head and neck into its body (Figure 11.8).

It is best to evaluate facial symmetry from the front and from the side when the patient is in a seated or standing position (Figure 11.9).

The presence of a head tilt or drooped lips, ears, and eyelids, especially when asymmetric, are concerning in that they may be the result of neurologic dysfunction and as such should be noted in the medical record [38, 39]. Note that aural asymmetry, on the other hand, is not necessarily pathologic and may be considered normal for the patient (Figure 11.10).

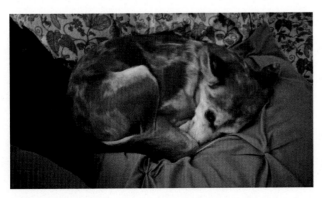

Figure 11.8 The patient that is hunched makes it difficult to assess facial symmetry. Source: Courtesy of Arielle Hatcher.

11.3 The Eyes and Accessory Visual Structures

11.3.1 A Systematic Approach to the Eye Examination

Both eyes and their adnexa should be examined in every patient using a systematic approach even in the absence of an ocular presenting complaint [40–43].

When ocular concerns are raised, the following are among the most commonly reported clinical signs in canine and feline patients [44–46]:

- "red eye";
- "cloudy eye";
- "bulging eye";
- vision loss;
- ocular discharge;
- blepharospasm (squinting);
- photophobia (light sensitivity);
- pawing at one or both eyes;
- rubbing one or both sides of the face on the carpet.

The history is an important starting point [47]. Owners often present pets for the concerns listed above, and they may have tremendous insight into the duration and/or progression of the symptom. If the client is new to the practice, the clinician must rely upon them to provide pertinent information such as whether this is a new or recurrent problem, and what diagnostics and/or therapeutics have been attempted [47]. Moreover, the clinician must recognize that the eyes do not exist in isolation from the rest of the patient. It is possible that the client has identified concurrent symptoms that, together with the ocular presenting complaint, paint a picture of systemic disease. It is critical that the clinician be open to considering additional presenting complaints as opposed to just the eyes so that he does not misdiagnose ocular manifestations of systemic disease [47].

11.3.2 Evaluating the Adnexa of the Eye

After taking a thorough history, the adnexa of the eye should be examined first. The adnexa include the eyelids, lacrimal apparatus, the nictitating membrane, and the conjunctiva [48–50] (Figure 11.11).

The incidence of eyelid disease is high in dogs [48], so when considering the eyelids, it is important that the clinician evaluates for:

- entropion;
- ectropion;
- redness;
- blepharospasm;
- masses.

When the upper or lower eyelid rolls inward, either as a whole or as a fraction, the patient is said to have entropion. More often than not, entropion in dogs involves the lower

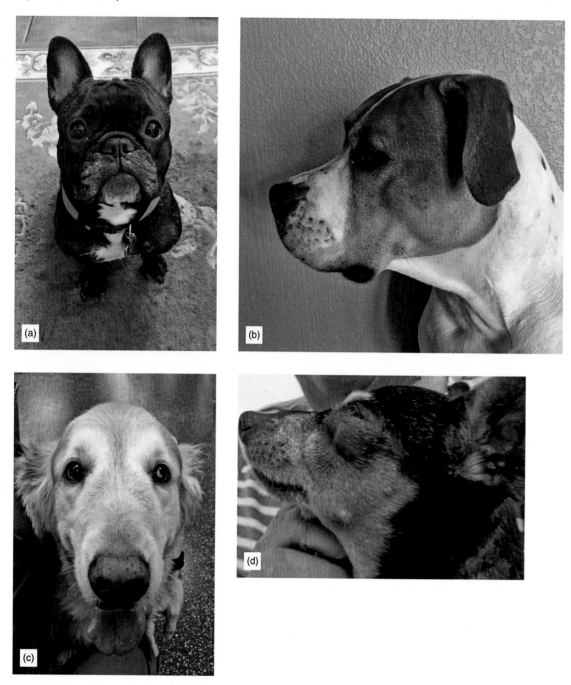

Figure 11.9 (a) This head-on view of a French Bulldog makes for an easy assessment of facial symmetry. Source: Courtesy of Cailin McElhenny. (b) The profile view of an American Bulldog also assists with the clinician's assessment of facial symmetry. Source: Courtesy of Kiefer Hazard. (c) When viewed from the front, this geriatric patient has bilaterally symmetrical atrophy of the temporal muscles and also a bilaterally symmetrical prominent dorsal muzzle as if a swelling or mass effect were present. (d) When viewed from the side, this patient has pronounced left buccal and left peri-ocular swelling secondary to facial bite wounds. Source: Courtesy of Patricia Bennett, DVM.

eyelid and typically the lateral rather than the medial half. However, it is also seen in the lateral aspect of the upper eyelid in certain breeds such as the Saint Bernard, Boxer, Chow Chow, and Rottweiler. Rarely does it occur at the medial aspect of the eyelids. When it does, it is more typically seen in the Pekingese, Pug, English Bulldog, and the King Charles Cavalier Spaniel. Entropion is thought to be inherited in the dog. Entropion may also be transient when induced by pain and blepharospasm, as from a corneal ulcer [48, 51].

Entropion is a diagnosis made through direct observation. Facial hairs extend to the lid margin, which is abnormal. Because this fur then comes into contact with the cornea, corneal irritation with secondary epiphora often results [48].

Ectropion, on the other hand, refers to the rolling out of one or both of the lower eyelids. In certain breeds, such as hounds, ectropion is considered normal. In other breeds, such as hunters and setters, it may be present transiently following exercise or during relaxation. When it occurs in

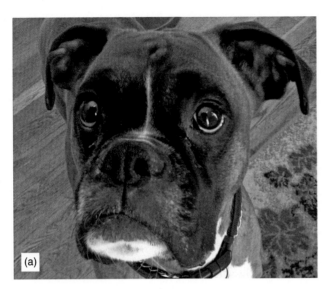

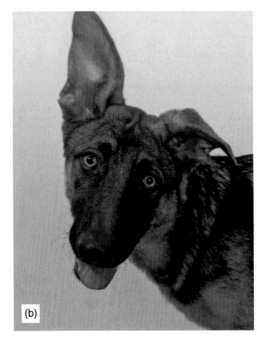

Figure 11.10 (a) Aural symmetry in a Boxer dog. Source: Courtesy of Symmantha Page. (b) Asymmetric ear carriage in a normal German Shepherd dog. Source: Courtesy of Jule Schweighoefer.

breeds other than those listed, it is considered common, but abnormal. The client may report a "saggy" appearance to one or both eyes, and the associated conjunctiva may become progressively red from irritation [48].

The eyelids themselves should be evaluated for redness (Figure 11.12). Blepharitis is common and may be triggered by an underlying dermatopathy such as allergic skin disease [48]. In addition to having red eyelids, the patient may be "squinty." Ocular pain should be considered in any patient that is exhibiting blepharospasm [48] (Figure 11.13).

While evaluating the adnexa of both eyes, the astute clinician should also note if ocular discharge is present

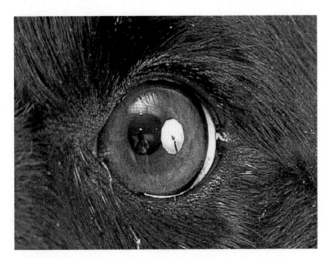

Figure 11.11 Close-up of the adnexa of the canine eye. Source: Courtesy of the Media Resources Department at Midwestern University.

and, if so, whether it is considered "normal" for the patient. For some patients, epiphora is the norm: they have experienced tear overflow for their entire life. For example, American Cocker Spaniels, Bedlington Terriers, and Golden Retrievers may have inherited defects that cause atresia of the lacrimal punctum. When this occurs, it is typically unilateral and only involves the lower punctum. The result is that these patients are prone to lifelong tear overflow. Accordingly, these patients may have "tear stripes," a dark discoloration of fur that starts at the medial canthus and tracks ventrally (Figure 11.14) [50].

Alternatively, the American Cocker Spaniel may have inherited a displaced lacrimal punctum: tears do not flow into the ventral canaliculi because the anatomy is not properly aligned to facilitate tear drainage [50].

Toy breeds often have tear overflow, not because of an anatomic defect involving a lacrimal punctum, but because their "bug-eyed" appearance results in taut eyelids against the globes. These reduce the size of the lacrimal lake so tears are likely to spill over the edge of the eyelid while waiting to be drained through the nasolacrimal duct [50].

Patients that have trichiasis, normal cilia (eyelashes) or hairs, as from nasal folds, that are abnormally directed toward the cornea may also present with epiphora. In this case, excessive tearing is a reflex in response to corneal irritation. Similarly, patients with distichia, an extra row of cilia on the eyelid margin, may have increased corneal contact by the cilia that is sufficiently irritating to trigger lacrimation [48].

Other patients develop epiphora secondary to a plugged nasolacrimal duct or ocular irritation. In this case, the

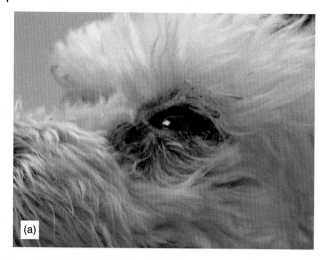
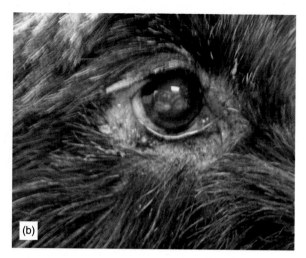

Figure 11.12 (a) Blepharitis (eyelid inflammation) in a dog. Note the redness associated with the left upper and lower eyelids and also the surrounding fur being crusted over with discharge. Source: Courtesy of Patricia Bennett, DVM. (b) Blepharitis with associated peri-ocular alopecia. Note that the upper and lower right eyelids are also associated with crusting secondary to ocular discharge. Source: Courtesy of Elizabeth Robbins, DVM.

onset of epiphora is more acute and more typically seen in an adult patient without a previous history of tear over-flow. These patients benefit from nasolacrimal irrigation to determine whether or not the puncta, the canaliculi, and the nasolacrimal duct are patent. An alternative test of nasolacrimal duct patency is to administer topical flu-orescein stain to both eyes. If both nasolacrimal ducts are patent, then fluorescein should appear on the nares, sug-gesting that tear drainage is adequate [50].

Epiphora refers to overflow of otherwise normal tears. There are, however, other types of ocular discharge. When a patient presents with ocular discharge, it is important that the clinician notes the color and consistency of the discharge and also its origin: is it unilateral or bilateral?

Clear ocular discharge may indicate irritation, inflam-mation, allergies, or viral infection. As ocular discharge becomes more opaque and takes on a color such as white, yellow, or green, it may be indicative of an underlying bac-terial infection. It may also indicate a change in the com-position of tear film, as is evident in keratoconjunctivitis

sicca (KCS). Typically, KCS refers to a deficiency in the watery component of tears; however, some dogs may also have deficiencies in mucin [50, 52, 53] (Figure 11.15).

The clinician should also note the presence of any eye-lid masses (Figure 11.16). Although eyelid masses are common in the dog, the majority are benign meibomian gland tumors [48]. If the patient is a young dog, viral pap-illomas and histiocytomas are prioritized in terms of dif-ferential diagnosis. The former may occur simultaneously with oral viral papillomas. Both viral papillomas arise and resolve spontaneously. Of the 25% of eyelid masses that are malignant, it is rare to see metastasis [48, 54].

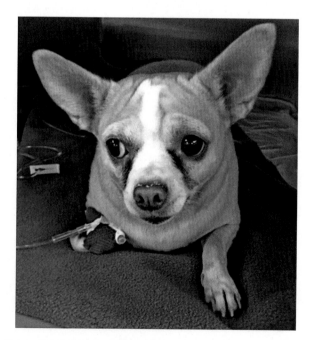

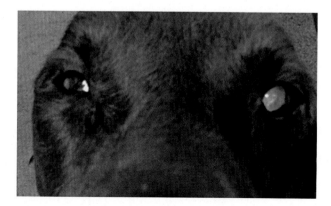

Figure 11.13 Unilateral blepharospasm of the left eye. Source: Courtesy of Elizabeth Robbins, DVM.

Figure 11.14 Note the bilateral "tear stripes" that have resulted from chronic epiphora in this Chihuahua.

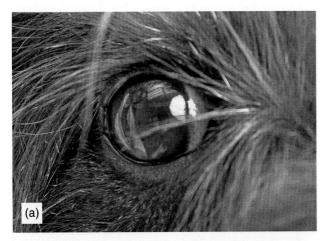

(a)

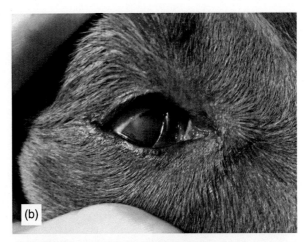

(b)

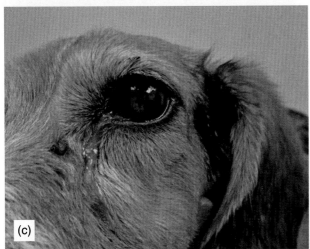

(c)

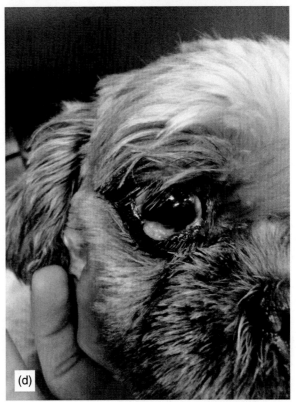

(d)

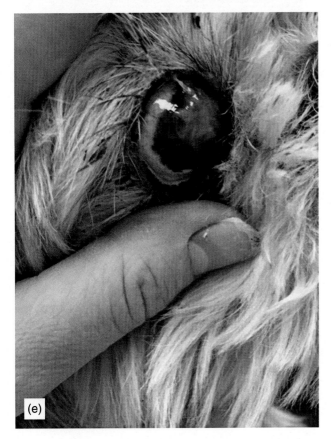

(e)

Figure 11.15 (a) Note the presence of trichiasis in this canine patient. Because nasal fold fur is coming into contact with the patient's right eye, the right eye historically has exhibited tear overflow. In this case, the excess tearing is triggered by corneal contact by the fur. Trimming the fur as needed so that it does not touch the cornea will solve the issue. Source: Courtesy of the Media Resources Department at Midwestern University. (b) Serous ocular discharge secondary to glaucoma. Note the visible wetness associated with the right lower eyelid. Source: Courtesy of Jess Darmofal. (c) Note the left-sided mucoid ocular discharge in this canine patient. Source: Courtesy of Patricia Bennett, DVM. (d) Note the right-sided mucopurulent ocular discharge. Source: Courtesy of Andrew Weisenfeld, DVM. (e) Note the crusts associated with the peri-ocular fur. These crusts commonly occur when ocular discharge dries.

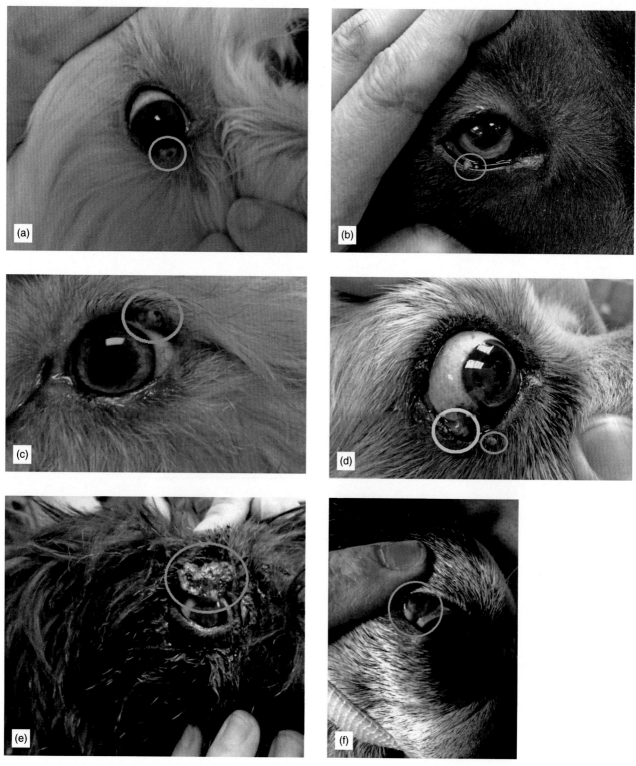

Figure 11.16 (a) Lower eyelid mass associated with OD. Source: Courtesy of Patricia Bennett, DVM. (b) Two lower eyelid masses associated with OD. Source: Courtesy of Kate Anderson, DVM. (c) Upper eyelid mass associated with OS. Source: Courtesy of Patricia Bennett, DVM. (d) Two lower eyelid masses associated with OD. The one circled in orange is arising along the deep margin of the eyelid whereas that circled in blue is arising from the surface of the eyelid. Source: Courtesy of Patricia Bennett, DVM. (e) Expansive, irritated, and ulcerated upper eyelid mass associated with OD. (f) Meimobian gland adenoma of the right upper eyelid protruding onto the conjunctival surface. Source: Courtesy of Amanda Maltese, DVM.

Compared with viral papillomas, cutaneous papillomas are eyelid masses that are more commonly seen in older dogs, especially Cocker Spaniels and Kerry Blue Terriers. These may also be localized to other areas of the head and the feet. They typically remain small at less than 0.5 cm in diameter. They vary in color, are often alopecic, and may either be smooth-surfaced or display fronds [55].

Cutaneous papillomas should not be confused with canine oral papillomatosis, an affliction of young dogs with cauliflower-like lesions in or around the oral cavity that may extend to the lips (Figure 11.17). These lesions typically regress within 3 months whereas cutaneous papillomas do not.

Note that eyelid growths are not always neoplastic – they may also result from inflammation. For example, when one or more of the eyelid's meibomian glands abscesses, a focal hordeolum or stye develops. This acute and painful swelling may look like a mass when in fact it is merely an eyelid swelling caused by a bacterial infection that is responsive to topical antibiotic therapy (Figure 11.18).

After the eyelids have been thoroughly assessed, the clinician may look deeper into the conjunctiva. The conjunctiva

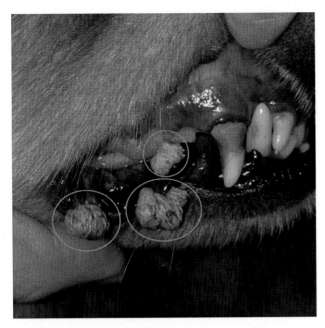

Figure 11.17 Canine oral papillomatosis. Source: Courtesy of Paola Bazan Steyling, DVM.

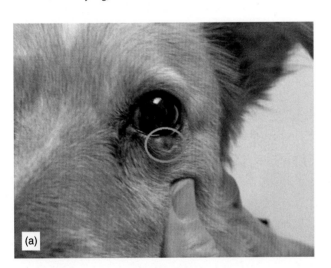

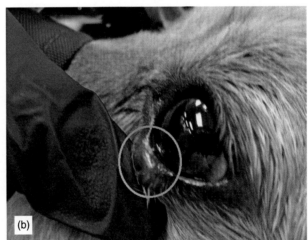

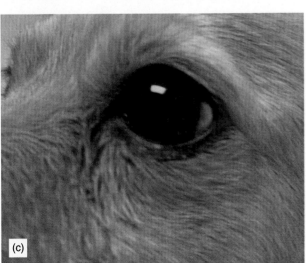

Figure 11.18 Stye associated with the left lower eyelid as viewed (a) head-on and (b) from the side. (c) Resolution of the stye associated with the left lower eyelid following antibiotic topical therapy.

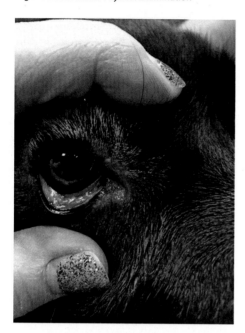

Figure 11.19 Chemosis of the palpebral conjunctiva OD.

should be evaluated for color and symmetry. A normal conjunctiva is a homogenous, healthy pink in color. As the conjunctiva become inflamed, as in conjunctivitis, conjunctival hyperemia is apparent; the conjunctiva takes on a reddened, irritated appearance [49, 56].

The conjunctiva should also evaluated for chemosis, conjunctival edema. Chemosis typically goes hand-in-hand with conjunctivitis and frequently causes the conjunctiva to take on a glossy, prominent, "puffy" appearance (Figure 11.19) [49, 56]. Note that it is not abnormal for the Shar Pei breed of dog to exhibit chemosis without concurrent conjunctivitis. It is thought that this occurs in the breed because they have increased mucin in the conjunctival stroma [49].

If conjunctival irritation is chronic, the conjunctiva may take on a cobblestone appearance due to the prominence of lymphoid follicles. When these follicles are visible, they are not pathognomonic for one particular causative agent. They simply denote conjunctivitis of long-standing duration [49].

In the dog, conjunctivitis may have an allergic or immune-mediated component, or it may be due to viral infections such as canine distemper virus and canine adenovirus types 1 and 2. More frequently, conjunctivitis in the dog has a bacterial origin. The difficulty in definitively diagnosing bacterial conjunctivitis in the dog is that 91% of conjunctiva of healthy dogs without conjunctivitis produce positive bacterial cultures. The majority of bacteria that are swabbed from normal and abnormal canine conjunctiva are Gram-positive isolates such as *Streptococci* and *Staphylococci*. Therefore, diagnosis may initially be made based upon presenting complaint and physical examination findings rather than culture, and the patient's response to topical antibiotic therapy may be used to judge clinical success [49, 57–61].

The incidence of fungal conjunctivitis within the canine population is difficult to appreciate because 22% of dogs will have their conjunctiva culture positive for fungi [62].

In addition to being evaluated for inflammatory and infectious disease, the conjunctiva should be assessed for masses. Compared with large animals, companion animals tend to present with conjunctival neoplasia less frequently. However, when it occurs, it may be locally aggressive and may metastasize, as is typically seen in cases of conjunctival melanoma [49, 63].

In addition to the conjunctiva, the nictitating membrane associated with each orbit should be evaluated. To do so, the clinician must manipulate the soft tissue over each orbit to get the nictitating membrane to come into view. Pushing down gently, but firmly, over the upper palpebra will facilitate visualization of this structure (Figure 11.20).

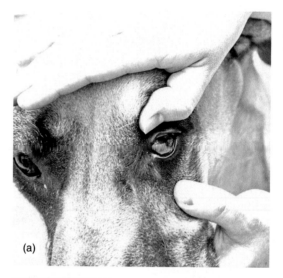

(a)

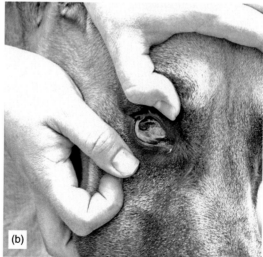

(b)

Figure 11.20 (a) Inspecting the nictitating membrane associated with OS by pushing down with firm pressure over the left globe. (b) Inspecting the nictitating membrane associated with OD by pushing down with firm pressure over the right globe.
Source (a), (b): Courtesy of the Media Resources Department at Midwestern University.

Patients that present with ocular complaints may have prominent nictitating membranes that do not require as much effort on the veterinarian's part to extrude them completely. These nictitating membranes may already be prominently exposed. In kittens and puppies, their prominence has been assumed to relate to heavy gastrointestinal parasite burden. More often, when nictitating membranes are prominent without manipulation on the part of the clinician, they are reflective of ocular pain or irritation as from a corneal ulcer [56].

Nictitating membranes may also become prominent if there is a foreign body in the orbit. Plant material, especially seeds, can become lodged beneath the nictitating membrane and is a common source of corneal abrasion and ulceration.

Topical ophthalmic anesthetics such as proparacaine must be used to numb the affected eye. This allows for the insertion of a cotton-tip applicator, moistened with saline, under the nictitating membrane to see if there is indeed a foreign body trapped underneath. Because topical ophthalmic anesthetics delay corneal healing, they are inappropriate for use on an outpatient basis to maintain comfort of the eye. However, their one-time use is necessary in this instance [56].

Nictitating membranes may also become prominent if they prolapse (Figure 11.21). Prolapse of the gland of the third eyelid is colloquially referred to as "cherry eye." When it occurs, it is typically in a young adult dog that presents for acute development of a red "mass" in the medial canthus of one or both eyes. Owners may notice

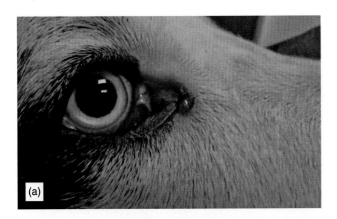

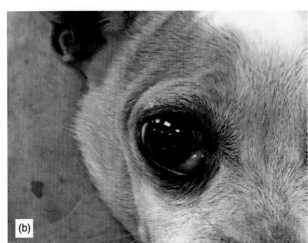

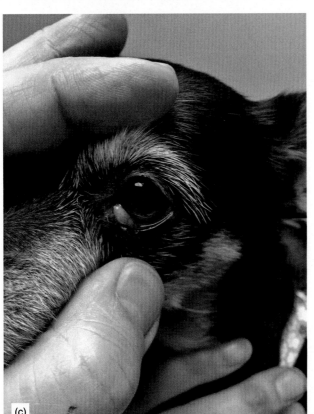

Figure 11.21 (a) Everted T-shaped hyaline cartilage associated with the third eyelid. Source: Courtesy of Patricia Bennett, DVM.
(b) "Cherry eye" OD. Source: Courtesy of Samantha Thurman, DVM.
(c) "Cherry eye" OS. Source: Courtesy of Frank Isom, DVM.

initially that the apparent growth comes and goes. Eventually, it becomes permanently visible. Certain dog breeds are more likely to be affected, including Cocker Spaniels, Boston Terriers, Shih Tzus, Beagles, and Pekingese. Cats are rarely affected, except for the Burmese [49, 64–67].

Orbital neoplasia and orbital cellulitis have also been linked to cases of prolapse of the gland of the third eyelid [49].

11.3.3 Evaluating the Globe

With regard to the globe, the following should be assessed [56]:

- how the globe sits within the orbit;
- whether the globe can be retropulsed;
- whether or not strabismus is present.

In addition, the clinician should examine the following:

- sclera;
- cornea;
- iris;
- pupil;
- lens;
- fundus.

The globe should be well seated within the orbit, a bony case comprised of the maxilla and the frontal, lacrimal, zygomatic, presphenoid, basisphenoid, and palatine bones (Figure 11.22a) [56, 68]. The type of skull that the dog has influences the size of both the orbit and the globe, and also the globe's position within the orbit [3, 5, 68]. Because of their shallow orbits and large palpebral fissures, brachycephalic breeds exhibit conformational exophthalmos, meaning that they naturally have a "bug-eyed" or "bulgy" eye appearance: the globes appear to protrude more than would typically be considered normal [68].

By contrast, pathological exophthalmos is often the result of orbital disease: a space-occupying lesion is present within the orbit, pushing the globe forward. Masses

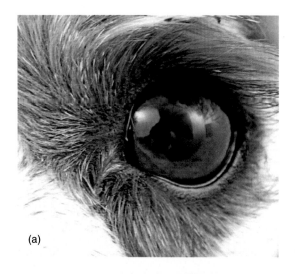
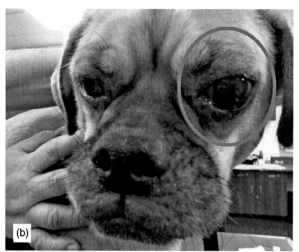
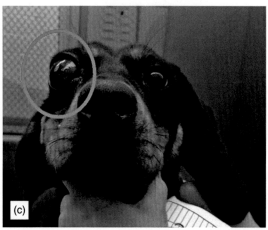
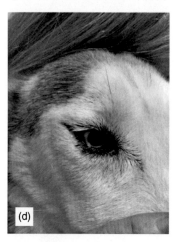

Figure 11.22 (a) Normal anatomic positioning of the globe within the orbit. Source: Courtesy of the Media Resources Department at Midwestern University. (b) Moderate buphthalmos OS in a Boxer dog secondary to glaucoma. Source: Courtesy of Elizabeth Robbins, DVM. (c) Severe buphthalmos OD secondary to glaucoma. Source: Courtesy of Tradel Harris, DVM. (d) Microphthalmia in a Husky dog. This patient also has a presumptive cutaneous papilloma along the rim of the lower right eyelid. Source: Courtesy of Samantha Thurman, DVM.

involving the masticatory muscles or the zygomatic salivary gland may also cause pathological exophthalmos [68].

The appearance of buphthalmos, eye enlargement due to glaucoma, bears a striking resemblance to exophthalmos because the enlarged globe becomes just as prominent [68, 69] (Figure 11.22b and c). A key difference between buphthalmos and exophthalmos is that patients that present with the former tend to have additional changes to the appearance of the globe. For example, the glaucoma patient tends to present with corneal edema, congestion of episcleral vessels, and a dilated pupil in addition to buphthalmos [69].

If extreme, both buphthalmos and exophthalmos can prevent eyelid closure. When the lids are unable to close, the cornea is inadequately protected by tear film and may dry out. Exposure keratitis with subsequent corneal ulceration is probable [56].

However, exophthalmos and buphthalmos are not always as obvious as is depicted in Figure 11.22b and c. When the patient is in the early stages of disease, exophthalmos and buphthalmos may be less overt. In these cases, retropulsion of each globe can help to identify retro-orbital disease before pathology is grossly visible [68]. Retropulsion is a technique that requires the clinician to apply firm, even pressure to the globe through closed eyelids. An orbit that is devoid of disease should allow for some "give": the globe should be able to be balloted gently because there is nothing to obstruct the globe's movement in the retro-orbital space. By contrast, the presence of a retro-orbital mass will create an obstruction that prevents ballottement: there will be resistance to retropulsion. The ability of both eyes to be retropulsed should be evaluated at each visit, and both eyes should be equal in their response. Ultrasonography of the retrobulbar region can be a helpful diagnostic tool when a space-occupying mass is suspected [56, 68].

The normal globe should also not retract into the orbit, a condition called enophthalmos. Enophthalmos is distinct from microphthalmos, a condition that is characterized by a decreased globe size, although both present with a similar appearance (Figure 11.22d). When enophthalmos occurs, it may be secondary to dehydration or cachexia. In both of these circumstances, there will be bilateral involvement. Enophthalmos can also result from the atrophy of orbital fat or the loss of function of the orbitalis muscle, in which case one or both globes are affected. In addition, conditions such as tetanus, which increases retractor tone in the extraocular muscles, will result in bilateral enophthalmos [56]. By contrast, microphthalmos is a congenital rather than an acquired condition. Dogs with both merle genes and blue eyes are often affected [68, 70–72].

In addition to assessing globe position, the astute clinician should evaluate the patient for strabismus. Recall from Section 3.2.3 that strabismus is an umbrella term for several forms of misalignment between the eyes so that the eyes are prevented from directing their gaze at the same point in space at the same time. When strabismus is present in a veterinary patient, there is typically an underlying neuropathy [43, 46, 73, 74].

Recall that the direction of the strabismus implies which cranial nerve is involved [38, 39]:

- ventrolateral strabismus: cranial nerve III – the oculomotor nerve;
- medial strabismus: cranial nerve VI – the abducent nerve;
- rotatory strabismus: cranial nerve IV – the trochlear nerve.

Strabismus can occur in one or both eyes. In addition to being common in Siamese cats [44, 75–77], strabismus is common in brachycephalic and toy breeds of dogs [68]. Strabismus is also common following the replacement of a globe after traumatic proptosis (Figure 11.23). It may result from damaged ventral and medial rectus muscles or their associated nerves. Although this type of strabismus will improve over 1–2 months, it will never fully resolve [58].

The astute clinician should also recognize if there is nystagmus, involuntary eye movement of one or both eyes that may be physiologic or pathologic, congenital or acquired. Acquired nystagmus results from systemic or central nervous system disease, toxicosis [78], or pharmacotherapy [79–81].

11.3.4 Evaluating the Sclera

The sclera should be inspected for hyperemia, hemorrhage, icterus, other forms of pigmentation, and masses (Figure 11.24).

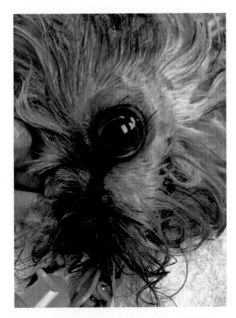

Figure 11.23 Canine patient with a proptosed OS. This patient is likely to experience strabismus following replacement of the globe within the orbit. Source: Courtesy of Amanda Maltese, DVM.

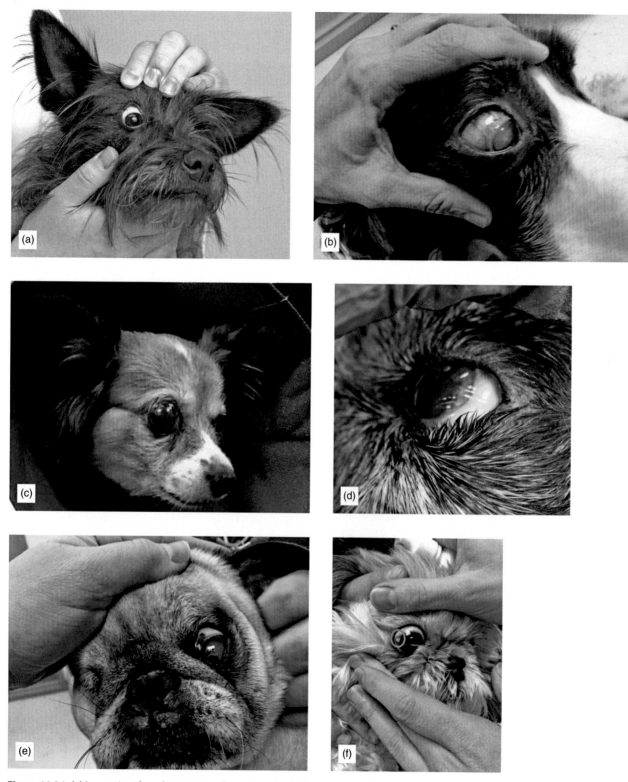

Figure 11.24 (a) Inspecting the sclera as part of a routine physical examination. (b) Injected sclera in a patient that also has a concurrent cataract and glaucoma. Source: Courtesy of Patricia Bennett, DVM. (c) Diffuse scleral hemorrhage secondary to proptosis. Source: Courtesy of Frank Isom, DVM. (d) Icteric sclera. Source: Courtesy of Ali Brower, DVM, DACVP. (e) Pigmentation of the sclera in a pug. (f) Scleral mast cell tumor. Source: Courtesy of Amanda Maltese, DVM.

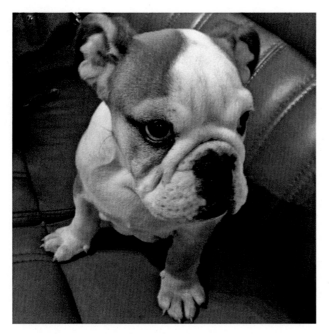

Figure 11.25 English Bulldog puppy demonstrating "eye white," a desirable trait in this brachycephalic breed. Source: Courtesy of Shirley Yang, DVM.

Note that the sclera is frequently prominent in brachycephalic breeds and that in certain breeds this feature is valued as it is written into the breed standard (Figure 11.25). In order for this to occur, the patient must have over-sized palpebral fissures or very shallow orbits [30].

Brachycephalic breeds also commonly acquire brown pigment at the sclera, limbus, or medial cornea (Figure 11.24e). When this focal deposition of pigment occurs, it is typically the result of long-term irritation as from trichiasis or entropion. This is opposed to cases involving diffuse pigmentary keratitis (Figure 11.26), in which pigment spreads completely over the cornea and may result in blindnes [82].

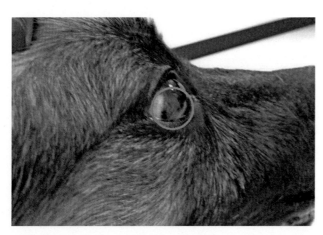

Figure 11.26 Note that pigmentary keratitis is more diffuse in this patient: brown pigment has taken over approximately two-thirds of the patient's ocular surface.

11.3.5 Evaluating the Cornea

The cornea should be evaluated for integrity and transparency. Some corneal defects are so catastrophic that they are visible with the naked eye without additional diagnostic tests. Other corneal defects are invisible to the eye without the use of sodium fluorescein stain and a cobalt blue light [82] (Figure 11.27).

Corneal ulcers may result from traumatic injury to the surface of the eye such as physical contact by foreign bodies, thermal damage secondary to fire exposure, and chemical irritation from shampoos that are incompletely rinsed from the coat during bathing. In addition, corneal ulcers may result from infectious disease, inadequate lubrication of the cornea with tear film, or systemic diseases that compromise wound healing [82].

When they occur, corneal ulcers may vary in depth from superficial to deep. Indolent ulcers are complicated ulcers that are slow to heal. These are commonly seen in Boxers; however, other breeds are not immune [82–85].

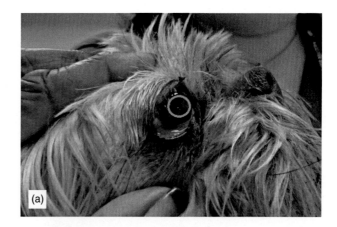

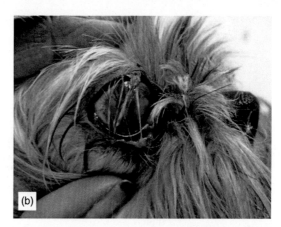

Figure 11.27 (a) Note the corneal defect OD of this patient that is visible to the naked eye without sodium fluorescein staining. (b) Note that the corneal defect in (a) is much more extensive than was initially thought once sodium fluorescein staining was used to outline its margins. Source (a), (b): Courtesy of Patricia Bennett, DVM.

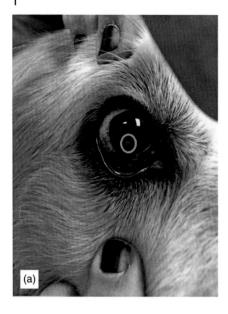
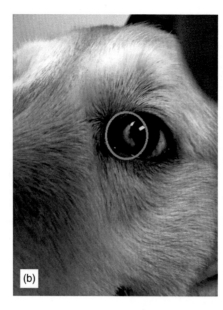

Figure 11.28 (a) Lipid keratopathy is just beginning to develop OD. (b) Note that lipid keratopathy is more advanced OS in the same patient as depicted in (a).

In addition to being intact, the cornea should be transparent. Traumatic injuries to the eye, including corneal ulcers, can compromise this transparency [82]. Transparency of the cornea may also be reduced by lipid keratopathy, the corneal deposition of lipid (Figure 11.28). This condition is inherited in Siberian Huskies [86], but is not unique to Huskies and several other breeds have been reported. In most cases, lipid keratopathy is unrelated to metabolic concerns such as hyperlipidemia [87]. An exception is the Fox Terrier, a breed with a familial lipid storage disease that tends to lay down lipid in a circular ring next to the limbus [82].

Corneal edema may reduce corneal translucency (Figure 11.29). This may occur in the absence of an inflammatory response. For example, acquired corneal endothelial degeneration is a non-inflammatory cause of corneal edema, as also is systemic pharmacologic toxicity. For example, when tocainide is prescribed to Doberman Pinschers for extended periods of time to manage cardiomyopathy, corneal edema is a common sequela [82, 88, 90].

More commonly, the clinician detects corneal edema secondary to an underlying inflammatory process such as corneal trauma or pannus (Figure 11.30). Pannus refers to a typically bilateral superficial keratitis with a presumptive immune-mediated basis. It is most commonly seen in the German Shepherd, but has since been recognized in other breeds [82, 91–93].

An early sign of pannus is conjunctivitis, followed by the progressive deposition of a gray to red opacity along the entire corneal surface. Over time, this heavy pigmentation leads to blindness. Treatment is aimed at suppressing corneal inflammation using topical glucocorticoids. Therapy is palliative and requires long-term commitment to treatment on the part of the owner [82].

11.3.6 Evaluating the Iris

The iris is the part of the eye that we refer to when describing eye color. Compared with the cat, the dog's iris tends to have a narrower range of color, from rich browns to light blues (Figure 11.31).

Heterochromic irises are present when one iris or at least a portion of it lacks pigment compared with the contralateral iris [94]. Heterochromic irises are commonly seen in dogs that carry the merle gene because it suppresses melanocytes. This causes white or diluted pigment within the skin and coat, blue irises, and potentially deafness [95]. In affected patients with heterochromic irises, deafness is typically unilateral and occurs on

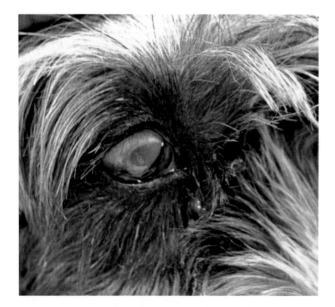

Figure 11.29 Note the loss of corneal translucency due to widespread corneal edema. Source: Courtesy of Patricia Bennett, DVM.

Figure 11.30 (a) Note the loss of corneal translucency due to superficial keratitis, characterized by an irregularly raised corneal surface OS with red–gray patches along the cornea. (b) Note the improvement in the same patient after using topical prednisolone acetate and cyclosporine therapy. Source (a), (b): Courtesy of Andrew Weisenfeld, DVM.

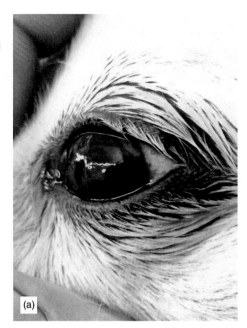
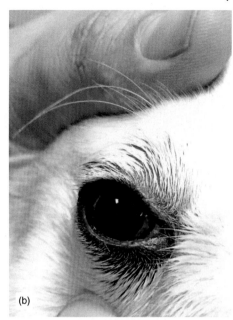

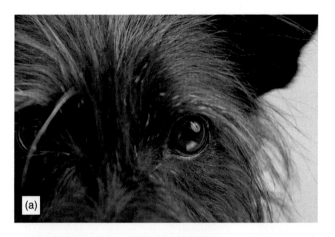
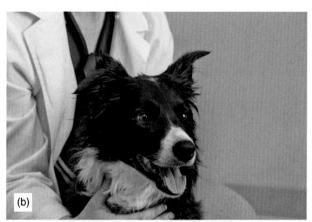

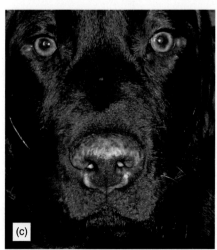
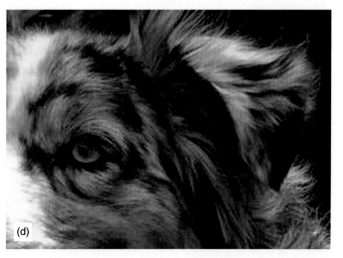

Figure 11.31 (a) Deep brown iris in a canine patient. Source: Courtesy of the Media Resources Department at Midwestern University (b) Medium brown irises in a dog. Source: Courtesy of the Media Resources Department at Midwestern University. (c) Hazel irises in a canine patient. Source: Courtesy of Jackie Kucskar, DVM. (d) Crystal blue iris in a dog.

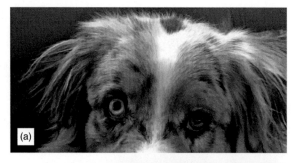

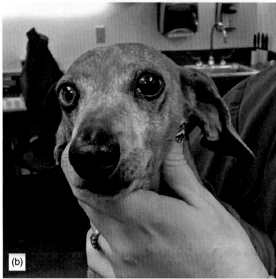

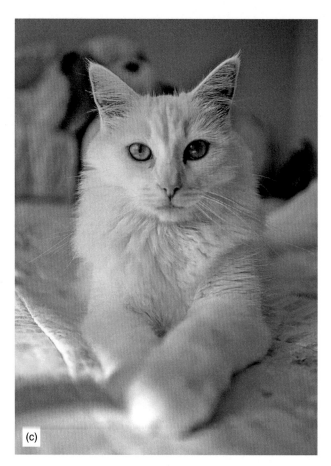

Figure 11.32 (a) Heterochromic irises in a dog with OD blue and OS brown. Source: Courtesy of Amanda Rappaport. (b) Heterochromic irises in a dog with OD blue–gray and OS deep brown. (c) Heterochromic irises in a cat with OD blue and OS hazel. Source: Courtesy of Kat Mackin.

the side of the blue eye [94] (Figure 11.32a and b). Dogs are not the only species that have heterochromic irises, and cats may also display this feature (Figure 11.32c). When they do, they are also more likely to be deaf if they are white-coated with at least one blue eye [94].

Like cats, dogs may also develop iris nevi, iris melanomas, persistent pupillary membranes, and colobomas. See Section 3.2.6 for more information on identifying these on the physical examination.

11.3.7 Evaluating the Pupils

The pupil is an intentional defect in the iris, the muscles of which control its size and shape [94]. Different species have different pupil shapes at rest. Dogs, for instance, have round pupils compared with the vertical slit of the cat's pupil. (Figure 11.33).

As ambient lighting dims, pupils dilate to increase the amount of light that enters the eye [94] (Figure 11.34).

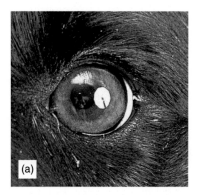

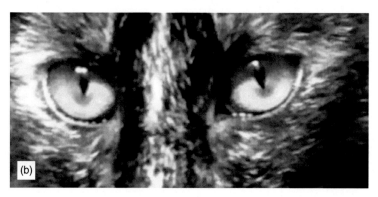

Figure 11.33 (a) Normal rounded shape of a dog pupil. Source: Courtesy of the Media Resources Department at Midwestern University. (b) Normal vertical slit shape of a cat pupil. Source: Courtesy of Leigh Ann Howard.

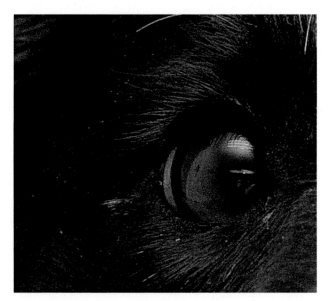

Figure 11.34 Mydriatic pupil in a dog due to decreased ambient lighting. Compare the pupil size of this patient with that in Figure 11.33a. Source: Courtesy of the Media Resources Department at Midwestern University.

Pupils also dilate when the sympathetic nervous system is activated [94], although in the author's experience, this sympathetic drive is much less apparent in a dog than cat.

Pupils should be symmetrical. When they are not, the patient is said to have anisocoria [94] (Figure 11.35a). The presence of anisocoria may indicate underlying neurologic dysfunction [38, 39, 94]. However, anisocoria can also be non-pathologic, induced by a patient's positioning relative to a light source. For example, anisocoria may be present in a dog that is seated beside a window in broad daylight: the pupil nearest the window may appear slightly smaller than the contralateral one (Figure 11.35b) [94, 96].

11.3.8 Assessing Ocular Reflexes

See Section 3.2.8 to review how to perform the following tests [44, 96]:

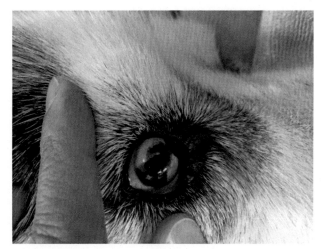

Figure 11.36 This patient presented for hyphema following a traumatic event in which it sustained blunt force trauma to the head. Source: Courtesy of Shirley Yang.

- the pupillary light reflex (PLR): cranial nerves II and III (the optic and oculomotor nerves);
- the palpebral reflex: cranial nerves V and VII (the trigeminal and facial nerves);
- the menace response: cranial nerves II and VII (the optic and facial nerves).

11.3.9 Assessing the Anterior Chamber

The anterior chamber of the eye is a fluid-filled space between the cornea and the lens. Because aqueous humor is a clear fluid, the anterior chamber should appear transparent when a slit lamp is used to shine a light beam through it. Any opacities typically indicate underlying pathology such as the introduction of abnormal fluid within that space [94].

Blunt force trauma to the eye may cause hyphema, blood within the anterior chamber [97] (Figure 11.36). Hyphema may also result from coagulopathies or vasculitis, as from tick-borne diseases [94]. When hyphema is present, it may partially or completely fill the anterior

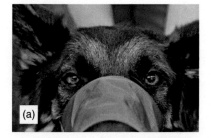

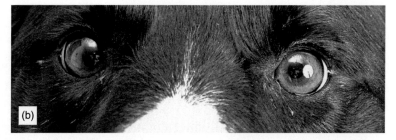

Figure 11.35 (a) This patient presented to the clinic with anisocoria. Note that the pupil associated with OS is larger than that associated with OD. Primary neurological disease was suspected. (b) Note the asymmetry in pupil size. The right pupil is larger than the left pupil. In this patient, anisocoria was not due to underlying neuropathy. Anisocoria was induced by the angle of the camera and the position of the light source, which came from the patient's left side. Source: Courtesy of the Media Resources Department at Midwestern University.

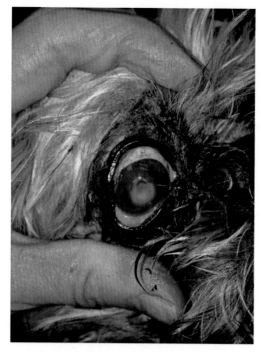

Figure 11.37 This patient presented for a fluorescein stain-positive corneal ulcer with hypopyon. Note the creamy material deep to the cornea around the perimeter of the corneal defect. Source: Courtesy of Paola Bazan Steyling, DVM.

chamber. The larger the quantity of the hemorrhage, the more likely it is that the blood will be clotted [94].

Blood is not the only substance that can accumulate within the anterior chamber. White blood cells may also accumulate (Figure 11.37). When hypopyon occurs, it is typically the result of intraocular sepsis as from progressive corneal ulceration or uveitis. Although hypopyon is typically bacterial in origin, it can be sterile, as occurs with certain types of ocular neoplasia, such as lymphoma. [94, 98, 99].

In addition to the abnormal accumulation of fluid and cells within the anterior chamber, adhesions may develop that can be seen with the naked eye. For example, adhesions called anterior synechiae frequently form between the cornea and the iris following a bout of uveitis [44, 46, 56, 98, 99].

11.3.10 Assessing the Lens

The lens should be evaluated for the presence of opacities called cataracts (Figure 11.38). See Section 3.2.10 to review how cataracts are named. Cataracts occur more frequently in dogs than cats. In particular, their onset tends to be acute in diabetic dogs owing to the accumulation of sorbitol within the lens [100–103].

In addition to cataracts, each lens should also be evaluated for subluxations. Traumatic injuries such as blunt force trauma to the head can displace the lens, which can in turn obstruct the outflow tract of aqueous humor [43].

11.3.11 Introduction to Fundoscopy

See Section 3.2.11 to review the purpose of fundoscopy and the basic fundic anatomy.

Recall that the tapetum lucidum is a hemispherical zone that is dorsal to the optic disc. It intensifies the light that falls upon the photoreceptors, improving vision when ambient lighting is dim. This is what creates "eyeshine," the apparent glow of the pupils when light is directed at patients with this built-in feature (Figure 11.39) [43, 44, 46]. The tapetum lucidum of the adult dog varies in color from blue–green to yellow–green to yellow–tan. It is purple–blue in puppies less than 2–4 months of age [43, 44, 46].

In addition to appreciating the tapetum lucidum during fundoscopy, the clinician should assess the retinal

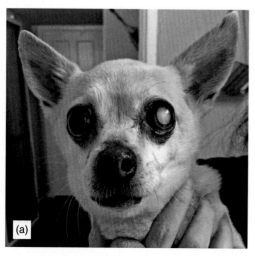
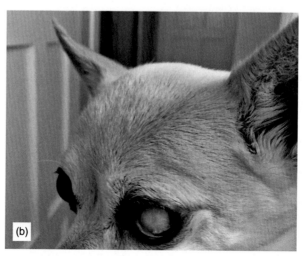

Figure 11.38 (a) Mature cortical cataract OS, viewed head-on. Source: Courtesy of Lai-Ting Torres. (b) Mature cortical cataract OS, viewed from the side. Source: Courtesy of Lai-Ting Torres. (Continued)

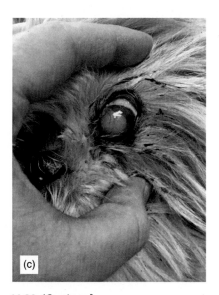
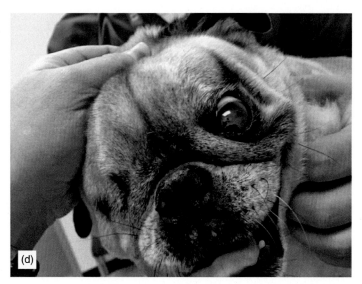

Figure 11.38 (*Continued*)
(c) Mature cortical cataract OS. Note that this patient also has concurrent corneal neovascularization OS that is unrelated to the cataract.
(d) Mature cortical cataract OS. Note that this patient also has concurrent pigmentary keratitis OS that is unrelated to the cataract.

vasculature. Dogs typically have 3–5 retinal veins and several smaller retinal arteries. The former may course over the optic disc; the latter may partially join a ring near its center [46, 104]. The clinician should consider the thickness of the vasculature. If vessels that are thinner than anticipated, retinal atrophy may be present [46, 104, 105]. Similarly, the clinician should pay attention to the course that the vasculature takes. Vessels should not be tortuous. When they are, the patient should be evaluated for systemic hypertension [46, 104, 105].

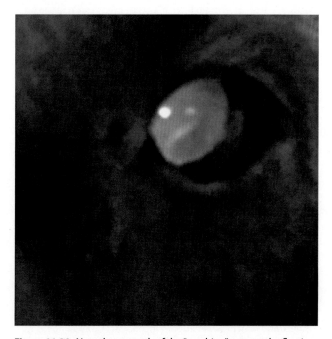

Figure 11.39 Note the strength of the "eyeshine" or tapetal reflection in this patient's left eye. Source: Courtesy of Elizabeth Robbins, DVM

11.3.12 Fundoscopy and Direct Ophthalmoscopy

See Section 3.2.12 to review the concept of direct ophthalmoscopy [105, 106].

To perform direct ophthalmoscopy, recall that the clinician should stand at a flexed arm's length from the patient and direct the light into the patient's eye. He may then look through the viewing aperture to catch the tapetal reflection. Once this reflection is captured, he should move in with the ophthalmoscope until approximately 5 cm away from the patient's eye [105–109] (Figure 11.40).

Recall the limitations of direct ophthalmoscopy: only a fraction of the fundus will be visible: typically the central optic disc. As needed, the clinician may adjust the diopter setting 1–3 diopters each way from zero to crisp up the view [105, 106, 108].

For safety purposes, the clinician should get used to evaluating the patient's right eye with his right eye and the patient's left eye with his left eye. This minimizes "nose to nose" contact, which increases the chance that the clinician will sustain a bite to the face.

11.3.13 Fundoscopy and Indirect Ophthalmoscopy

See Section 3.2.13 to review the concept of indirect ophthalmoscopy [106].

To perform indirect ophthalmoscopy, recall that the clinician begins by standing at a flexed arm's length from the patient. The clinician then places a strong light source at eye level alongside his head. With the light source maintaining its position alongside his head, the clinician should direct the light at the patient's eye to catch the tapetal reflection. Once the tapetal reflection is captured, the clinician must bring the lens in between himself and

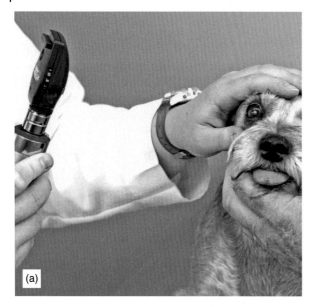
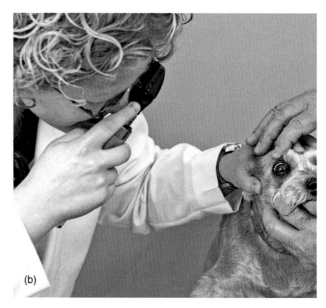

Figure 11.40 (a) Using direct ophthalmoscopy to begin the eye examination. Note that the clinician starts the examination by directing the light source into the patient's eye from a distance. (b) Once the tapetal reflex is captured, it is appropriate for the clinician to move in toward the patient with the ophthalmoscope. Ultimately, the clinician will be standing cheek-to-cheek with the patient with the ophthalmoscope in between. Good restraint is important to protect the clinician from injury in the event that the patient becomes spooked. Source (a), (b): Courtesy of the Media Resources Department at Midwestern University.

the patient. For stability, the clinician may rest the hand that is holding the lens against the patient's brow [106, 108, 109] (Figure 11.41).

With the lens in place and perpendicular to the light source, the fundic image should be visible, albeit inverted [106]. The clinician may then adjust his view by moving the lens toward and away from the eye until the eyelids and iris disappear from view, allowing the fundic image to fill the lens [106].

Recall that a distinct advantage of indirect ophthalmoscopy is that it provides the clinician with a larger field of view. This allows the clinician to perform a more thorough examination of the fundus [106].

11.4 The Ears

The ears consist of the pinnae, the external ear canal, the tympanic membrane, and the middle and inner ear, all of which work in concert with the central nervous system through a series of intricate signaling pathways to confer the special sense of hearing [44, 110, 111].

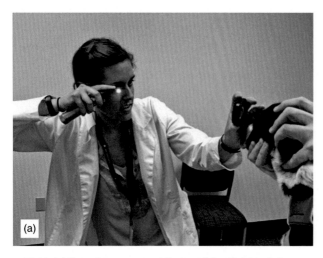
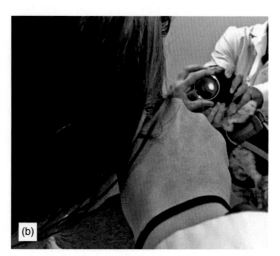

Figure 11.41 (a) Note the proper positioning of the clinician, light source, lens, and patient when attempting indirect ophthalmoscopy. (b) An over-the-shoulder angle to demonstrate the proper positioning of the clinician, light source, lens, and patient when attempting indirect ophthalmoscopy.

Dogs have a fairly broad range for hearing, from 67 Hz to 45 kHz. This is a smaller range than in cats, but is better than in humans, whose range is from 64 Hz to 23 kHz. Dogs are therefore able to detect higher frequency sounds than people, but with little difference between the two species when evaluating sounds at low frequency [112].

Recall from Section 3.3 that in order to assess hearing in the dog objectively, the patient must undergo electrodiagnostic testing such as the brain-stem auditory evoked response (BAER) [44, 113–116]. This can be performed as early as 5–6 weeks of age. If deafness is confirmed, the client should be instructed to remove that patient from the breeding pool because congenital deafness is often hereditary [95].

When examining the external ear of any new patient, the clinician should get into the habit of documenting ear carriage. Recall from Section 9.7 that ears represent one form of body language that dogs may use to communicate both inter- and intraspecies. However, ear carriage is also often breed-dependent (Figure 11.42).

In addition to assessing the patient's ear carriage, the clinician should evaluate each pinna for integrity and note if any wounds or lacerations are present. Superficial curvilinear lacerations are likely to be self-induced scratches that, if present, may indicate pruritus associated with ear canal disease.

The clinician should also palpate each pinna for warmth. If one ear is palpably warmer than the other, then the warmer ear may be inflamed, as from an underlying infection.

The dorsal and ventral aspects and also the margins of both pinnae should be evaluated (Figure 11.43a–c). In particular, the clinician should look for hypotrichosis, alopecia, and/or crusting (Figure 11.43d). Crusting may indicate fungal or parasitic diseases such as ringworm or sarcoptic mange [117, 118].

Next, the clinician inspects the external ear canal (Figure 11.44). In certain breeds of dog, such as the Poodle and Schnauzer, the entrance to the external ear canal tends to be obstructed by fur (Figure 11.45) [44]. This is considered normal for these breeds. However, this abundance of fur may contribute to otitis externa by decreasing aeration of the ear canal and by helping to retain moisture and debris. To avoid these concerns, some clients elect to have both ear canals plucked prophylactically.

When examining the external ear canal, the clinician should take note of any of the following as they may be signs that there is underlying aural pathology:

- redness (Figure 11.46a);
- stenosis (narrowing) of the entrance into the external ear canal (Figure 11.46b);
- aural discharge (Figure 11.46c and d);
- aural odor.

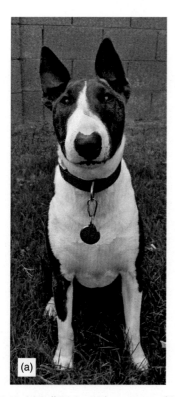
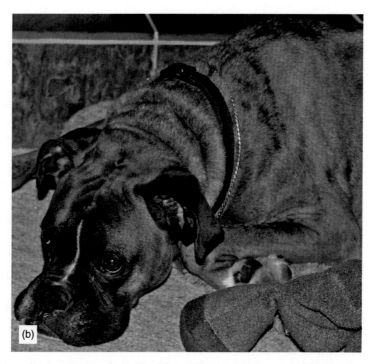

Figure 11.42 (a) Bull Terrier with erect ears. (b) Natural ear carriage in a boxer dog. The ears have not been cropped. Source: Courtesy of Symmantha Page. (Continued)

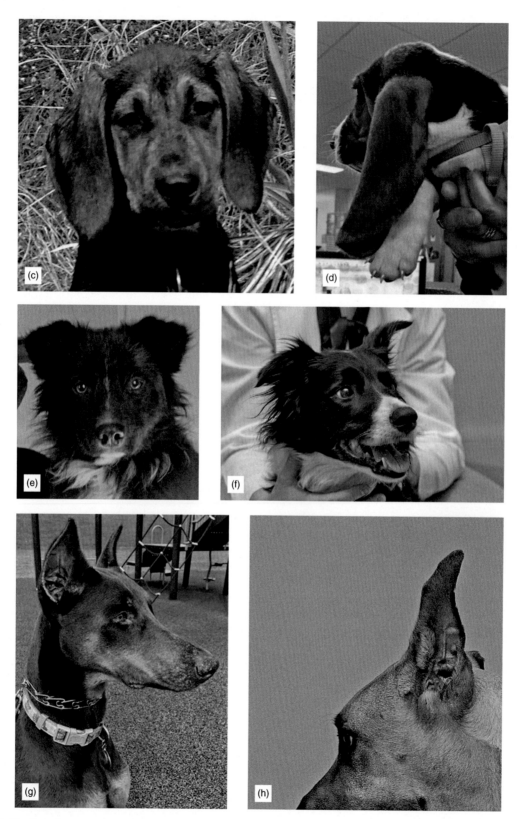

Figure 11.42 *(Continued)*
(c) Floppy ears are typically seen in Beagles. Source: Courtesy of Lauren Beren. (d) This Basset Hound puppy also has breed-characteristic floppy ears. Note that, during puppyhood, the ears are nearly as long as the limbs. (e) This patient is demonstrating "button ears." This is commonly seen in terrier breeds and in terrier crosses. Source: Courtesy of Lauren Beren. (f) This Border Collie is demonstrating the cocked or semi-pricked ear carriage that is typical for the breed. Source: Courtesy of the Media Resources Department at Midwestern University. (g) This Doberman Pinscher has cropped ears, which are written into the breed standard. Source: Courtesy of Courtney Keller. (h) This Great Dane is also sporting the cropped ear look.

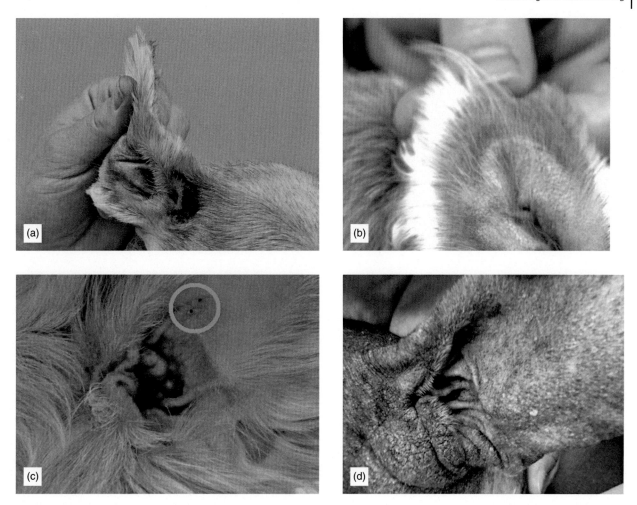

Figure 11.43 (a) Evaluating the margins of a normal ear, devoid of lesions. Source: Courtesy of the Media Resources Department at Midwestern University. (b) Evaluating the ventral aspect of a normal ear, devoid of lesions. Source: Courtesy of the Media Resources Department at Midwestern University. (c) Note these two subtle punctate lesions on the ventral aspect of a pinna. (d) Note the appreciable amount of crusting along the ventral aspect of this pinna. The crusts encircle the entrance to the external ear canal.

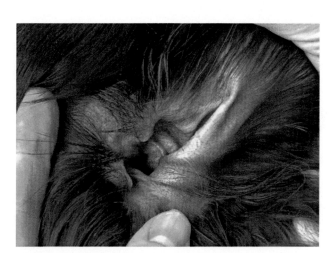

Figure 11.44 Evaluating the external ear canal of a normal ear. Source: Courtesy of the Media Resources Department at Midwestern University.

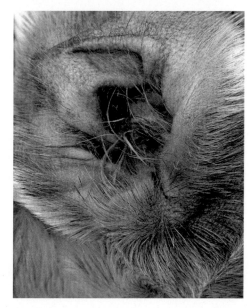

Figure 11.45 Excess fur at the entrance to the external ear canal in a Miniature Schnauzer. Source: Courtesy of the Media Resources Department at Midwestern University.

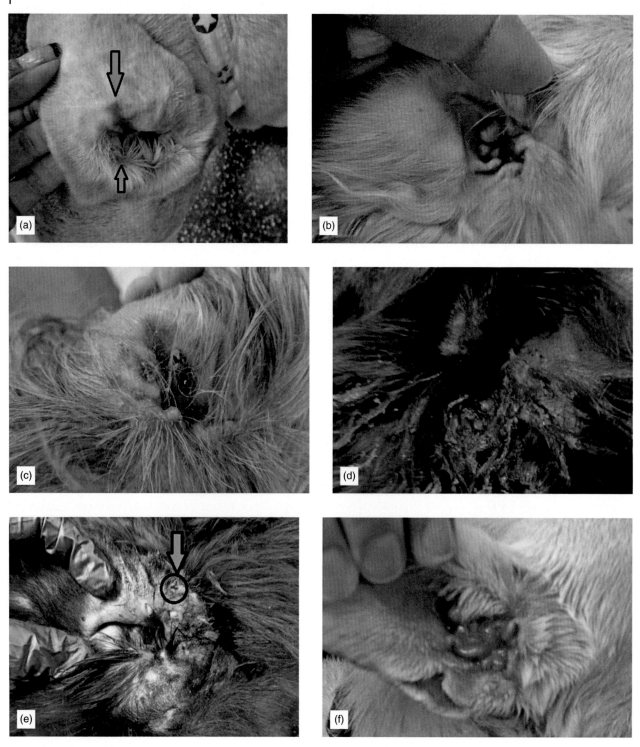

Figure 11.46 (a) Note the redness associated with the entrance to the external ear canal. Source: Courtesy of Patricia Bennett, DVM. (b) Note the stenosis associated with the entrance to the external ear canal. (c) Moderate amount of chunky tan exudate arising from the external ear canal. (d) Copious amount of brown exudate that is clumped in mats to the fur surrounding the external ear canal. (e) Freshly bleeding superficial erosion along the ventrolateral margin of the pinna. (f) Copious purulent discharge associated with a stenotic ear canal.

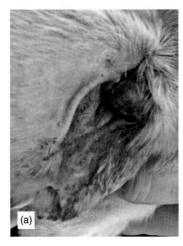 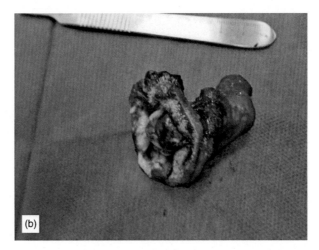

Figure 11.47 (a) Grossly visible mass occluding the entrance to the external ear canal. (b) Post-operative view of the excised aural mass depicted in (a). Note how extensive it is. Source (a), (b): Courtesy of Samantha Thurman, DVM.

Small amounts of cerumen can be normal. However, the following types of discharge should not be observed:

- frank blood (Figure 11.46e);
- purulent material (Figure 11.46f);
- dark brown, "coffee-ground" debris.

Although more commonly seen in kittens, ear mites can be a presenting complaint in canine patients, particularly those that have been in close living quarters with an infected cat [119].

The author has made it a habit to smell each ear even if it looks clean. This has allowed her to appreciate the typical scent that she associates with different types of infection. In no way does the author's olfaction preclude the need for otic cytology; however, it provides a starting point in terms of the anticipated outcome. In the author's experience, yeast otitis smells slightly sweet compared with the rancid, rotting odor associated with bacterial otitis.

The vertical ear canal should be palpated to assess for erythema, pain, and compressibility. A normal vertical canal should not be painful on palpation, yet should be slightly compressible, without eliciting a squishing or sloshing sound. If the vertical canal is not compressible, it may indicate the presence of a space-occupying mass. Sometimes these masses are visible at the entrance to the external ear canal (Figure 11.47); sometimes they are not. If compression of the vertical canal elicits a whooshing sound, then the ear canal is likely to contain fluid, which is abnormal [44].

It is impossible to examine the horizontal ear canal without an otoscope. There is an approximately 75° bend between the vertical and horizontal ear canals that leads to the tympanic membrane [120]. Recall that the patient needs to be restrained effectively by the veterinary team in order to perform the otoscopic examination successfully. The restrainer should avoid the tendency to tilt the head and neck to the side, because doing so can "crimp" the external ear canal, in effect obstructing the view.

Each pinna should be gently lifted cranio-dorso-laterally to straighten the bend between the vertical and horizontal ear canals. At that point, an otoscope can be placed in the entrance to the external ear canal, taking care to have it equipped with a cone of the correct tip diameter and length. The patient should be given a moment to acclimate. At that point, the otoscope can be advanced while continuing to maintain gentle but firm traction on the pinna [106, 111] (Figure 11.48). The horizontal ear canal can be assessed for discharge, erythema, pain, and stenosis.

The tympanic membrane should be transparent and intact. It consists of a grayish blue pars tensa and a more dorsal, pinkish, elastic pars flaccida [106, 111]. In cases of chronic otitis media, the tympanic membrane may become an opaque, cloudy white. If there is fluid build-up in the middle ear, the tympanic membrane may also bulge forward into the horizontal ear canal. A ruptured ear drum is visible as an overt tear in the tympanic membrane [111, 121]. The novice may have difficulty visualizing the tympanum and should refer to Section 3.3 to troubleshoot potential problem areas.

If ear cleaning is required to obtain a better view, the clinician should take care to collect any and all ear samples prior to cleaning. If the ear drum cannot be visualized prior to cleaning, sterile saline should be used as a cleaning agent because it is safe to come into contact with the middle or inner ear in the event that the tympanic membrane has ruptured.

11.5 The Nose

The nose plays an important role in respiration and olfaction, and should be evaluated at each visit. Each patient should have two symmetrical nares, and a cobblestone appearance to the nasal planum (Figure 11.49).

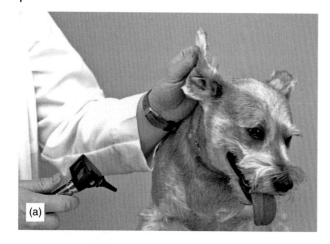

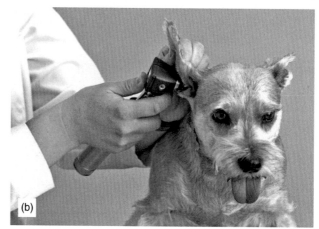

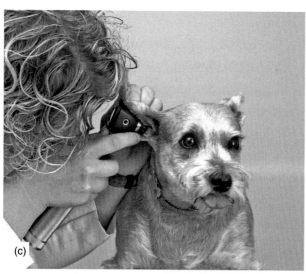

Figure 11.48 (a) Beginning the otoscopic examination by lifting the pinna. (b) Gently applying traction on the pinna to straighten the ear canal. (c) Straightening the ear canal to visualize the tympanum. Note that this is an unusually cooperative patient. It is not typically safe to perform an otoscopic examination without restraint. Source (a)–(c): Courtesy of the Media Resources Department at Midwestern University.

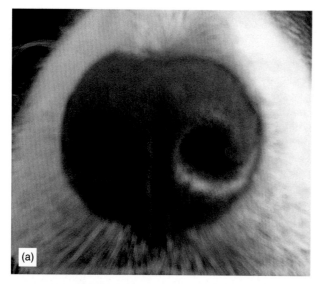

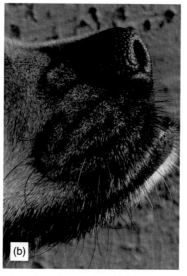

Figure 11.49 (a) Note the normal appearance of two symmetrical nares in a dog. Source: Courtesy of the Media Resources Department at Midwestern University. (b) Note the normal appearance of the nose when observed in the profile view. Source: Courtesy of Kara N. Jones.

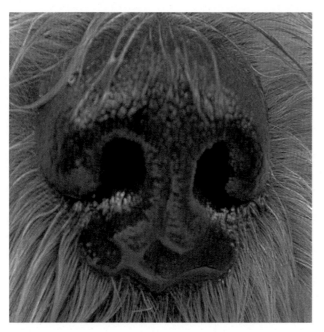

Figure 11.50 Bilateral serous nasal discharge in a canine patient. Source: Courtesy of the Media Resources Department at Midwestern University.

A palpably moist nose is considered normal. However, the nares themselves should be evaluated for gross discharge. The presence of discharge can be normal or abnormal, unilateral or bilateral (Figure 11.50). Serous discharge may be the result of allergic rhinitis. Bilaterally symmetrical serous discharge could also indicate the development of volume overload in a

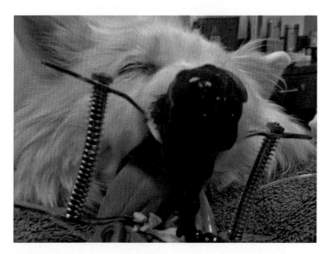

Figure 11.51 Severe epistaxis in a patient under general anesthesia. The patient had previously presented for intermittent epistaxis due to aggressive nasal tumors that were subsequently biopsied. Source: Courtesy of Elizabeth Robbins, DVM.

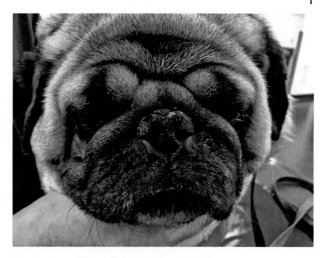

Figure 11.52 Bilaterally stenotic nares in a Pug.

hospitalized patient that is receiving an excess of intravenous fluids [122, 123]. It is abnormal to see mucoid, mucopurulent, and hemorrhagic nasal discharges (Figure 11.51).

Airflow through each nostril should be assessed by placing a glass slide in front of the nose. Assuming that the patient is breathing through its nostrils rather than panting, the breath should fog up the slide in two concentric circles, one per nare. If one side lacks a circle of fog on the slide, then airflow is minimal to nonexistent through that side of the upper respiratory tract. Alternatively, the clinician may hold a tuft of cotton in front of each nostril and assess for movement of the cotton [122]. Certain breeds of dogs, in particular the brachycephalic breeds, are known for having reduced airflow through the nostrils due to stenotic nares [122] (Figure 11.52).

The bridge of the nose should also be assessed for asymmetry and pain on palpation (Figure 11.53). The clinician should evaluate the mucocutaneous junction where the nasal planum meets the bridge of the nose. Any depigmentation, abrasion, or ulceration should be noted. Solar dermatosis, especially in white dogs, along with squamous cell carcinoma, pemphigus, systemic and discoid lupus erythematosis, and dermatophytosis can yield abnormal physical examination findings in this location.

11.6 The Extra-Oral Examination

The clinician should begin the extra-oral examination by evaluating the patient for facial symmetry (Figure 11.54).

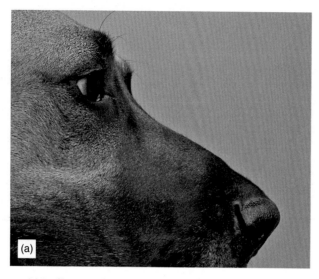
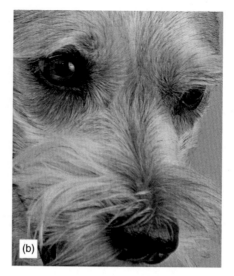

Figure 11.53 (a) Profile view of a Great Dane, demonstrating its grossly normal bridge of the nose. (b) Head-on view of a Miniature Schnauzer, demonstrating its grossly normal bridge of the nose. Source (a), (b): Courtesy of the Media Resources Department at Midwestern University.

In addition, the clinician should determine the structural stability of the skull and facial bones by the following (Figure 11.55):

- palpating over the maxilla;
- palpating over the zygomatic arches;
- palpating over the temporomandibular joints;
- palpating the angular processes of the mandible;
- palpating the ventral aspect of the left and right bodies of the mandible for fractures and/or symphyseal instability;
- palpating the intermandibular space.

Further, the clinician should palpate the submandibular lymph nodes and the mandibular salivary glands. The submandibular lymph nodes are caudoventral to the angle of the mandible. In order to feel them, the clinician should slide his fingers down the angle of the mandible to the ventrolateral neck. Grasping a generous amount of skin bilaterally between the thumb and index fingers, the clinician should then slide his fingers from deep to superficial. This should allow the submandibular lymph nodes to "slip" through his fingers [124] (Figure 11.56).

There are normally two, and sometimes three, submandibular lymph nodes on each side. Rarely, up to five nodes per side have been documented. [125] When two submandibular lymph nodes are present, typically the smaller of the two is dorsal to the linguofacial vein. Ventral to this vein is the second node, which typically measures 2.0 cm long and 1.0 cm wide [125]. When more than two submandibular lymph nodes are present, the single ventral node is most often the one that becomes a multiple [125].

Note that the groupings and numbers of nodes may vary from the left to the right side of the patient: groupings are

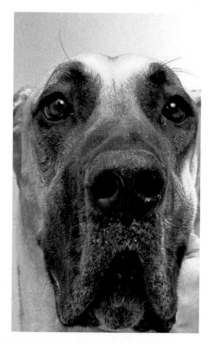

Figure 11.54 Evaluating the head and face for symmetry. There is no apparent facial asymmetry in this patient that would suggest myopathies or neuropathies. Source: Courtesy of the Media Resources Department at Midwestern University.

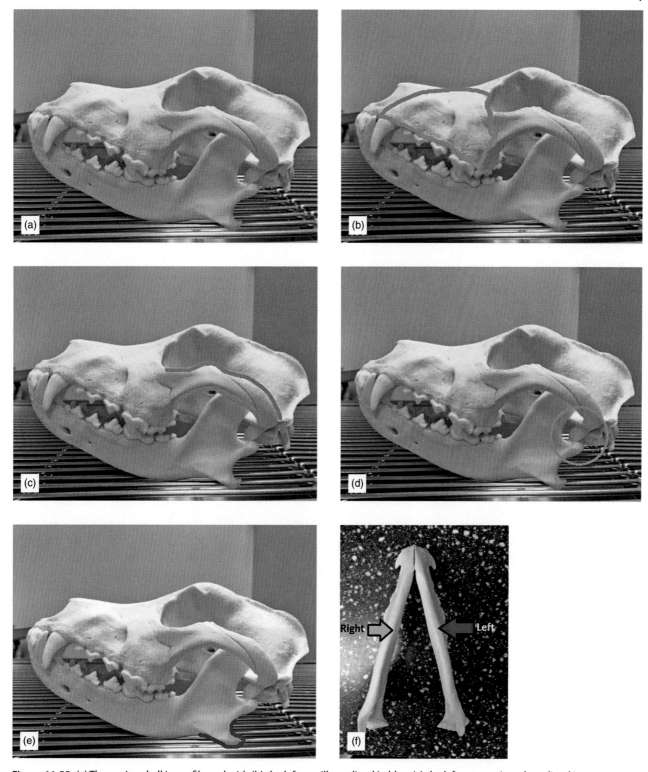

Figure 11.55 (a) The canine skull in profile and with (b) the left maxilla outlined in blue, (c) the left zygomatic arch outlined in orange, (d) the left temporomandibular joint circled in blue, and (e) the left angular process of the mandible outlined in dark blue. Ventral aspect of the canine mandible with (f) the left and right bodies identified and (Continued)

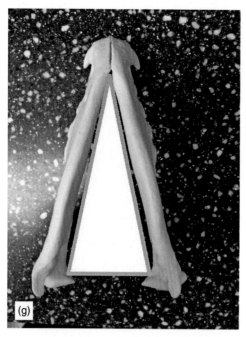

bilaterally identical in only 44.4% of specimens examined [125]. Regardless of the number of submandibular lymph nodes, all are located cranial to the mandibular salivary gland, which is also palpable in the normal dog. Finding one or more enlarged submandibular lymph nodes may raise the clinician's suspicion that there is underlying pathology. Dental disease, for instance, commonly results in lymphadenomegaly.

Like the submandibular lymph nodes, the mandibular salivary gland should be discrete, smooth, and supple. Changes in size, texture, and consistency, especially when asymmetric, should be a red flag that underlying pathology is probable.

Another important aspect of the extra-oral examination is to evaluate the lip folds (Figure 11.57). In particular, the clinician should assess for swelling, crusting, erosions, or ulcerations.

Only after all of the above have been evaluated and documented is the clinician ready to lift the lips and dive into the intra-oral examination.

Figure 11.55 (*Continued*)
(g) the intermandibular space outlined by a triangle.

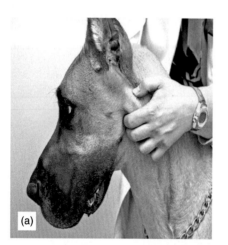

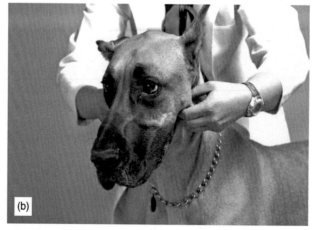

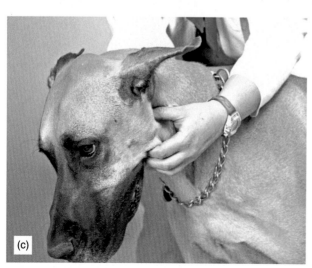

Figure 11.56 (a) Side view and (b) front view of grasping a skin fold caudoventral to the angle of the mandible. (c) Digging out the submandibular lymph nodes and allowing them to "blip" through the clinician's fingers. Source (a)–(c): Courtesy of the Media Resources Department at Midwestern University.

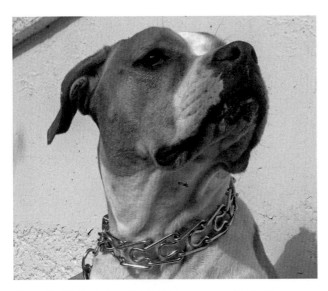

Figure 11.57 Evaluating the lip folds in a normal patient. Source: Courtesy of Kiefer Hazard.

11.7 The Intra-Oral Examination

The ultimate goal of the intra-oral examination is to open the patient's mouth. However, the intra-oral examination encompasses much more than that: it is designed to assess the mucous membranes, dentition, gingiva, mucosa, tongue, sublingual space, palate, and oropharynx.

11.7.1 Assessing Mucous Membrane Color

Mucous membrane color assists with the clinician's assessment of circulatory status. Normal mucous membranes are a healthy pink color (Figure 11.58a); however, some patients with lentigo have mottled black pigment throughout (Figure 11.58b) – this is also considered normal. By contrast, white or pale mucous membranes indicate that the patient may be experiencing shock or that it is significantly anemic (Figure 11.58c). Cyanotic mucous membranes typically confer hypoxia. Cherry red mucous membranes are classic for carbon monoxide toxicosis, and icteric mucous membranes reflect

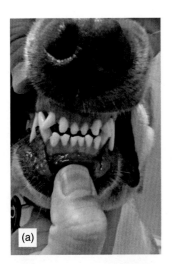

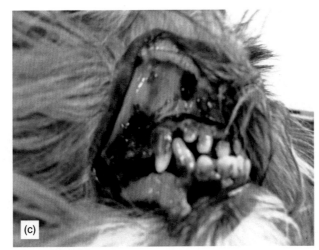

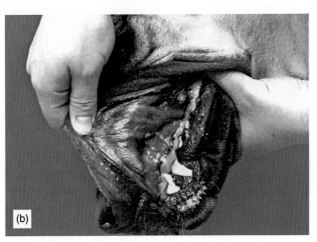

Figure 11.58 (a) Note the healthy pink color that is associated with normal mucous membranes. (b) Lifting the lips with fingertips to display another version of normal pigmentation of the gums of this Great Dane. Note also that changes in pigment can extend to the buccal mucosa. Source: Courtesy of the Media Resources Department at Midwestern University. (c) Note the abnormal pale pink color associated with abnormal mucous membranes. This patient also has evidence of petechiations and blood clots that are suggestive of an underlying coagulopathy.

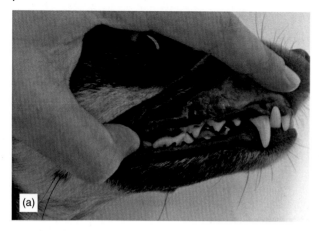

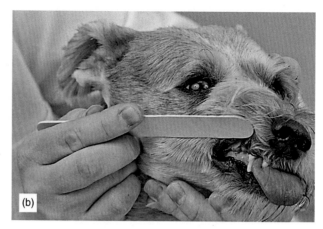

Figure 11.59 (a) Evaluating mucous membrane color in this tolerant patient by the clinician lifting its lips with his fingertips. (b) Lifting the lips with a tongue depressor in a dog of unknown temperament. This is an easy way to spare fingertips from being nipped if the patient objects to having its gums assessed. Source: Courtesy of the Media Resources Department at Midwestern University.

underlying hyperbilirubinemia as from intravascular hemolysis or hepatopathy. If there are petechiations or ecchymoses within the mucous membranes, coagulopathies are a potential concern.

Mucous membranes should be moist. If they are tacky or stick to the clinician's fingers, then the patient is likely to be dehydrated. See Section 10.3 to review additional methods by which dehydration may be assessed.

Depending upon the patient's temperament, the clinician may use fingers or a tongue depressor to lift the lip folds to assess mucous membrane color and moistness (Figure 11.59).

11.7.2 Assessing Capillary Refill Time

See Section 3.6.2 to review the appropriate technique for assessing capillary refill time (CRT). A normal CRT is

1–2 seconds on average. If a patient is in shock or dehydrated, the CRT will be prolonged.

11.7.3 Examining the Mucosa

The clinician should assess the buccal and alveolar mucosa for redness, erosions, ulcerations, and masses (Figure 11.60).

11.7.4 Examining the Gingiva

The clinician should evaluate for gingivitis. If present, the clinician should note whether the distribution is focal or generalized (Figure 11.61).

During an intra-oral examination, gingivitis is typically classified as focal versus generalized. However, during dental charting under general anesthesia, each individual

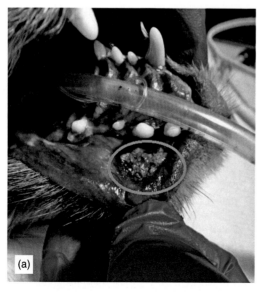

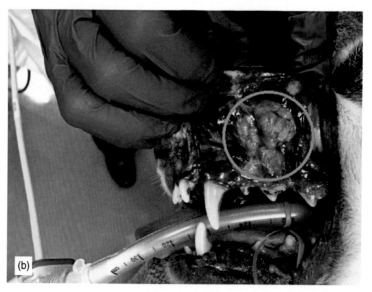

Figure 11.60 Lesions buccal to (a) the left maxillary canine tooth and (b) the left maxillary second premolar tooth. Source (a), (b): Courtesy of Samantha Thurman, DVM.

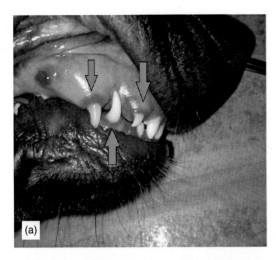

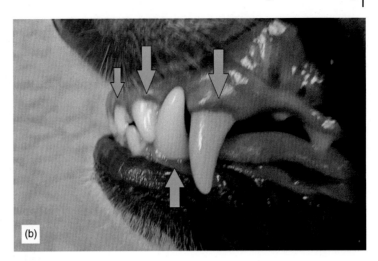

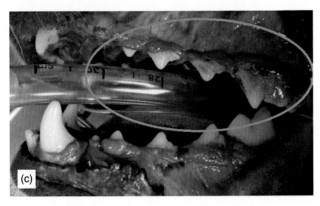

Figure 11.61 (a) Focal gingivitis associated with teething. Source: Courtesy of Jule Schweighoefer. (b) Focal gingivitis in an adult dog secondary to dental disease. Source: Courtesy of Sarah Ciamello. (c) Generalized gingivitis associated with the left maxillary dental arcade. Source: Courtesy of Patricia Bennett, DVM.

tooth can be assigned a gingival index (GI) score. There is no universal standardization in veterinary medicine with regard to the gingival index score. However, the author has adapted the following based upon others' approaches that have been documented in the human and veterinary medical literature [126, 127]:

- GI 0: Normal gingiva.
- GI 1: Mild inflammation. Slight color change and edema. No bleeding on probing.
- GI 2: Moderate inflammation. Redness. Moderate edema. Bleeding on probing.
- GI 3: Severe inflammation, marked redness, edema and ulceration. Tendency for spontaneous bleeding.

Note that in order to assign the GI score, the clinician is required to probe the gum line surrounding each tooth. Because this is not a procedure that awake patients will tolerate, the GI score is typically reserved for dental charting under anesthesia. This allows the veterinary team to keep track of trends and progress for each individual tooth.

The gingiva should also be evaluated for gingival hyperplasia (Figure 11.62a). This may be breed-related: boxers have been overreported in the literature compared with other breeds. Gingival hyperplasia can also be due to pharmacologic therapy: it has been triggered by the use of amlodipine [128, 129] and cyclosporine [130].

Sometimes it is difficult to distinguish gingival hyperplasia from other forms of gingival tumors, including malignancies. Biopsies are often indicated (Figure 11.62b and c).

11.7.5 Assessing the Dentition

The clinician should also assess the dentition. In order to evaluate the dentition properly, the clinician needs first to understand the dental formula for the canine patient:

- The dental formula for an immature dog, meaning one with deciduous dentition, is [131–134]

$$2 \times (I3/3, C1/1, P3/3) = 28 \text{ teeth total}$$

- The dental formula for an adult dog, meaning one with permanent dentition, is [131–134]

$$2 \times (I3/3, C1/1, P4/4, M2/3) = 42 \text{ teeth total}$$

Deciduous teeth tend to be smaller than permanent teeth (Figure 11.63). In the dog, the deciduous incisors and canines erupt between 3 and 4 weeks of age and the deciduous premolars between 4 and 12 weeks of age. Eruption of permanent teeth begins with the permanent incisors and canine teeth between 3 and 4 months of age. Eruption of the permanent premolars takes place between 4 and 6 months of age and eruption of permanent molars between 5 and 7 months of age [135].

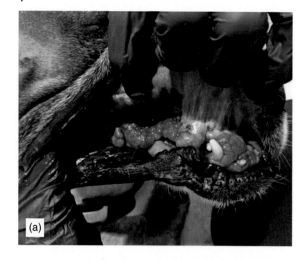

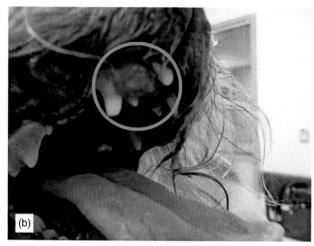

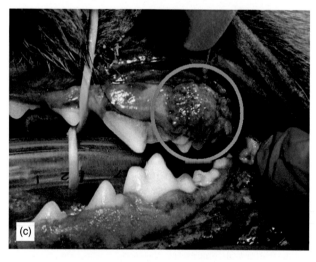

Figure 11.62 (a) Extensive gingival hyperplasia. Source: Courtesy of Elizabeth Robbins, DVM. (b) Gingival mass between this patient's right maxillary canine and third premolar tooth. Source: Courtesy of Patricia Bennett, DVM. (c) Extensive, ulcerated gingival growth. Source: Courtesy of Elizabeth Robbins, DVM.

Because eruption of permanent teeth is gradual, it is typical for puppies to exhibit age-appropriate mixed dentition: both deciduous and permanent teeth can be present in the mouth simultaneously (Figure 11.64).

To facilitate the identification of teeth in veterinary medicine, the modified Triadan system of nomenclature was developed [132, 134, 136, 137]. Each tooth is given a three-digit identification number. The dental arcade that the tooth is in dictates what the first digit in the three-digit identification number will be:

- Every tooth in the right maxillary arcade has an identification number that starts with 1.

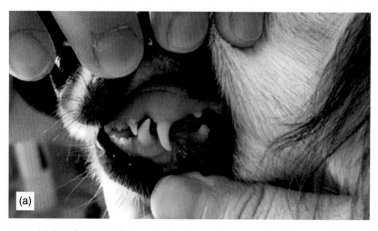

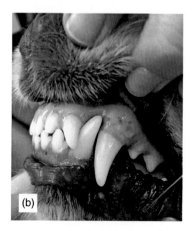

Figure 11.63 (a) Deciduous teeth in a puppy. Source: Courtesy of Shirley Yang, DVM. (b) Permanent teeth in an adult dog. Source: Courtesy of Elizabeth Robbins, DVM.

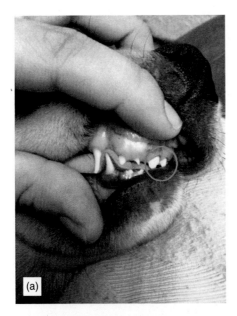

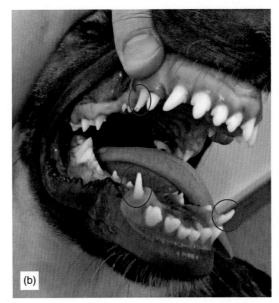

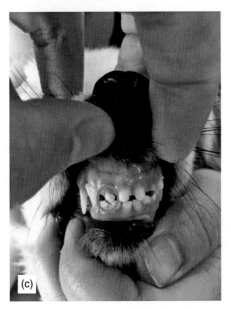

Figure 11.64 Age-appropriate mixed dentition. (a) The permanent maxillary incisors are circled in blue. Source: Courtesy of Lauren Beren. (b) The deciduous canine teeth are circled in blue. Source: Courtesy of Jule Schweighoefer. (c) Note that the deciduous maxillary incisor that is circled in blue is loose and is about to become dislodged. Source: Courtesy of Shirley Yang, DVM.

- Every tooth in the left maxillary arcade has an identification number that starts with 2.
- Every tooth in the left mandibular arcade has an identification number that starts with 3.
- Every tooth in the right mandibular arcade has an identification number that starts with 4.

The teeth are then numbered beginning from midline. For instance, each arcade has three incisors. So, in the right maxillary arcade, the incisor nearest midline is given the identification number 101, the middle incisor is 102, and the third incisor from midline is 103 [136].

The canine teeth are always number 4. So, in the right maxillary arcade, the canine tooth is given the identification number 104, the canine tooth in the left maxillary arcade is 204, the canine tooth in the left mandibular arcade is 304, and the canine tooth in the right mandibular arcade is 404 [136].

The last tooth in the maxillary arcade for the dog is given the number 10. So, in the right maxillary arcade, the second of two molars is 110, and in the left maxillary arcade, the second of two molars is 210 [136].

The last tooth in the mandibular arcade for the dog is given the number 11. So, in the left mandibular arcade, the third of three molars is 311, and in the right mandibular arcade, the third of three molars is 411 [136].

The remainder of teeth (the premolars) are filled in numerically, counting down from the last molar [136] (Figure 11.65).

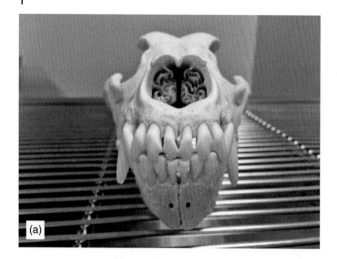

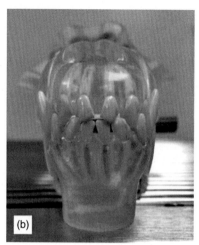

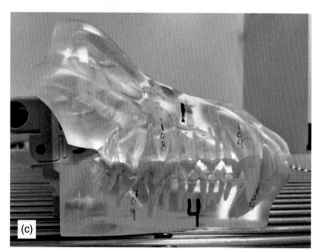

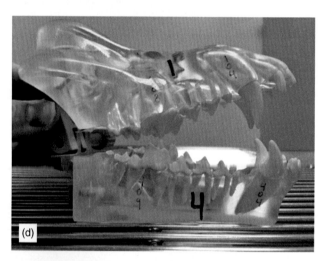

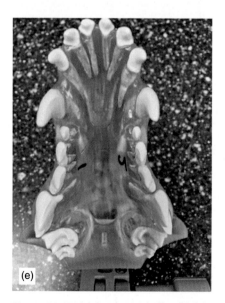

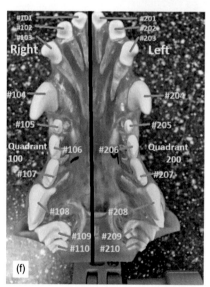

Figure 11.65 (a) Synthetic skull model demonstrating adult dentition in a dog, viewed head-on. Dental models showing adult dentition in a dog: (b) viewed head-on; (c) viewed from the side, with the mouth closed; (d) viewed from the side, with the mouth open; (e) in the maxillary arcades only; (f) in the maxillary arcades only, with the teeth labeled using the modified Triadan system; (Continued)

Figure 11.65 (*Continued*)
(g) in the mandibular arcades only;
(h) in the mandibular arcades only, with the teeth labeled using the modified Triadan system.

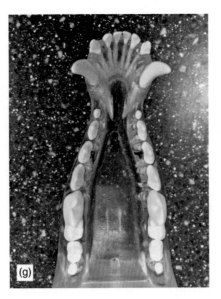

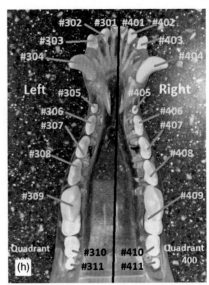

The modified Triadan system allows the clinician to identify lesions in specific teeth, such as when a tooth is missing, fractured, extracted, or in the process of resorption. Clinicians can also identify if there are supernumerary teeth such as retained deciduous teeth [132, 138] (Figure 11.66).

11.7.6 Assessing the Occlusion

In addition to numbering the dentition, the clinician should assess the occlusion by asking whether or not the bite is normal [132, 134, 138]. A "scissors bite" represents normal occlusion: there is a space between the upper canines and the adjacent incisor into which the lower canines should naturally fit [133, 134] (Figure 11.67).

A malocclusion occurs when there is misalignment of the teeth. This may be a primary dental issue or may be due to a primary skeletal issue. Class 1 malocclusions are the result of the former whereas Class 2 and 3 malocclusions are due to the latter [132, 139]. See Section 3.6.6 to review types of Class 1 malocclusions.

Overcrowding is a common Class 1 malocclusion that is seen in toy and small breed dogs (Figure 11.68).

A Class II malocclusion occurs when the mandible is shorter than expected. This results in an overbite: the maxillary dental arcades protrude beyond the mandibular arcades (Figure 11.69). This is sometimes referred to as "parrot mouth." If this is severe, the mandibular canine

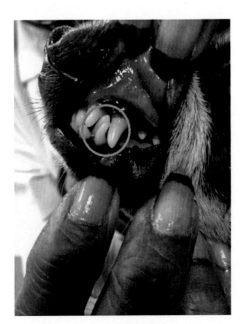

Figure 11.66 Retained deciduous left mandibular canine tooth. Source: Courtesy of Patricia Bennett, DVM.

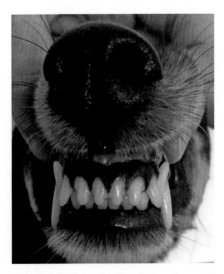

Figure 11.67 Normal "scissors bite" occlusion. Source: Courtesy of Jule Schweighoefer.

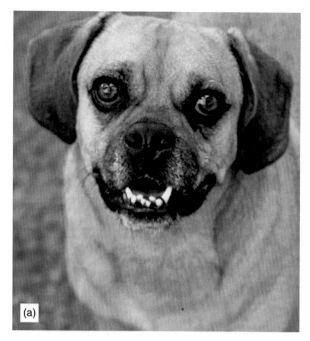
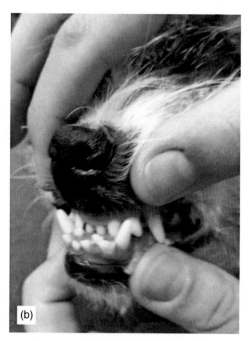

Figure 11.68 (a) Crowding of the teeth in this brachycephalic patient has led to irregularly spaced mandibular incisors. Source: Courtesy of Shelby Newton. (b) Note the irregular spacing between #301 and #303. Source: Courtesy of David May.

teeth may come into contact with the hard palate. Irritation or ulceration may result. In worst-case scenarios, an oronasal fistula may develop due to penetration of the mandibular canines through the hard palate [132, 134, 139].

A Class III malocclusion occurs when the mandible is too long (mandibular prognathism) or the maxilla is too short (maxillary brachygnathism). This results in an underbite, characterized by the mandibular dental arcades protruding beyond the maxillary dental arcades (Figure 11.70). This is sometimes referred to as "monkey mouth" [134, 139].

11.7.7 Assessing for Calculus

Recall from Section 3.6.7 that calculus is a hardened deposit of dead microorganisms encased in calcium salts. Calculus forms when plaque, a sticky substance that intra-oral bacteria produce, binds to the teeth. Like gingivitis, calculus distribution may be non-existent, focal, or generalized (Figure 11.71).

Just as each individual tooth can be assigned a gingival index (GI) score during dental charting, each individual tooth can also be assigned a calculus index (CI)

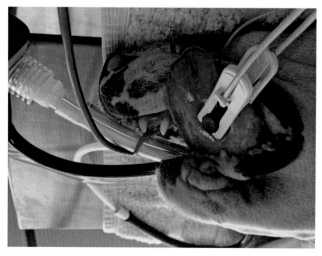

Figure 11.69 This patient has a prominent overbite. Source: Courtesy of Jeana E. Barrow, MS.

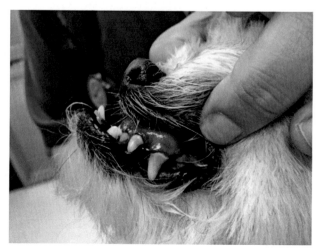

Figure 11.70 This patient has a prominent underbite.

Figure 11.71 (a) Focal calculus associated with #203 and #204. Source: Courtesy of Lai-Ting Torres. (b) Generalized distribution of severe calculus. Source: Courtesy of Samantha Thurman, DVM.

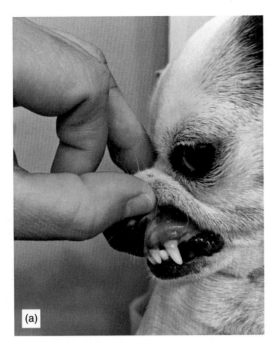
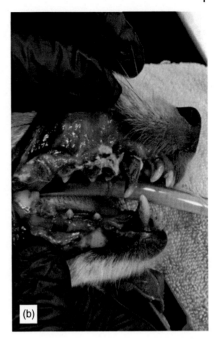

score. As with the GI score, there is no universal standardization in veterinary medicine with regard to the CI score; however, the author has adapted the following based upon others' approaches that have been documented in the human and veterinary medical literature [138, 140–144]:

- CI 0: No observable calculus present.
- CI 1: Scattered calculus covering less than one-third of the buccal surface of the tooth.
- CI 2: Calculus covering between one- and two-thirds of the buccal surface of the tooth with minimal subgingival calculus.

- CI 3: Calculus covering greater than two-thirds of the buccal surface of the tooth and extending subgingivally.

11.7.8 Miscellaneous Acquired Tooth-Related Defects

When teeth are constantly chewing against external objects such as rocks, metal bars of crates and kennels, and tennis balls, the constant friction of the teeth against the offending objects can cause appreciable wear and tear on the teeth. This can result in abrasions: the affected teeth are worn down over time (Figure 11.72) [132]. Attrition has a similar appearance; however, this is due to wear and tear caused by teeth grinding against each other [132].

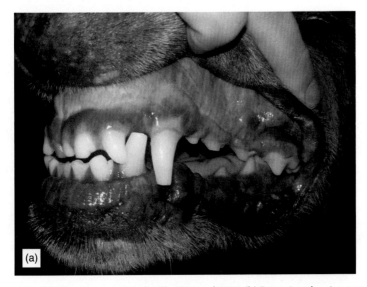
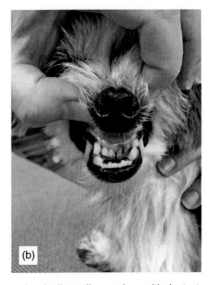

Figure 11.72 (a) Abrasion associated with #204 and #304. (b) Extensive abrasion associated with all maxillary and mandibular incisors.

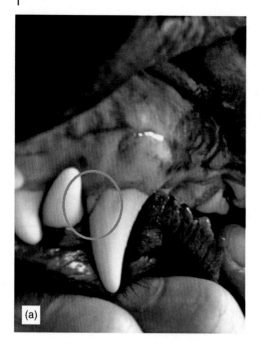
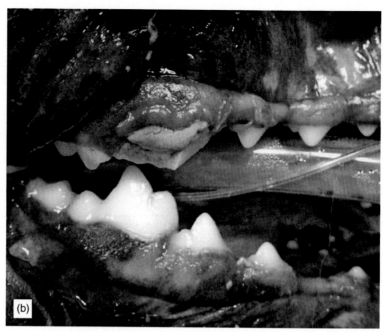

Figure 11.73 (a) Fracture associated with the base of #204. (b) Slab fracture associated with #108. Source: Courtesy of Elizabeth Robbins, DVM.

Fractures of one or more teeth are also possible sequelae of chewing against hard objects (Figure 11.73). In addition, fractures may be sustained from traumatic events such as being hit by a car. When they occur, fractures may involve the crown and/or the root, with or without exposure of the pulp cavity [132].

If trauma to one or more teeth does not result in a fracture, it can cause pulpitis. When inflammation of the pulp is irreversible, pulpal hemorrhage results. This leads to increased pressure within the tooth, causing the death of cells lining the pulp chamber and also cells guarding dentinal tubules. Without this cellular barrier intact, erythrocytes are able to enter the tooth. Initially, the affected tooth appears pink in color. Eventually, the tooth discolors to purple and eventually tan. Root canal therapy is the ideal treatment for this defect (Figure 11.74) [132].

11.7.9 Opening the Mouth

Only after all of the above data have been gathered is it essential to complete the final step of the intra-oral examination, opening the mouth. See Section 3.6.8 to review the best approaches for opening the patient's mouth.

To Review:

- In a small- to medium-breed dog, the clinician may cup the patient's head with one hand such that his thumb and index finger grasp the zygomatic arches.
- In a large-breed dog, the clinician may cup the patient's head with one hand so that his thumb and

index finger grasp on either side behind both maxillary canine teeth.

The clinician is then able to raise the dog's head to the ceiling. Using the index finger or the middle finger of the other hand, the clinician may then push down on the mandibular incisors to open the mouth (Figure 11.75).

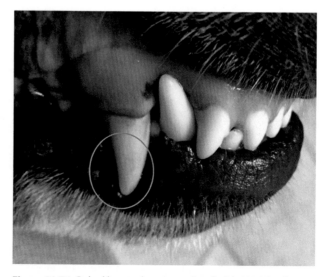

Figure 11.74 Pulpal hemorrhage associated with #104, leading to a purplish discoloration of the distal crown. Source: Courtesy of Kim Wallitsch.

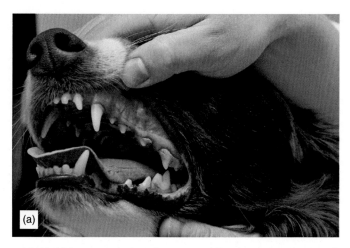
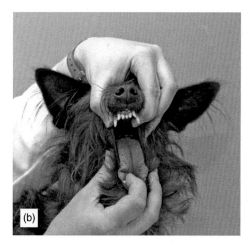

Figure 11.75 (a) Proper technique for approaching the patient to open the mouth. Note how the clinician's hand is cupping over the bridge of the nose. (b) Proper technique for opening the mouth fully. Note how the clinician's fingertips of the hand that is cupping the bridge of the nose are located behind the maxillary canines for safety purposes. Note how the index finger of the contralateral hand is being used to help pry the jaw open. Source (a), (b): Courtesy of the Media Resources Department at Midwestern University.

Once the patient's mouth is open, the clinician should be able to smell the patient's breath [138] and ask:

- Does it smell like ketones, indicating an underlying metabolic pathology?
- Does it smell fetid, as if there is oral necrosis?

With the mouth open, the clinician may evaluate the hard palate for clefts, masses, or asymmetry (Figure 11.76).

The clinician should evaluate the pharyngeal region as able for masses and other lesions. Using an otoscope or ophthalmoscope to illuminate the region can be very helpful. Sedation may be required.

11.7.10 Examining the Tongue

The surface of the tongue should be assessed for normal anatomy and also for erosions or ulcerations [138] (Figure 11.77). These could result from:

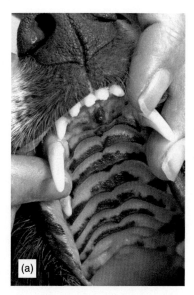
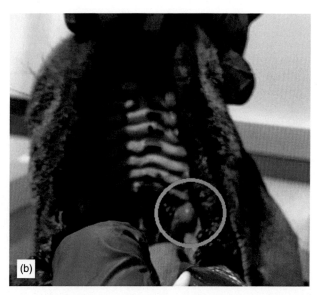

Figure 11.76 (a) Examining the hard palate. This represents a variation of normal in terms of pigmentation. Not every hard palate is mottled pink and black like the one depicted here, which is a variation of normal. Source: Courtesy of the Media Resources Department at Midwestern University. (b) Note the lesion that is present on the hard palate of this patient. This lesion is visible to the observer only when the mouth is fully opened. Source: Courtesy of Elizabeth Robbins, DVM.

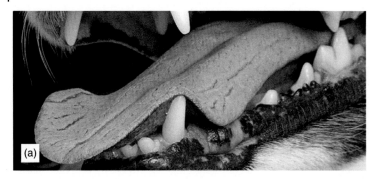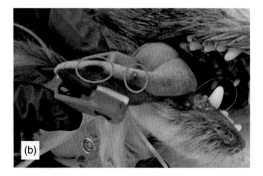

Figure 11.77 (a) Visually inspecting a normal tongue. Source: Courtesy of the Media Resources Department at Midwestern University. (b) This canine tongue is abnormal. Note the two erosions along its outer margins. Source: Courtesy of Samantha Thurman, DVM.

- electrocution burns, as from the dog biting a wire;
- uremic syndrome in a patient with kidney disease.

Although it more commonly occurs in cats than dogs, the clinician should always remember to look under the tongue for string foreign bodies [44]. When dogs and cats eat string, it may catch around the frenulum. It is equally important to look for sublingual masses.

11.7.11 Assessing for Periodontal Disease

See Section 3.6.10 for the definition and typical progression of periodontal disease.

Recall that assessing cats and dogs for periodontal disease requires a more extensive oral examination than can be accomplished in the awake patient

(Figure 11.78). Assessing for periodontal disease involves extensive dental charting, probing, and imaging of the alveolar bone. Periodontal disease cannot be definitively staged without whole-mouth radiographs to augment gross physical examination findings [132, 133, 145].

When periodontal disease is diagnosed, it may involve one or more teeth. Different teeth can be at different stages of periodontal disease, which is yet another reason why dental charting is so important. It allows the veterinary team to track the progression of disease and identify patient-appropriate areas of intervention for each individual tooth.

To standardize the language that is used to describe periodontal disease, the American Veterinary Dental College developed a classification system [132, 133, 139,

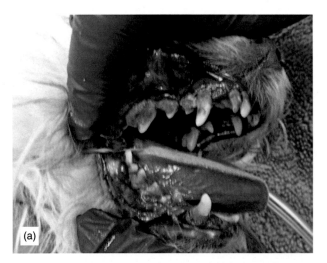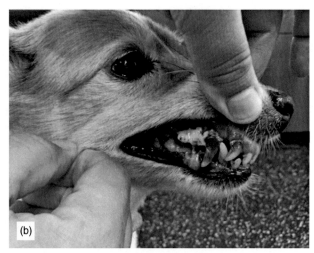

Figure 11.78 (a) This patient has severe dental disease and is very likely to have periodontal disease. However, the clinician is unable to stage the periodontal disease without more thorough dental charting and probing that involves general anesthesia, and also full mouth radiographs. Source: Courtesy of Elizabeth Robbins, DVM. (b) This patient also has severe dental disease and is very likely to have periodontal disease. However, staging this patient requires more thorough dental charting and probing that involves general anesthesia, and also full mouth radiographs. Source: Courtesy of Samantha Thurman, DVM.

146]. This system allows for the staging of periodontal disease in a way that is universally understood among the veterinary profession and minimizes confusion:

- PD 0: Negative for gingivitis, with radiographically normal peridontium.
- PD 1: Gingivitis is present as the only indication of periodontal disease. The peridontium is radiographically normal.
- PD 2: Gingivitis is present, and radiographic signs of periodontal disease are present: at most there is 25% loss of periodontal attachment.
- PD 3: Gingivitis is present, and radiographic signs are progressive: there is between 25 and 50% loss of periodontal attachment.
- PD 4: Periodontal disease is advanced, with greater than 50% loss of periodontal attachment.

When periodontal disease is advanced, there is often visible exposure of the furcation, the area that joins the crown to the root. There also may be bone destruction to the degree that a fistula develops as an open track that spans the oral and nasal cavities (Figure 11.79) [132].

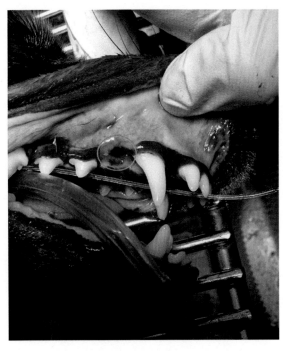

Figure 11.79 Oronasal fistula due to advanced periodontal disease. Source: Courtesy of Paola Bazan Steyling, DVM.

References

1 Stone, H.R., McGreevy, P.D., Starling, M.J., and Forkman, B. (2016) Associations between domestic-dog morphology and behaviour scores in the dog mentality assessment. *PLoS One*, **11** (2), e0149403.

2 Sisson, S., Grossman, J.D., and Getty, R. (1975) *Sisson and Grossman's The Anatomy of the Domestic Animals*, 5th edn., Saunders, Philadelphia.

3 McGreevy, P., Grassi, T.D., and Harman, A.M. (2004) A strong correlation exists between the distribution of retinal ganglion cells and nose length in the dog. *Brain, Behavior and Evolution*, **63** (1), 13–22.

4 Schoenebeck, J.J. and Ostrander, E.A. (2013) The genetics of canine skull shape variation. *Genetics*, **193** (2), 317–325.

5 Peichl, L. (1992) Topography of ganglion cells in the dog and wolf retina. *Journal of Comparative Neurology*, **324** (4), 603–620.

6 McGreevy, P.D., Georgevsky, D., Carrasco, J. et al. (2013) Dog behavior co-varies with height, bodyweight and skull shape. *PLoS One*, **8** (12), e80529.

7 Larson, G., Karlsson, E.K., Perri, A. et al. (2012) Rethinking dog domestication by integrating genetics, archeology, and biogeography. *Proceedings of the National Academy of Sciences of the United States of America*, **109** (23), 8878–8883.

8 Wilcox, B. and Walkowicz, C. (1995) *The Atlas of Dog Breeds of the World*, 5th edn., TFH Publications, Neptune City, NJ.

9 McGreevy, P.D. and Nicholas, F.W. (1999) Some practical solutions to welfare problems in dog breeding. *Animal Welfare*, **8** (4), 329–341.

10 Miller, P.E. and Murphy, C.J. (1995) Vision in dogs. *Journal of the American Veterinary Medical Association*, **207** (12), 1623–1634.

11 Karjalainen, L., Ojala, M., and Vilva, V. (1996) Environmental effects and genetic parameters for measurements of hunting performance in the Finnish Spitz. *Journal of Animal Breeding and Genetics*, **113** (6), 525–534.

12 Liinamo, A.E., Karjalainen, E., Ojala, M., and Vilva, V. (1997) Estimates of genetic parameters and environmental effects for measures of hunting performance in Finnish Hounds. *Journal of Animal Science*, **75** (3), 622–629.

13 Schmutz, S.M. and Schmutz, J.K. (1998) Heritability estimates of behaviors associated with hunting in dogs. *Journal of Heredity*, **89** (3), 233–237.

14 Coppinger, R. and Schneider, R. (1995) Evolution of working dogs, in *The Domestic Dog: Its Evolution, Behaviour, and Interactions with People* (ed. J. Serpell), Cambridge University Press, Cambridge, pp. 21–50.

15 Coppinger, R. and Coppinger, L. (2001) *Dogs: A Startling New Understanding of Canine Origin, Behavior, and Evolution*, Scribner, New York.

16 Zeder, M.A. (2012) Pathways to animal domestication, in *Biodiversity in Agriculture: Domestication, Evolution, and Sustainability* (eds. P. Gepts, R.R. Famula, R.L. Bettinger et al.), Cambridge University Press, Cambridge, pp. 227–259.

17 Trut, L.N. (1999) Early canid domestication: the farm-fox experiment. *American Scientist*, **87** (2), 160–169.

18 Drake, A.G. (2011) Dispelling dog dogma: an investigation of heterochrony in dogs using 3D geometric morphometric analysis of skull shape. *Evolution & Development*, **13** (2), 204–213.

19 Drake, A.G. and Klingenberg, C.P. (2010) Large-scale diversification of skull shape in domestic dogs: disparity and modularity. *American Naturalist*, **175** (3), 289–301.

20 Gould, S.J. (1977) *Ontogeny and Phylogeny*, Belknap Press, Cambridge, MA.

21 The Kennel Club (2016) *History of the Kennel Club*, http://www.thekennelclub.org.uk/our-resources/about-the-kennel-club/history-of-the-kennel-club/ (accessed 10 June 2016).

22 Fogle, B. (1995) *The Encyclopedia of the Dog*, 1st American edn., Dorling Kindersley, New York.

23 Wayne, R.K. and Jenks, S.M. (1991) Mitochondrial-DNA analysis implying extensive hybridization of the endangered red wolf *Canis rufus. Nature*, **351** (6327), 565–568.

24 Wayne, R.K., Lehman, N., Allard, M.W., and Honeycutt, R.L. (1992) Mitochondrial-DNA variability of the gray wolf – genetic consequences of population decline and habitat fragmentation. *Conservation Biology*, **6** (4), 559–569.

25 Roberts, T., McGreevy, P., and Valenzuela, M. (2010) Human induced rotation and reorganization of the brain of domestic dogs. *PLoS One*, **5** (7), e11946.

26 Haworth, K.E., Islam, I., Breen, M. *et al.* (2001) Canine TCOF1; cloning, chromosome assignment and genetic analysis in dogs with different head types. *Mammalian Genome*, **12** (8), 622–629.

27 Wayne, R.K. (1986) Cranial morphology of domestic and wild canids – the influence of development on morphological change. *Evolution*, **40** (2), 243–261.

28 Young, A. and Bannasch, D. (2006) Morphological variation in the dog, in *The Dog and Its Genome* (eds. E.A. Ostrander, U. Giger, and K. Lindblad-Toh), Cold Spring Harbor Laboratory Press, Cold Spring Harbor, NY, pp. 47–65.

29 Hecht, J. and Horowitz, A. (2015) Seeing dogs: human preferences for dog physical attributes. *Anthrozoos*, **28** (1), 153–163.

30 Packer, R.M., Hendricks, A., and Burn, C.C. (2015) Impact of facial conformation on canine health: corneal ulceration. *PLoS One*, **10** (5), e0123827.

31 Coren, S. (1994) *The Intelligence of Dogs*, Bantam, New York.

32 Ley, J.M., Bennett, P.C., and Coleman, G.J. (2009) A refinement and validation of the Monash Canine Personality Questionnaire (MCPQ). *Applied Animal Behaviour Science*, **116** (2–4), 220–227.

33 Rooney, N.J. and Bradshaw, J.W.S. (2004) Breed and sex differences in the behavioural attributes of specialist search dogs – a questionnaire survey of trainers and handlers. *Applied Animal Behaviour Science*, **86** (1–2), 123–135.

34 Serpell, J.A. and Hsu, Y.Y. (2005) Effects of breed, sex, and neuter status on trainability in dogs. *Anthrozoos*, **18** (3), 196–207.

35 Helton, W.S. (2009) Cephalic index and perceived dog trainability. *Behavioural Processes*, **82** (3), 355–358.

36 Georgevsky, D., Carrasco, J.J., Valenzuela, M., and McGreevy, P.D. (2014) Domestic dog skull diversity across breeds, breed groupings, and genetic clusters. *Journal of Veterinary Behavior*, **9** (5), 228–234.

37 Drake, A.G. and Klingenberg, C.P. (2008) The pace of morphological change: historical transformation of skull shape in St Bernard dogs. *Proceedings. Biological Sciences*, **275** (1630), 71–76.

38 Thomas, W.B. and Dewey, C.W. (2008) Performing the neurological examination, in *A Practical Guide to Canine and Feline Neurology*, 2nd edn. (ed. C.W. Dewey), Wiley-Blackwell, Ames, IA, pp. 53–74.

39 de Lahunta, A. and Glass, E. (2009) The neurologic examination, in *Veterinary Neuroanatomy and Clinical Neurology*, 4th edn. (eds. A. de Lahunta, E Glass, and M. Kent), Saunders Elsevier, St. Louis, pp. 487–501.

40 Harvey, A. and Tasker, S. (2013) *BSAVA Manual of Feline Practice: A Foundational Manual*, 2nd edn., British Small Animal Veterinary Association, Gloucester.

41 Gould, D. and McLellan, G. (2015) *BSAVA Manual of Canine and Feline Ophthalmology*, 2nd edn., British Small Animal Veterinary Association, Gloucester.

42 Gelatt, K.N. (2014) *Essentials of Veterinary Ophthalmology*, 3rd edn., Wiley-Blackwell, Ames, IA.

43 Maggs, D.J., Miller, P.E., and Ofri, R. (2013) *Slatter's Fundamentals of Veterinary Ophthalmology*, 5th edn., Saunders Elsevier, St. Louis.

44 Rijnberk, A. and van Sluijs, F.S. (eds.) (2009) *Medical History and Physical Examination in Companion Animals*, 2nd edn., Saunders Elsevier, St. Louis.

45 Dziezyc, J. and Millichamp, N.J. (2004) *Color Atlas of Canine and Feline Ophthalmology*, Saunders Elsevier, St. Louis.

46 Ketring, K.L. and Glaze, M.B. (2012) *Atlas of Feline Ophthalmology*, 2nd edn., Wiley-Blackwell, Ames, IA.

47 Martin, C.L. (2005) Anamnesis and the ophthalmic examination, in *Ophthalmic Disease in Veterinary Medicine*, Manson, London, pp. 11–40.

48 Martin, C.L. (2005) Eyelids, in *Ophthalmic Disease in Veterinary Medicine*, Manson, London, pp. 145–182.

49 Martin, C.L. (2005) Conjunctiva and third eyelid, in *Ophthalmic Disease in Veterinary Medicine*, Manson, London, pp. 205–209.

50 Martin, C.L. (2005) Lacrimal system, in *Ophthalmic Disease in Veterinary Medicine*, Manson, London, pp. 219–240.

51 Rubin, L. (1989) *Inherited Eye Diseases in Purebred Dogs*, Williams and Wilkins, Baltimore.

52 Moore, C.P. and Collier, L.L. (1990) Ocular surface disease associated with loss of conjunctival goblet cells in dogs. *Journal of the American Animal Hospital Association*, **26** (5), 458–466.

53 Martin, C.L. (2005) Problem-based management of ocular emergencies, in *Ophthalmic Disease in Veterinary Medicine*, Manson, London, pp. 93–104.

54 Krehbiel, J.D. and Langham, R.F. (1975) Eyelid neoplasms of dogs. *American Journal of Veterinary Research*, **36** (1), 115–119.

55 Medleau, L. and Hnilica, K.A. (2006) Papillomas, in *Small Animal Dermatology: A Color Atlas and Therapeutic Guide*, 2nd edn. (eds. L. Medleau and K.A. Hnilica), Saunders Elsevier, St. Louis, pp. 141–143.

56 Lim, C.C. (2015) *Small Animal Ophthalmic Atlas and Guide*, Wiley-Blackwell, Ames, IA.

57 Urban, M., Wyman, M., Rheins, M., and Marraro, R.V. (1972) Conjunctival flora of clinically normal dogs. *Journal of the American Veterinary Medical Association*, **161** (2), 201–206.

58 Bistner, S.I., Roberts, S.R., and Anderson, R.P. (1969) Conjunctival bacteria: clinical appearances can be deceiving. *Modern Veterinary Practice*, **50**, 45–47.

59 McDonald, P.J. and Watson, A.D.J. (1976) Microbial flora of normal canine conjunctiva. *Journal of Small Animal Practice*, **17**, 809–812.

60 Hacker, D.V., Jensen, H.E., and Selby, L.A. (1979) Comparison of conjunctival culture techniques in the dog. *Journal of the American Animal Hospital Association*, **15** (2), 223–225.

61 Gerding, P.A., Cormany, K., Weisiger, R., and Kakoma, I. (1993) Survey and topographic distribution of bacterial and fungal microorganisms in eyes of clinically normal dogs. *Canine Practice*, **18** (2), 34–38.

62 Samuelson, D.A., Andresen, T.L., and Gwin, R.M. (1984) Conjunctival fungal flora in horses, cattle, dogs, and cats. *Journal of the American Veterinary Medical Association*, **184** (10), 1240–1242.

63 Collins, B.K., Collier, L.L., Miller, M., and Linton, L. (1993) Biologic behavior and histologic characteristics of canine conjunctival melanoma. *Veterinary and Comparative Ophthalmology*, **3**, 135–140.

64 Albert, R.A., Garrett, P.D., Whitley, R.D., and Thomas, K.L. (1982) Surgical correction of everted third eyelid in two cats. *Journal of the American Veterinary Medical Association*, **180** (7), 763–766.

65 Koch, S.A. (1979) Congenital ophthalmic abnormalities in the Burmese cat. *Journal of the American Veterinary Medical Association*, **174** (1), 90–91.

66 Christmas, R. (1992) Surgical correction of congenital ocular and nasal dermoids and third eyelid gland prolapse in related Burmese kittens. *Canadian Veterinary Journal/Revue Vétérinaire Canadienne*, **33** (4), 265–266.

67 Schoofs, S.H. (1999) Prolapse of the gland of the third eyelid in a cat: a case report and literature review. *Journal of the American Animal Hospital Association*, **35** (3), 240–242.

68 Martin, C.L. (2005) Orbit and globe, in *Ophthalmic Disease in Veterinary Medicine*, Manson, London, pp. 132–133.

69 Martin, C.L. (2005) Glaucoma, in *Ophthalmic Disease in Veterinary Medicine*, Manson, London, pp. 337–368.

70 Lucas, D.R. (1954) Ocular associations of dappling in the coat colour of dogs. II. Histology. *Journal of Comparative Pathology*, **64** (3), 260–266.

71 Gelatt, K.N. and McGill, L.D. (1973) Clinical characteristics of microphthalmia with colobomas of the Australian Shepherd dog. *Journal of the American Veterinary Medical Association*, **162** (5), 393–396.

72 Bauer, B.S., Sandmeyer, L.S., and Grahn, B.H. (2015) Diagnostic ophthalmology. Microphthalmos and multiple ocular anomalies (MOA) OU consistent with merle ocular dysgenesis (MOD). *Canadian Veterinary Journal/Revue Vétérinaire Canadienne*, **56** (7), 767–768.

73 Gunton, K.B., Wasserman, B.N., and DeBenedictis, C. (2015) Strabismus. *Primary Care*, **42** (3), 393–407.

74 Campos, E.C. (2008) Why do the eyes cross? A review and discussion of the nature and origin of essential infantile esotropia, microstrabismus, accommodative esotropia, and acute comitant esotropia. *Journal of AAPOS*, **12** (4), 326–331.

75 Rengstorff, R.H. (1976) Strabismus measurements in the Siamese cat. *American Journal of Optometry and Physiological Optics*, **53** (10), 643–646.

76 Blake, R. and Crawford, M.L. (1974) Development of strabismus in Siamese cats. *Brain Research*, **77** (3), 492–496.

77 Hyde, J.E. (1962) Cross-eyedness: a study in Siamese cats. *American Journal of Ophthalmology*, **53**, 70–75.

78 Fitzgerald, K.T., Bronstein, A.C., and Newquist, K.L. (2013) Marijuana poisoning. *Topics in Companion Animal Medicine*, **28** (1), 8–12.

79 Rossmeisl, J.H., Jr. (2010) Vestibular disease in dogs and cats. *Veterinary Clinics of North America: Small Animal Practice*, **40** (1), 81–100.

80 Thomas, W.B. (2000) Vestibular dysfunction. *Veterinary Clinics of North America: Small Animal Practice*, **30** (1), 227–249, viii.

81 Kornegay, J.N. (1991) Ataxia, head tilt, nystagmus. Vestibular diseases. *Problems in Veterinary Medicine*, **3** (3), 417–425.

82 Martin, C.L. (2005) Cornea and sclera, in *Ophthalmic Disease in Veterinary Medicine*, Manson, London, pp. 241–297.

83 Roberts, S. (1965) Superficial indolent ulcer of the cornea in Boxer dogs. *Journal of Small Animal Practice*, **6**, 111–115.

84 Gelatt, K.N. and Samuelson, D.A. (1982) Recurrent corneal erosions and epithelial dystrophy in the Boxer dog. *Journal of the American Animal Hospital Association*, **18** (3), 453–460.

85 Kirschner, S.E., Niyo, Y., and Betts, D.M. (1989) Idiopathic persistent corneal erosions – clinical and pathological findings in 18 dogs. *Journal of the American Animal Hospital Association*, **25** (1), 84–90.

86 Waring, G.O., Macmillan, A., and Reveles, P. (1986) Inheritance of crystalline corneal-dystrophy in Siberian huskies. *Journal of the American Animal Hospital Association*, **22** (5), 655–658.

87 Roth, A.M., Ekins, M.B., Waring, G.O. *et al.* (1981) Oval corneal opacities in beagles. III. Histochemical demonstration of stromal lipids without hyperlipidemia. *Investigative Ophthalmology and Visual Science*, **21** (1), 95–106.

88 Gratzek A.T., Calvert C.A., Martin C.L., and Kaswan, R.L. (1993) Corneal edema in dogs treated with tocainide. *Progress in Veterinary and Comparative Ophthalmology*, **3**, 47–51.

89 Gwin, R.M., Polack, F.M., Warren, J.K. *et al.* (1982) Primary canine corneal endothelial-cell dystrophy – specular microscopic evaluation, diagnosis and therapy. *Journal of the American Animal Hospital Association*, **18** (3), 471–479.

90 Martin, C.L. and Dice, P.F. (1982) Corneal endothelial dystrophy in the dog. *Journal of the American Animal Hospital Association*, **18** (2), 327–336.

91 Slatter, D.H., Lavach, J.D., Severin, G.A., and Young, S. (1977) Uberreiter's syndrome (chronic superficial keratitis) in dogs in the Rocky Mountain area – a study of 463 cases. *Journal of Small Animal Practice*, **18** (12), 757–772.

92 Chavkin, M.J., Roberts, S.M., Salman, M.D. *et al.* (1994) Risk factors for development of chronic superficial keratitis in dogs. *Journal of the American Veterinary Medical Association*, **204** (10), 1630–1634.

93 Bedford, P.G. and Longstaffe, J.A. (1979) Corneal pannus (chronic superficial keratitis) in the German Shepherd dog. *Journal of Small Animal Practice*, **20** (1), 41–56.

94 Martin, C.L. (2005) Anterior uvea and anterior chamber, in *Ophthalmic Disease in Veterinary Medicine*, Manson, London, pp. 298–336.

95 Strain, G.M. (2012) Canine deafness. *Veterinary Clinics of North America: Small Animal Practice*, **42**, 1209–1224.

96 deLahunta, A., Glass, E., and Kent, M. (eds.) *Veterinary Neuroanatomy and Clinical Neurology*, 4th edn., Saunders Elsevier, St. Louis.

97 Telle, M.R. and Betbeze, C. (2015) Hyphema: considerations in the small animal patient. *Topics in Companion Animal Medicine*, **30** (3), 97–106.

98 Townsend, W.M. (2008) Canine and feline uveitis. *Veterinary Clinics of North America: Small Animal Practice*, **38** (2), 323–346, vii.

99 Colitz, C.M. (2005) Feline uveitis: diagnosis and treatment. *Clinical Techniques in Small Animal Practice*, **20** (2), 117–120.

100 Torrance, A.G. and Mooney, C.T. (eds.) (1998) *BSAVA Manual of Small Animal Endocrinology*, 2nd edn., British Small Animal Veterinary Association, Cheltenham.

101 Salgado, D., Reusch, C., and Spiess, B. (2000) Diabetic cataracts: different incidence between dogs and cats. *Schweizer Archiv für Tierheilkunde*, **142** (6), 349–353.

102 Basher, A.W. and Roberts, S.M. (1995) Ocular manifestations of diabetes mellitus: diabetic cataracts in dogs. *Veterinary Clinics of North America: Small Animal Practice*, **25** (3), 661–676.

103 Peiffer, R.L. and Gelatt, K.N. (1974) Cataracts in the cat. *Feline Practice*, **4**, 34–38.

104 Martin, C.L. (2005) Vitreous and ocular fundus, in *Ophthalmic Disease in Veterinary Medicine*, Manson, London, pp. 401–470.

105 Boevé, M.H., Stades, F.C., and Djajadiningrat-Laanen, S.C. (2009) The eyes, in *Medical History and Physical Examination in Companion Animals*, 2nd edn. (eds. A. Rijnberk and F.S. van Sluijs), Saunders Elsevier, St. Louis, pp. 175–201.

106 Welch Allyn (2016) *Direct and Indirect Veterinary Eye and Ear Examination Instructions*, https://www.welchallyn.com/content/dam/welchallyn/documents/sap-documents/LIT/80020/80020547LITPDF.pdf (accessed 14 June 2016).

107 Gramlich, J.L. (2009) Routine canine ocular exam. *Lab Animal*, **38** (5), 151–152.

108 Eaton, J.S. (2016) *Facing Your Fundic Fears: Examination of the Ocular Fundus*, http://www.cuvs.org/pdf/pdflinks/Examination%20of%20the%20Ocular%20Fundus%20Lab.pdf (accessed 14 June 2016).

109 Brooks, D.E. (2008) Examination of the ocular fundus – Part 2: indirect and direct ophthalmoscopy. *Clinician's Brief*, December, 37–39.

110 Heine, P.A. (2004) Anatomy of the ear. *Veterinary Clinics of North America: Small Animal Practice*, **34** (2), 379–395.

111 Cole, L.K. (2004) Otoscopic evaluation of the ear canal. *Veterinary Clinics of North America: Small Animal Practice*, **34** (2), 397–410.

112 Strain, G.M. (2012) Canine deafness. *Veterinary Clinics of North America: Small Animal Practice*, **42** (6), 1209–1224.

113 Bach, J.P., Lupke, M., and Wefstaedt, P. (2013) Deafness in the dog and cat: aetiology, diagnostics and treatment. *Tierarztliche Praxis, Ausgabe K, Kleintiere/Heimtiere*, **41** (6), 421–427; quiz, 8 (in German).

114 Sims, M.H. (1988) Electrodiagnostic evaluation of auditory function. *Veterinary Clinics of North America: Small Animal Practice*, **18** (4), 913–944.

115 Dijkshoorn, N.A. and van der Wel, T. (1997) Screening for deafness in companion animals. *Tijdschrift voor Diergeneeskunge*, **122** (6), 168–169 (in Dutch).

116 Cook, L.B. (2004) Neurologic evaluation of the ear. *Veterinary Clinics of North America: Small Animal Practice*, **34** (2), 425–435, vi.

117 Medleau, L. and Hnilica, K.A. (eds.) (2006) *Small Animal Dermatology: A Color Atlas and Therapeutic Guide*, 2nd edn., Saunders Elsevier, St. Louis.

118 Matousek, J.L. (2004) Diseases of the ear pinna. *Veterinary Clinics of North America: Small Animal Practice*, **34** (2), 511–540.

119 Medleau, L. and Hnilica, K.A. (2006) Ear mites, in *Small Animal Dermatology: A Color Atlas and Therapeutic Guide*, 2nd edn. (eds. L. Medleau and K.A. Hnilica), Saunders Elsevier, St. Louis, pp. 118–119.

120 Angus, J.C. (2004) Diseases of the ear, in *Small Animal Dermatology Secrets* (ed. K.L. Campbell), Hanley & Belfus, Philadelphia, pp. 364–384.

121 Gotthelf, L.N. (2004) Diagnosis and treatment of otitis media in dogs and cats. *Veterinary Clinics of North America: Small Animal Practice*, **34** (2), 469–487.

122 Stokhof, A.A. and Venker-van Haagen, A.J. (2009) Respiratory system, in *Medical History and Physical Examination in Companion Animals*, 2nd edn. (eds. A. Rijnberk and F.S. van Sluijs), Saunders Elsevier, St. Louis, pp. 63–74.

123 Mathews, K.A. (2006) Monitoring fluid therapy and complications of fluid therapy, in *Fluid, Electrolyte, and Acid–Base Disorders in Small Animal Practice*, 3rd edn. (ed. S.P. DiBartola), Saunders Elsevier, St. Louis, pp. 377–391.

124 Rijnberk, A. and Stokhof, A.A. (2009) General examination, in *Medical History and Physical Examination in Companion Animals*, 2nd edn. (eds. A. Rijnberk and F.S. van Sluijs), Saunders Elsevier, St. Louis, pp. 47–62.

125 Bezuidenhout, A.J. (1993) The lymphatic system, in *Miller's Anatomy of the Dog*, 3rd edn. (eds. H.E. Evans and M.E. Miller), Saunders, Philadelphia, pp. 717–757.

126 Mestrinho, L.A., Runhau, J., Braganca, M., and Niza, M.M. (2013) Risk assessment of feline tooth resorption: a Portuguese clinical case control study. *Journal of Veterinary Dentistry*, **30** (2), 78–83.

127 Silness, J. and Loe, H. (1964) Periodontal disease in pregnancy. II. Correlation between oral hygiene and periodontal condtion. *Acta Odontologica Scandinavica*, **22**, 121–135.

128 Thomason, J.D., Fallaw, T.L., Carmichael, K.P. *et al.* (2009) Gingival hyperplasia associated with the administration of amlodipine to dogs with degenerative valvular disease (2004–2008). *Journal of Veterinary Internal Medicine*, **23** (1), 39–42.

129 Pariser, M.S. and Berdoulay, P. (2011) Amlodipine-induced gingival hyperplasia in a Great Dane. *Journal of the American Animal Hospital Association*, **47** (5), 375–376.

130 Nam, H.S., McAnulty, J.F., Kwak, H.H. *et al.* (2008) Gingival overgrowth in dogs associated with clinically relevant cyclosporine blood levels: observations in a canine renal transplantation model. *Veterinary Surgery*, **37** (3), 247–253.

131 Evans, H.E. (1993) The digestive apparatus and abdomen, in *Miller's Anatomy of the Dog*, 3rd edn. (eds. H.E. Evans and M.E. Miller), Saunders, Philadelphia, pp. 385–462.

132 Holmstrom, S.E. (2013) *Veterinary Dentistry: A Team Approach*, 2nd edn., Saunders Elsevier, St. Louis.

133 Lobprise, H.B. and Wiggs, R.B. (2000) *The Veterinarian's Companion for Common Dental Procedures*, AAHA Press, Lakewood, CO.

134 Shipp, A.D. and Fahrenkrug, P. (1992) *Practitioners' Guide to Veterinary Dentistry*, Dr. Shipp's Laboratories, Beverly Hills, CA.

135 Fulton, A.J., Fiani, N., and Verstraete, F.J. (2014) Canine pediatric dentistry. *Veterinary Clinics of North America: Small Animal Practice*, **44** (2), 303–324.

136 Floyd, M.R. (1991) The modified Triadan system: nomenclature for veterinary dentistry. *Journal of Veterinary Dentistry*, **8** (4), 18–19.

137 Reiter, A.M. and Soltero-Rivera, M.M. (2014) Applied feline oral anatomy and tooth extraction techniques: an illustrated guide. *Journal of Feline Medicine and Surgery*, **16** (11), 900–913.

138 Clarke, D.E. and Caiafa, A. (2014) Oral examination in the cat: a systematic approach. *Journal of Feline Medicine and Surgery*, **16** (11), 873–886.

139 American Veterinary Dental College (2016) *AVDC Nomenclature*, http://www.avdc.org/Nomenclature.pdf (accessed 16 April 2016).

140 Logan, E.I. and Boyce, E.N. (1994) Oral health assessment in dogs: parameters and methods. *Journal of Veterinary Dentistry*, **11** (2), 58–63.

141 Hennet, P. (1999) Review of studies assessing plaque accumulation and gingival inflammation in dogs. *Journal of Veterinary Dentistry*, **16** (1), 23–29.

142 Fischman, S.L. (1998) Clinical index systems used to assess the efficacy of mouthrinses on plaque and gingivitis. *Journal of Clinical Periodontology*, **15** (8), 506–510.

143 Gunsolley, J.C., Chinchilli, V.M., Koertge, T.E. *et al.* The use of repeated measures analysis of variance for plaque and gingival indices. *Journal of Clinical Periodontology*, **16** (3), 156–163.

144 Fischman, S.L. (1986) Current status of indexes of plaque. *Journal of Clinical Periodontology*, **13** (5), 371–374.

145 Lemmons, M. (2013) Clinical feline dental radiography. *Veterinary Clinics of North America: Small Animal Practice*, **43** (3), 533–554.

146 Holmstrom, S.E. (2012) Veterinary dentistry in senior canines and felines. *Veterinary Clinics of North America: Small Animal Practice*, **42** (4), 793–808, viii.

12

Examining the Endocrine and Lymphatic Systems of the Dog

12.1 Thyroid Gland Neoplasia in the Dog

Endocrine organs are largely inaccessible to the clinician despite the best efforts to perform a comprehensive physical examination. Only in the intact male are normal endocrine organs readily palpable. All other endocrine organs are either too internal to appreciate, such as the endocrine pancreas, or, in the case of the thyroid gland, are palpable only in certain diseased states.

Recall from Section 4.1 that the thyroid gland consists of two lobes. The right lobe is seated more cranial in the cervical region than the left [1, 2].

In health, the thyroid gland is covered by muscle. It is also intimately associated with key vascular, gastrointestinal, and nervous system landmarks. The right lobe lies in close apposition to the common carotid artery, internal jugular vein, and the vagosympathetic trunk. The left lobe abuts the esophagus and the caudal laryngeal nerve. The vascular supply to this region is quite rich, and is capable of supporting aggressive invasion of thyroid-associated tumors into local tissue [1, 3].

The normal thyroid gland is not typically palpable on the physical examination [3]. The abnormal thyroid gland may or may not be appreciated, depending upon the type of pathology. In senior dogs, the two most common diseased states of the thyroid are acquired hypothyroidism and thyroid neoplasia [4]. Of these, only the latter is palpable.

Thyroid tumors represent 1.1–3.8% of all canine neoplasias [5–8]. Neither sex is predisposed to thyroid neoplasia [9–15]. However, the Beagle, Boxer, Golden Retriever, and Husky breeds appear to be at increased risk within the United States [4, 9, 10, 14, 15]. By contrast, the breeds that are over-represented in Scotland are the Shetland Collie, Old English Sheepdog, and Cairn Terrier [16].

When thyroid tumors develop in the dog, they are more likely to be malignant [6, 9, 10]. Only 9% are adenomas [5]. Thyroid tumors also tend to be large and invasive [4]. The regional anatomy supports expansion of the growing tumor by way of the local blood supply. Because the trachea, larynx, esophagus, and neurovascular structures are neighbors of the thyroid, these vital structures are likely to be compromised [1, 3, 6, 7].

In stark contrast to cats, canine thyroid tumors tend not to be functional [1]. Fewer than one-quarter of canine patients with thyroid tumors present with clinical or biochemical data that support a hyperthyroid state [6, 10, 11, 17, 18]. It is even less likely to see clinical hypothyroidism secondary to thyroid neoplasia [1, 6, 8]. The risk of developing one or more thyroid tumors increases with age: the incidence is 1.1% in 8–12-year-old dogs compared with 4.0% in 12–15-year-old dogs [3].

The etiology of thyroid tumors is better understood in people than in our canine patients [3]. In people, there is a definitive link between excessive exposure to radiation and the development of thyroid cancer [3, 19–21]. Although the possibility of this link in veterinary medicine has been explored experimentally in the laboratory, it has been difficult to extrapolate conclusions to the general canine population [22].

The role of dietary iodine in inducing thyroid cancer has also been studied in people: both deficiencies and excesses of iodine may contribute to thyroidal illness and subsequent neoplasia [3, 23]. However, whether or not this concern is valid in veterinary medicine remains to be determined [3].

Dietary iodine has been researched less extensively in the dog with regard to thyroid cancer and more extensively with regard to feline hyperthyroidism. When it was discovered during the late 1970s that the majority of commercial cat foods contained up to 10 times the recommended level of iodine [24], it was thought that this excess could explain hyperthyroidism. Recommendations for dietary iodine have since been reduced [25], yet hyperthyroidism persists.

Just as more research is necessary to understand the missing links in the etiology of feline hyperthyroidism, so is necessary to explore the causes of thyroid cancer in the dog. Much remains unknown in terms of canine risk factors other than breed. What is known about canine thyroid cancer is that follicular carcinomas predominate [6].

Performing the Small Animal Physical Examination, First Edition. Ryane E. Englar.
© 2017 John Wiley & Sons, Inc. Published 2017 by John Wiley & Sons, Inc.

Two-thirds to three-fourths of these malignancies are unilateral [1, 10, 26]. When tumors are bilateral, it is challenging to discern whether each tumor arose independently of the other or whether one tumor was the by-product of the other's metastasis [1].

The rate of metastasis is high in dogs with thyroid carcinomas [1]. At the time of diagnosis, one-third of dogs have detectable metastatic disease [1]. At necropsy, metastasis is recognized in 6–9 out of every 10 dogs [9–11, 14]. The major metastatic sites for thyroid cancer in the dog are the regional lymph nodes and the lungs [6, 7]. Because the nodes cranial to the thyroid are responsible for draining lymph, the submandibular, parotid, and medial retropharyngeal nodes are most commonly implicated [2]. Pulmonary metastasis occurs when neoplastic cells invade the neighboring cranial and caudal thyroid veins [1, 14].

12.2 The Typical Presentation of Thyroid Gland Neoplasia in the Dog

Rarely is thyroid gland neoplasia an incidental finding on physical examination [3, 9, 27]. More often than not, veterinary clients are the ones responsible for identifying a cervical swelling [9, 11, 16, 26–28] and presenting the dog to a veterinarian for evaluation within 1–2 months [3]. Clients typically report rapid growth of a firm, yet apparently non-painful mass that may or may not be freely moveable within the cervical region, depending on how aggressively invasive the tumor is at the time of initial diagnosis [3].

To confirm the presence of a ventral cervical mass, all the clinician needs to do is to firmly cup a hand and guide it down the ventral midline of the neck. To facilitate this motion, the thumb should be on one side of the neck and the fingers should be against the other. The palm is what cups the ventral midline. The author then concentrates on applying firm pressure to the thumb and fingertips to appreciate the ventrolateral structures of the neck. If one or both of the thyroid gland lobes are involved, one or more firm masses should be evident in the region of the throat. An exception would be if the thyroid tumor(s) arose from ectopic thyroid tissue, which may extend well into the thoracic inlet and out of reach of the clinician's fingertips [1, 2, 6, 7].

Because of their tendency to metastasize to regional lymph nodes, thyroid carcinomas may also present for one or more swellings under the angle of the mandible due to submandibular lymphadenopathy [2, 4]. See Section 11.6 to review the proper technique for palpating the submandibular lymph nodes of a dog.

The patient may be otherwise asymptomatic. However, as the enlarging mass begins to compress surrounding soft tissue structures, additional clinical signs may develop that raise the client's level of concern. When the upper airway or the pharynx is compressed, the patient may present with cough or dysphonia [9, 11, 13, 14]. As the lower airway becomes involved, dyspnea may develop. Compression of the esophagus may lead to dysphagia and retching [1, 11, 14, 26]. Over time, this may cause anorexia and result in weight loss [4]. Rarely, venous and lymphatic drainage are compromised [9]. When this occurs, cervical swelling is exacerbated and the patient may appear to be edematous in the face and throat [3, 4, 9].

Functional thyroid tumors may induce hyperthyroid-associated clinical signs; however, these are not typically as pronounced in the dog as they are when present in the hyperthyroid cat [7, 8, 18]. See Section 4.1.1 to review the typical clinical presentation of a hyperthyroid state.

When the clinician confirms the client's concern that a mass is present along the throat, he should prioritize thyroid tumors as a differential diagnosis given the location. However, until a diagnostic work-up is performed to confirm these suspicions, additional differentials must be considered. Abscesses and granulomas secondary to foreign bodies such as a stick ingestion gone awry cannot be ruled out by palpation alone. Less common, but possible differentials include salivary mucoceles, carotid body tumors, and soft tissue sarcomas [1, 3].

The utility of imaging, particularly ultrasound, as a diagnostic modality is that it helps to differentiate thyroid tumors from aforementioned differentials [1]. Ultrasound is also advantageous because it allows the clinician to make an assessment about the vascularity of the tumor as well as its invasiveness. In addition, ultrasound may facilitate fine needle aspiration (FNA) of samples although biopsies are indicated for definitive diagnosis owing to the low yield and blood contamination that are frequently associated with FNAs [1, 14, 29].

Because of the rapid rate with which thyroid carcinomas expand and the high likelihood of invasion into surrounding soft tissue structures, a rapid diagnosis is critical. The prognosis for untreated patients is poor: median survival time is 3 months following the diagnosis [28] compared with more than 3 years when treated with surgical excision [1, 26], and up to nearly 4 years with radiation therapy [30, 31].

12.3 The Pathophysiology of Hypothyroidism

Acquired hypothyroidism is a frequent occurrence in senior dogs [4]. It results from underproduction of thyroxine (T4) and triiodothyronine (T3). In theory, this could arise as a primary disorder (originating from the thyroid gland itself), secondary disorder [origi-nating from impaired stimulation of the thyroid gland by the pituitary gland via thyroid-stimulating hor-mone (TSH)], or tertiary disorder [originating from impaired stimulation of the thyroid gland indirectly by the hypothalamus via thyrotropin-releasing hormone (TRH)] [32].

In reality, 95% of the cases of canine hypothyroidism are due to dysfunction at the level of the thyroid itself [32]. Of these cases, 50% are caused by lymphocytic thy-roiditis [33], an immune-mediated condition marked by progression destruction of thyroid gland architecture [32]. The remaining 50% of cases of primary hypothy-roidism in dogs are caused by idiopathic atrophy: thy-roid parenchyma is subsequently replaced by adipose tissue [32].

In health, thyroid hormones contribute to metabolic rate, oxygen consumption, and heart rate. Thyroid hormones act as inotropes and chronotropes, thereby enhancing the response of the heart to catecholamines [32].

Across all age groups of dogs, puppies have the highest T4 concentrations, and as they mature, the levels steadily decline. Dogs older than 6 years of age have total thy-roxine (TT4) concentrations that are 21% lower than in young adult dogs [34], and old dogs have TT4 concen-trations that are 40% lower than in young adults [4, 32, 35]. This age-related decline in thyroid hormone concen-trations is poorly understood. It may be that the thyroid gland becomes less sensitive to TSH or that the thyroid gland degenerates with age [4].

In addition to age, other variables such as pharmaceuticals can adversely impact the hypothalamic–pituitary–thyroid axis. Glucocorticoids, for example, affect the way in which the body metabolizes thyroid hormones. In addition, glucocorticoids inhibit the secretion of TSH. Sulfonamides block the synthesis of thyroid hormones by inhibiting iodination, and pheno-barbital decreases TT4 and free T4 (FT4) [4].

Concurrent non-thyroidal illnesses such as hypoadren-ocorticism, diabetic ketoacidosis, and organ failure can also suppress the hypothalamic–pituitary–thyroid axis [4, 36–39]. The decline in total thyroid hormone is pro-portional to the severity of the illness; severe decreases are associated with higher mortality rates [4, 40, 41].

Breed is yet another factor that impacts the hypothalamic–pituitary–thyroid axis. In a study by Shiel *et al.*, 91% of young, healthy Greyhounds were found to have TT4 concentrations either below or at the low end of the normal reference range [42].

However, despite the influence of these factors – age, pharmacologic agents, and breed – some middle-aged to older dogs do in fact develop clinically relevant hypo-thyroidism.

12.4 The Typical Presentation of a Hypothyroid Dog

The challenge of canine hypothyroidism is that the pathology within the thyroid gland cannot be detected on physical examination. Unlike thyroid neoplasia, in which there is a palpable, sometimes even grossly vis-ible cervical mass, dogs with hypothyroidism palpate as being normal, that is, the clinician is unable to feel the thyroid gland to detect that something is amiss.

At first glance, it may strike the reader as unusual for hypothyroidism to be included in a physical examination textbook, given that the thyroid of a hypothyroid dog is not palpable. However, it is important to mention the hypothyroid dog with regard to the physical examination because very often these patients present with classic historical or examination-related findings.

The typical canine patient with hypothyroidism is a purebred dog [43, 44]. Specifically, the breeds considered at an increased risk for developing this endocrinopa-thy are Golden Retrievers, Doberman Pinschers, Lab-rador Retrievers, and Cocker Spaniels [4, 32]. Boxers, Dachshunds, Miniature Schnauzers, Great Danes, and Old English Sheepdogs are also overrepresented in the literature [45, 46].

With the exception of congenital hypothyroidism, which has been reported in the juvenile Giant Schnauzer [47], Boxer [48], and Scottish Deerhound [49], the majority of hypothyroid patients are middle- to older-aged [33].

Because thyroid hormones regulate metabolism and hypothyroidism implies a sluggish metabolic rate, clients may report unusually sloth-like behavior. The patient may be inactive or sedentary. Initially clients may liken this to a normal by-product of aging; how-ever, its persistence may become concerning. Clients may also report decreased mental stimulation: the patient may be less engaged with the client and/or its surroundings. Both the client and veterinarian may remark upon the patient's weight gain despite the cli-ent's insistence that there has been no change in diet [4, 45, 50].

On physical examination, 60–80% of hypothyroid dogs display a classic dermatopathy [51, 52]: bilaterally sym-metrical, non-pruritic truncal alopecia with an alopecic "rat tail." The head and distal limbs tend to remain unaf-fected compared with the areas of wear along the body. What coat remains tends to be dull, coarse, and/or brit-tle. In some cases, the undercoat may be lost altogether, with or without the loss of primary guard hairs, giving the patient the appearance of having retained its puppy coat [4, 32, 45, 50].

Because the anagen phase of hair growth requires thyroid hormones, the lack thereof may cause a patient not to regrow its fur post-clipping. As a result, many patients present for coat-related concerns following grooming [4, 50].

The skin itself may be normal or it may become excessively flaky and/or greasy. In areas of wear where the coat has thinned, the underlying skin may exhibit hyperpigmentation or even hyperkeratosis [50].

Other hypothyroid patients may present for recurrent bacterial skin infections [50]: 20–30% of dogs with hypothyroidism are diagnosed with pyoderma [51, 52]. Systemic *Malassezia* overgrowth is also not uncommon [50]. When these secondary infections develop, hypothyroid patients become pruritic [50].

Rarely does myxedema, the deposition of hyaluronic acid in the dermis, causing edema, occur [50]. Hyaluronic acid is in excess in these patients because the lack of thyroid hormone reduces the metabolic breakdown of glycosaminoglycans [53]. The result is thickened, puffy skin over the forehead, eyelids, and cheeks [50]. Vesicles develop on the surface of the affected skin [50, 54]. Mucin may be expressed digitally from these vessels as a clear, stringy substance [50].

When a canine patient of the "right" age and breed presents with a history and/or physical examination findings that mirror the above, then a diagnosis of hypothyroidism should be considered until proven otherwise.

12.5 The Atypical Presentation of a Hypothyroid Dog

Hypothyroid dogs may also present, albeit rarely, with neurologic signs in the absence of dermatopathy [4, 55–58]. Although the etiology remains unknown in dogs, it has been demonstrated in rats that hypothyroid-induced reduction in axonal transport leads to peripheral neuropathy [59]. The mechanism underlying cranial nerve dysfunction secondary to hypothyroidism is even more unclear; however, it has been hypothesized that the deposits of mucin compress the cranial nerves where they exit the skull [60, 61]. Of all cranial nerves, the trigeminal, facial, and vestibulocochlear nerves are most likely to be impacted [55, 60].

Although the canine neurologic examination will be reviewed in detail in Chapter 16, it should be recognized that endocrinopathy can result in peripheral neuropathy or peripheral vestibular syndrome, and that a patient that presents with either may not have a primary neurologic disease [55].

In particular, a middle-aged to older, middle- to large-sized breed that presents for slowly progressive neurologic deficits may in fact be hypothyroid. These patients tend to show mild gait deficits that then develop into paraparesis or tetraparesis. They may or may not be ataxic. Spinal reflexes may be reduced in all four limbs, although the hind limbs tend to be the most impaired. Although these patients necessitate a full orthopedic and neurologic work-up to rule out potential pathology that could require surgery, it is important that the clinician not wear blinders and be cognizant that hypothyroidism is a possibility. When hypothyroidism is implicated in neurologic disease, the patient can recover: neurologic signs are reversible after 2–3 months of supplementing the patient with thyroxine [55, 59, 62].

Atypical hypothyroid patients may also exhibit intermittent or constant forelimb lameness that is responsive to treatment with thyroxine [55, 58, 59]. In addition, hypothyroid-induced facial paralysis and vestibular dysfunction, characterized by a head tilt, ataxia, circling, strabismus, and nystagmus, are responsive to thyroxine supplementation [55, 56, 60, 61].

Although these clinical signs represent atypical presentations of hypothyroidism, they serve as good reminders that a systems-based approach to the physical examination, although effective in teaching the novice clinician to be comprehensive, must ultimately integrate physical examination findings, given the overlap between systems. The astute clinician must learn to construct the isolated details into a complete clinical picture. Neurologic disease may not simply be neurologic disease; dermatologic disease may not simply be dermatologic disease; endocrinopathy may not simply be straightforward endocrinopathy. In other words, they may be inextricably linked. It is up to the clinician to recognize that link if diagnosis and treatment are to be facilitated.

12.6 Assessing the Lymphatic System

Just as the clinician is limited by which components of the endocrine system are palpable on the physical examination, the clinician is granted few opportunities to evaluate the lymphatic system.

As discussed in Section 4.2, the lymphatic system neighbors the vasculature. Its series of lymph vessels exist to collect fluid and proteins that are forced out of blood vessels by hydrostatic pressure. The vessels then return this excess fluid to the general circulation via lymphatic ducts. Without this network, peripheral tissues would rapidly drown in edema [63].

With the exception of lymphatic obstruction, which causes grossly visible edema, the clinician is unable to evaluate the lymphatic vasculature individually. The only structures of the lymphatic system that the clinician is able to assess at each visit are the lymph nodes.

Think of the lymph nodes as filters of lymph as well as sites for lymphocytes to proliferate and differentiate [63].

Lymph nodes are positioned in the body where they interfere least with mobility and the circulation [63]. The peripheral lymph nodes tend to be paired. Three sets are typically palpable in the normal patient [64]:

- the submandibular lymph nodes;
- the superficial cervical lymph nodes, otherwise referred to as pre-scapular lymph nodes;
- the popliteal lymph nodes.

These sets of lymph nodes should be palpated at each visit, with the clinician noting their size, shape, consistency, and symmetry, and whether palpation is painful. Lymph nodes should feel rubbery [65], like scallops. They should not be tender to the touch.

12.7 Examining the Submandibular Lymph Nodes

See Section 11.6.

12.8 Examining the Superficial Cervical or Pre-Scapular Lymph Nodes

The superficial cervical or pre-scapular lymph nodes are located at the cranial border of each scapula, covered by the cleidocervical and omotransversarius muscles. These nodes are oval, flat, and typically paired when comparing the left and right sides of the body. There may be as few as one and as many as four on each side, the right and the left. They collectively drain the neck, shoulder, and corresponding forelimb [63, 66].

To palpate the superficial cervical or pre-scapular lymph nodes, the clinician may stand directly behind the patient or immediately in front. The author prefers the former approach, using her left hand to palpate the left nodes and the right hand to palpate the right nodes. Both hands are used simultaneously to appreciate significant differences in symmetry, size, and consistency between sides.

The patient can be seated or standing for this exercise. The clinician simply follows his fingertips up from the humerus to the point of the shoulder. At the point of the shoulder, the clinician's thumb and index finger should grasp deep to the scapular border. As the clinician then moves his thumb and index finger from deep to superficial, the lymph nodes should "slip" through, much like a thyroid nodule can be felt to "slip" through the fingertips upon ventral neck palpation (Figure 12.1).

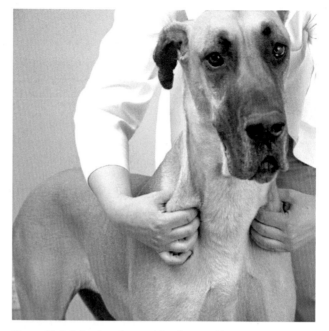

Figure 12.1 Palpating the superficial cervical lymph nodes by grasping deep to the scapular border at the point of the shoulder. Source: Courtesy of the Media Resources Department at Midwestern University.

12.9 Examining the Popliteal Lymph Nodes

The popliteal lymph nodes are located at the caudal aspect of each stifle, sandwiched between the biceps femoris and semitendinosus muscles. These nodes are more round than the superficial cervical lymph nodes. They are paired structures, with typically one on each side, the right and the left. They collectively drain the distal hind limbs [63, 66].

To palpate the popliteal lymph nodes, the clinician should stand behind the patient with the patient facing in the same direction as the clinician. The clinician should pinch the thumb and index finger of each hand together as if crimping pie crust. Together, the thumb and index finger of the left hand are placed over the left caudal thigh; the thumb and index finger of the right hand are placed over the right caudal thigh. Beginning at the caudal thigh, the thumb and index finger are then progressively slid down the thigh to the caudal stifle, applying firm and constant pressure all the way. At the level of the caudal stifle, the clinician can grasp deep to the skin. As the clinician's fingertips move from deep to superficial, the lymph nodes should "slip" through (Figure 12.2).

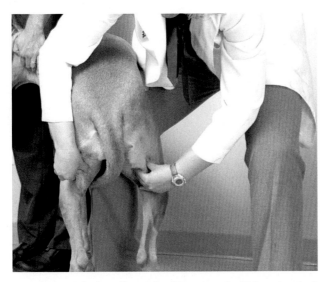

Figure 12.2 Palpating the popliteal lymph nodes. This patient had a tendency to want to sit down, so the clinician has supported the dog's weight to keep it standing by placing her knee under the dog's caudal abdomen. Source: Courtesy of the Media Resources Department at Midwestern University.

12.10 Feeling for Lymph Nodes That Should Not Be Present

Compared with the submandibular, superficial cervical, and popliteal lymph nodes, which should be appreciated at every visit, there are two sets of lymph nodes that are not typically palpable in health:

1) the axillary lymph nodes;
2) the superficial inguinal lymph nodes.

The axillary lymph nodes are located, as their name implies, within the arm pit, caudal to the shoulder joint. The teres major muscle forms its lateral boundary, and the rectus thoracis muscle forms its medial boundary. The axillary lymph nodes are disc-shaped and deeper than expected, which is why they are not normally palpable. They drain the thoracic wall and the thoracic limbs and also the thoracic and cranial abdominal mammary glands [63, 66].

Even though the axillary lymph nodes are not typically palpable, the clinician should feel for their presence at each visit. The only way that the clinician will know if they are enlarged is if he feels for them. By including this palpation in each examination, the clinician develops consistency in his approach to the physical examination and is less likely to miss them on the rare occasion when they are enlarged and in need of a more extensive work-up.

To feel for the axillary lymph nodes, the clinician should stand behind the patient with the patient facing in the same direction as the clinician. The clinician should take flattened hands with fingers pressed together and slide them into the axilla: the left palm against the left axillary and the right palm against the right axilla. Using his fingertips as a paddle, the clinician should start by reaching rostrally and then moving caudally. The act of strumming one's fingers back and forth should allow the lymph nodes to "blip" past the clinician's fingertips if they are indeed enlarged.

The superficial inguinal lymph nodes are located where the caudoventral abdominal wall meets the medial thighs. There are one to two nodes per side, and their shape is typically oval. These drain the abdominal and inguinal mammary glands. They also receive drainage from the popliteal nodes, ventral pelvis, tail, and the medial thigh, stifle, and crus. In the male, drainage includes the penis, prepuce, and scrotum [63, 66].

To palpate for the superficial inguinal lymph nodes, which are appreciated only in diseased states involving lymph drainage, the clinician should stand behind the patient with the patient facing in the same direction as the clinician. The clinician should take flattened hands with fingers pressed together and slide them into the crease between the medial thigh and the abdominal wall: the left palm against the left crease and the right palm against the right crease. Using his fingertips as a paddle, the clinician should feel dorsolateral to the last mammary gland. The act of strumming one's fingers back and forth should allow the lymph nodes to "blip" past the clinician's fingertips if they are indeed enlarged. Alternatively, the clinician may palpate this region one side at a time with the patient in lateral recumbency and each hind limb gently abducted.

References

1 Liptak, J.M. (2007) Canine thyroid carcinoma. *Clinical Techniques in Small Animal Practice*, **22** (2), 75–81.

2 Hullinger, R.L. (1979) The endocrine system, in *Miller's Anatomy of the Dog*, 2nd edn. (eds. H.E. Evans and G.C. Christensen), Saunders, Philadelphia, pp. 602–631.

3 Barber, L.G. (2007) Thyroid tumors in dogs and cats. *Veterinary Clinics of North America: Small Animal Practice*, **37** (4), 755–773, vii.

4 Scott-Moncrieff, J.C. (2012) Thyroid disorders in the geriatric veterinary patient. *Veterinary Clinics of North America: Small Animal Practice*, **42** (4), 707–725, vi–vii.

5 Wucherer, K.L. and Wilke, V. (2010) Thyroid cancer in dogs: an update based on 638 cases (1995–2005). *Journal of the American Animal Hospital Association*, **46** (4), 249–254.

6 Page, R.L. (2001) Tumors of the endocrine system, in *Small Animal Clinical Oncology*, 3rd edn. (eds. S.J. Withrow and E.G. MacEwen), Saunders, Philadelphia, pp. 423–427.

7 Capen, C.C. (2002) Tumors of the endocrine glands, in *Tumors in Domestic Animals*, 4th edn. (ed. D.J. Meuten), Iowa State Press, Ames, IA, pp. 638–664.

8 Mooney, C.T. (2005) Hyperthyroidism, in *Textbook of Veterinary Internal Medicine: Diseases of the Dog and Cat*, 6th edn. (eds. S.J. Ettinger and E.C. Feldman), Saunders Elsevier, St. Louis, pp. 1544–1560.

9 Brodey, R.S. and Kelly, D.F. (1968) Thyroid neoplasms in the dog. A clinicopathologic study of 57 cases. *Cancer*, **22** (2), 406–416.

10 Leav, I., Schiller, A.L., Rijnberk, A. *et al.* (1976) Adenomas and carcinomas of the canine and feline thyroid. *American Journal of Pathology*, **83** (1), 61–122.

11 Carver, J.R., Kapatkin, A., and Patnaik, A.K. (1995) A comparison of medullary thyroid carcinoma and thyroid adenocarcinoma in dogs: a retrospective study of 38 cases. *Veterinary Surgery*, **24** (4), 315–319.

12 Patnaik, A.K. and Lieberman, P.H. (1991) Gross, histologic, cytochemical, and immunocytochemical study of medullary thyroid carcinoma in sixteen dogs. *Veterinary Pathology*, **28** (3), 223–233.

13 Birchard, S.J. and Roesel, O.F. (1981) Neoplasia of the thyroid-gland in the dog – a retrospective study of 16 cases. *Journal of the American Animal Hospital Association*, **17** (3), 369–372.

14 Harari, J., Patterson, J.S., and Rosenthal, R.C. (1986) Clinical and pathologic features of thyroid tumors in 26 dogs. *Journal of the American Veterinary Medical Association*, **188** (10), 1160–1164.

15 Hayes, H.M., Jr. and Fraumeni, J.F., Jr. (1975) Canine thyroid neoplasms: epidemiologic features. *Journal of the National Cancer Institute*, **55** (4), 931–934.

16 Sullivan, M., Cox, F., Pead, M.J., and Mcneil, P. (1987) Thyroid tumors in the dog. *Journal of Small Animal Practice*, **28** (6), 505–512.

17 Marks, S.L., Koblik, P.D., Hornof, W.J., and Feldman, E.C. (1994) 99mTc-pertechnetate imaging of thyroid tumors in dogs: 29 cases (1980–1992). *Journal of the American Veterinary Medical Association*, **204** (5), 756–760.

18 Kent, M.S., Griffey, S.M., Verstraete, F.J. *et al.* (2002) Computer-assisted image analysis of neovascularization in thyroid neoplasms from dogs. *American Journal of Veterinary Research*, **63** (3), 363–369.

19 Ron, E., Lubin, J.H., Shore, R.E. *et al.* (1995) Thyroid cancer after exposure to external radiation: a pooled analysis of seven studies. *Radiation Research*, **141** (3), 259–277.

20 Hancock, S.L., Cox, R.S., and McDougall, I.R. (1991) Thyroid diseases after treatment of Hodgkin's disease. *New England Journal of Medicine*, **325** (9), 599–605.

21 Robbins, J. and Schneider, A.B. (2000) Thyroid cancer following exposure to radioactive iodine. *Reviews in Endocrine and Metabolic Disorders*, **1** (3), 197–203.

22 Benjamin, S.A., Saunders, W.J., Lee, A.C. *et al.* (1997) Non-neoplastic and neoplastic thyroid disease in beagles irradiated during prenatal and postnatal development. *Radiation Research*, **147** (4), 422–430.

23 Carling, T. and Udelsman, R. (2004) Cancer of the endocrine system. Section 2. Thyroid tumors, in *Cancer: Principles and Practice of Oncology*, 7th edn. (eds. V.T. DeVita, S. Hellman, and S.A. Rosenberg), Lippincott Williams & Wilkins, Philadelphia, pp. 1727–1840.

24 Mumma, R.O., Rashid, K.A., Shane, B.S. *et al.* (1986) Toxic and protective constituents in pet foods. *American Journal of Veterinary Research*, **47** (7), 1633–1637.

25 Dzanis, D.A. (1994) The Association of American Feed Control Officials Dog and Cat Food Nutrient Profiles: substantiation of nutritional adequacy of complete and balanced pet foods in the United States. *Journal of Nutrition*, **124** (12 Suppl.), 2535S–2539S.

26 Klein, M.K., Powers, B.E., Withrow, S.J., *et al.* (1995) Treatment of thyroid-carcinoma in dogs by surgical resection alone – 20 cases (1981–1989). *Journal of the American Veterinary Medical Association*, **206** (7), 1007–1009.

27 Mitchell, M., Hurov, L.I., and Troy, G.C. (1979) Canine thyroid carcinomas: clinical occurrence, staging by means of scintiscans, and therapy in 15 cases. *Veterinary Surgery*, **8**, 112–118.

28 Worth, A.J., Zuber, R.M., and Hocking, M. (2005) Radioiodide (^{131}I) therapy for the treatment of canine thyroid carcinoma. *Australian Veterinary Journal*, **83** (4), 208–214.

29 Thompson, E.J., Stirtzinger, T., Lumsden, J.H., and Little, P.B. (1980) Fine needle aspiration cytology in the diagnosis of canine thyroid carcinoma. *Canadian Veterinary Journal/Revue Vétérinaire Canadienne*, **21** (6), 186–188.

30 Theon, A.P., Marks, S.L., Feldman, E.S., and Griffey, S. (2000) Prognostic factors and patterns of treatment failure in dogs with unresectable differentiated thyroid carcinomas treated with megavoltage irradiation. *Journal of the American Veterinary Medical Association*, **216** (11), 1775–1779.

31 Pack, L., Roberts, R.E., Dawson, S.D., and Dookwah, H.D. (2001) Definitive radiation therapy for infiltrative thyroid carcinoma in dogs. *Veterinary Radiology & Ultrasound*, **42** (5), 471–474.

32 Feldman, E.C. and Nelson, R.W. (2004) Hypothyroidism, in *Canine and Feline Endocrinology and Reproduction*, 3rd edn. (eds. E.C. Feldman and R.W. Nelson), Saunders, St. Louis, pp. 86–151.

33 Graham, P.A., Refsal, K.R., Nachreiner, R.F. (2007) Etiopathologic findings of canine hypothyroidism. *Veterinary Clinics of North America: Small Animal Practice*, **37** (4), 617–631, v.

34 Reimers, T.J., Lawler, D.F., Sutaria, P.M. *et al.* (1990) Effects of age, sex, and body size on serum concentrations of thyroid and adrenocortical hormones in dogs. *American Journal of Veterinary Research*, **51** (3), 454–457.

35 Gonzalez, E., and Quadri, S.K. (1998) Effects of aging on the pituitary–thyroid axis in the dog. *Experimental Gerontology*, **23** (3), 151–160.

36 Kantrowitz, L.B., Peterson, M.E., Melian, C., and Nichols, R. (2001) Serum total thyroxine, total triiodothyronine, free thyroxine, and thyrotropin

concentrations in dogs with nonthyroidal disease. *Journal of the American Veterinary Medical Association*, **219** (6), 765–769.

37 Nelson, R.W., Ihle, S.L., Feldman, E.C., and Bottoms, G.D. (1991) Serum free-thyroxine concentration in healthy dogs, dogs with hypothyroidism, and euthyroid dogs with concurrent illness. *Journal of the American Veterinary Medical Association*, **198** (8), 1401–1407.

38 Panciera, D.L. and Refsal, K.R. (1994) Thyroid function in dogs with spontaneous and induced congestive heart failure. *Canadian Journal of Veterinary Research*, **58** (3), 157–162.

39 Vail, D.M., Panciera, D.L., and Ogilvie, G.K. (1994) Thyroid hormone concentrations in dogs with chronic weight-loss, with special reference to cancer cachexia. *Journal of Veterinary Internal Medicine*, **8** (2), 122–127.

40 Elliott, D.A., King, L.G., and Zerbe, C.A. (1995) Thyroid hormone concentrations in critically ill canine intensive care patients. *Journal of Veterinary Emergency and Critical Care*, **5**, 17–23.

41 Mooney, C.T., Shiel, R.E., and Dixon, R.M. (2008) Thyroid hormone abnormalities and outcome in dogs with non-thyroidal illness. *Journal of Small Animal Practice*, **49** (1), 11–16.

42 Shiel, R.E., Brennan, S.F., Omodo-Eluk, A.J., and Mooney, C.T. (2007) Thyroid hormone concentrations in young, healthy, pretraining greyhounds. *Veterinary Record*, **161** (18), 616–619.

43 Bellumori, T.P., Famula, T.R., Bannasch, D.L. *et al.* (2013) Prevalence of inherited disorders among mixed-breed and purebred dogs: 27,254 cases (1995–2010). *Journal of the American Veterinary Medical Association*, **242** (11), 1549–1555.

44 Oberbauer, A.M., Belanger, J.M., Bellumori, T. *et al.* (2015) Ten inherited disorders in purebred dogs by functional breed groupings. *Canine Genetics and Epidemiology*, **2**, 9.

45 Merchant, S.R. and Taboada, J. (1997) Endocrinopathies. Thyroid and adrenal disorders. *Veterinary Clinics of North America: Small Animal Practice*, **27** (6), 1285–1303.

46 Kemppainen, R.T.J., and MacDonald, J.M. (1993) Canine hypothyroidism, in *Current Veterinary Dermatology; The Science and Art of Therapy* (eds. C.E. Griffin, K.W. Kwochka, and J.M. MacDonald), Mosby Year Book, St. Louis, pp. 265–272.

47 Greco, D.S., Feldman, E.C., Peterson, M.E. *et al.* (1991) Congenital hypothyroid dwarfism in a family of Giant Schnauzers. *Journal of Veterinary Internal Medicine*, **5** (2), 57–65.

48 Mooney, C.T. and Anderson, T.J. (1993) Congenital hypothyroidism in a boxer dog. *Journal of Small Animal Practice*, **34** (1), 31–35.

49 Robinson, W.F., Shaw, S.E., Stanley, B., and Wyburn, R.S. (1988) Congenital hypothyroidism in Scottish Deerhound puppies. *Australian Veterinary Journal*, **65** (12), 386–389.

50 Scott-Moncrieff, J.C. (2007) Clinical signs and concurrent diseases of hypothyroidism in dogs and cats. *Veterinary Clinics of North America: Small Animal Practice*, **37** (4), 709–722, vi.

51 Panciera, D.L. (1994) Hypothyroidism in dogs: 66 cases (1987–1992). *Journal of the American Veterinary Medical Association*, **204** (5), 761–767.

52 Dixon, R.M., Reid, S.W., and Mooney, C.T. (1999) Epidemiological, clinical, haematological and biochemical characteristics of canine hypothyroidism. *Veterinary Record*, **145** (17), 481–487.

53 Doliger, S., Delverdier, M., More, J. *et al.* (1995) Histochemical study of cutaneous mucins in hypothyroid dogs. *Veterinary Pathology*, **32** (6), 628–634.

54 Miller, W.H., Jr. and Buerger, R.G. (1990) Cutaneous mucinous vesiculation in a dog with hypothyroidism. *Journal of the American Veterinary Medical Association*, **196** (5), 757–759.

55 Fors, S. (2006) Neuromuscular manifestations of hypothyroidism in dogs. *Svensk Veterinartidning*, **14**, 11–17.

56 Bichsel, P., Jacobs, G., and Oliver, J.E., Jr. (1988) Neurologic manifestations associated with hypothyroidism in four dogs. *Journal of the American Veterinary Medical Association*, **192** (12), 1745–1747.

57 Braund, K.G., Dillon, A.R., August, J.R., and Ganjam, V.K. (1981) Hypothyroid myopathy in two dogs. *Veterinary Pathology*, **18** (5), 589–598.

58 Budsberg, S.C., Moore, G.E., and Klappenbach, K. (1993) Thyroxine-responsive unilateral forelimb lameness and generalized neuromuscular disease in four hypothyroid dogs. *Journal of the American Veterinary Medical Association*, **202** (11), 1859–1860.

59 Jaggy A., Oliver J.E., Ferguson D.C. *et al.* (1994) Neurological manifestations of hypothyroidism: a retrospective study of 29 dogs. *Journal of Veterinary Internal Medicine*, **8** (5), 328–336.

60 Cuddon, P.A. (2002) Acquired canine peripheral neuropathies. *Veterinary Clinics of North America: Small Animal Practice*, **32** (1), 207–249.

61 Jaggy, A. and Oliver, J.E (1994). Neurologic manifestations of thyroid disease. *Veterinary Clinics of North America: Small Animal Practice*, **24** (3), 487–494.

62 Indrieri, R.J., Whalen, L.R., Cardinet, G.H., and Holliday, T.A. (1987) Neuromuscular abnormalities associated with hypothyroidism and lymphocytic thyroiditis in three dogs. *Journal of the American Veterinary Medical Association*, **190** (5), 544–548.

63 Bezuidenhout, A.J. (1993) The lymphatic system, in *Miller's Anatomy of the Dog*, 3rd edn. (eds. H.E. Evans and M.E. Miller), Saunders, Philadelphia, pp. 717–757.

64 Rijnberk, A. and Stokhof, A.A. (2009) General examination, in *Medical History and Physical Examination in Companion Animals*, 2nd edn. (eds. A. Rijnberk and F.J. vanSluijs), Saunders Elsevier, St. Louis, pp. 47–62.

65 Rijnberk, A. and vanSluijs, F.S. (eds.) (2009) *Medical History and Physical Examination in Companion Animals*, 2nd edn., Saunders Elsevier, St. Louis.

66 Dyce, K.M., Sack, W.O., and Wensing, C.J.G. (1996) *Textbook of Veterinary Anatomy*, 2nd edn., Saunders, Philadelphia.

13

Examining the Cardiovascular and Respiratory Systems of the Dog

13.1 Congenital Heart Disease in the Dog

Congenital heart disease occurs more frequently in the dog than in the cat: its incidence is 6.8–8 per 1000 canine patients compared with 0.2–1.0 per 1000 feline patients that present to university clinics annually [1, 2]. In dogs, these number translate to one affected patient out of every 15 litters [2].

Of canine patients that present to cardiology referral centers, congenital heart disease occurs with even greater frequency, being identified in roughly 21.7% of all cases [3].

Congenital defects may cause volume overload, such as patent ductus arteriosus (PDA). The ductus arteriosus is a normal fetal structure. Because the fetal lung is ordinarily collapsed, blood is shunted away from the lungs, from the pulmonary artery to the descending aorta. After the patient is born and takes its first breath, the lungs begin to function. As they do, blood needs to travel through them in order to become oxygenated, and the only way this occurs is via closure of the ductus arteriosus. This begins within hours of birth; the ductus arteriosus is effectively closed 48 hours after birth, and within 1 month of life all that remains of the ductus arteriosus is a conglomeration of elastic fibers, the ligamentum arteriosum [2, 4].

When this closure does not occur, the ductus arteriosus is said to be patent, and this congenital defect is referred to as a PDA. Depending upon the resource consulted, PDAs are the number one or number two congenital defect in dogs [4, 5]. In a left-to-right PDA, which is most typical, high pressure within the aorta causes blood to shunt inappropriately into the pulmonary circulation. This additional volume overwhelms the pulmonary vasculature, which is already receiving blood from the pulmonary artery. As a result, an excess of blood returns from the lungs to the left atrium. Over time, volume overload of the left atrium into the left ventricle causes both chambers of the heart to respond by dilation and hypertrophy. Ultimately, left-sided heart failure develops, with resultant pulmonary congestion [2, 4].

Less commonly, a right-to-left PDA occurs. The increased volume to the pulmonary vasculature causes increased pressure within the pulmonary vasculature. When this increase in vascular resistance within the pulmonary tree exceeds systemic vascular resistance, blood is shunted inappropriately from the pulmonary artery to the aorta in the same manner as occurred during fetal life. The unoxygenated blood from the pulmonary artery in effect dilutes the oxygenated blood within the aorta, causing poor systemic oxygenation, caudal cyanosis, and polycythemia as a compensatory mechanism in the body's attempt to increase perfusion to tissues [2, 4].

Breeds at increased risk of PDA include the Miniature Poodle, Chihuahua, Maltese, Bichon Frise, Cocker Spaniel, English Springer Spaniel, Keeshond, and Shetland Sheepdog. Regionally, Labrador Retrievers, Newfoundlands, and German Shepherds may be predisposed based upon their gene pool [2, 4].

Congenital defects may also cause pressure overload, such as subaortic stenosis (SAS) or pulmonic stenosis (PS). SAS is the most common type of aortic stenosis in the dog. It occurs when left ventricular emptying is discouraged by the presence of a fibrous band just below the aortic semilunar valves. This results in incomplete emptying of the left ventricle and pressure overload in an attempt by the ventricle to improve its pumping efficiency. In order to pump out more blood, the left ventricular wall thickens. However, this complicates the situation because it increases the myocardial oxygen demand, yet the left ventricle is no more efficient. The inheritance pattern of this condition has been established in the Newfoundland, a breed commonly at risk. Other predisposed breeds include the Boxer, English Bulldog, German Shepherd, Golden Retriever, Great Dane, and Bull Terrier. Depending upon the resource consulted, SAS is the number one or number two congenital defect in dogs [2, 4, 5].

The pathophysiology of PS is similar to that of SAS with the exception of location: in PS, the outflow obstruction is at the level of the pulmonic valve. This impinges on the ejection of blood from the right ventricle. Over time, the right ventricle hypertrophies in an attempt to compensate for pressure overload. The inheritance pattern in the Beagle has been established; other predisposed breeds include the Cocker Spaniel, English Bulldog, Bull

Performing the Small Animal Physical Examination, First Edition. Ryane E. Englar.
© 2017 John Wiley & Sons, Inc. Published 2017 by John Wiley & Sons, Inc.

Mastiff, Samoyed, Schnauzer, and West Highland White Terrier. PS is one of the top three congenital defects in the dog [2, 4, 5].

Other congenital defects such as Tetralogy of Fallot primarily cause cyanosis due to an assortment of lesions that collectively complicate perfusion. Tetralogy of Fallot involves a combination of the following [2, 4]:

- PS;
- right ventricular hypertrophy;
- ventricular septal defect, causing oxygenated blood to be shunted to the right side of the heart;
- dextroposition/overriding of the aorta.

The English Bulldog, Miniature Poodle, and Miniature Schnauzer are predisposed. These patients present with polycythemia and generalized cyanosis in addition to generalized malaise, perceived weakness, and shortness of breath. These patients may be presented with a history of collapse. When ausculted, they have a classic "washing machine" murmur [2, 4].

Less commonly seen congenital heart defects include peritoneopericardial diaphragmatic hernias. In addition to causing vascular compromise, these also adversely impact respiration. Inappropriately maintained communication between the thoracic and abdominal cavities causes abdominal contents to migrate into the chest, in effect encroaching upon the lungs' ability to inflate. The result is a patient that cannot fully expand its lungs (see Figure 5.10a and b) [2].

When it comes to congenital heart disease overall, purebred dogs are more likely to be affected than mixed breeds [1, 6–8]. As mentioned, breed predispositions vary by disease [2]. So, too, do sex predispositions. Female dogs, for instance, are more likely to develop PDA [1, 2].

Dogs with congenital heart disease may present on physical examination with no known history of cardiac disease. A heart murmur or arrhythmia may well be incidental findings on the cardiothoracic component of the physical examination, as is typical of cats with cardiac disease [2].

Puppies may also be clinically normal, yet have an innocent, functional, non-pathologic murmur identified on their initial wellness or vaccination follow-up examinations [9–12]. These murmurs are fairly common findings at the initial wellness examination [13]: in a 2015 study by Szatmári *et al.*, 28% of 195 puppies had an innocent murmur [14]. Innocent murmurs tend to be systolic, low-grade, musical, and loudest along the left sternal border. They result from turbulence within the heart and vessels as the heart is still developing, and they tend to resolve by 5 months of age. They may also result from physiologic anemia [2, 14].

Based upon auscultation alone, it is challenging for the general practitioner to discern which murmurs in puppies are innocent versus those which are reflective of underlying cardiac pathology [15–19]. Referral to a veterinary cardiologist is ideal [9, 10, 14] for follow-up echocardiography, which is superior to survey radiography for the detection of congenital heart disease [13, 20].

Clients may elect the "wait and see" approach, hoping for the murmur to dissipate with age. This is appropriate and acceptable in many circumstances, without harm to the patient. However, the following signs indicate that cardiac findings on the physical examination are less likely to be innocent and are therefore in much greater need of diagnostic intervention [13]:

- a continuous murmur as occurs with PDA;
- the presence of additional abnormal heart sounds;
- the presence of abnormal or missing pulses;
- the patient is otherwise clinical.

Dogs that are clinical for heart disease may present for failure to thrive, weakness, cyanosis, or collapse. Patients may also develop exercise intolerance and labored breathing. Sudden death may occur in cases of SAS [2].

13.2 Acquired Heart Disease in the Dog

When heart disease is acquired in the dog, it may be due to structural or functional issues. With regard to the former, there are two main categories to consider:

- acquired valvular diseases [21];
- acquired cardiomyopathy, in which the heart muscle itself becomes diseased [22].

Valvular disease is common in the dog, accounting for 75–80% of cases [21, 23, 24]. Specifically, mitral valve disease (MVD) has the greatest frequency of occurrence, especially in male small-breed dogs such as Miniature Poodles, Pomeranians, Yorkshire Terriers, Chihuahuas, and King Charles Cavalier Spaniels [21]. In MVD, there is progressive degeneration of the valve. Nodules develop on valve leaflets, distorting valvular anatomy. If the nodules become sufficiently numerous or prominent, they will hinder coaptation of the leaflets, causing a "leaky" valve through which backward flow of blood travels. Every time the heart beats in a patient with MVD, there is inappropriate regurgitation of blood back through the mitral valve into the left atrium. Over time, this increases left atrial pressure. In response, the left atrium dilates. Eventually, there is so much additive backflow of blood that pulmonary vein pressure increases and pulmonary edema may ensue [21].

In moderate to severe cases of MVD, left atrium dilation may be evident on thoracic radiographic study. The prominent left atrium may in fact cause dorsal displacement of the trachea or compression of the mainstem bronchus, causing the patient to present for a chronic cough [21] (Figure 13.1).

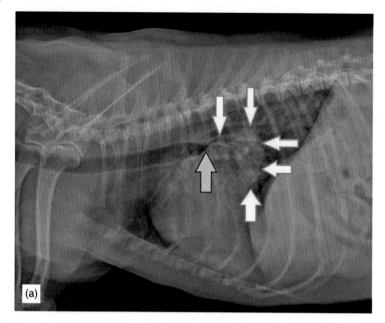 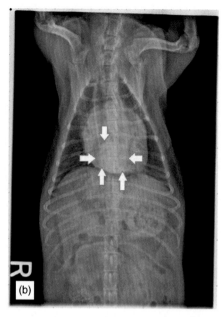

Figure 13.1 (a) Lateral thoracic radiograph of a canine patient with MVD that has resulted in left-sided congestive heart failure. The white arrows denote an enlarged left atrium and the yellow arrow depicts compression of the mainstem bronchus. This compression is likely to blame for the patient's development of a cough. (b) Orthogonal view of the same patient as in (a). The white arrows denote an enlarged left atrium. Source (a), (b): Courtesy of Daniel Foy, MS, DVM, DACVIM, DACVECC.

Canine cardiomyopathy is also common in dogs [22, 23, 25]. In particular, dilated cardiomyopathy (DCM) is overrepresented in Doberman Pinschers and Irish Wolfhounds, with males at increased risk for development of DCM [22]. Unlike cats, in which DCM has been primarily linked to taurine deficiency [26], the etiology in dogs is unknown [22]. Dogs that are affected develop progressive left ventricular dilation. As disease worsens, the left atrium also dilates and ventricular contractility is compromised. The result is an enlarged, yet comparatively flaccid heart, the contractions of which are inefficient and incomplete. Aortic blood flow is at decreased velocity. Blood backs up from the left ventricle into the left atrium. When regurgitation is sufficient, congestive heart failure ensues. Ventricular arrhythmias are common and sudden death occurs in one-third to half of Doberman Pinschers that acquire this disease [22].

Obesity may increase the risk of acquired heart disease in the dog [23]. In people, there is a proven link between obesity and heart failure [27–29]. Although atherogenic coronary heart disease is rare in dogs compared with people [23], in large part due to dogs' high high-density lipoprotein (HDL) to low-density lipoprotein (LDL) ratio [30], obesity in dogs does increase heart rate and blood pressure [31–34]. In addition, obese dogs develop concentric cardiac hypertrophy [35] and the thickness of their left ventricular free wall increases [36].

Much remains to be learned about canine cardiomyopathy. However, a key message is that canine cardiac patients tend to be more varied than feline patients. Whereas feline patients do not typically present with a cardiac complaint [13], dogs may do so, especially

when the patient has acquired cardiac disease. Dobermans with DCM, for example, will frequently present for syncope or exercise intolerance [22]. It is up to the astute clinician to pair breed and historical findings with key physical examination findings in order to assess the likelihood that the patient has true cardiac disease.

13.3 Assessing the Cardiovascular System Prior to Auscultation

An assessment of the cardiovascular system begins with observation of the patient in the examination room.

13.3.1 Attitude

The clinician should observe the patient's attitude, mentation, and emotional status as soon as he enters the examination room. In particular, he should ask the following two questions:

1) Is the patient alert and responsive?
2) Is the patient visibly distressed?

Within an unfamiliar setting such as a veterinary clinic, canine patients may be fearful. If the degree of fear is extreme, the patient may glue itself to the floor or hunch against the wall as if "frozen" with fear. See Figure 9.7b for a visual depiction of a clinic-anxious canine patient. However, keep in mind that a patient may also be "frozen" due to respiratory distress: a dog may be so focused on labored breathing to survive that it takes little else into consideration. Recall that labored breathing is not uncommon in severe cases of SAS and PS [2]. In these situations, attention to the dog's body language (ears, eyes, and posture) may help the clinician to decide if the patient is acting out of fear or due to disease.

13.3.2   Respiratory Rate

Compared with a cat's respiratory rate of 20–40 breaths per minute, the respiratory rate for a typical dog is 10–30 breaths per minute. Larger breeds of dogs tend to have respiratory rates that are toward the lower end and smaller breeds toward the higher end of the normal range [37].

Note that respiratory rate is not the same parameter as respiratory depth. A patient could be tachypneic with very shallow breaths or a bradypneic patient could have very deep breaths.

Note also that patients may make an assessment of respiratory rate difficult by sniffing excessively in an attempt to explore their environment. Sniffing is not the same as tachypnea. In a patient that is sniffing, the clinician should delay the assessment of respiratory rate until the patient has settled so as not to obtain artificially a "respiratory rate" of 50–100 that could imply that the patient is in respiratory distress as from significant respiratory or cardiac disease.

Respiratory rate tends to be elevated in very anxious patients [38], and may also be elevated in patients with cardiac disease [39].

13.3.3   Respiratory Effort

Recall from Section 5.2.3 that the respiratory cycle is one round of inspiration and expiration [37]. Inspiration is a typically active process compared with expiration, which is passive.

Dyspnea occurs when there is difficulty getting air in, getting air out, or both, creating effort on the part of the patient to complete the respiratory cycle [40, 41]. Inspiratory dyspnea results when the upper airway narrows. It takes more effort to draw air into the body, and the body may require the use of the auxiliary respiratory muscles, the scalenus and the sternocephalicus, to complete the process. In addition, the alar folds of the nostrils may flare and the lips may retract to increase airflow [40].

When the lungs are inelastic, the ribcage is non-compliant, or the bronchi are narrowed, expiratory dyspnea results. It takes more effort to push air out of the body. Abdominal pressure is engaged against the diaphragm to expel air forcibly by increasing intrathoracic pressure. However, this process may narrow smaller bronchi, exacerbating respiratory distress [40, 41]. Increased respiratory effort is visible and should cue the clinician to either respiratory, cardiac, or mixed respiratory and cardiac disease.

13.3.4   Respiratory Route

Unlike cats, which are not built to sustain long periods of open-mouth breathing [42], dogs are nasal and mouth breathers. Whereas an open-mouth breathing cat can easily become a respiratory or cardiac emergency [26], a panting dog is not necessarily abnormal. Panting is in fact normal for dogs as a means by which they blow off excess heat [37]. Via a process called thermal polypnea [43], dogs acclimate to high ambient temperatures by taking in air through the nose and exhaling it through the mouth [44]. As hot air is inspired, the lateral nasal gland increases the amount of fluid it secretes to saturate the air with moisture prior to exhalation [45]. Because that air is subsequently expelled through the mouth, the heat that it contains does not have the opportunity to warm up the nasal mucosa. It simply is forced through the mouth into the environment.

It is important to remember that excitement and anxious energy can also lead to increased body heat production. In other words, the environment is not the only potential source of heat stress for the patient. With a patient that is overly excited or overly anxious within the veterinary setting, care must be taken to allow it the opportunity to utilize thermal polypnea. A patient's ability to blow off heat should not be compromised because if it is, the patient may panic and become increasingly resistant to restraint [46].

For this reason, the author prefers basket muzzles to nylon muzzles for in-clinic use because the patient's ability to pant is not hindered. Figure 9.21a and b illustrate the appearance of a basket muzzle and how it allows the patient to open its mouth without becoming a safety hazard to the veterinary team.

13.3.5   Mucous Membrane Color

See Section 11.7.1. Recall that the oral mucous membranes are the most commonly used tissues to assess mucous membrane color. However, when the gums are not accessible on account of patient temperament, the clinician can assess the color of the conjunctival sac (Figure 13.2). The conjunctival sac is reliable in terms of its color and will appear pale, for example, if a patient is anemic.

As an alternative to the conjunctival sac, the clinician may also evaluate a dog's mucous membrane color by assessing the color of the vulvar lips or the inner lining of the prepuce. In the case of females, this is only reliable when the patient is not actively cycling because mucous membrane color of the vulvar lip folds may change in relation to the stage of the reproductive cycle (Figure 13.3) [37].

13.3.6   Capillary Refill Time (CRT)

See Section 11.7.2.

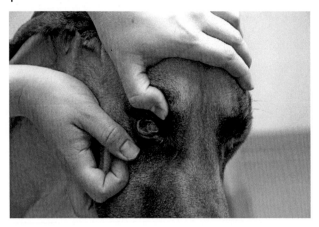

Figure 13.2 Evaluating mucous membrane color of the conjunctival sac in combination with an assessment of the nictitating membrane. Source: Courtesy of the Media Resources Department at Midwestern University.

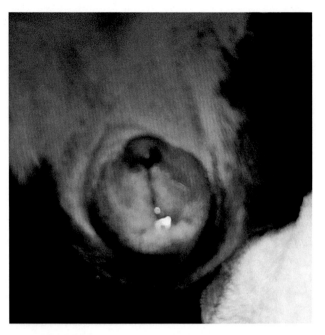

Figure 13.3 Evaluating mucous membrane color of this patient's vulvar lips would be inappropriate because the patient is actively in estrus. The stage of the reproductive cycle will alter mucous membrane color of this region of the body in such a way that makes it unreliable. Source: Courtesy of Shannon Carey, DVM.

13.3.7 Jugular Pulse

The jugular vein is the largest vein on either side of the neck. Although it is used frequently to sample blood in dogs, the veterinary team often forgets that it is equally useful, if not more so, as an indicator of venous return and central venous pressure [40].

In the normal standing patient that is staring straight ahead, the jugular vein cannot be seen or felt. This does not hold true if venous return to the heart is obstructed [40, 47].

In right-sided heart failure, there is a back-up of blood returning to the right-side of the heart because the right side of the heart is inefficient, ineffective, or both. This overload of blood distends the jugular veins so that the jugular veins become visible, palpable, or both. Sometimes the jugular veins become so distended that they may pulse visibly with each heartbeat [40, 47, 48].

Other places to look for evidence of poor venous return in dogs are the ventral thorax and abdomen, the prepuce, and at or proximal to the tarsal joint. These areas may "stock up" in situations involving poor venous return, meaning that they may appear rather edematous. Stocking up of the abdomen is often referred to as ascites. Ascites occurs more frequently in dogs than cats, which more typically present in respiratory distress [40, 47].

13.3.8 Assessing Femoral Pulses

The arterial pulse is the palpable wave generated by ventricular systole whereby blood forcibly passes from the left ventricle of the heart to the aorta. What is felt as the pulse is essentially the stretch of an artery to accommodate the blood [47].

The femoral arteries are the most common site of pulse detection in the dog. Every heartbeat should be associated with a pulse [47]. To appreciate the femoral pulse, the clinician should position himself behind the patient, with the patient facing away from the clinician. With fingers together and curled palms, the clinician may feel for the femoral arteries, which are located in the groin at the crease where the pelvic limbs attach to the body. Using the fingertips as opposed to the thumbs will increase the clinician's sensitivity in detecting pulses. Using the fingertips will also reduce the chance that the pulse that is felt is not the clinician's own digital pulse and is instead truly the patient's. If there is any doubt, the clinician may auscult the heart at the same time he is feeling for the pulse. The patient's pulse and heart rate should match (Figure 13.4a and b).

Once the clinician gets used to where to feel for the femoral pulse, he should practice palpating both the left and right femoral arteries at the same time. As the clinician develops sound technical skills, feeling both arteries simultaneously will help in assessing the symmetry of the pulses. The presence of asymmetrical pulses may help to facilitate a diagnosis of underlying cardiac compromise.

The following information can be obtained from the pulse:

- pulse rate;
- perfusion;
- pulse quality.

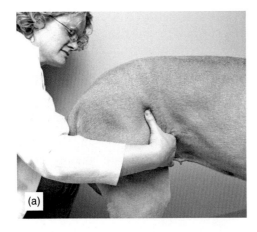

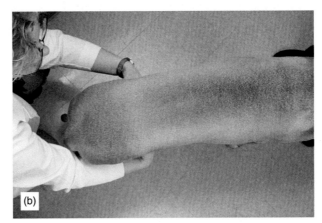

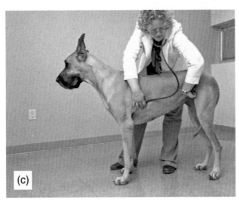

Figure 13.4 (a) Proper positioning for palpation of the femoral pulses, viewed from the side. (b) Proper positioning for palpation of the femoral pulses, viewed from above. (c) Pairing auscultation with femoral pulse palpation to be certain that each heart beat is associated with a pulse. Source (a)–(c): Courtesy of the Media Resources Department at Midwestern University.

As mentioned, the pulse rate should match the heart rate. For each heartbeat that is ausculted, there should be a corresponding pulse. To determine if the pulse rate matches the heart rate, the clinician should simultaneously auscult the heart and palpate the femoral pulses (Figure 13.4c).

If the pulses are not synchronous with heart rate, then there are so-called "dropped beats" of the heart as can occur with cardiac arrhythmias. When contraction of the heart occurs prematurely due to the electrical activity of an ectopic focus, the ventricles may not have had a chance to fill such that ventricular output is reduced. The resultant stroke volume may be insufficient to translate into a palpable pulse. The pulse is therefore absent despite cardiac contraction [49].

Absent pulses can also reflect lack of perfusion, although aortic thromboembolisms are much more commonly seen in the cat than in the dog [26, 47, 48, 50].

How strong or weak a pulse is depends upon the difference between the systolic and diastolic blood pressures. The greater the difference, the stronger is the pulse; the weaker the difference, the poorer is the pulse [47].

- "Bounding" pulses are stronger than normal and result from either a reduced diastolic pressure, an elevated systolic pressure, or both [47].

- "Thready" pulses are weaker than normal and result from either a reduced systolic pressure, an elevated diastolic pressure or both [47].
- Erratic pulses may reflect underlying atrial fibrillation [47].

Assessing the pulse is an imperfect science. See Section 5.2.10 to review the shortcomings associated with its evaluation.

13.4 Cardiothoracic Auscultation

When considering the cardiovascular system, it is important to review the pathway of blood through the body as this is the foundation for understanding cardiac parameters, heart sounds, and the various points in the cycle at which dysfunction can arise. See Section 5.3.1 to review the cardiac cycle.

13.4.1 Normal Heart Sounds

"Lub-dub" is what often comes to mind when students are asked to describe normal heart sounds. The first heart sound, S1, represents the "lub" and the second heart sound, S2, represents the "dub." More specifically,

S1 occurs as the atrioventricular valves close and the ventricles contract, whereas S2 occurs as the pulmonic and aortic valves close and the heart fills [51].

13.4.2 Abnormal Heart Sounds

Murmurs are specific types of cardiac sounds that are not heard in the normal patient and are the result of turbulent blood flow. Whereas S1 and S2 are typically crisp, discrete sounds, murmurs may be described as a "whoosh" as from turbulence [47].

When murmurs are ausculted, they should be described by their location in the cardiac cycle [47]:

- Systolic murmurs occur between S1 and S2.
- Diastolic murmurs occur between S2 and S1.

Murmurs should also be described by their intensity. Intensity is typically described in terms of grade [47, 51]:

- Grade 1 murmurs are low-intensity sounds that are difficult to pick up immediately, often because they are highly focal. They are often indistinct in that they may blend into S1 such that the only indication of their presence is a seemingly prolonged S1.
- Grade 2 murmurs are also soft sounds but, unlike Grade 1 murmurs, they are distinct. They are also more readily identified despite tending to be focal.
- Grade 3 murmurs are of moderate intensity and are easily heard as soon as the stethoscope is applied to the chest.
- Grade 4 murmurs are loud and tend to be more diffuse.
- Grade 5 murmurs are very loud and diffuse, and are characterized by a palpable thrill – that is, turbulence is so great as to create a vibration that is palpable across the chest wall.
- Grade 6 murmurs are very loud and do not require the use of a stethoscope to hear.

Murmurs should also be described by the so-called point of maximum intensity – that is, the valve corresponding to the loudest region of the murmur [51]. This may help to prioritize the list of differential diagnoses based on the location(s) where one or more valves appear to be dysfunctional.

13.4.3 Other Heart Sounds

Both S1 and S2 are typically audible on cardiothoracic auscultation of the normal patient. However, in addition to S1 and S2, there are certain heart sounds that are not typically heard in health but that may arise with cardiac pathology [51]:

- S3 occurs on the coattails of S2 as blood flows from the atria into the now relaxed, partially filled ventricles. S3 is heard in pathologic situations involving ventricular dilation such as dilated cardiomyopathy (DCM).

- S4 occurs as the atria contract, just prior to S1. S4 is heard in pathologic situations involving atrial dilation, such as hypertrophic cardiomyopathy, which is rare in dogs and more commonly seen in cats. S4 is also appreciated in third-degree atrioventricular block.

When heard, S3 and S4 result in "gallop rhythms" [51]. When S3 is present, the gallop rhythm that is created is

$$1 \quad 23 \quad 1 \quad 23 \quad 1 \quad 23 \quad 1 \quad 23$$

When S4 is present, the gallop rhythm that is created is

$$41 \quad 2 \quad 41 \quad 2 \quad 41 \quad 2 \quad 41 \quad 2$$

13.4.4 Ausculting the Heart

The dog has a much larger thorax than the cat [51] (Figure 13.5).

When evaluating the left lateral thorax, the clinician may use the acronym P–A–M to recall the valves that may be ausculted in this region of the chest (Figure 13.6a and b) [40, 47]:

- The **pulmonic** valve: auscult over the left second to third intercostal space, seated dorsal to the sternum at approximately one-third of the distance between the sternum and vertebral column.
- The **aortic** valve: auscult over the left second to third intercostal space.
- The **mitral** valve: auscult over the left fifth to sixth intercostal space, near the sternum.

When evaluating the right lateral thorax, the clinician may use the acronym R–A–T to recall that the **right atrial** valve is the **tricuspid**, which may be ausculted over the fourth to fifth intercostal space near the sternum [40, 47] (Figure 13.6c and d).

To appreciate auscultation in a live patient, see Figure 13.7.

13.4.5 Understanding How the Stethoscope Is Built to Facilitate Auscultation

See Section 5.3.6.

13.4.6 Understanding the Limitations of Cardiothoracic Auscultation

Cardiothoracic auscultation constitutes an important part of every physical examination: it allows for the detection of murmurs and arrhythmias that could be pathologic and may therefore reflect underlying cardiac disease.

The primary limitation of cardiothoracic auscultation is that it cannot discern physiologic from pathologic murmurs unless the grade of the murmur is fairly severe, in which case the latter can be assumed [15–19]. Given that 15% of clinically healthy puppies between 20 and 108 days old were found to have a murmur on cardiothoracic

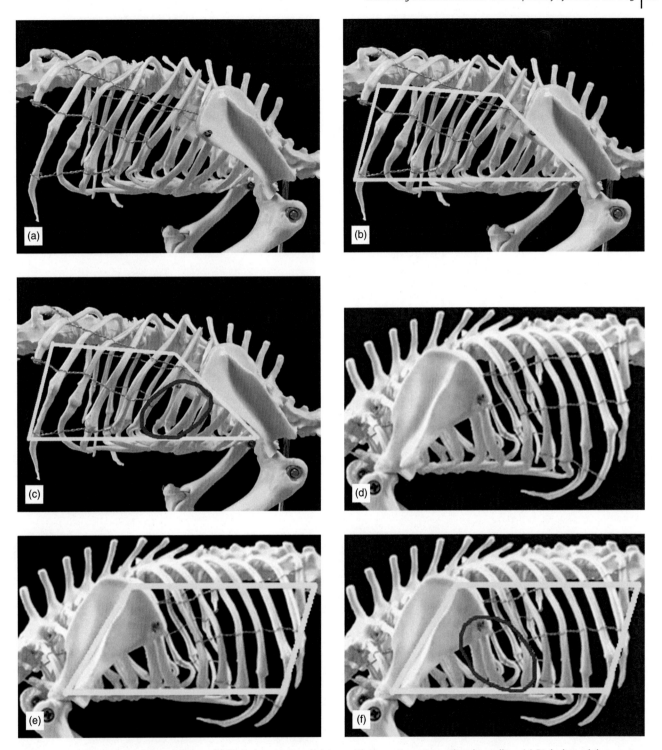

Figure 13.5 (a) Right lateral dog skeleton. (b) Right lateral dog skeleton with thoracic cavity outlined in yellow. (c) Right lateral dog skeleton with thoracic cavity outlined in yellow and rudimentary heart drawn in, in red. (d) Left lateral dog skeleton. (e) Left lateral dog skeleton with thoracic cavity outlined in yellow. (f) Left lateral dog skeleton with thoracic cavity outlined in yellow and rudimentary heart drawn in, in red. (*Continued*)

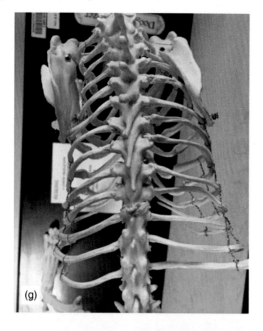

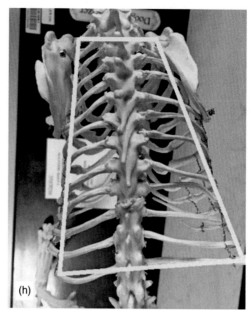

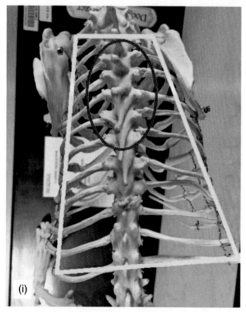

Figure 13.5 (*Continued*)
(g) Aerial view of dog skeleton. (h) Aerial view of
dog skeleton with thoracic cavity outlined in yellow.
(i) Aerial view of dog skeleton with thoracic cavity
outlined in yellow and rudimentary heart drawn in,
in red.

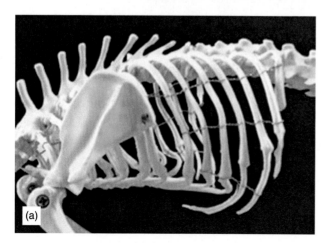

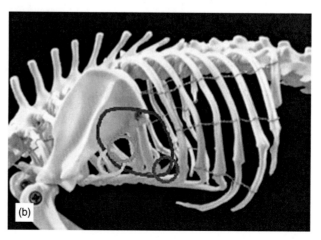

Figure 13.6 (a) Left lateral dog skeleton, close-up. (b) Left lateral dog skeleton, close-up, with rudimentary heart valves drawn in: yellow–orange = pulmonic valve; blue = aortic valve; purple = mitral valve. (*Continued*)

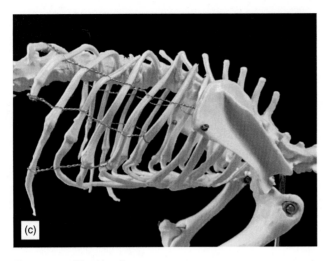

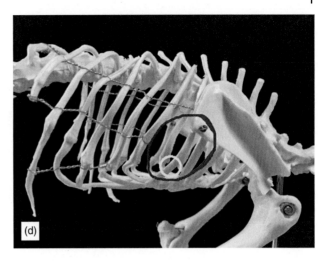

Figure 13.6 (*Continued*)
(c) Right lateral dog skeleton, close-up. (d) Right lateral dog skeleton, close-up, with rudimentary heart valve drawn in: yellow = tricuspid valve.

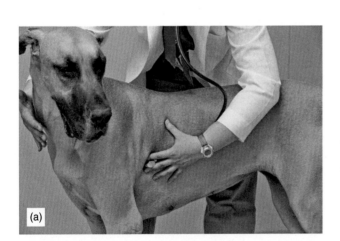

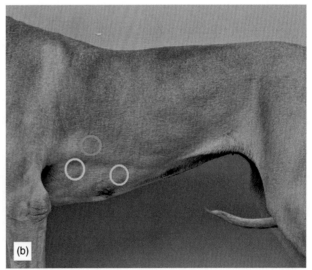

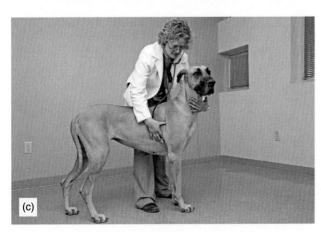

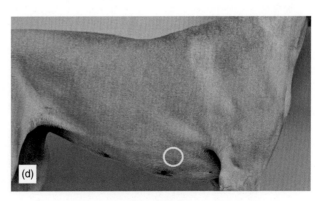

Figure 13.7 (a) Left lateral thoracic auscultation in a live patient. (b) Left lateral view of live patient detailing proper locations for cardiac auscultation: yellow–orange = pulmonic valve; blue = aortic valve; purple = mitral valve. (c) Right lateral thoracic auscultation in a live patient. (d) Right lateral view of live patient detailing proper locations for cardiac auscultation: yellow = tricuspid valve.
Source (a)–(d): Courtesy of the Media Resources Department at Midwestern University.

examination in a 2015 study by Szatmári *et al.*, there is a need for additional follow-up to classify the murmur definitively as something to be or not to be concerned about [14]. Echocardiography is the ideal imaging modality to confirm the location(s) of the faulty valve(s), and to establish whether true pathology is present [9, 10, 14].

A second limitation of cardiothoracic auscultation is that the murmur's point of maximum intensity as determined through auscultation is not always accurate in identifying the likely cause of the murmur [13]. In other words, auscultation has very low specificity when it comes to murmur identification. In a study of Whippets with murmurs, a presumptive diagnosis of mitral regurgitation, based upon auscultation alone, was incorrect in 166 of 186 dogs [52].

A third limitation of cardiothoracic auscultation is that it cannot identify cardiomegaly with the exception of severe pericardial effusion, in which case heart sounds are typically muffled and the patient may present with concurrent pulsus paradoxus: pulse quality varies with respiration [53]. Cardiomegaly may precipitate congestive heart failure. Identification of which chambers of the heart are enlarged on survey radiography may contribute to the development of a workable diagnosis for the clinician. For example, in a small-breed patient with an enlarged left atrium, as evident on orthogonal thoracic radiographs, the clinician is more likely to consider mitral valve degeneration (see Figure 13.1). Similarly, if a clinician were to see an enlarged cardiac silhouette on survey chest films in an asymptomatic patient (Figure 13.8), the films may spur

him to recommend referral to a veterinary cardiologist even if cardiothoracic auscultation is unremarkable.

The bottom line is that cardiothoracic auscultation is useful as a starting point. However, additional diagnostic tests may need to be performed in order to secure an accurate diagnosis that then allows for appropriate medical management of the patient.

13.5 The Respiratory Patient

The canine respiratory patient typically has one of four presentations: disease of the upper airway, the larynx, lower airway, and/or the thoracic cavity.

13.5.1 The Upper Airway Patient

Upper airway disease is less commonly seen in dogs than in cats, which tend to be affected in communal settings such as shelters and catteries [54–60]. However, dogs, too, are most at risk when housed in high-density conditions such as boarding and breeding kennels, pet shops, research facilities, and shelters [61–64].

When upper airway disease occurs in dogs, several potential causes should be considered, including, but not limited to, the following [61, 64–67]:

- Infectious disease:
  - Bacterial
    - *Bordetella bronchiseptica*
    - *Mycoplasma* spp.
    - Secondary invaders
      - *Streptococcus* spp.
      - *Pasteurella* spp.
      - *Pseudomonas* spp.
  - Viral
    - Canine distemper virus (CDV)
    - Canine adenovirus type 2 (CAV-2]
    - Canine parainfluenza virus (CPIV)
    - Canine herpesvirus-1 (CHV)
    - Canine respiratory coronavirus
    - Canine influenza virus
  - Fungal
    - *Aspergillus fumigatus.*
- Structural disease:
  - Chronic hyperplastic rhinitis, secondary to infectious disease
  - Brachycephalic airway syndrome
  - Intranasal neoplasia
    - Adenocarcinoma
    - Fibrosarcoma
    - Chondrosarcoma
    - Osteosarcoma
    - Squamous cell carcinoma
    - Rarely, lymphoma
    - Rarely, benign intranasal polyps.

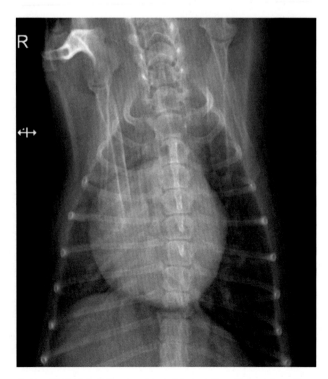

Figure 13.8 This Chihuahua has evidence of cardiomegaly on its V/D thoracic radiograph. Source: Courtesy of Patricia Bennett, DVM.

- Aspiration reflex/reverse or inspiratory sneezing:
  - Normal response of nasal mucosa to mechanical irritation.
- Foreign bodies:
  - Grass awn.

When one or more infectious agents colonizes the upper respiratory tract of a dog, the patient is said to have canine infectious respiratory disease (CIRD). Colloquially, this is referred to as infectious tracheobronchitis or kennel cough [61, 67, 68], and it has been identified globally [63].

Patients with CIRD typically present with mild, self-limiting signs of nasal discharge and a paroxysmal dry cough [61, 63]. Nasal discharge is typically serous but may become mucopurulent once upper airway inflammation is sufficient and/or if opportunistic secondary bacterial infections take root. Co-infections are common and increase morbidity, as do secondary infections: the lower airway may become involved and medical intervention may be required [63, 64, 67].

See Section 3.4 for images of nasal discharge. Although these images pertain to cats, nasal discharge in a dog would look similar.

Dogs that recover from CIRD, in particular Whippets and Dachshunds, may be predisposed to chronic hyperplastic rhinitis. The upper respiratory tract becomes so compromised by severe primary viral infection that secondary infection of the upper airway with one or more species of bacteria occurs. There is less nasal turbinate damage than is seen in cats following severe bouts of feline herpesvirus (FHV); however, the nasal mucosa is visibly thickened when viewed via advanced imaging modalities. This hyperplastic mucosa is responsible for producing persistent, copious nasal discharge for which long-term antibiotics are indicated. Relapse is common once antibiotic therapy is discontinued [65].

Compared with cats, dogs have a higher incidence of fungal rhinitis. When fungal rhinitis occurs in the dog, *Aspergillus fumigatus* is more commonly implicated than *Cryptococcus neoformans*, which is more typical in the cat. Dolichocephalic dogs tend to be affected more than breeds with other skull shapes. In particular, the German Shepherd appears to be predisposed. Nasal discharge may involve one or both nostrils, and is typically mucoid, mucopurulent, or honey-like in color and consistency. As the condition progresses, a destructive rhinitis ensues and epistaxis may result. Facial distortion is a possibility although airflow through both nares typically remains normal [65].

Non-infectious causes of upper airway disease in dogs infrequently include nasopharyngeal polyps, which occur primarily in young cats [55, 69–71]. Of greater concern to dogs is a condition due to conformation that is referred to as the brachycephalic upper airway syndrome [72–79].

Brachycephalic upper airway syndrome is unique to brachycephalic breeds and is the direct result of a foreshortened facial skeleton for aesthetic purposes [78]. Recall from Section 11.1 that brachycephalic breeds have a high cephalic index and broad, short skulls that give their muzzle a "pushed in" appearance [80–83]. This shorter, wider skull predisposes brachycephalic breeds to respiratory disorders [73] due to any combination of the following anatomical abnormalities [72]:

- Stenotic nares [74, 75, 84, 85].
- Narrowed nasal passages [74, 86].
- Malformed and/or oversized rostral and caudal nasal turbinates [76, 87, 88].
- Hyperplastic tongue [77, 79].
- Elongated soft palate [74, 89–91].
- Inappropriate thickening of the soft palate [77, 92–96].
- Chondromalacia of the arytenoid cartilages, causing protrusion into the laryngeal lumen [74, 97].
- Everted laryngeal saccules [92, 97].
- Laryngeal collapse due to increased airway resistance [78, 97–99].
- Hypoplastic trachea [74, 88, 90, 100].
- Bronchial collapse [74, 101].

Of the anatomic deviations listed, certain brachycephalic breeds are affected the most: Pugs, English Bulldogs, and French Bulldogs [77, 93, 101–104]. Of these three breeds, Pugs tend to have the most aberrant nasal turbinates, meaning that the turbinates abnormally continue to grow throughout life [88, 92]. Hypoplastic tracheas are most common in English Bulldogs, whereas Pugs are more often affected by bronchial collapse [74], with the cranial left bronchus most often involved [101].

With regard to upper airway disease that stems from the brachycephalic airway syndrome, affected patients typically present for progressive disease that may be severe by the time the patient reaches 12 months of age [75, 105].

Because many of the anatomic defects that comprise the brachycephalic syndrome tend to cause upper airway obstruction during the inspiratory part of the respiratory cycle, clients may report stertor, a snoring sound. This is typically pronounced when the patient is asleep, however, it may persist when the patient is awake [55, 74, 75].

Patients with concurrent laryngeal disease as a feature of their brachycephalic syndrome may also present with stridor, in which a harsh, high-pitched sound materializes during inspiration [55, 74, 75].

Patients with brachycephalic syndrome are often heat and exercise intolerant. If overly stressed, their mucous membranes may easily become cyanotic and they may be prone to syncopal collapse [75, 104, 106].

Other less common, non-infectious, structural causes of upper airway disease in the dog include intranasal neoplasia, of which the most common type is adenocarcinoma [65, 107, 108].

13.5.2 The Patient with Laryngeal Disease

Laryngeal disease in dogs as it pertains to brachycephalic syndrome was reviewed in brief in Section 13.5.1. However, laryngeal disease is not limited to cases of brachycephalic syndrome. In addition, canine laryngeal paralysis is a chronic, progressive syndrome most notably observed in large-breed dogs. Certain breeds are predisposed to congenital disease, including the Bouvier des Flandres [109], Dalmatian [110], Bull Terrier, Siberian Husky [111, 112], and white-coated German Shepherd [113, 114].

Alternatively, the majority of dogs acquire laryngeal paralysis as from underlying polyneuropathy, polymyoypathy, trauma, immune-mediated, neoplastic, and/or metabolic disease, such as hypothyroidism. More often than not, the cause of the condition is never identified [114, 115].

Labrador Retrievers are overrepresented in cases of acquired laryngeal paralysis, as are Golden Retrievers, Newfoundlands, and Irish Setters [115].

When laryngeal paralysis occurs, the abductor muscles of the larynx fail to abduct the arytenoid cartilages during inspiration. This may occur unilaterally or bilaterally depending upon whether one or both of the recurrent laryngeal nerves are implicated. The result is upper airway obstruction, characterized by stridorous breathing, exercise intolerance, respiratory distress, and, potentially, collapse [114, 115].

13.5.3 The Lower Airway Patient

Lower airway disease in the canine patient may be due to the following [116]:

- Bronchopneumonia:
  - Infectious
    - Secondary to infectious tracheobronchitis
    - Secondary to damage to the lower airway from smoke inhalation
  - Aspiration induced, as from megaesophagus.
- Allergic airway disease:
  - Pulmonary infiltration with eosinophilia.
- Left-sided congestive heart failure.
- Parasites:
  - *Oslerus osleri*
  - *Dirofilaria immitis*, the heartworm
  - *Pneumocystis carinii*

- Tracheal collapse
- Bronchial collapse
- Pulmonary neoplasia.

Bronchopneumonia occurs when there is bronchial constriction and flooding of the alveoli. This handicaps the efficiency of gas exchange with resulting hypoxemia. Risk factors for the development of bronchopneumonia include a history of infectious tracheobronchitis and/or an underlying anatomic anomaly such as megaesophagus, which raises the likelihood of aspiration pneumonia (Figure 13.9) [116].

Patients with bronchopneumonia tend to be systemically ill. Depression, decreased appetite, and dehydration are common and the patient may be febrile [116].

Bronchopneumonia may be suspected when the following abnormal lung sounds are ausculted [116]:

- Crackles.
  Crackles are "popping" sounds that occur when airways that were obstructed finally open. The presence of crackles usually indicates that there is an abundance of airway secretion.
- Wheezes.
  Wheezes are "musical" sounds that occur when airways that had been collapsed open during inspiration or close during expiration. They result when there is decreased airway lumen diameter, as in reactive airways that have thickened, or airway collapse due to neighboring pulmonary disease.

Bronchopneumonia may be confirmed with thoracic radiography. Survey films of the chest may demonstrate areas of consolidation or air bronchograms [116].

Allergic airway disease is less commonly seen in the dog than in the cat. When it occurs in the dog, as in allergic bronchitis, it is poorly understood. A relatively new syndrome, pulmonary infiltration with eosinophilia, has been identified in the dog and is thought to be a hypersensitivity reaction to inhaled allergens such as fungal spores or systemic antigens such as heartworm microfilariae. These patients may have a complete blood count that reflects systemic eosinophilia, or the eosinophils may be compartmentalized to the respiratory tree, to be discovered via cytology from samples obtained through bronchoscopy [116].

Sections 13.1 and 13.2 briefly reviewed that pulmonary congestion can result from left-sided congestive heart failure (Figure 13.10). Typically, these patients have radiographic evidence of left-sided heart enlargement, such as an enlarged left atrium that is causing dorsal displacement or pinching of the trachea, engorged pulmonary vasculature, and a peri-hilar to caudodorsal interstitial pattern [116].

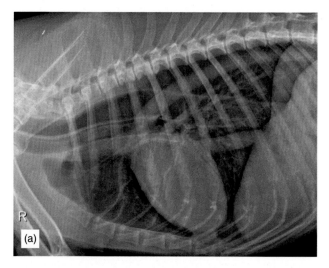
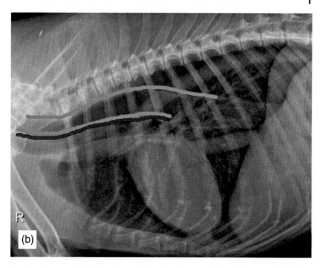

Figure 13.9 (a) This canine patient has radiographic evidence of megaesophagus. (b) The same patient as in (a) with the borders of the esophagus been outlined in blue. The classic "tracheal stripe" sign that is confirmatory for megaesophagus is outlined in red. The "tracheal stripe" sign is created by summation of the dorsal tracheal wall with the ventral wall of the esophagus. Source (a), (b): Courtesy of Jason Eberhardt, DVM, DACVIM.

Tracheal and bronchial collapse in dogs as they pertain to brachycephalic syndrome were reviewed in brief in Section 13.5.1. However, tracheal collapse is not limited to cases of brachycephalic syndrome. In addition, they may result from tracheobronchomalacia, softening of the tracheal cartilage, for which there is no known etiology in people or dogs [117–120]. Because the tracheal rings are softer than expected, they do not maintain their shape in a dog with tracheomalacia. Instead, the tracheal rings flatten dorsoventrally, causing the tracheal membrane to prolapse into the tracheal lumen. This causes tracheal collapse at one or more locations along the windpipe. The result is a patient with varying degrees of tracheal sensitivity that is prone to cough with a characteristic "goose-honk." Toy and small-breed dogs are predisposed, including Chihuahuas, Yorkshire Terriers, Pomeranians, Poodles, and Maltese [121], and roughly one in four patients demonstrates clinical signs by 6 months of age [122], although mid-life to older presentations are not uncommon [117].

Primary lung cancer occurs infrequently in dogs [123]. More often, lung cancer in dogs is the by-product of metastasis [124, 125]. When lung cancer is primary, adenocarcinoma is the most frequent type [126]. Radiographically, these lesions are typically solitary and spherical, and arise from the caudal lung lobes [123].

13.5.4 The Patient with Thoracic Cavity Disease

Recall from Section 5.4.3 that thoracic cavity disease results when there is either an accumulation of fluid, air, or solid tissue within the pleural space. This reduces the ability of the lungs to expand. The patient typically presents in respiratory distress, with head and neck extended in an attempt to gasp air.

When fluid accumulates within the pleural space, the dog is said to have pleural effusion. This effusion can be secondary to the following [127, 128]:

- Congestive heart failure, in which case the fluid is clear to pale yellow.
  More common to see CHF-induced pleural effusion in cats than in dogs.

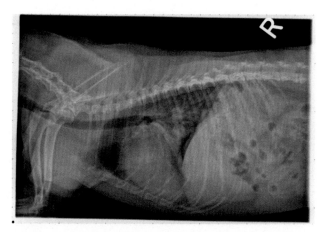

Figure 13.10 Radiographic evidence of left-sided congestive heart in a canine patient. Source: Courtesy of Daniel Foy, MS, DVM, DACVIM, DACVECC.

- Pyothorax, in which case the fluid is opaque and cream colored.
  Most commonly seen in young to middle-aged sporting and gun dog breeds.
- Hemothorax, in which case the fluid is hemorrhagic.
  Commonly seen secondary to trauma or coagulopathy.
- Chylothorax, in which case the fluid is milky white to pink [127].
  More commonly seen in Springer Spaniels and Afghan Hounds.

Regardless of the fluid type, its presence causes the lungs to float up to the dorsocaudal margin of the thoracic cavity, resulting in muffled heart and lung sounds cranioventrally [127, 128]. This is evident radiographically although not all dogs with pleural effusion are stable enough for diagnostic imaging: they may be so severely compromised and dyspneic that the stress of radiographs could easily cause them to decompensate into respiratory arrest [127, 128].

When dogs with pleural effusion can tolerate a radiographic examination, one can appreciate the rounding or scalloping of lung margins, the separation of the lung from the thoracic wall, the increased haziness of the cardiac silhouette, and classic interlobar fissure lines. (See Figure 5.9 to visualize the appearance of this as seen in feline thoracic radiographs.)

In addition to fluid, air can accumulate inappropriately within the pleural cavity. When this occurs, it is usually the result of a traumatic chest wound (an open pneumothorax) or a ruptured bronchus (a closed pneumothorax). The entry of air into the pleural cavity causes the lung lobes to collapse. The patient typically presents in respiratory distress. On survey films of the chest, the lung lobes are retracted from the thoracic wall and they appear more opaque. Typically, pneumothorax is bilateral [128].

Solid tissue can also accumulate inappropriately within the pleural space. This may be the result of trauma, as in the case of diaphragmatic hernias [129–131], congenital malformations, as in the case of peritoneopericardial hernias [132], and neoplastic disease. As with fluid accumulation within the pleural space, tissue accumulation encroaches upon the lung fields, taking away the lungs' ability to expand maximally. The net result is a patient with compromised ability to inflate its lungs fully.

13.6 Assessing the Respiratory System Prior to Auscultation

An assessment of the respiratory system begins with observation of the patient in the examination room. Review the following characteristics from Sections 13.3.1–13.3.6:

- attitude;
- respiratory rate;
- respiratory effort;
- respiratory route;
- mucous membrane color;
- Capillary refill time (CRT).

As when assessing the cardiovascular system, these same characteristics should be observed and documented for every physical examination, especially when a patient presents with a respiratory complaint.

In addition, the clinician should note whether or not the patient is observed to sneeze or cough. If either action is observed, the clinician should follow up with the owner as to duration, frequency, progression, and also if the action, in particular coughing, occurs at a particular time of day or night.

Both sneezing and coughing are non-specific signs involving the respiratory system. Sneezing may be a protective response to allergens or other irritants [40]. Sneezing could also be the body's response to inflammation or a foreign body, tumor or otherwise [40].

Coughing is a second protective reflex that may be stimulated by the larynx, trachea, or bronchi. A laryngeal-induced cough tends to be episodic. It may be so harsh as to trigger gagging that may or may not be productive [40].

13.6.1 The Nose

The clinician should note whether or not the patient has nasal discharge. If nasal discharge is present, the following should be considered:

- Is it unilateral or bilateral?
- Is it fresh or dry?
- Is it copious?
- Is it serous, mucoid, mucopurulent, or hemorrhagic?

See Section 3.4 for images of nasal discharge. Although these images pertain to cats, nasal discharge in a dog would look similar.

The clinician should check for airflow. Review the glass slide technique of assessing airflow that was discussed in Section 3.4.

The clinician should listen for audible upper airway noise, in particular stertor. Recall that stertor is an abnormal sound that is associated with the passage of air through a narrowed upper airway.

13.6.2 The Larynx and the Trachea

The larynx should be palpated to assess for symmetry. To facilitate this examination, the clinician may lift the patient's head and neck. Note that the larynx is very sensitive. Firm pressure may elicit a cough in a normal patient.

The trachea should also be palpated, beginning distal to the larynx and ending at the thoracic inlet. It is important to note if doing so elicits a reproducible cough. A cough on tracheal palpation is not normal and typically indicates tracheal sensitivity.

13.6.3 Thoracic Compliance

Unlike the feline patient, the canine patient is not routinely assessed for thoracic compliance. Medium, large, and giant-sized breeds have low chest compliance: their walls tend to be stiff. Assessing for thoracic compliance would therefore be of limited value.

13.6.4 Thoracic Percussion

See Section 5.5.4 to review the technique of thoracic percussion.

Recall that normal lung fields should sound sonorous when percussed. This sound is low and resonant. When there is a space-occupying mass, percussion yields a duller sound because solid tissue does not contain gas.

Not every primary care clinician uses percussion as a standard aspect of the physical examination. In fact, some clinicians do not make use of it at all because the smaller the patient, the more difficult it is to distinguish normal from abnormal resonance. However, with practice, percussion can corroborate physical examination findings that are suggestive of thoracic cavity disease. For instance, in cases of pneumothorax, percussion should yield increased resonance dorsally; in cases of pyo- or hemothorax, resonance should be decreased ventrally; and in cases of infiltrate within a particular lung lobe, the affected area should be less resonant [40, 127].

13.7 Understanding Normal Airway Sounds

Airway sounds occur when airflow through an air space creates vibrations within that air space. The speed with which the air flows and also the degree of turbulence within the air current influence the type of vibrations that can be heard [40].

Recall that ausculted airway sounds can be normal or adventitious (abnormal). Normal airway sounds include bronchial and vesicular sounds [40]:

- Bronchial sounds arise from the caudal trachea and larger bronchi. These sound harsh, like wind on a stormy day, due to expected turbulence of airflow in these regions.
- Vesicular sounds arise from the periphery of the thoracic cavity. They are soft sounds, like leaves rustling on an autumn day. Their presence confirms that there is air-filled lung between the chest wall and the more turbulent larger airways such as the trachea.

Bronchovesicular sounds are sandwiched between bronchial and vesicular in terms of their location, tone, and loudness. Decreases in these sounds may indicate abnormal tissue or fluid accumulation between the chest wall and the airspace [40].

Note that normal airway sounds are dynamic. For example [40]:

- Normal airway sounds tend to be louder on inspiration than expiration.
- Normal airway sounds may also be increased or decreased. For instance, normal airway sounds are accentuated in patients that are tachypneic.

13.8 Ausculting the Airway

The upper and lower airways should be ausculted in every patient to appreciate airway sounds. Ausculting the trachea should yield bronchial sounds; ausculting the lower airway should yield vesicular and bronchovesicular sounds [40].

It is important to auscult the entire lower airway: the right and left thoracic cavity and also the cranial and the caudal borders of the lung fields (Figure 13.11).

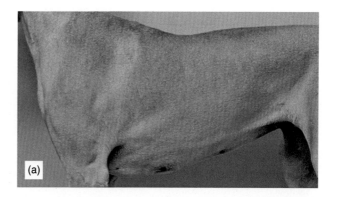

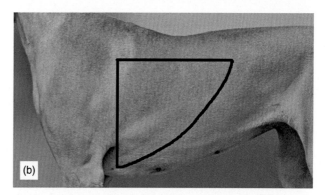

Figure 13.11 (a) Left lateral thorax of a live dog. (b) Left lateral thorax of a live dog with the estimated borders of the lung fields drawn in. Source (a), (b): Courtesy of the Media Resources Department at Midwestern University.

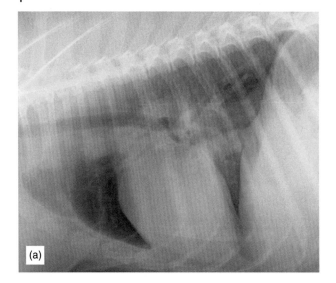

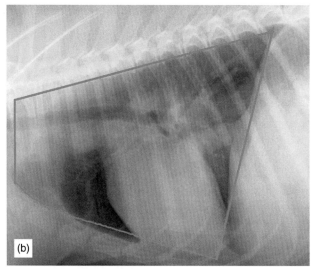

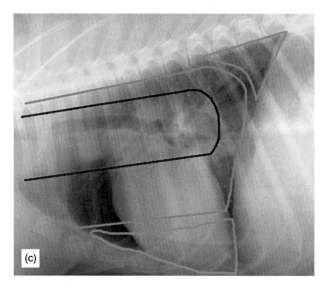

Figure 13.12 (a) Left lateral thoracic radiograph. (b) Left lateral thoracic radiograph with the borders of the lung field outlined in blue. (c) Left lateral thoracic radiograph demonstrating rudimentary diagramming of the lung fields based upon where one might expect to auscult normal airway sounds. Bronchial sounds are heard within the region outlined by red. Bronchovesicular sounds are heard within the region bordered by the blue and red lines. Vesicular sounds are heard within the green triangles.

The novice clinician should consider comparing the clinical anatomy in a live dog with what is seen on a lateral thoracic radiograph to broaden their understanding of respiratory anatomy relative to the cardiovascular system (Figure 13.12a and b). The novice clinician might also consider taking it a step further and attempt to conceptualize the lung field in terms of where they would expect to auscult the normal airway sounds (Figure 13.12c).

13.9 Understanding Adventitious Airway Sounds

Adventitious airway sounds are abnormal. See Section 13.5.3 to review the two most commonly ausculted adventitious airway sounds in veterinary medicine: crackles and wheezes.

As always, the clinician should take care to auscult the entire lung field, including the left and right thoracic cavities and the cranial and caudal borders. Respiratory sounds, whether they are normal and adventitious, are not always symmetrical. Unilateral changes in airflow can result in unilateral changes in respiratory sounds.

13.10 Panting as an Obstruction to Auscultation

Panting can complicate auscultation of the respiratory system: the loudness of panting obscures the quieter respiratory noises that are of interest to the veterinarian (Figure 13.13).

The clinician may decrease sounds attributed to panting by gently closing the patient's mouth and keeping it closed during auscultation. The patient is now forced to breathe through its nose, which should lessen the noise interference. If the clinician makes use of this approach, he should explain to the client why he is closing the dog's mouth so that the client does not feel that he is handling the patient roughly.

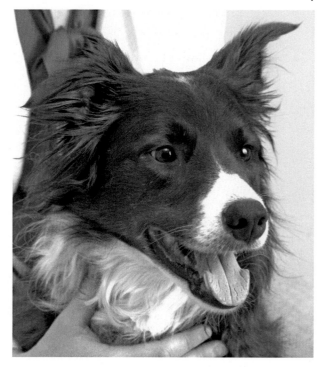

Figure 13.13 A panting dog. Source: Courtesy of the Media Resources Department at Midwestern University.

References

1 Patterson, D.F. (1968) Epidemiologic and genetic studies of congenital heart disease in the dog. *Circulation Research*, **23** (2), 171–202.

2 Strickland, K.N. (2008) Congenital heart disease, in *Manual of Canine and Feline Cardiology*, 4th edn. (eds. L.P. Tilley, F.W.K. Smith, M.A. Oyama, and M.M. Sleeper), Saunders, Philadelphia, pp. 215–239.

3 Oliveira, P., Domenech, O., Silva, J. *et al.* (2011) Retrospective review of congenital heart disease in 976 dogs. *Journal of Veterinary Internal Medicine*, **25** (3), 477–483.

4 Bulmer, B.J. (2011) The cardiovascular system, in *Small Animal Pediatrics: The First 12 Months of Life* (eds. M.E. Peterson and M.A. Kutzler), Saunders Elsevier, St. Louis, pp. 289–304.

5 Schrope, D.P. (2015) Prevalence of congenital heart disease in 76,301 mixed-breed dogs and 57,025 mixed-breed cats. *Journal of Veterinary Cardiology*, **17** (3), 192–202.

6 Bellumori, T.P., Famula, T.R., Bannasch, D.L. *et al.* (2013) Prevalence of inherited disorders among mixed-breed and purebred dogs: 27,254 cases (1995–2010). *Journal of the American Veterinary Medical Association*, **242** (11), 1549–1555.

7 Karlsson, E.K. and Lindblad-Toh, K. (2008) Leader of the pack: gene mapping in dogs and other model organisms. *Nature Reviews Genetics*, **9** (9), 713–725.

8 Oberbauer, A.M., Belanger, J.M., Bellumori, T. *et al.* (2015) Ten inherited disorders in purebred dogs by functional breed groupings. *Canine Genetics and Epidemiology*, 2, 9.

9 Dennis, S. (2013) Sound advice for heart murmurs. *Journal of Small Animal Practice*, **54** (9), 443–444.

10 Fonfara, S. (2015) Listen to the sound: what is normal? *Journal of Small Animal Practice*, **56** (2), 75–76.

11 Tavel, M.E. (2006) Cardiac auscultation: a glorious past – and it does have a future! *Circulation*, **113** (9), 1255–1259.

12 Bavegems, V.C., Duchateau, L., Polis, I.E. *et al.* (2011) Detection of innocent systolic murmurs by auscultation and their relation to hematologic and echocardiographic findings in clinically normal Whippets. *Journal of the American Veterinary Medical Association*, **238** (4), 468–471.

13 Cote, E., Edwards, N.J., Ettinger, S.J. *et al.* (2015) Management of incidentally detected heart murmurs in dogs and cats. *Journal of Veterinary Cardiology*, **17** (4), 245–261.

14 Szatmári, V., van Leeuwen, M.W., and Teske, E. (2015) Innocent cardiac murmur in puppies: prevalence, correlation with hematocrit, and auscultation characteristics. *Journal of Veterinary Internal Medicine*, **29** (6), 1524–1528.

15 Abbott, J. (2001) Auscultation: what type of practice makes perfect? *Journal of Veterinary Internal Medicine*, **15** (6), 505–506.

16 Mackie, A.S., Jutras, L.C., Dancea, A.B. *et al.* (2009) Can cardiologists distinguish innocent from pathologic murmurs in neonates? *Journal of Pediatrics*, **154** (1), 50–54.e1.

17 Naylor, J.M., Yadernuk, L.M., Pharr, J.W., and Ashburner, J.S. (2001) An assessment of the ability of diplomates, practitioners, and students to describe and interpret recordings of heart murmurs and arrhythmia. *Journal of Veterinary Internal Medicine*, **15** (6), 507–515.

18 Pyle, R.L. (2000) Interpreting low-intensity cardiac murmurs in dogs predisposed to subaortic stenosis. *Journal of the American Animal Hospital Association*, **36** (5), 379–382.

19 Shub, C. (2003) Echocardiography or auscultation? How to evaluate systolic murmurs. *Canadian Family Physician/Médecin de Famille Canadien*, **49**, 163–167.

20 Tse, Y.C., Rush, J.E., Cunningham, S.M. *et al.* (2013) Evaluation of a training course in focused echocardiography for noncardiology house officers. *Journal of Veterinary Emergency and Critical Care*, **23** (3), 268–273.

21 Abbott, J.A. (2008) Acquired valvular disease, in *Manual of Canine and Feline Cardiology*, 4th edn. (eds. L.P. Tilley, F.W.K. Smith, M.A. Oyama, and M.M. Sleeper), Saunders, Philadelphia, pp. 110–138.

22 Oyama, M.A. (2008) Canine cardiomyopathy, in *Manual of Canine and Feline Cardiology*, 4th edn. (eds. L.P. Tilley, F.W.K. Smith, M.A. Oyama, and M.M. Sleeper), Saunders, Philadelphia, pp. 139–150.

23 Chandler, M.L. (2016) Impact of obesity on cardiopulmonary disease. *Veterinary Clinics of North America: Small Animal Practice*, **46** (5), 817–830.

24 Olson, L.H., Haggstrom, J., and Henrik, D.P. (2010) Acquired valvular heart disease, in *Textbook of Veterinary Internal Medicine*, 7th edn. (eds. S.J. Ettinger and E.C. Feldman), Saunders Elsevier, St. Louis, pp. 1299–1319.

25 Meurs, K.M. (2010) Myocardial disease; canine, in *Textbook of Veterinary Internal Medicine*, 7th edn. (eds. S.J. Ettinger and E.C. Feldman), Saunders Elsevier, St. Louis, pp. 1320–1327.

26 Kienle, R.D. (2008) Feline cardiomyopathy, in *Manual of Canine and Feline Cardiology*, 4th edn. (eds. L.P. Tilley, F.W.K. Smith, M.A. Oyama, and M.M. Sleeper), Saunders, Philadelphia, pp. 151–175.

27 Habbu, A., Lakkis, N.M., and Dokainish, H. (2006) The obesity paradox: fact or fiction? *American Journal of Cardiology*, **98** (7), 944–948.

28 Pi-Sunyer, X. (2009) The medical risks of obesity. *Postgraduate Medicine*, **121** (6), 21–33.

29 Kenchaiah, S., Evans, J.C., Levy, D. *et al.* (2002) Obesity and the risk of heart failure. *New England Journal of Medicine*, **347** (5), 305–313.

30 Boynosky, N.A. and Stokking, L. (2014) Atherosclerosis associated with vasculopathic lesions in a golden retriever with hypercholesterolemia.

Canadian Veterinary Journal/Revue Vétérinaire Canadienne, **55** (5), 484–488.

31 Van Vliet, B.N., Hall, J.E., Mizelle, H.L. *et al.* (1995) Reduced parasympathetic control of heart rate in obese dogs. *American Journal of Physiology*, **269** (2 Pt. 2), H629–H637.

32 Truett, A.A., Borne, A.T., Poincot, M.A., and West, D.B. (1996) Autonomic control of blood pressure and heart rate in obese hypertensive dogs. *American Journal of Physiology*, **270** (3 Pt. 2), R541–R549.

33 Bouthegourd, J.C., Kelly, M., Clety, N. *et al.* (2009) Effects of weight loss on heart rate normalization and increase in spontaneous activity in moderately exercised overweight dogs. *International Journal of Applied Research in Veterinary Medicine*, **7** (4), 153–164.

34 Slupe, J.L., Freeman, L.M., and Rush, J.E. (2008) Association of body weight and body condition with survival in dogs with heart failure. *Journal of Veterinary Internal Medicine*, **22** (3), 561–565.

35 Pelosi, A., Rosenstein, D., Abood, S.K., and Olivier, B.N. (2013) Cardiac effect of short-term experimental weight gain and loss in dogs. *Veterinary Record*, **172** (6), 153.

36 Mehlman, E., Bright, J.M., Jeckel, K. *et al.* (2013) Echocardiographic evidence of left ventricular hypertrophy in obese dogs. *Journal of Veterinary Internal Medicine*, **27** (1), 62–68.

37 Rijnberk, A. and Stokhof, A.A. (2009) General examination, in *Medical History and Physical Examination in Companion Animals*, 2nd edn. (eds. A. Rijnberk and F.J. van Sluijs), Saunders Elsevier, St. Louis, pp. 47–62.

38 Overall, K.L. (1997) Fears, anxieties, and stereotypies, in *Clinical Behavioral Medicine for Small Animals* (ed. K.L. Overall), Mosby, St. Louis, p. 213.

39 Strickland, K.N. (2008) Pathophysiology and therapy of heart failure, in *Manual of Canine and Feline Cardiology*, 4th edn. (eds. L.P. Tilley, F.W.K. Smith, M.A. Oyama, and M.M. Sleeper), Saunders, Philadelphia, pp. 288–314.

40 Rijnberk, A. and van Sluijs, F.S. (eds.) (2009) *Medical History and Physical Examination in Companion Animals*, 2nd edn., Saunders Elsevier, St. Louis.

41 Dyce, K.M., Sack, W.O., and Wensing, C.J.G. (2010) *Textbook of Veterinary Anatomy*, 4th edn. Saunders Elsevier, St. Louis.

42 Hunt, G.B. and Foster, S.F. (2009) Nasopharyngeal disorders, in *Kirk's Current Veterinary Therapy*, vol. XIV (eds. J.D. Bonagura and D.C. Twedt), Saunders Elsevier, St. Louis, pp. 622–626.

43 Stokhof, A.A. and Venker-van Haagen, A.J. (2009) Respiratory system, in *Medical History and Physical Examination in Companion Animals*, 2nd edn. (eds. A. Rijnberk and F.J. van Sluijs), Saunders Elsevier, St. Louis, pp. 63–74.

44 Schmidt-Nielsen, K., Bretz, W.L., and Taylor, C.R. (1970) Panting in dogs – unidirectional air flow over evaporative surfaces. *Science*, 169 (3950), 1102.

45 Blatt, C.M., Taylor, C.R., and Habal, M.B. (1972) Thermal panting in dogs – lateral nasal gland, a source

of water for evaporative cooling. *Science*, **177** (4051), 804.

46 van Dongen, A.M. and Robben, J.H. (2009) Positions and restraint, in *Medical History and Physical Examination in Companion Animals*, 2nd edn. (eds. A. Rijnberk and F.J. van Sluijs), Saunders Elsevier, St. Louis, pp. 227–231.

47 Gompf, R.E. (2008) The history and physical examination, in *Manual of Canine and Feline Cardiology*, 4th edn. (eds. L.P. Tilley, F.W.K. Smith, M.A. Oyama, and M.M. Sleeper), Saunders, Philadelphia, pp. 2–23.

48 Cole, S.G. and Drobatz, K.J. (2008) Emergency management and critical care, in *Manual of Canine and Feline Cardiology*, 4th edn. (eds. L.P. Tilley, F.W.K. Smith, M.A. Oyama, and M.M. Sleeper), Saunders, Philadelphia, pp. 342–355.

49 Cote, E. and Harpster, N.K. (2009) Feline cardiac arrhythmias, in *Kirk's Current Veterinary Therapy*, vol. XIV (eds. J.D. Bonagura and D.C. Twedt), Saunders Elsevier, St. Louis, pp. 731–739.

50 Hogan, D.F. (2006) Prevention and management of thromboembolism, in *Consultations in Feline Internal Medicine*, vol. 5 (ed. J.R. August), Saunders Elsevier, St. Louis, pp. 331–345.

51 Stokhof, A.A. and De Rick, A. (2009) Circulatory system, in *Medical History and Physical Examination in Companion Animals*, 2nd edn. (eds. A.Rijnberk and F.J. van Sluijs), Saunders Elsevier, St. Louis, pp. 75–85.

52 Stepien, R.L., Kellihan, H., and Fuentes, L. (2011) Accuracy of auscultation alone to identify mitral insufficiency in adult whippets. *Journal of Veterinary Internal Medicine*, **25**, 1480.

53 Tobias, A.H. and McNiel, E.A. (2008) Pericardial disorders and cardiac tumors, in *Manual of Canine and Feline Cardiology*, 4th edn. (eds. L.P. Tilley, F.W.K. Smith, M.A. Oyama, and M.M. Sleeper), Saunders, Philadelphia, pp. 200–214.

54 Sykes, J.E. (2014) Pediatric feline upper respiratory disease. *Veterinary Clinics of North America: Small Animal Practice*, 44 (2), 331–342.

55 Quimby, J. and Lappin, M.R. (2012) The upper respiratory tract, in *The Cat: Clinical Medicine and Management* (ed. S.E.Little), Saunders Elsevier, St. Louis, pp. 846–861.

56 McManus, C.M., Levy, J.K., Andersen, L.A. *et al.* (2014) Prevalence of upper respiratory pathogens in four management models for unowned cats in the southeast United States. *Veterinary Journal*, **201** (2), 196–201.

57 Dinnage, J.D., Scarlett, J.M., and Richards, J.R. (2009) Descriptive epidemiology of feline upper respiratory tract disease in an animal shelter. *Journal of Feline Medicine and Surgery*, **11** (10), 816–825.

58 Binns, S.H., Dawson, S., Speakman, A.J. *et al.* (2000) A study of feline upper respiratory tract disease with reference to prevalence and risk factors for infection with feline calicivirus and feline herpesvirus. *Journal of Feline Medicine and Surgery*, **2** (3), 123–133.

59 Bannasch, M.J. and Foley, J.E. (2005) Epidemiologic evaluation of multiple respiratory pathogens in cats in animal shelters. *Journal of Feline Medicine and Surgery*, 7 (2), 109–119.

60 Di Martino, B., Di Francesco, C.E., Meridiani, I., and Marsilio, F. (2007) Etiological investigation of multiple respiratory infections in cats. *New Microbiologica*, **30** (4), 455–461.

61 Mochizuki, M., Yachi, A., Ohshima, T. *et al.* (2008) Etiologic study of upper respiratory infections of household dogs. *Journal of Veterinary Medicine and Science*, **70** (6), 563–569.

62 Appel, M,J, and Binn, L.N. (1987) Canine infectious tracheobronchitis, in *Virus Infections of Carnivores* (ed. M.J. Appel), Elsevier, Amsterdam, pp. 201–211.

63 Buonavoglia, C. and Martella, V. (2007) Canine respiratory viruses. *Veterinary Research*, **38** (2), 355–373.

64 Sykes, J.E. (2013) Canine viral respiratory infections, in *Canine and Feline Infectious Diseases*, Saunders Elsevier, St. Louis pp. 170–181.

65 Herrtage, M.E. and Jones, B.R. (2010) Respiratory disorders: diseases of the upper respiratory tract, in *Clinical Medicine of the Dog and Cat* (ed. M. Schaer), CRC Press, Boca Rato n , FL, pp. 187–193.

66 Kuehn, N.F. (2009) Rhinitis in the dog, in *Kirk's Current Veterinary Therapy*, vol. XIV (eds. J.D. Bonagura and D.C. Twedt), Saunders Elsevier, St. Louis, pp. 609–616.

67 Schulz, B.S., Kurz, S., Weber, K. *et al.* (2014) Detection of respiratory viruses and *Bordetella bronchiseptica* in dogs with acute respiratory tract infections. *Veterinary Journal*, 201 (3), 365–369.

68 Ford, R.B. (2006) Canine infectious tracheobronchitis, in *Infectious Diseases of the Dog and Cat*, 3rd edn. (ed. C.E. Greene). Saunders Elsevier, St. Louis, pp. 54–61.

69 Henderson, S.M., Bradley, K., Day, M.J. *et al.* (2004) Investigation of nasal disease in the cat – a retrospective study of 77 cases. *Journal of Feline Medicine and Surgery*, **6** (4), 245–257.

70 Schmidt, J.F. and Kapatkin, A. (1990) Nasopharyngeal and ear canal polyps in the cat. *Feline Practice*, **18** (4), 16–19.

71 Kapatkin, A.S., Matthiesen, D.T., Noone, K.E. *et al.* (1990) Results of surgery and long-term follow-up in 31 cats with nasopharyngeal polyps. *Journal of the American Animal Hospital Association*, **26** (4), 387–392.

72 Pope, E.R. and Constantinescu, G.M. (2009) Brachycephalic upper airway syndrome in dogs, in *Kirk's Current Veterinary Therapy*, vol. XIV (eds. J.D. Bonagura and D.C. Twedt), Saunders Elsevier, St. Louis, pp. 619–621.

73 Asher, L., Diesel, G., Summers, J.F. *et al.* (209) Inherited defects in pedigree dogs. Part 1. *Disorders related to breed standards. Veterinary Journal*, **182** (3), 402–411.

74 Dupré, G. and Heidenreich, D. (2016) Brachycephalic syndrome. *Veterinary Clinics of North America: Small Animal Practice*, **46** (4), 691–707.

75 Roedler, F.S., Pohl, S., and Oechtering, G.U. (2013) How does severe brachycephaly affect dog's lives? Results of a structured preoperative owner questionnaire. *Veterinary Journal*, **198** (3), 606–610.

76 Oechtering, G.U., Pohl, S., Schlueter, C. *et al.* (2016) A novel approach to brachycephalic syndrome. 1. Evaluation of anatomical intranasal airway obstruction. *Veterinary Surgery*, **45** (2), 165–172.

77 Heidenreich, D., Gradner, G., Kneissl, S., and Dupré G. (2016) Nasopharyngeal dimensions from computed tomography of Pugs and French Bulldogs with brachycephalic airway syndrome. *Veterinary Surgery*, **45** (1), 83–90.

78 Packer, R.M., Hendricks, A., Tivers, M.S., and Burn, C.C. (2015) Impact of facial conformation on canine health: brachycephalic obstructive airway syndrome. *PLoS One*, **10** (10), e0137496.

79 Liu, N.C., Sargan, D.R., Adams, V.J., and Ladlow, J.F. (2015) Characterisation of brachycephalic obstructive airway syndrome in French Bulldogs using whole-body barometric plethysmography. *PLoS One*, **10** (6), e0130741.

80 Haworth, K.E., Islam, I., Breen, M. *et al.* (2001) Canine TCOF1; cloning, chromosome assignment and genetic analysis in dogs with different head types. *Mammalian Genome*, **12** (8), 622–629.

81 Wayne, R.K. (1986) Cranial morphology of domestic and wild canids – the influence of development on morphological change. *Evolution*, **40** (2), 243–261.

82 Young, A. and Bannasch, D. (2006) Morphological variation in the dog, in *The Dog and Its Genome* (eds. E.A. Ostrander, U. Giger, and K. Lindblad-Toh), Cold Spring Harbor Laboratory Press, Cold Spring Harbor, NY, pp. 47–65.

83 Schoenebeck, J.J. and Ostrander, E.A. (2013) The genetics of canine skull shape variation. *Genetics*, **193** (2), 317–325.

84 Trader, R.L. (1949) Nose operation. *Journal of the American Veterinary Medical Association*, **114** (865), 210–211.

85 Leonard, H.C. (1956) Surgical relief for stenotic nares in a dog. *Journal of the American Veterinary Medical Association*, **128** (11), 530.

86 Schuenemann, R. and Oechtering, G.U. (2014) Inside the brachycephalic nose: intranasal mucosal contact points. *Journal of the American Animal Hospital Association*, **50** (3), 149–158.

87 Oechtering, T.H., Oechtering, G.U., and Noller, C. (2007) Structural characteristics of the nose in brachycephalic dog breeds analysed by computed tomography. *Tierarztliche Praxis, Ausgabe K, Kleintiere/Heimtiere*, **35** (3), 177 (in German).

88 Ginn, J.A., Kumar, M.S.A., McKiernan, B.C., and Powers, B.E. (2008) Nasopharyngeal turbinates in brachycephalic dogs and cats. *Journal of the American Animal Hospital Association*, **44** (5), 243–249.

89 Harvey, C.E. (1989) Inherited and congenital airway conditions. *Journal of Small Animal Practice*, **30** (3), 184–187.

90 Riecks, T.W., Birchard, S.J., and Stephens, J.A. (2007) Surgical correction of brachycephalic syndrome in dogs: 62 cases (1991–2004). *Journal of the American Veterinary Medical Association*, **230** (9), 1324–1328.

91 Torrez, C.V. and Hunt, G.B. (2006) Results of surgical correction of abnormalities associated with brachycephalic airway obstruction syndrome in dogs in Australia. *Journal of Small Animal Practice*, **47** (3), 150–154.

92 Dupré, G., Findji, L., and Oechtering, G. (2012) Brachycephalic airway syndrome, in *Small Animal Soft Tissue Surgery* (ed. E. Monnet), Wiley-Blackwell, Ames, IA, pp. 167–183.

93 Grand, J.G. and Bureau, S. (2011) Structural characteristics of the soft palate and meatus nasopharyngeus in brachycephalic and non-brachycephalic dogs analysed by CT. *Journal of Small Animal Practice*, **52** (5), 232–239.

94 Crosse, K.R., Bray, J.P., Orbell, G., and Preston, C.A. (2015) Histological evaluation of the soft palate in dogs affected by brachycephalic obstructive airway syndrome. *New Zealand Veterinary Journal*, **63** (6), 319–325.

95 Pichetto, M., Arrighi, S., Gobbetti, M., and Romussi, S. (2015) The anatomy of the dog soft palate. III. Histological evaluation of the caudal soft palate in brachycephalic neonates. *Anatomical Record*, **298** (3), 618–623.

96 Pichetto, M., Arrighi, S., Roccabianca, P., and Romussi, S. (2011) The anatomy of the dog soft palate. II. Histological evaluation of the caudal soft palate in brachycephalic breeds with grade I brachycephalic airway obstructive syndrome. *Anatomical Record*, **294** (7), 1267–1272.

97 Leonard, H.C. (1960) Collapse of the larynx and adjacent structures in the dog. *Journal of the American Veterinary Medical Association*, **137**, 360–363.

98 White, R.N. (2012) Surgical management of laryngeal collapse associated with brachycephalic airway obstruction syndrome in dogs. *Journal of Small Animal Practice*, **53** (1), 44–50.

99 Wykes, P.M. (1991) Brachycephalic airway obstructive syndrome. *Problems in Veterinary Medicine*, **3** (2), 188–197.

100 Coyne, B.E. and Fingland, R.B. (1992) Hypoplasia of the trachea in dogs: 103 cases (1974–1990). *Journal of the American Veterinary Medical Association*, **201** (5), 768–772.

101 De Lorenzi, D., Bertoncello, D., and Drigo, M. (2009) Bronchial abnormalities found in a consecutive series of 40 brachycephalic dogs. *Journal of the American Veterinary Medical Association*, **235** (7), 835–840.

102 Poncet, C.M., Dupré, G.P., Freiche, V.G., and Bouvy, B.M. (2006) Long-term results of upper respiratory syndrome surgery and gastrointestinal tract medical treatment in 51 brachycephalic dogs. *Journal of Small Animal Practice*, **47** (3), 137–142.

103 Poncet, C.M., Dupré, G.P., Freiche, V.G. *et al.* (2005) Prevalence of gastrointestinal tract lesions in 73 brachycephalic dogs with upper respiratory syndrome. *Journal of Small Animal Practice*, **46** (6), 273–279.

104 Fasanella, F.J., Shivley, J.M., Wardlaw, J.L., and Givaruangsawat, S. (2010) Brachycephalic airway obstructive syndrome in dogs: 90 cases (1991–2008). *Journal of the American Veterinary Medical Association*, **237** (9), 1048–1051.

105 Knecht, C.D. (1979) Upper airway obstruction in brachycephalic dogs. *Compendium: Continuing Education for the Practicing Veterinarian*, **1**, 25–31.

106 Lorinson, D., Bright, R.M., and White, R.A.S. (1997) Brachycephalic airway obstruction syndrome – a review of 118 cases. *Canine Practice*, **22** (5–6), 18–21.

107 Turek, M.M. and Lana, S.E. (2007) Tumors of the respiratory system: Section D: Canine nasosinal tumors, in *Withrow & MacEwen's Small Animal Clinical Oncology*, 4th edn. (ed. S.J. Withrow and D.M. Vail), Saunders Elsevier, St. Louis, pp. 525–539.

108 Madewell, B.R., Priester, W.A., Gillette, E.L., and Snyder, S.P. (1976) Neoplasms of the nasal passages and paranasal sinuses in domesticated animals as reported by 13 veterinary colleges. *American Journal of Veterinary Research*, **37** (7), 851–856.

109 Venkervanhaagen, A.J., Bouw, J., and Hartman, W. (1981) Hereditary transmission of laryngeal paralysis in Bouviers. *Journal of the American Animal Hospital Association*, **17** (1), 75–76.

110 Braund, K.G., Shores, A., Cochrane, S. *et al.* (1994) Laryngeal paralysis–polyneuropathy complex in young Dalmatians. *American Journal of Veterinary Research*, **55** (4), 534–542.

111 Polizopoulou, Z.S., Koutinas, A.F., Papadopoulos, G.C., and Saridomichelakis, M.N. (2003) Juvenile laryngeal paralysis in three Siberian Husky × Alaskan Malamute puppies. *Veterinary Record*, **153** (20), 624–627.

112 O'Brien, J.A. and Hendriks, J. (1986) Inherited laryngeal paralysis – analysis in the Husky Cross. *Veterinary Quarterly*, **8** (4), 301–302.

113 Ridyard, A.E., Corcoran, B.M., Tasker, S. *et al.* (2000) Spontaneous laryngeal paralysis in four white-coated German shepherd dogs. *Journal of Small Animal Practice*, **41** (12), 558–561.

114 Herrtage, M. and Jones, B.R. (2009) Respiratory disorders: diseases of the larynx and pharynx, in *Clinical Medicine of the Dog and Cat*, 2nd edn. (ed. M. Schaer), CRC Press, Boca Raton, FL, pp. 194–196.

115 MacPhail, C. (2014) Laryngeal disease in dogs and cats. *Veterinary Clinics of North America: Small Animal Practice*, **44** (1), 19–31.

116 Herrtage, M. and Jones, B.R. (2009) Respiratory disorders: diseases of the lower respiratory tract, in *Clinical Medicine of the Dog and Cat*, 2nd edn. (ed. M. Schaer), CRC Press, Boca Raton, FL, pp. 197–211.

117 Maggiore, A.D. (2014) Tracheal and airway collapse in dogs. *Veterinary Clinics of North America: Small Animal Practice*, **44** (1), 117–127.

118 Bottero, E., Bellino, C., De Lorenzi, D. *et al.* (2013) Clinical evaluation and endoscopic classification of bronchomalacia in dogs. *Journal of Veterinary Internal Medicine*, **27** (4), 840–846.

119 Mair, E. and Parsons, D.S. (1992) Pediatric tracheomalacia and major airway collapse. *Annals of Otology, Rhinology and Laryngology*, **101**, 300–309.

120 Fiest, J.H., Johnson, T.H., and Wilson, R.J. (1975) Acquired tracheomalacia: etiology and differential diagnosis. *Chest*, **68**, 340–345.

121 Macready, D.M., Johnson, L.R., and Pollard, R.E. (2007) Fluoroscopic and radiographic evaluation of tracheal collapse in dogs: 62 cases (2001–2006). *Journal of the American Veterinary Medical Association*, **230** (12), 1870–1876.

122 Herrtage, M.J. (2009) Medical management of tracheal collapse, in *Kirk's Current Veterinary Therapy*, vol. XIV (eds. J.D. Bonagura and D.C. Twedt), Saunders Elsevier, St. Louis, pp. 630–635.

123 Withrow, S.J. (2007) Tumors of the respiratory system: Section C: Lung cancer, in *Withrow & MacEwen's Small Animal Clinical Oncology*, 4th edn. (ed. S.J. Withrow and D.M. Vail), Saunders Elsevier, St. Louis, pp. 517–539.

124 Moulton, J.E., von Tscharner, C., and Schneider, R. (1981) Classification of lung carcinomas in the dog and cat. *Veterinary Pathology*, **18** (4), 513–528.

125 Ramos-Vara, J.A., Miller, M.A., and Johnson, G.C. (2005) Usefulness of thyroid transcription factor-1 immunohistochemical staining in the differential diagnosis of primary pulmonary tumors of dogs. *Veterinary Pathology*, **42** (3), 315–320.

126 Hahn, F.F., Muggenburg, B.A., and Griffith, W.C. (1996) Primary lung neoplasia in a beagle colony. *Veterinary Pathology*, **33** (6), 633–638.

127 Baral, R.M. (2012) The thoracic cavity, in *The Cat: Clinical Medicine and Management* (ed. S.E. Little), Saunders Elsevier, St. Louis, pp. 892–913.

128 Herrtage, M. and Jones, B.R. (2009) Respiratory disorders: conditions causing a reduction in thoracic capacity, in *Clinical Medicine of the Dog and Cat*, 2nd edn. (ed. M. Schaer), CRC Press, Boca Raton, FL, pp. 212–219.

129 Voges, A.K., Bertrand, S., Hill, R.C. *et al.* (1997) True diaphragmatic hernia in a cat. *Veterinary Radiology & Ultrasound*, **38** (2), 116–119.

130 Worth, A.J. and Machon, R.G. (2005) Traumatic diaphragmatic herniation: pathophysiology and management. *Compendium: Continuing Education for the Practicing Veterinarian*, **27** (3), 178.

131 Schmiedt, C.W., Tobias, K.M., and Stevenson, M.A. (2003) Traumatic diaphragmatic hernia in cats: 34 cases (1991–2001). *Journal of the American Veterinary Medical Association*, **222** (9), 1237–1240.

132 Fossum, T.W. (2000) Pleural and extrapleural diseases, in *Textbook of Veterinary Internal Medicine* (eds. S.J. Ettinger and E.C. Feldman), Saunders, Philadelphia, p. 1098.

14

Examining the Abdominal Cavity of the Dog

14.1 Overview of the Digestive Tract

Recall that the gastrointestinal system consists of the upper and lower digestive tracts. The upper digestive tract consists of the oral cavity, oropharynx, salivary glands, esophagus, stomach, and duodenum, and the lower digestive tract consists of the ileum, jejunum, ascending, transverse, and descending colons, rectum, and anus. In close proximity to the upper digestive tract, the hepatobiliary system engages with the small bowel to create a loop of enterohepatic circulation that is vital to metabolic and biotransformation pathways. Together, the digestive tract functions to metabolize food into absorbable nutrients that can then be used as energy with which to fuel the body [1].

Chapter 11 reviewed the components of the canine digestive tract up to the oropharynx. This chapter covers all aspects of the digestive tract distal to that region.

Because dysfunction within the digestive tract tends to be symptomatic, history-taking plays an important role in the medical work-up of any gut-related presenting complaint. In particular, history-taking should elucidate the timeline and progression of clinical signs.

Recall from Section 6.1 that the clinician should take care to ask the following of the client [1]:

- What is the client observing that is concerning?
- When were clinical signs first apparent?
- What is the duration of the clinical signs?
- Are clinical signs associated with a particular time of day?
- Are clinical signs associated with a particular type of food?
- Are clinical signs associated with a particular type of activity?
- Are clinical signs progressing? If so, in what way?

A comprehensive physical examination then proceeds. In the author's experience, the abdominal cavity challenges veterinary students. It is difficult for students to appreciate structures that they cannot see, especially when the majority of abdominal structures are not palpable in

health. Students should first learn which organs are palpable in the normal patient and which are not.

In the healthy dog, the following digestive tract structures should be palpable [1]:

- small intestinal loops;
- descending colon.

Depending upon the patient, the following digestive tract structures may be palpable in a healthy dog [1]:

- liver;
- spleen.

The following digestive tract structures are palpable only in a diseased state, if at all [1]:

- esophagus;
- gall bladder;
- pancreas;
- mesenteric lymph nodes;
- colonic lymph nodes.

14.2 The Esophagus

See Section 6.2 to review esophageal anatomy.

In a normal patient, the esophagus is hidden under muscle and is neither visible nor palpable [1]. The esophagus becomes palpable when obstructed, as occurs in dogs that swallow foreign bodies [1]. Bones are most commonly implicated [2]. However, rawhide, dental chews, fishhooks, sewing needles, plastic, wooden sticks, and metal have been reported in the medical literature [3–11]. The distal esophagus is the most common site of obstruction in dogs, followed by the level of the heart base [2, 3, 7–10, 12, 13]. Small-breed dogs appear to be overrepresented [2, 14], particularly terriers, Shih Tzus, and Chihuahuas [7–10, 12, 13].

Patients with esophageal obstructions tend to present for gagging and regurgitation [2, 14]. Regurgitation is a passive process by which there is retrograde movement of food from the esophagus out through the oral cavity. It is the hallmark of esophageal disease, and typically lacks the

Performing the Small Animal Physical Examination, First Edition. Ryane E. Englar.
© 2017 John Wiley & Sons, Inc. Published 2017 by John Wiley & Sons, Inc.

prodromal signs that accompany vomiting: lip-licking and hypersalivation [15]. The patient may continue to exhibit these clinical signs in the examination room. In addition, the patient may show pain when asked to extend its neck or when pressure is applied over the left thoracic inlet [1].

It is therefore important that the clinician gets into the habit of feeling for the esophagus: doing so routinely will better prepare him for the next case of esophageal obstruction that walks through the door. To feel for the esophagus, the clinician should stand in front of the patient and encourage it to raise its head. As the clinician runs his hand down the ventrolateral left neck, he should look and feel for any bulge, particularly at the level of the thoracic inlet, that may be suggestive of esophageal dilation. When esophageal obstruction is severe, causing a back-up of food and water orad to the obstruction, the clinician may even be able to feel sloshing of esophageal contents beneath the skin [1].

Only in some cases of esophageal obstruction is the esophagus palpable. In most other cases of esophageal disease, such as esophagitis, esophageal strictures, and megaesophagus, physical examination of the esophageal region is unremarkable. Megaesophagus was first introduced in Section 13.5.3 as a risk factor for the development of aspiration pneumonia. Megaesophagus can be congenital [16–18], as in the Irish Setter, Great Dane, German Shepherd, Labrador Retriever, and Newfoundland [16], or it can be acquired, secondary to myasthenia gravis [19–21], hypoadrenocorticism, lead poisoning, and potentially hypothyroidism [16]. In these circumstances, the clinician must rely upon historical findings to guide him to consider esophageal disease, in which case contrast esophagrams and/or endoscopy are indicated [15].

14.3 Visual Inspection of the Abdomen

Before the clinician palpates the abdomen, he should observe the abdominal silhouette for size, shape, and symmetry. Bilaterally symmetrical, diffuse enlargement of the abdomen could be physiologic, as in the case of pregnancy, or could be pathologic, as from ascites (Figure 14.1).

By contrast, focal enlargement of the abdomen may reflect organ-associated pathology. For example, cranial abdominal enlargement may indicate hepatomegaly [1].

In addition to looking for abdominal distension, the clinician should observe the patient for other clinical signs that may be suggestive of abdominal pain, what is colloquially referred to as "acute abdomen" [22, 23]. In particular, clinicians should note the presence of a "prayer posture" in which the forelimbs are extended, the ventral chest is lowered to the floor, and the rump is elevated [24, 25]. This posture mirrors that of a "play bow" (see Figure 9.5) except that the patient characteristically is being presented for malaise.

Other visual cues that the patient may demonstrate to convey abdominal discomfort are pacing, restlessness, and an inability to settle. The patient may be reluctant to sit or lie down. The patient is less likely to "flank watch," as is done routinely by colicky horses, and is more likely to splint or guard the abdomen upon any form of physical contact [24].

These cues are not pathognomonic for any particular organ dysfunction. In fact, the "acute abdomen" presentation can involve digestive, urogenital, musculoskeletal, nervous, cardiovascular, and respiratory systems.

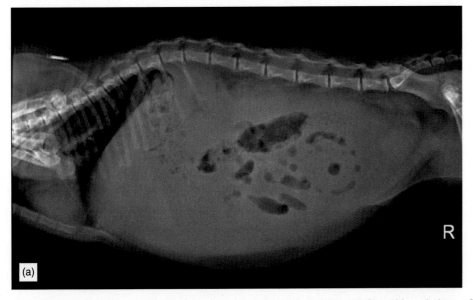
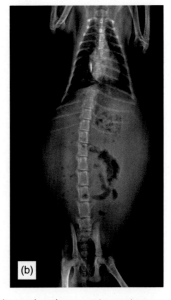

Figure 14.1 Radiographic evidence of ascites in (a) a lateral film and (b) a V/D film. Although this is a feline rather than a canine patient, the appearance of ascites on radiographs is the same: note the diffusely increased density of the abdominal contents, with poor definition of soft tissue structures, which have been obscured by the fluid.

Back pain, for instance, can mirror abdominal pain because in both circumstances, the patient is presented for hunching [22, 24].

Regardless of system involvement, whenever a clinician is presented with an "acute abdomen" patient, he should take care to ease into abdominal palpation. Being too aggressive with the initial approach to the abdominal palpation may reinforce the patient's tendency to guard the abdomen. The clinician would do better to start with superficial palpation of the abdomen before the application of deep pressure [22–25].

14.4 Auscultion and Superficial Palpation of the Abdomen

14.4.1 Auscultation of the Abdomen

Auscultation of the abdomen is an essential part of the comprehensive physical examination because it can provide important information regarding the motility of the digestive tract. When a clinician auscults the abdominal cavity, he is listening for gut sounds. These are classically referred to as borborygmi. In order for borborygmi to be audible, the bowel must contain some fluid and gas, and be motile. If borborymi are not heard, then the bowel is either empty or not moving, or both [1].

It has been suggested that auscultation of the abdomen should precede abdominal palpation because the latter may shift the intestinal loops within the abdominal cavity and, in so doing, alter gut sounds [22, 23].

Auscultation of the abdomen requires patience. In patients with delayed gut motility, it may take 2–3 minutes to appreciate borborygmi. For example, gut sounds are frequently decreased in anorectic patients. Were a clinician to rush through auscultation of the abdomen, he might miss that gut sounds are indeed present, just diminished [22, 23].

In addition to anorexia, ileus can result from peritonitis or ascites [23].

At the opposite end of the spectrum are increased borborygmi, which can be the result of acute enteritis or acute intestinal obstruction [23].

14.4.2 Superficial Palpation of the Abdomen

The purpose of superficial abdominal palpation is to detect and localize pain, determine if there is a palpable fluid wave, and assess for hernias [22].

14.4.2.1 Fluid Waves

The presence of a fluid wave is suggestive of abdominal effusions [1]. Abdominal effusions could be hemorrhagic, as from trauma. Effusions also result from uroabdomen and septic peritonitis, as from leakage of gastrointestinal contents from a bowel perforation [24].

To assess for a fluid wave, the clinician typically stands behind the patient with the patient facing away from the clinician. The palm of the left hand is placed flush against the left side of the abdomen and the palm of the right hand is placed loosely against the right side of the abdomen. The clinician then performs ballottement: with the fingertips of his right hand, he taps the right abdominal wall to bounce internal structures off of the opposite wall. He then repeats this by balloting the left abdominal wall to feel for any response against the right abdominal wall. If there is appreciable fluid within the peritoneal cavity, the clinician will feel a wave of fluid against the wall opposite to the one that was tapped. This is not appreciated in a healthy patient, only in a patient with abdominal effusion [1]. If there is a palpable fluid wave, further diagnostic intervention is warranted to determine the fluid's source.

Abdominocentesis, sometimes referred to as abdominal paracentesis, with or without peritoneal lavage, may be performed to sample the free-floating fluid [24, 26].

Cytology of the free-floating fluid allows the clinician to rule in or out inflammatory processes and septicemia [24]. Emergency laparotomy is indicated when degenerate neutrophils and bacteria are identified [24].

The free-floating fluid can also be analyzed to help narrow down the list of differential diagnoses [24]. For instance, if the concentration of glucose in the free-floating fluid is less than 50 mg/dL or if the concentration of lactate exceeds 5.5 mmol/L, then septicemia is likely [27]. In addition, if the free-floating abdominal fluid contains potassium or creatinine at levels that exceed the concentration contained within peripheral blood, then the urinary tract has ruptured and urine is spilling into the abdominal cavity [24].

Note that there are limits to the clinician's ability to palpate free-floating fluid within the abdominal cavity. These limits may be related to the time frame in the disease process or be due to the quantity of fluid.

For example, hemoperitoneum secondary to hepatic or splenic injury is not instantaneous: it may take 3 hours or more after the traumatic event for hemoperitoneum to be detectable on physical examination [26, 28]. For this reason, the physical examination alone only has a 50% accuracy in detecting when emergency surgery is indicated for a trauma patient [26, 28, 29].

The quantity of free-floating fluid may also handicap the clinician's assessment: if too little fluid is present, then the clinician will not detect a fluid wave. For this reason, abdominal ultrasound is increasingly of value in an emergency room setting. It is much better equipped to identify small volumes of fluid than the clinician's fingertips. To be exact, abdominal ultrasound is capable of detecting as little as 4 mL/kg body weight of free fluid [24, 30].

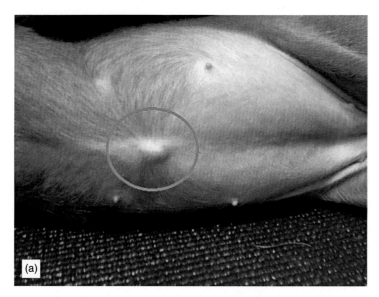
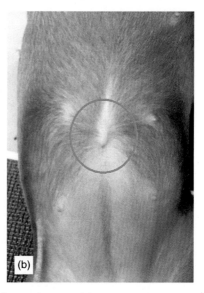

Figure 14.2 Umbilical hernia evident on visual inspection of a canine patient (a) in lateral recumbency and (b) supported in a standing position.

14.4.2.2 Hernias

See Section 6.4 to review the anatomy of the abdominal wall.

Recall that an abdominal hernia represents a defect in the abdominal wall, and that this defect can occur at any point. However, most common sites of herniation are at the umbilicus along the ventral midline, paracostally at the caudal rib margin, scrotallly, and inguinally. At these locations, hernias tend to be congenital in origin rather than traumatically induced [31–34].

Hernias vary in size and reducibility. When they occur at the umbilicus, they are often the result of an over-wide linea alba or hypoplastic rectus muscles [31].

Some umbilical hernias are visible without palpation (Figure 14.2). Others are so small and/or reducible that they require midline palpation to appreciate their presence as a soft swelling at the umbilicus. Some patients may need to be supported so that they are standing upright on their two back feet in order for these small hernias to become apparent visually.

Most umbilical hernias remain soft and contain falciform fat, if anything [31]. The majority that are identified measure less than 2–3 mm and patients are not rushed to surgery immediately because there is a possibility of spontaneous closure in puppies up to 6 months of age [35]. Typically, tincture of time is provided to see if the hernia self-resolves. If not, then the hernia is conveniently repaired surgically at the same time as the elective ovariohysterectomy or orchiectomy.

The primary risk associated with a persistent hernia is that intra-abdominal contents may slip through the defect in the abdominal wall and become trapped between the skin and the muscle layer of the abdominal wall. The most common organs to become entrapped are the intestine, uterus, and urinary bladder. Entrapped tissues may become incarcerated. This is exquisitely painful and can be lethal within hours owing to devitalization of tissues secondary to compromised circulation [31].

When a hernia, umbilical or otherwise, is identified on superficial palpation of the integrity of the abdominal wall, the clinician should note the following:

- Size of hernia [36].
  Hernias that allow one human finger to slip through are at increased risk for bowel entrapment because the small intestine is roughly equal in size [31].
- Consistency of the hernia [36].
  If abdominal contents are palpably poking through the defect in the abdominal wall, they ought to be soft and non-painful to the touch. If abdominal contents ever become firm or tender, there is an increased risk of entrapment [31].
- Reducibility.
  Non-reducible hernias involve tissue that is poking through the defect in the abdominal wall and cannot readily be replaced within the abdomen. This means that the tissue has become entrapped and, if entrapped long enough, adhesions may form. Entrapment and adhesions increase the risk that the patient will present for a surgical emergency because incarcerated tissues are often irreducible [31, 34].

In addition to umbilical defects, defects in the abdominal wall may be present caudally as inguinal hernias that may or may not be reducible (Figure 14.3).

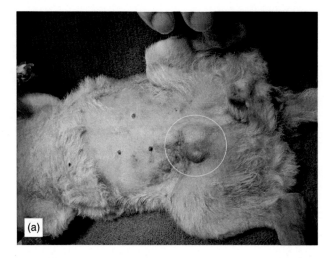

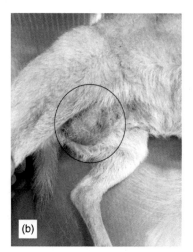

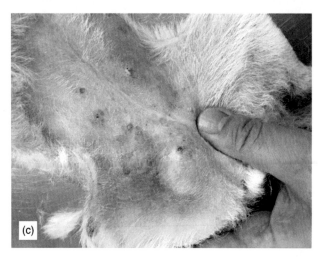

Figure 14.3 (a) Non-reducible inguinal hernia evident on visual inspection of a canine patient in dorsal recumbency. (b) Reducible inguinal hernia evident on visual inspection of a canine patient in left lateral recumbency. The reducibility of this hernia was not evident until the patient was placed in dorsal recumbency: see (c) for comparison. (c) Same patient as in (b), but in dorsal recumbency. Note that the patient's inguinal hernia is reducible. Source (a)–(c): Courtesy of Frank Isom, DVM.

Recall that inguinal hernias represent a defect in the inguinal ring. See Section 6.4 to review the anatomy associated with the inguinal ring.

If an inguinal hernia is sufficiently large, it is possible for the uterus, urinary bladder, or jejunum to become entrapped. Although it may not be possible to diagnose the entrapped organ definitively by palpation alone, ultrasound can be used to augment the physical examination findings [31, 34, 37].

Few studies have examined the incidence of hernias in dogs. In the author's experience, hernias occur more commonly in dogs than cats, but with what frequency is unclear. A 1993 study by Ruble and Hird examined pet-store puppies ranging in age from 6 to 18 weeks and found that 1.3% of pups sold over a 2-year span had inguinal hernias compared with 0.6% with umbilical hernias [38].

In spite of their apparent infrequency, hernias should be felt for at each new puppy visit. If one is identified on physical examination, its presence paves the way for a critical conversation between the client and the veterinary team as to if, when, and how to correct the defect surgically. It also raises the issue of genetics: because the bulk of congenital umbilical hernias are believed to be inherited [34], puppies that are born with or subsequently develop umbilical hernias should not be bred once they reach sexual maturity.

14.5 Deep Palpation of the Abdomen

Following superficial palpation, the clinician should perform deep palpation of the abdomen to define further the intra-abdominal architecture [22, 23]. As mentioned, deep palpation of the abdomen presents a challenge for most beginners because students must learn to trust what they feel rather than what they see. In many cases, their attempts may also be thwarted by a tensing patient [22, 23, 25].

The best way for novices to refine physical examination techniques is to practice on patients that are under general anesthesia. Because their abdominal muscles are relaxed, these patients are much easier candidates on which to appreciate normal versus abnormal abdominal structures.

Students can also experiment with different techniques for abdominal palpation to see which works best for them:

- One technique requires the use of both hands at the same time. The clinician can start out with flat hands, one on either side of the abdomen, as when assessing for the presence or absence of a palpable fluid wave. One hand can serve as a "table," against which the other hand can direct abdominal structures (see Figure 6.3a, which depicts the same process in a cat).

- An alternative technique is to use one hand only to palpate by cupping the hand, palm up toward the patient. This works best in small dogs or cats (see Figure 6.3b, which depicts the same process in a cat).

As students gain confidence in performing deep abdominal palpation in anesthetized patients, they may graduate to performing deep abdominal palpation in awake patients.

The author finds deep abdominal palpation in a dog to be easiest if the patient remains standing. The clinician can then stand behind the patient, with the patient facing away from her. There is no one "right" approach to deep abdominal palpation. The author tends to start cranially and move caudally; some of her colleagues do the examination in reverse. It is less important which approach is used and more that the clinician develops his own systematic way to be certain that no region of the abdomen is missed.

It may help the novice to break the abdomen into the following three compartments (Figure 14.4a and b) [1]:

1) Cranial abdomen:
   The cranial abdomen contains the liver, stomach, pancreas, spleen, and kidneys.

2) Mid-abdomen:
   The mid-abdomen contains the small intestine, ureters, and ovaries (females only).

3) Caudal abdomen:
   The caudal abdomen contains the urinary bladder, prostate (males only), urethra, descending colon, and rectum.

Once these three compartments of the abdomen can be visualized based upon their location in space, some clinicians further subdivide them into dorsal, medial, and ventral quadrants (Figure 14.4c) [1]:

- Craniodorsal abdomen:
  The craniodorsal abdomen contains the kidneys.
- Craniomedial abdomen:
  The craniomedial abdomen contains the liver and pancreas.
- Cranioventral abdomen:
  The cranioventral abdomen contains the liver, stomach, and spleen.
- Dorsal mid-abdomen:
  The dorsal mid-abdomen contains the ureters and ovaries.
- Medial mid-abdomen:
  The medial mid-abdomen contains the small intestine.
- Ventral mid-abdomen:
  The ventral mid-abdomen contains the small intestine.

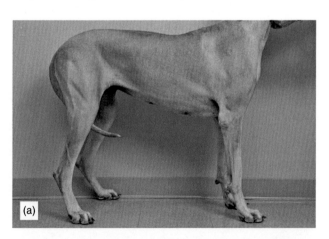

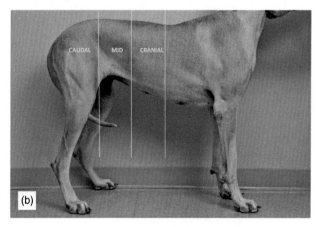

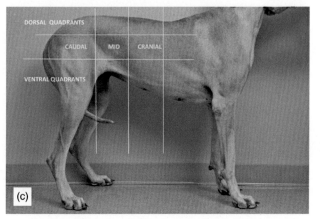

Figure 14.4 (a) Right lateral view of a live canine patient. (b) Right lateral view of a live canine patient, with the abdominal cavity artificially divided into cranial, mid (MID), and caudal compartments. (c) Right lateral view of a live canine patient, with the abdominal cavity artificially divided into cranial, mid (MID), and caudal compartments. In addition, the dorsal and ventral quadrants have been drawn in. Source (a)–(c): Courtesy of the Media Resources Department at Midwestern University.

- Dorsal caudal abdomen:
  The dorsal caudal abdomen contains the descending colon and rectum.
- Medial caudal abdomen:
  The medial mid-abdomen contains the urinary bladder and prostate.
- Ventral caudal abdomen:
  The ventral caudal abdomen contains the urethra.

Note that there is overlap between some quadrants when this approach to the abdomen is used. For example, the liver falls in both the craniomedial and cranioventral quadrants.

For those who are detail oriented, dividing up the abdomen into quadrants may be effective as a learning tool. For those who are not, dividing up the abdomen in this way may be overwhelming. Student clinicians need to determine for themselves which approach is best and know that compartmentalization of the abdomen is an option, not a requirement.

14.5.1 The Liver

The liver lies within the costal arch and is not typically palpable in deep-chested dogs. However, a portion of the liver may be accessible in dogs with broad thoracic cavities [1].

To feel for the liver within the cranioventral quadrant of the abdomen, it may help to elevate the patient's front end. This allows gravity to work on the organs of the cranial abdomen, in effect, causing them to "drop" slightly lower in the abdomen, where they may be easier to access.

When the liver is enlarged, typically the right side is more easily appreciated than the left [1]. This is because the liver, although centrally located, is biased slightly to the right of midline as a result of its right-sided caudate process, which cups the right kidney [33].

Hepatomegaly is a non-specific finding. When it occurs, it may be due to the following:

- Chronic glucocorticoid or phenobarbital use [39, 40].
- Endocrine disease, such as hyperadrenocorticism [41] and diabetes mellitus [42].
- Infectious disease [43]:
  - bacterial
  - viral, such as canine adenovirus I [44]
  - fungal [45]
  - protozoal, such as babesiosis [46]
  - parasitic, such as heartworm disease, leading to secondary vena cava syndrome.
- Familial disease:
  - canine hepatic amyloidosis in the Shar Pei [47, 48]
  - inherited disorder of copper metabolism [49].
- Inflammatory disease, such as hepatitis [45].
- Immune-mediated disease, such as immune-mediated hemolytic anemia [43].
- Hepatic abscess (Figure 14.5) [43].

- Neoplasia, such as hepatic carcinoma or bile duct carcinoma [43].
- Toxin, such as aflatoxin [50].

Patients with hepatomegaly may be otherwise healthy or they may present with non-specific clinical signs: lethargy, decreased appetite, and vomiting [43].

When vomiting occurs, it may be because the enlarged liver is pushing on the upper gastrointestinal tract, inducing nausea, or because toxins are not being efficiently cleared by the liver, causing direct stimulation of the chemoreceptor trigger zone [43].

If patients have concurrent hyperbilirubinemia, they may also display icterus [43] (see Figure 11.24d).

Unlike cats, polydipsia and polyuria frequently develop in dogs with hepatopathy [43]. Dogs may also develop acholic feces [43].

Note that clinical signs of hepatopathy may be acute in onset. However, because the liver has enormous potential for regeneration, clinical signs are typically delayed: hepatic disease is often subclinical unless hepatic reserves are exhausted. Even then, when hepatomegaly is appreciated on physical examination, the patient requires a more extensive diagnostic work-up to obtain a definitive diagnosis [43].

14.5.2 The Stomach

The stomach is positioned in the abdominal cavity caudal to the liver. Both the fundus and body of the stomach are predominantly associated with the left side of the cranial abdomen; however, the ventral aspect of the body crosses to the right as it merges with the pylorus [33].

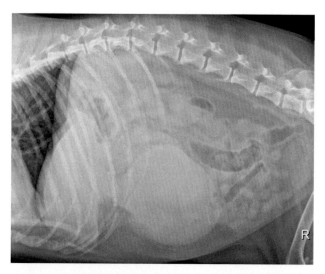

Figure 14.5 Right lateral radiograph. Note the rounded mass that is present in the mid-abdomen. The mass is displacing the small intestine caudally. This mass was surgically resected during an exploratory laparotomy. The pathology report confirmed that it was a hepatic abscess.

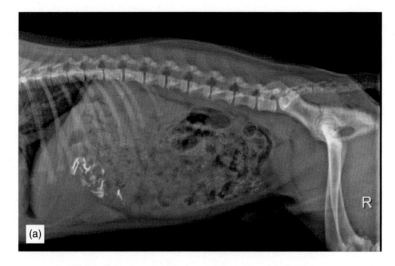
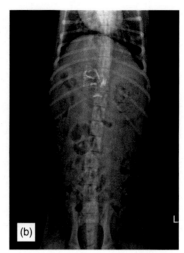

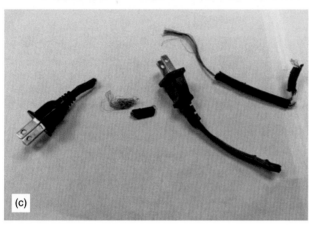

Figure 14.6 (a) Right lateral radiograph and (b) V/D radiograph of the abdomen. Note the multiple irregular fragments of a foreign body within the stomach of this puppy. (c) This is the uneaten portion of the foreign body that the patient in (a) and (b) had consumed. The puppy consumed electrical cords. Source (a)–(c): Courtesy of Patricia Bennett, DVM.

The stomach as a whole is typically not palpable [1, 51]. When the stomach is palpable just beyond the costal margin, most notably on the left-hand side of the abdomen, it may be because either [1]:

- the liver is enlarged, causing displacement of the stomach caudally;
- the stomach is significantly distended.

The potential causes of hepatomegaly were reviewed in Section 14.5.1. When the stomach itself is distended, it may be the result of [1]:

- overeating;
- ingestion of a foreign body (Figure 14.6);
- accumulation of gas and/or fluid (Figure 14.7).

Puppies are prone to overeating if granted free access to food. Eating more than is typical at one sitting forces the stomach to stretch. The patient may present to the veterinary clinic with a visibly swollen cranial abdomen that is palpable, doughy in consistency, and compressible just beyond the costal margins on the left side of the cranial abdomen.

Alternatively, many dogs – adults included – are notorious for ingesting non-food items. Foreign bodies are common among dogs that present to emergency clinics [13, 52, 53], with clinical signs developing hours to days post-ingestion [53, 54]. Pedigreed dogs are over-represented, especially Labrador Retrievers, Golden Retrievers, American Pit Bull Terriers, Staffordshire Bull Terriers, Border Collies, and Jack Russell Terriers [52, 53].

Unlike cats, dogs typically ingest non-linear foreign bodies [52], which result in higher survival rates compared with linear foreign bodies [53]. Linear foreign bodies are especially problematic because they tend to anchor either at the tongue base or pylorus, causing plication of the intestinal loops as peristalsis of the digestive tract unsuccessfully attempts to advance the foreign body into the intestine [55]. In these patients, a thorough oral examination may reveal the entrapped string or thread around the base of the tongue, or the experienced clinician may appreciate the abnormal bunching of intestines within the abdominal cavity on deep palpation [55].

More often than not, however, presenting signs are non-specific for malaise: vomiting, anorexia, lethargy, and abdominal pain [52]. Survey radiographs of the abdomen may be unremarkable, and the clinician may require advanced imaging modalities such as ultrasonography to make the diagnosis [56–60].

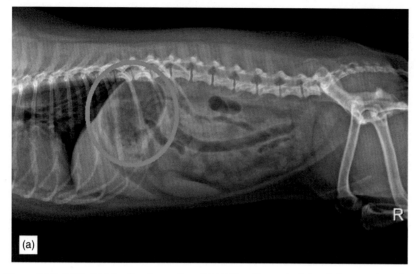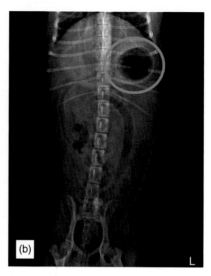

Figure 14.7 (a) Right lateral radiograph and (b) V/D radiograph of the abdomen. Note the gas-filled stomach.

In addition to foreign body ingestion, accumulation of gas and/or fluid within the stomach, as occurs in gastric dilatation–volvulus (GDV), also leads to gastric stretch [61]. However, this stretch is usually quite extreme. The stomach is not only palpable just beyond the costal margins of the cranial abdomen, it is visibly distended [61]. When the patient is viewed from behind, its abdominal silhouette typically billows out like the outline of a cow. Unlike overindulgence in food, which leads to a doughy stomach on palpation, the stomach of a patient with GDV will palpate as taut and painful [61].

GDV most commonly occurs in large-breed dogs with deep chests [62–64].

Several risk factors have been identified; however, the exact cause is unclear [61–63, 65–68]:

- Type of diet:
  Commercial cereal- and/or soy-based diets may increase risk.
- Amount fed at one sitting:
  Eating large meals may encourage repeated stretch of the hepatogastric and hepatoduodenal ligaments, increasing the risk of volvulus.
- Delayed gastric emptying.
- Exercising heavily after eating.
- Postprandial stress.
- Body condition:
  Underweight dogs are thought to be at increased risk.
- Age:
  Older animals are thought to be at increased risk.
- Prior splenectomy.

When volvulus occurs, the stomach migrates from its normal anatomic position. The right-sided pylorus becomes cranioventral relative to the body of the stomach.

The pylorus then moves to the left of midline. Eventually, the pylorus is positioned dorsal to the esophagus and the fundus, still to the left of midline [61].

This change in position crimps inflow and outflow to the digestive tract. As a result, there is nowhere for the build-up of gas to dissipate: the stomach progressively inflates. As it does, the patient is prompted to vomit. However, all attempts to do so are unsuccessful. At the time of presentation, the patient is typically hypersalivating and unproductively retching [61, 69].

Concurrently, GDV reduces venous return to the heart through the compression of the portal vein and vena cava. As a result, cardiac output tanks, as does arterial pressure. Cardiac arrhythmias are commonly seen as the patient decompensates. The patient most typically presents in a state of hypovolemic shock: tachycardic and tachypneic [61, 70–73]. These patients are critically ill upon presentation: they do not simply present with a distended abdomen.

14.5.3 The Spleen

In the dog, the spleen is a triangular or wedge-shaped organ that is housed within the cranial-to-mid abdomen. Its body abuts the left abdominal wall and its tail curls along the ventrolateral abdomen [33, 74, 75]. The spleen is not typically palpable in dogs: it is housed within the costal arch [1]. However, when the spleen is enlarged, it sinks ventrally and caudally relative to its normal anatomical position, allowing it to be palpable [1] (Figure 14.8).

Students occasionally express difficulty discerning that the enlarged organ is in fact the spleen as opposed to the liver. What helps in these instances is to attempt

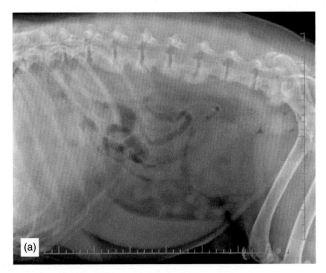
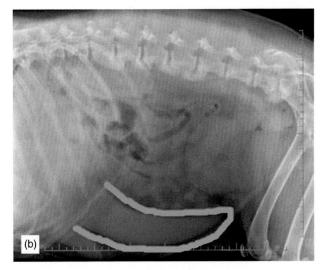

Figure 14.8 (a) Right lateral radiograph of the abdomen. Note the enlarged spleen against the ventral body wall. (b) Right lateral radiograph of the abdomen. The enlarged spleen is highlighted in blue, adjacent to the ventral body wall. Source (a), (b): Courtesy of Daniel Foy, MS, DVM, DACVIM, DACVECC.

to displace the organ caudally. The liver will not displace caudally via digital palpation because it is in a sense anchored to its position. However, because the spleen is just loosely attached to the stomach by means of the gastrosplenic ligament, it is more mobile and can be caudally displaced [1].

Splenomegaly may be due to the following [76–78]:

- Pharmacotherapy, such as anesthetic drug protocols:
  - Medetomidine, diazepam, and ketamine [79].
- Infectious disease:
  - Parasitic.
    o Babesiosis [80].
    o Leishmaniasis [81].
- Hematoma [82].
- Nodular hyperplasia.
- Immune-mediated disease.
- Splenic torsion [83]:
  This is a rare event in the canine patient. When it occurs, deep-chested, large-breed dogs are overrepresented, especially German Shepherds and Great Danes [83–85].
- Malignant neoplasia:
  Hemangiosarcoma predominates as a cause of splenic neoplasia in the dog. [86, 87].
  Lymphoma has also been implicated in splenic cancer in the dog [88, 89].

Note from this list that splenomegaly may be generalized or focal. When the spleen is focally enlarged, a regional mass effect may be palpable. This may be the result of a non-neoplastic lesion such as a splenic hematoma as from a traumatic event, an abscess, or nodular hyperplasia.

A typical spleen feels smooth. When nodular hyperplasia is present, the surface of the spleen takes on an undulated texture. Less commonly, neoplastic disease effects focal changes in the splenic architecture.

14.5.4 The Pancreas

Recall from Section 6.5.4 that the pancreas consists of two lobes or limbs. The left lobe of the pancreas tracks caudomedially from the neighboring pylorus. It then crosses the median plane behind the stomach. The right lobe of the pancreas tracks caudodorsally from the neighboring pylorus and follows the descending duodenum. It is positioned lateral to the ascending colon [33, 90].

Neither limb of the pancreas is palpable in the normal canine patient [1]. Even in disease, the pancreas is difficult to palpate [1].

Exocrine pancreatic neoplasia is rare in dogs, with an incidence of less than 1% [91, 92]. When it occurs, adenocarcinoma is most common [92], with Airedales, Boxers, Labrador Retrievers, and Cocker Spaniels overrepresented [93]. Rarely is a mass palpable on physical examination [91]. As was the case with cats, the majority of canine patients are definitively diagnosed with pancreatic cancer on necropsy, with evidence of metastatic disease in the liver, omentum, mesentery, lungs, thyroid, heart, and duodenum [91, 92].

Rather than a palpable abdominal mass, canine patients with exocrine pancreatic neoplasia tend to present with non-specific signs of malaise: lethargy, anorexia, vomiting, depression, and weakness. Clinical signs frequently wax and wane over the course of several months, during which time weight loss is progressive [91–93].

Rarely seen is multifocal necrotizing steatitis, secondary to pancreatic carcinoma through an unknown mechanism. This results in subcutaneous and/or soft tissue swellings from which a purulent discharge may drain [94].

Other pancreatic diseases in canine patients are equally challenging to diagnose based upon physical examination alone because they are not characterized by organ enlargement that can be appreciated externally. For example, pancreatitis is more commonly diagnosed than exocrine pancreatic neoplasia in the canine patient, yet the most that physical examination typically yields is cranial abdominal pain and/or dehydration secondary to vomiting [95]. The clinician must rely upon a diagnostic work-up for a definitive diagnosis [95]. Because abdominal radiographs are typically unremarkable, abdominal ultrasonography is often employed [95]. The hypoechoic pancreas may reflect ongoing necrosis whereas the hyperechoic pancreas may reflect fibrosis secondary to inflammation [96]. Either deviation from normal echogenicity, in addition to the confirmed presence of peripancreatic fluid via ultrasound, may facilitate a diagnosis in a patient whose clinical signs are supportive [96, 97].

As was mentioned in Section 6.5.4, students have asked the author why it is necessary to feel for a pancreas if normal and diseased pancreases are so rarely identified on the physical examination. The goal is less about finding the pancreas and more about learning what the normal cranial abdomen feels like so that on those rare occasions when an abnormal finding exists, a trigger goes off and the student recognizes pathology.

A secondary goal in having students feel for the pancreas is to assess for evidence of pancreatic discomfort. Although physical examination findings in dogs with pancreatitis tend to be non-specific, as already mentioned, cranial abdominal pain is present in 58% of patients [96]. Although it is true that cranial abdominal pain is not pathognomonic for pancreatitis, its presence supports it as a potential diagnosis and should encourage the savvy clinician to launch a more extensive diagnostic investigation.

14.5.5 The Small Intestine

See Section 6.5.5 to review the anatomy of the small bowel.

Recall that the small intestine is dynamic: at any given point in time, some sections may be filled with ingesta while neighboring segments may be empty. This changes frequently as peristaltic waves continue to move ingesta aborad to maintain gut transit time and regularity [33].

The clinician is able to examine only a portion of the small bowel – primarily the jejunum. This represents a snapshot of the health of the intestines. To make the most of that snapshot, the clinician should appreciate [1, 98]:

- the texture of the intestinal loops;
- the thickness of the intestinal loops;
- the contents of the lumen;
- whether or not palpation is distressing to the patient.

The normal texture of the dog's small bowel is slightly less firm than the cat's and its loops are generally smooth. They should blip through the clinician's fingers with ease, without causing discomfort to the patient [1].

The small bowel should not be diffusely thickened. Diffuse thickening commonly occurs in puppies that are overloaded with gastrointestinal parasites such as ascarids. These puppies tend to be bloated. They present with a classic "Buddha belly" and a doughy feel to their gut [99–101]. Diffuse thickening of the small bowel may also be the result of food intolerance and/or dietary indiscretion causing enteritis [98–100].

In addition, the small bowel should not exhibit focal thickening. As was reviewed in Section 6.5.5, focal thickening of the small bowel could be attributed to [1, 98]:

- inflammatory bowel disease (IBD);
- foreign body;
- neoplasia.

Although large-scale epidemiologic studies have not been performed [102], IBD is believed to be a common chronic enteropathy in the dog [103–107], especially those which are young to middle-aged [102, 104, 108]. IBD is not a one-size-fits-all condition: there are several broad categories of IBD, including the following [102]:

- Lymphocytic–plasmacytic enteritis (LPE):
  - German Shepherds and Shar-Peis are overrepresented.
  - There is also an extreme version of LPE in Basenjis that is inherited through unknown mechanisms.
- Eosinophilic enteritis (EE):
  - Boxers, German Shepherds, and Dobermans are predisposed.
- Familial protein-losing enteropathy and nephropathy of Soft Coated Wheaten Terriers [109].

Canine patients with IBD tend to present in poor body condition due to small bowel malabsorption, with or without dehydration, abdominal discomfort, and focally thickened bowel loops. If there is small intestinal bleeding, it may be evident on the rectal examination as melena [102]. Because none of these signs is pathognomonic for IBD, these patients require an extensive diagnostic work-up, including baseline bloodwork (hematology and clinical biochemistry), fecal analysis, diagnostic imaging, measurement of serum folate and

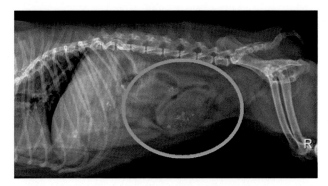

Figure 14.9 Right lateral radiograph of the abdomen. Note the presence of an intestinal mass in the mid-abdomen.

cobalamin, and histopathologic analysis of an intestinal biopsy [102].

In addition to IBD, foreign bodies may also cause focal thickening of the small bowel. See Section 14.5.2 for a review of foreign body ingestion in canine patients. When it comes to the intestinal tract, obstruction is most likely to occur with the ingestion of plastic or rubber balls and stones [53, 110] by young, large-breed dogs [110, 111]. The foreign body can be palpated in many cases [53]. Alternatively, the clinician may appreciate focal thickening of the bowel to which pain is localized [110].

In worst-case scenarios, a portion of the small bowel telescopes inside itself, causing an intussusception. Typically, proximal bowel telescopes into distal bowel. In dogs, the ileocolic junction and jejunojejunum are the most common sites of intussusception [110, 112, 113]. Note that intussusception is often triggered by ingestion of a foreign body. However, it also can be induced by viral enteritis as from canine parvovirus [110, 114].

Neoplasia can also cause focal thickening of the small bowel that may be palpable in 20–50% of dogs

[115–120] or, at the very least, radiographically evident (Figure 14.9).

The incidence of intestinal neoplasia is roughly 10% [121–124] and represents one-fifth of all canine tumors in the digestive tract [125]. Lymphoma, adenocarcinoma, and leiomyosarcoma predominate, with males being overrepresented in most tumor types [115–119, 126, 127]. Collies and German Shepherd dogs may also be predisposed, particularly when it comes to developing adenocarcinoma [115, 128, 129].

In addition to feeling for distinct masses, the clinician should tactilely assess the luminal contents. There may be palpable gas distension (Figure 14.10) [1].

In the majority of patients that present with small bowel disease, luminal contents will be fluid. Fluid palpates as sloshing past the clinician's fingers and most typically represents diarrhea, the primary clinical sign associated with small bowel disease [98]. Small bowel diarrhea tends to be voluminous and associated with weight loss. It typically does not involve increased frequency of defecation, tenesmus, or dyschezia. Unlike large bowel diarrhea, small bowel diarrhea does not tend to involve large amounts of fecal mucus [130].

When it occurs, small bowel diarrhea may be due to gastrointestinal and extragastrointestinal causes, including, but not limited to, the following [130]:

- dietary indiscretion;
- parasitic enteritis;
- viral enteritis;
- pancreatitis;
- exocrine pancreatic insufficiency;
- portosystemic shunt;
- hypoadrenocorticism;
- intestinal obstruction;
- toxicosis;

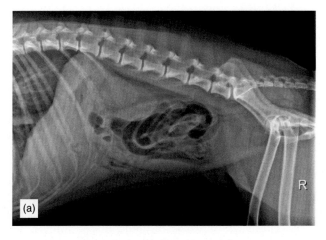

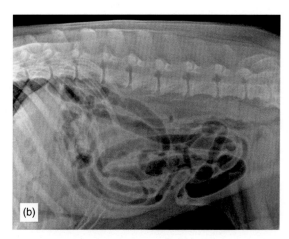

Figure 14.10 (a) Right lateral radiograph of the abdomen. Note the gas-distended small bowel in the mid-abdomen. (b) Right lateral radiograph of the abdomen. Note that the small bowel is diffusely gas filled and otherwise empty.

- small intestinal bacterial overgrowth (SIBO) as from malabsorptive small bowel disease.

When bacteria are implicated in small bowel diarrhea, the following species are most often blamed [131–134]:

- *Clostridium perfringens*
- *Clostridium difficile*
- *Campylobacter* spp.
- pathogenic *Escherichia coli*
- *Salmonella* spp.

14.5.6 The Mesenteric Lymph Nodes

Cranial mesenteric lymph nodes are dispersed throughout the root of the mesentery; there are also lymph nodes associated with the jejunum, cecum, and colon [33]. These nodes are not palpable in normal dogs [1].

Even in the abnormal dog, it is rare to be able to appreciate the mesenteric lymph nodes via palpation alone. More commonly, mesenteric lymphadenopathy is identified during exploratory laparotomy or via abdominal ultrasonography. In cats with alimentary lymphoma, for instance, mesenteric lymphadenopathy is evident via ultrasound in 33–50% of cases [135]. The author is uncertain of the equivalent percentage in canine patients.

14.5.7 The Large Intestine

See Section 6.5.7 to review the anatomic segmentation of the large bowel.

As in the cat, the descending colon is easily palpable in the dog, especially when it contains fecal matter. To differentiate normal fecal matter from a colonic mass, the clinician should try to compress the material. Barring obstipation, fecal matter should be compressible whereas masses tend not to be [33, 90].

Even when the descending colon lacks fecal material, it is palpable and distinguishable from the small intestine because the colonic wall is stiffer [33].

Foreign bodies may also be palpable within the large bowel if they have passed through the small bowel successfully without inducing obstruction; however, some foreign bodies are only visible on survey films of the abdomen (Figure 14.11).

14.5.8 The Anal Sacs

See Section 6.5.7 to review the anatomy of the anal sacs.

Anal sac impaction, anal sacculitis, and anal sac abscessation are relatively common in dogs, more so than cats, and are thought to affect up to 12% of the canine population at some point throughout life [136–138]. German Shepherd dogs are predisposed, which has been attributed to the increased depth of their anal sacs within perianal tissue [136, 139].

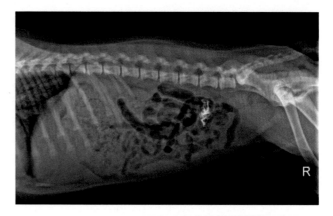

Figure 14.11 Right lateral radiograph of the abdomen of the same patient as in Figure 14.6. Note that the foreign body has successfully passed out of the stomach and small bowel and into the colon. This was not palpable on physical examination.

Small-breed dogs may also be overrepresented because their smaller ducts are more likely to become obstructed if anal gland secretions become thick and pasty [136, 139].

Unlike cats, the most common presentations for anal sacculitis in a dog are scooting, chewing at or around the anal area or tail base, avoidance of sitting, and tail-chasing [136, 139, 140]. Clients may even appreciate and present the patient for a visible swelling over the involved sac(s) [136].

Without medical management, in particular expression of the impacted and/or infected gland(s), anal sacs may rupture, creating a draining fistula (Figure 14.12) [136].

Sedation may be required to perform an internal rectal examination to assess the anal sacs, depending on the patient's pain level and tolerance [136]. The next section gives details of how to perform a rectal examination thoroughly, given that there are additional anatomic structures that should be evaluated per rectum.

When anal sacs are impacted, the clinician is typically able to express with difficulty a thick, pasty substance. Physical examination findings that are supportive of anal sac infection are expression of bloody and/or purulent discharge. When this type of discharge is expressed from one or both glands, infection should be confirmed via cytology. Because anal sacs naturally contain a mixed population of bacteria, the astute clinician should review the cytology of anal sac secretions to look for intracellular bacteria. When bacteria are identified within neutrophils, anal sac infection is confirmed and broad-spectrum antibiotics are indicated [136, 141, 142].

Anal sac tumors occur with less frequency than anal sacculitis and associated infections. However, when they do, they are typically malignant adenocarcinomas that have a high rate of metastasis to external iliac

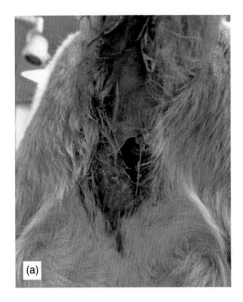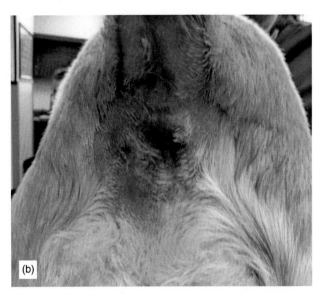

Figure 14.12 (a) This patient presented for scooting. Prior to clipping of the perineum, the clinician could appreciate the presence of an oozing blood-tinged, mucopurulent discharge in the region of the left anal sac. (b) Same patient as in (a). Clipping of the perineum revealed erythematous, abraded skin overlaying the left anal sac. There is also subtle swelling overlaying the same sac. Source (a), (b): Courtesy of Patricia Bennett, DVM.

(sublumbar) lymph nodes. The small size of these tumors may be distracting: many have already metastasized by the time they are identified on physical examination [143].

Anal sac adenocarcinomas are reported to cause hypercalcemia of malignancy: affected dogs may be clinical for signs of hypercalcemia such as polyuria/polydipsia (PU/PD), vomiting, constipation, and/or generalized muscle weakness [144, 145].

14.5.9 The Rectal Examination

The rectal exam should be performed in any adult dog that is presenting for the following [1]:

- tenesmus: straining to defecate;
- dyschezia: difficulty defecating;
- constipation;
- hematochezia: blood in the stool;
- diarrhea;
- dysuria;
- stranguria.

In addition, through the rectal examination, the experienced clinician may discover a [1]:

- perianal tumor;
- anal tumor;
- perineal swelling.

See Figure 14.13 and Figure 14.14.

Older, intact, male dogs [143] are overrepresented when it comes to benign perianal gland adenomas, as

are the following breeds: Cocker Spaniels, Bulldogs, Beagles, and Samoyeds [146–148]. These tumors are associated with the circumanal glands. Although they are non-invasive and non-metastatic, they can become ulcerative or necrotic. They can bleed extensively and cause intense anal pruritus [143]. Perianal gland adenomas need to be differentiated from invasive, metastatic anal squamous cell carcinomas and melanomas [143, 148].

In addition to perianal tumors, perineal swellings may be identified on the physical examination. These could be demonstrative of a perineal hernia, which occurs when the pelvic diaphragm becomes disrupted. The result is that abdominal cavity structures such as the rectum, urinary bladder, and/or prostate may become herniated into the ischiorectal fossa [143, 149, 150].

Patients with perineal hernias present with unilateral or bilateral swellings that are reducible. Additional clinical signs typically relate to which abdominal structures are entrapped. For instance, if the urinary bladder is herniated into the ischiorectal fossa, the patient may present for urinary obstruction. By contrast, primary rectal involvement may lead to tenesmus, dyschezia, constipation, and/or obstipation [143, 150].

The presence of a perineal hernia is confirmed by rectal examination. It is apparent when a rectal examination is indicated based on the aforementioned clinical signs. However, there is no consensus within the veterinary community when it comes to whether or not rectal examinations should be incorporated into the wellness appointment for healthy aclinical adults. In general, the author prefers to perform an annual rectal examination

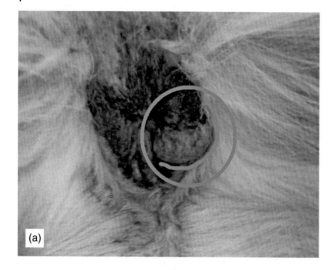

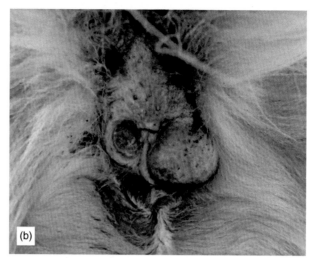

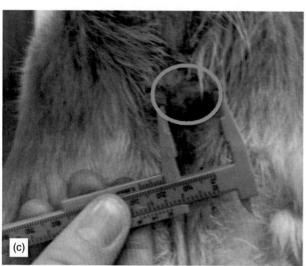

Figure 14.13 (a) This patient presented for subtle focal swelling at the right rim of the anus. Source: Courtesy of Patricia Bennett, DVM. (b) This patient presented with two anal rim-associated masses. Note that the left mass has already ruptured outwards and has a raw surface exposed to the elements whereas the right mass is encapsulated and therefore non-ulcerated. Source: Courtesy of Patricia Bennett, DVM. (c) Dorsal anal rim mass. Source: Courtesy of Elizabeth Robbins, DVM.

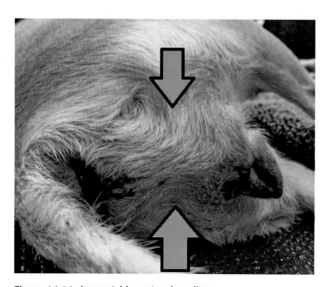

Figure 14.14 Appreciable perineal swelling.

in every adult dog so as not to miss early anal and rectal canal disease. A comprehensive rectal examination can provide a large quantity of information.

In anticipation of performing a rectal examination, the veterinary team should be prepared. The hand that will be examining the patient should be gloved and generously lubricated. With a gloved forefinger, the clinician may also apply some lubricant to the anal rim. The clinician should give the patient a moment to acclimate rather than just "diving in" [1]. Prior to advancing the gloved forefinger, the clinician should appreciate the perineum. Normal anal sacs are not palpable externally. However, enlarged or obstructed sacs may be palpable as a firm swelling or nodule. The clinician should also assess if there is anal tone. To determine this, the clinician can touch the anal rim with his gloved forefinger. An anus with normal tone will "wink" as the anal sphincters close. Decreased or absent tone suggests a problem with the innervation of the anus [1].

When the clinician is ready to advance a forefinger, he should do so gently, without force and without rapid turning or grinding motions. His motion should be smooth and fluid [1]. Recall from Section 6.5.8 that the clinician is feeling for the following [1]:

- the pelvic diaphragm: the muscles and bones that border and/or help to define the rectal canal;
- the prostate, in male dogs, along the ventral floor of the pelvis;
- the urethra along the ventral floor of the pelvis;
- the left and right anal sacs.

The clinician should not expect to feel [1]:

- abnormal thickening of the rectal wall;
- irregularities of the surface of the rectal mucosa;
- a defect in the pelvic diaphragm;
- the internal iliac lymph node;
- pelvic fractures.

As the clinician backtracks through the anal canal on the way out, he should feel for the left and right anal sacs to gain an appreciation for their shape and size. He should ask the following [1]:

- Are the anal sacs symmetrical?
- Are the anal sacs enlarged?
- Are the anal sacs painful?
- Are the anal sacs easy to express?

If anal sac expression is performed, the clinician should grossly evaluate the secretions of the anal sacs. As already mentioned, if the secretions are bloody or purulent, the clinician should create a slide imprint of his gloved finger post-expression to evaluate the contents of both anal sacs microscopically [1].

Finally, as the clinician exits the anal canal, he should remember to appreciate the rim of the rectal canal. It is possible to miss a mass or a hernia defect if the clinician is too focused on feeling deep inside.

14.6 The Upper Urinary Tract

See Section 6.6 to review the anatomy of the upper urinary tract.

As in the cat, the dog has a right kidney that is cranial to the left. However, unlike feline kidneys, canine kidneys are much less mobile and are therefore much more challenging to appreciate on the physical examination, especially in large and giant breed dogs. It is common for the clinician to feel neither kidney in a normal dog, or only the left kidney's caudal pole. As a result, it is very difficult to assess renal size based upon palpation alone. Imaging is more often than not required to detect renomegaly as may be associated with hydronephrosis, a tumor, or a cyst [33, 151].

Like the cat, the dog can be evaluated for renal size based upon survey radiographs that compare kidney length with the length of the vertebral body associated with L2 [152–154]. As determined in the ventrodorsal (V/D) view, this ratio of renal length to L2 vertebral body length ranges from 2.54 to 3.45 or, in the lateral view, from 2.38 to 3.19 [152–155].

Brachycephalic breeds appear to have a greater ratio of renal length to L2 vertebral body length than dolichocephalic breeds, meaning that Pugs and English Bulldogs, for instance, have longer than expected kidneys [154].

Unlike in cats, in dogs there is no definitive link between renal length and sexual status [151].

In veterinary medicine, ultrasonography is the preferred method of assessing renal length because it provides additional information about intra-renal architecture [156–158], even though it may underestimate renal size [159].

An additional challenge in dogs is determining which renal length is normal versus abnormal when comparing one individual with the population as a whole. Unlike cats, dogs are morphologically distinct: there is marked variation between breeds. Establishing a reliable normal range is difficult because it likely depends upon the breed more so than the species [160–162].

Rather than evaluating renal length alone to determine if kidneys are under- or oversized in a canine patient, the use of a ratio has been suggested, much like the renal length to L2 vertebral body length ratio as is measured in abdominal radiography. Renal length to aortic luminal diameter ration (K/Ao) as determined by ultrasonography has been tested. Using this ratio, renomegaly is said to be present when the K/Ao ratio is greater than 9.1. By contrast, canine kidneys are said to be undersized when the K/Ao ratio is less than 5.5 [162].

An alternative approach that uses ultrasonography is to determine the ratio of kidney length to the length of the vertebral body associated with L5 or L6, both of which are easier to access than L2 via ultrasound. Using this approach, renomegaly is said to be present when the ratio is >2.7. By contrast, canine kidneys are said to be undersized when the ratio is <1.3 [161].

Regardless of which approach is employed from an imaging perspective, the clinician should still attempt to palpate the kidneys in a live dog, even though the odds are significantly against success. Feeling for the kidneys is of value because some renal masses, such as leiomyoma, can be palpable if the kidney is sufficiently enlarged [163].

To attempt renal palpation in the dog, the clinician makes use of the same two techniques that are employed in the cat:

- Most commonly, the clinician examines a standing patient that is facing away from him:
  - The clinician takes his left hand and places it flattened against the left body wall.

- The clinician then applies firm pressure as if pushing into the abdomen with his left hand. What he is doing is creating a "table" against which organs from the opposite side can be pushed.
- Now, with his right hand, he curls his fingers slightly and pushes deeply into the right side of the cranial abdomen just caudal to the last rib.
- Applying firm pressure, he then moves his right hand caudally to catch the right kidney.
- He may then repeat the same technique for the contralateral side, using his flattened right hand as a "table," with the left hand curled to "catch" the left kidney.

- An alternative approach that works well for cat-sized dogs is to lift the small dog with one hand and support it at the level of its sternum so that the dog is in effect "standing" on his hind limbs:
  - This posture helps the kidneys to sink into a more accessible location.
  - The clinician can use his other hand to cup the abdomen to "catch" each kidney.
  - In order to evaluate both kidneys, the clinician will have to switch hands.

Remember that the majority of the time, the clinician will feel, at most, the caudal pole of the left kidney [151] in which case it should not be tender to the touch.

14.7 The Lower Urinary Tract

See Section 6.7 to review the anatomy of the lower urinary tract.

As in the cat, the dog has a urinary bladder that is typically palpable. The typical empty urinary bladder feels like a wad of balled-up tissue: soft, supple, and non-tender to the touch. As the urinary bladder fills a small amount, it feels like a very small water balloon: fluid surrounded by a stable, yet soft and pliable wall. Even when the bladder is moderately full, it still retains that water balloon-like quality, that is, it is compressible [151].

Like cats, dogs can also experience a urinary tract obstruction (UTO), which is typically unmistakable on abdominal palpation. The urinary bladder takes on a rock-hard feel: it is no longer compressible, and it is exceedingly painful.

However, unlike cats, in which UTO tends to be associated with a urethral plug [164, 165], UTO in the dog tends to be related to either:

- neoplasia of the urinary bladder, such as transitional cell carcinoma [166];
- neoplasia of the prostate, such as prostatic carcinoma [167];
- urolithiasis [168];
- urethrolithiasis [169, 170].

Urethral plugs can occur in dogs; however, they are much less likely than in cats. Only 42 canine urethral plugs were submitted to the Minnesota Urolith Center between 2006 and 2011 [171] compared with 618 feline urethral plugs that were submitted to the Canadian Veterinary Urolith Centre between 1998 and 2003 [172].

Of the urethral plugs that were submitted from canine patients, 83% were struvite in composition and 100% came from males, 71% of which were Pugs [171].

Because UTO is possible in dogs, the clinician should feel for the urinary bladder in all comprehensive physical examinations, but especially when the patient is presenting for the following urinary tract-related signs:

- dysuria;
- stranguria;
- hematuria;
- pollakiuria.

These clinical signs could signify an impending UTO or a urinary tract infection (UTI).

In addition, it is important that the clinician feels comfortable isolating the urinary bladder through palpation because this is an essential first step in blind cystocentesis, in which the urinary bladder is sampled via a needle inserted through the abdominal body wall without the aid of ultrasonography.

The urinary bladder is located within the caudoventral abdominal cavity, between the ventral body wall and the descending colon. However, if the descending colon is full, the colon can be displaced so that it sits lateral to the urinary bladder [151].

In order to palpate the urinary bladder, the clinician may position the patient as follows, depending upon his preference:

- The patient can be standing and facing away from the clinician. A two-handed approach to palpation will work best in large-breed dogs, whereas a one-handed approach is feasible for small- to medium-sized breeds.
- The patient can be facing away from the clinician with the front half of its body elevated in the same manner as was performed for kidney palpation. As above, a two-handed approach to palpation will work best in large-breed dogs, whereas a one-handed approach is feasible for small- to medium-sized breeds.
- The patient can be examined in lateral recumbency. In this position, the clinician cups his hand so that his thumb is on one side of the caudal abdomen and his fingers are on the other. The clinician then firmly brings his fingers and thumb together so that they practically touch, with the patient's body in between them. The clinician can now slide his hand cranially and then caudally, then back again until the urinary bladder "blips" through his hand.

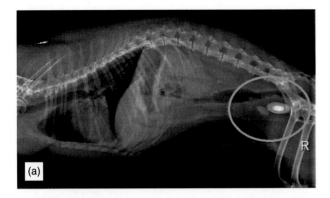

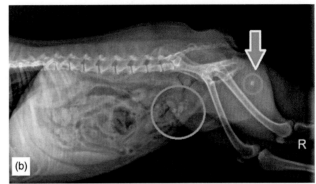

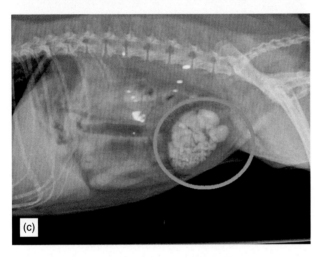

Figure 14.15 (a) Right lateral radiograph of the abdomen. Note the two ovoid stones in the urinary bladder. The more caudal of the two stones has a core that is more radiopaque than its periphery. (b) Right lateral radiograph of the abdomen. Note that uroliths are not the only type of urinary tract stone that is present. The arrow points to a sole urethrolith. (c) Right lateral radiograph of the abdomen. Note the large number of uroliths that are filling the urinary bladder. Source: Courtesy of Shirley Yang, DVM.

Some clinicians will place the patient in dorsal recumbency for blind cystocentesis; however, in this case, the clinician is less feeling for the urinary bladder and more using a blind-stick approach to cystocentesis by inserting the needle where a pool of alcohol forms when the clinician drizzles alcohol on the caudal ventrum.

The urinary bladder should be palpable in all dogs unless the patient is extraordinarily tense, in which case the urinary bladder will remain "hidden" beneath taut abdominal muscles [151].

The position of the urinary bladder within the abdomen will vary depending upon how distended it is with urine. If the urinary bladder is exceptionally full, it could potentially reach into the epigastrium [151].

Uroliths are palpable on physical examination in approximately 20% of canine patients [173]. Larger uroliths increase the odds of detection. So, too, does the presence of multiple stones, which may grate together in such a way that they feel like marbles rolling around in a sack.

Because urolithiasis is not detected by physical examination in the majority of patients [173], imaging is preferred to obtain a definitive diagnosis [168]. Survey radiographs of the abdomen are often the first line of approach in the detection of uroliths [168]. In addition to verifying their presence, abdominal radiographs provide details of the numbers of stones present and also whether or not stones

are present in other locations within the urinary tract such as the kidney (nephrolith), ureter (ureterolith), or urethra (urethrolith) [174, 175] (Figure 14.15).

One shortcoming of abdominal radiography is that only radiopaque uroliths are visible [176]. Calcium oxalate and silica stones are radiopaque, whereas ammonium urate and cystine stones tend to be radiolucent. Magnesium ammonium phosphate (struvite) stones trend toward being radiopaque; however, this depends largely upon the percentage of calcium phosphate that they contain [177, 178].

The more radiopaque the urolith, the more likely it will be detected by survey radiography. The false-negative detection rate is 5% for calcium oxalate dihydrate, calcium oxalate monohydrate, and silica, and 2% for magnesium ammonium phosphate, because most contain sufficient quantities of calcium phosphate to be detected. By contrast, ammonium urate has a 25% false-negative detection rate owing to its radiolucency [177].

In addition to confirming the presence of uroliths, the clinician needs to know the type(s) of urolith(s) to facilitate medical versus surgical management. Unfortunately, only laboratory analysis of uroliths is able to provide a definitive diagnosis.

It is an error to diagnose the type of urolith based upon their radiographic size. Although magnesium ammonium

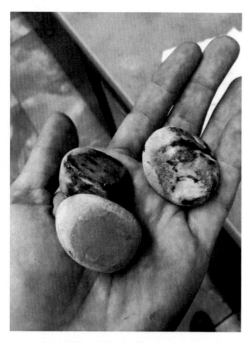

Figure 14.16 Three large ovoid uroliths in the palm of an adult man's hand, for size comparison. Based upon the odds for this type of urolith shape, there is a high likelihood that these stones are magnesium ammonium phosphate. However, there is no guarantee and the clinician would do best to send the stones to an outside laboratory for analysis. There is also no guarantee that the stone is not mixed in terms of mineral composition. Source: Courtesy of Andrew Weisenfeld, DVM.

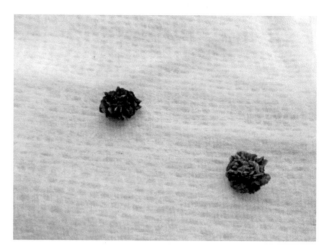

Figure 14.17 Two rosette-shaped uroliths. Based upon the odds for this type of urolith shape, there is a high likelihood that these stones are calcium oxalate. However, there is no guarantee and the clinician would do best to send the stones to an outside laboratory for analysis. There is also no guarantee that the stone is not mixed in terms of mineral composition.

phosphate stones are typically greater than 10 mm in diameter, smaller stones could be anything [177, 179].

It is equally an error to diagnose the type of urolith based upon their radiographic shape. Although 80% of magnesium ammonium phosphate stones are typically ovoid, the remaining 20% will be misidentified (Figure 14.16). Similarly, roughly 15% of calcium oxalate uroliths will appear to share the jackstone shape when viewed radiographically when in fact such a shape is classic for silica stones. Even rosettes, which represent calcium oxalate stones 95% of the time, do not typically demonstrate that shape when evaluated by radiographs (Figure 14.17). Furthermore, stone shapes may be in between two classic appearances such that when they are surgically removed, the clinician is at a loss to define the stones as a particular type without sending the stones off for analysis (Figure 14.18) [177, 179].

The history and clinicopathologic data may also help the clinician make an educated guess as to stone type to facilitate his recommendations for medical or surgical management. For example, struvite stones tend to be infection-induced in canine patients that are female and either less than 1 year old or greater than 10 years old [168, 180–182]. Infectious organisms such as *Staphylococcus*, *Enterococcus*, and *Proteus* spp. produce the enzyme urease, which produces ammonia

from the hydrolysis of urea [168, 183]. Ammonia contributes to alkaluria, which promotes the formation of struvites [184]. In these cases, the administration of an appropriate systemic antibiotic to target the source of the urinary tract infection, with or without an acidifying diet, and with or without oral urinary acidifiers such as D,L-methionine, is likely to lead to medical dissolution of struvite uroliths within 1–4 months in non-obstructed canine patients [185–187].

Calcium oxalate stones, on the other hand, tend to be associated with aciduria and certain breeds of small dogs: the Miniature Schnauzer, Lhasa Apso, Shih Tzu, Yorkshire Terrier, and Bichon Frise [168, 173, 188]. Prior to 2003, calcium oxalate stones in dogs and cats in the

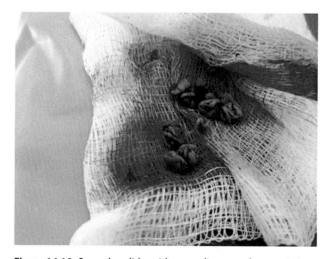

Figure 14.18 Several uroliths with a peculiar, non-characteristic shape. The clinician would do best to send the stones to an outside laboratory for analysis.

United States were rare in comparison with struvites: according to the Minnesota Urolith Center, only 5% of canine uroliths in 1997 were calcium oxalate. By 2003, the occurrence of calcium oxalate had risen to equal struvite, and calcium oxalate stones surpassed struvite in 2004. By 2005, 42% of canine urolith submissions were calcium oxalate. It has been hypothesized that the trend toward acidifying diets intended to prevent struvituria has fueled the increase in calcium oxalate stones, for which there is no means of medical dissolution and for which surgical retrieval is indicated [173, 189–192].

Dalmatians and English Bulldogs have extraordinarily increased risks of developing urate stones [193]:

- The chance that a urolith will be urate based in a Dalmatian is 228.9 times greater than in any other breed, with males being 16.4 times more at risk than females.
- The chance that a urolith will be urate based in an English Bulldogs is 43 times greater than in any other breed, with males being 14.3 times more at risk than females.

Likewise, English Bulldogs are at increased risk of developing cystine stones [193]:

- The chance that a urolith will cystine based in an English Bulldog is 32.3 times greater than in any other breed, with only males represented in a 1994 study by Bartges *et al.* [193].

14.8 The Male Reproductive Tract

The reproductive tract of the stud dog consists of both internal and external structures. The primary accessory sex gland in the stud dog is the prostate. Although the ampullae of the vas deferens are present in the dog, not all clinicians consider these to be important, given their small size [194].

Of the internal structures of the male dog, only the prostate is palpable per rectum. The prostate is most prominent in dogs that are intact and sexually mature; however, in most cases it is still palpable in castrated dogs [151, 194].

See Section 14.5.9 to review the technique for the rectal examination.

The prostate is bi-lobed; along its dorsal midline, a sulcus can be appreciated, which divides the right from the left side. It typically sits 1–2 cm caudal to the neck of the bladder, along the cranial aspect of the pubic symphysis, and blankets the cranial urethra. As dogs age, the prostate may sink out of the pelvic canal, cranially, making it more challenging to feel, especially in large-breed dogs. To facilitate palpation, especially in these patients, the clinician's free hand – the one that is not digitally exploring the rectum – may be used to cup the ventral abdomen firmly just cranial to the pelvic canal. When the clinician hikes the ventral abdomen up in this manner, the prostate has a

tendency to be lifted and raised back into the pelvic canal, where it is palpable digitally per rectum. Palpation over both lobes of the prostate should not elicit pain [151, 194].

As dogs age, prostatic enlargement is common [151, 194]: approximately 63% of dogs develop so-called prostatic hypertrophy or benign prostatic hyperplasia [195, 196]. These prostates palpate as being homogeneously enlarged, smooth-surfaced, and non-painful [195]. However, prostatic enlargement may lead to the development of tenesmus rather than the dysuria that is appreciated in human males with the same condition [195].

By contrast, prostatitis is characterized by a diffusely enlarged prostate that is exceedingly painful on digital palpation per rectum. Frequently, this condition is accompanied by clinical signs suggestive of systemic malaise, including fever, lethargy, depression, and/or anorexia [195].

Prostatic neoplasia is variable both in terms of gross appearance and, tactilely, by means of palpation per rectum. However, prostatic neoplasia is more likely than other prostatic conditions to cause multinodular, asymmetric lesions [195].

Both intact and castrated dogs may succumb to prostatic neoplasia, of which carcinoma is most likely [195, 197]. Some studies suggest equal risk regardless of sexual status [198], while others find the castrated male to be at increased risk [199, 200].

The external portion of the male reproductive tract that should be evaluated on every comprehensive physical examination includes the penis and the testicles. Unlike the tom cat, in which the penis is located in the perineum rather than the groin, the dog houses its penis between its thighs [33], which makes sexual determination of puppies very easy. Whereas male and female kittens have a tendency to look alike with regard to their genitalia shortly after birth, male and female puppies are readily distinguished. This distinction remains just as obvious in adulthood (Figure 14.19).

As demonstrated in Figure 14.19a, the penis of the dog is entirely sheathed by the prepuce except during excitement (Figure 14.20), sexual arousal, and manual inspection, which becomes especially important when there is a history of reported hematuria that may or may not be related to micturition [151].

Manual inspection of the penis is achieved by placing the canine patient in dorsal or lateral recumbency. The clinician then pushes against the skin fold that separates the prepuce from the abdominal wall to cause the penis to protrude from within the sheath. Manipulation of the penis in this way should not be met with resistance. If it is, it may signal the presence of a congenital anomaly such as a persistent penile frenulum or phimosis, characterized by an opening in the prepuce that is too narrow for the penis to glide through [151, 201, 202].

During manual inspection, the penis should be evaluated for structure and integrity. The canine penis is

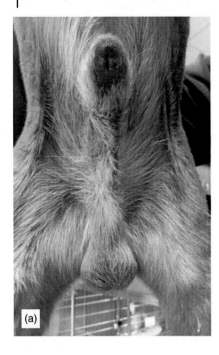

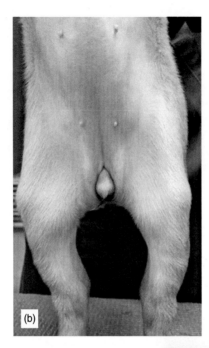

Figure 14.19 Ventral views of an intact adolescent (a) male and (b) female dog.

a vascular structure as opposed to the fibroelastic penis of the bull, boar, and ram. The caudal aspect of the canine penis is thickest; it tapers cranially until it terminates in a fibrocartilaginous tip. Penile tissue should be a healthy pink color and moist. The surface is by and large smooth, with the exception of lymphoid folllicles [151].

Occasionally, the mucosa takes on a visibly inflamed appearance that may or may not be associated with purulent material at the preputial opening and/or surrounding fur (Figure 14.21). This may be more promi-

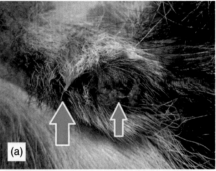

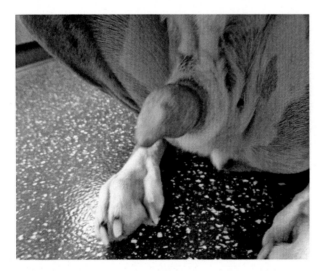

Figure 14.20 This patient's penis has naturally protruded from its sheath or prepuce due to excitement. This may or may not be accompanied by bilateral swellings at the base of the prepuce, representative of the penile bulbus glandis, which in the author's experience has led inexperienced clients to feel that their castrated male dog may not have been neutered after all because of the presence of what they feel are retained testicles.

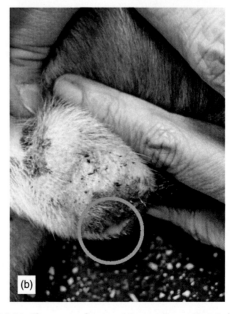

Figure 14.21 Close-ups of prepuce in a canine patient in left lateral recumbency. (a) Note the presence of mucoid discharge at the prepuce and also coated to peri-preputial fur. This is considered to be normal. (b) Note the presence of mucopurulent discharge at the preputial tip. This is considered to be normal.

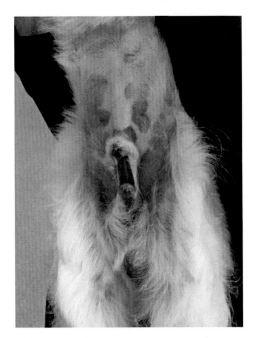

Figure 14.22 Hypospadias in a canine patient with an incompletely formed preputial sheath. Source: Courtesy of Michael Jaffe, DVM, DACVS-SA.

nent in intact males and is considered to be a variation of normal. No diagnostic work-up is indicated unless the patient presents with clinical signs such as obsessively licking at the prepuce with overt discomfort [151, 194].

The penis should also be evaluated in puppies for the opening of the urethra, which should ordinarily be located in a groove on the ventral side of the os penis,

the bone that develops in the septum that separates the corpora cavernosa [151, 194]. Hypospadias is a congenital condition in which the urethral folds fail to fuse, causing the urethra to open in an abnormal anatomic location (Figure 14.22) [203].

In addition to examining the penis, the clinician should assess each new and intact patient for the presence of two scrotal testicles. This is especially important at "new puppy" visits to establish whether or not testicular descent has occurred and if not, whether the patient is unilaterally or bilaterally cryptorchid.

See Section 6.8 to review embryonic development of the testes and their descent through the inguinal canal into the scrotal sac.

At birth, the testes are typically abdominal in puppies. Testes do not typically become scrotal until 3–10 days after birth. However, as in kittens, the testes may continue to pass in and out of the scrotum through the open inguinal canal until 10–14 weeks of age. Puppies also have a strongly effective cremaster muscle, which may challenge the clinician to find scrotal testes that are in fact present but have been hiked up high within the scrotal sac [204]. A puppy should not be considered unilaterally or bilaterally cryptorchid until 4–6 months old, when the inguinal canal closes, at which point the testes are either scrotally located or not [205–210].

Cryptorchidism occurs with greater frequency in dogs than cats: the incidence in canine patients ranges between 3.3 and 6.8% [211]. Unilateral, right-sided, inguinal cryptorchidism is the most common presentation in dogs, followed by unilateral, right-sided, abdominal (Figure 14.23) [195, 211–213].

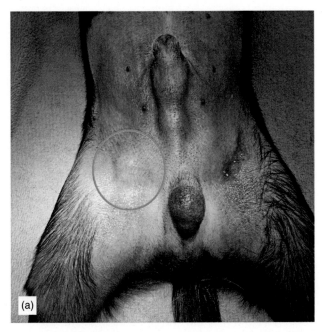

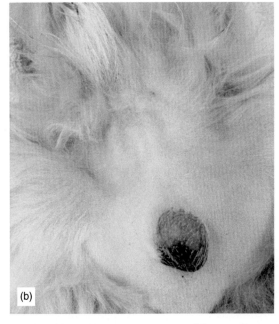

Figure 14.23 (a) Right-sided inguinal cryptorchid canine patient being prepped for orchiectomy. Source: Courtesy of Shannon Carey, DVM. (b) Right-sided abdominal cryptorchid canine patient. Source: Courtesy of Frank Isom, DVM.

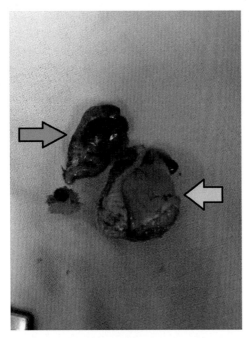

Figure 14.24 Size comparison of the cryptorchid testis (blue arrow) versus the normal, scrotal testis (orange arrow), post-orchiectomy. Note how the cryptorchid testis is appreciably smaller in size. Source: Courtesy of Shannon Carey, DVM.

Historically, pedigreed dogs have been overrepresented: in a study of 240 cryptorchid dogs, 77.5% were purebreds, especially German Shepherds, Boxers, and Chihuahuas [211]. The Toy, Miniature, and Standard Poodle, Yorkshire Terrier, Miniature Dachshund, English Bulldog, Maltese, and Pekingese are also overrepresented, whereas the following breeds are considered low risk: Beagle, Golden Retriever, Labrador Retriever, Saint Bernard, Great Dane, and English Setter [214].

When cryptorchidism occurs, the affected testicle is capable of producing testosterone via functional Leydig (interstitial) cells. However, in patients that present for abdominal cryptorchidism, spermatogenesis is impaired owing to testicular exposure to core body temperature. This causes degeneration of the germinal epithelium. The net result is impaired testicular size and texture: the cryptorchid testis is smaller and softer than expected (Figure 14.24) [195, 214].

Hormonal attempts to correct testicular descent are ineffective in the dog and should be discouraged by the veterinary team because even in the rare event that it is successful, the patient still carries a heritable trait [214]. The mode of inheritance for cryptorchidism is autosomal recessive [195, 207]. Because cryptorchidism is inherited, cryptorchid dogs should not be bred.

Even more important to the health of the affected patient is that it undergo orchiectomy. The cryptorchid testis is at increased risk of testicular cancer. Specifically, the chance that a cryptorchid will develop a Sertoli cell tumor is five times greater than in the general population;

the chance that a cryptorchid will develop a seminoma is three times greater [214]. In addition, the retained testis is more likely to experience torsion [195, 215–217].

14.9 The Female Reproductive Tract

The reproductive tract of the bitch consists of both internal and external structures. Of the internal structures, the normal ovaries are never palpable in the dog, nor is the non-pregnant uterus [218].

Ovaries could potentially be palpable when pathologically enlarged due to ovarian cysts or ovarian tumors [218]. However, the latter are rare and the former are more often identified at the time of ovariohysterectomy as incidental findings as anovulatory functional follicular cysts [219].

The uterus is palpable during the physiologic state of pregnancy [218, 220]. From mating to parturition, the gestation length in a dog ranges from 57 to 72 days, averaging 65.3 days [221]. Discrete uterine swellings, as from developing fetuses, may be detected via abdominal palpation between days 21 and 25 of gestation. These swellings continue to increase in size such that by days 33–35, uterine confluence makes diagnosis of pregnancy by palpation unreliable. It is not until at or after day 45 that pregnancy detection by palpation becomes possible again, owing to ossification of the fetuses, which allows for the fetal skeleton to be appreciated on the abdominal examination [218, 222].

The ability of the clinician to identify fetuses on palpation largely depends upon their level of experience and their digital sensitivity. For experienced ultrasonographers, pregnancy detection via ultrasound may be more accurate as early as 19–21 days post-LH peak or 30 days after the last recorded mating. As early as 23–25 days post-LH peak, fetal heartbeats can be identified by ultrasound. Although ultrasound is not reliable for establishing litter size, it is an appropriate means by which to assess fetal health and stress [222].

At or after day 45 of pregnancy, but most certainly within 5–10 days of anticipated delivery, a lateral abdominal radiograph should be obtained to estimate litter size by counting fetal skulls (Figure 14.25). Although it is possible to underestimate litter size in large litters, abdominal radiography helps the veterinary team and client plan for what is expected. It also helps with assessing the likelihood of fetopelvic disproportion, meaning that if fetal skulls well exceed the width of the maternal pelvic canal, a caesarian section will likely be indicated [222].

The uterus is also palpable during the pathologic state of pyometra. Pyometra is a common uterine disease in the dog that most notably affects mature bitches that have cycled previously. Although the youngest age reported in the literature is 4 months and the oldest is 16 years, the majority of canine patients with pyometra present between 2.4 and 7.25 years of age [223–229].

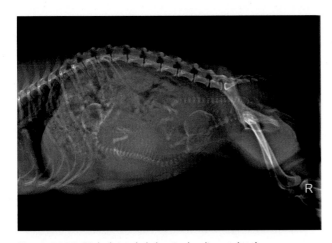

Figure 14.25 Right lateral abdominal radiograph taken pre-whelping to assess litter size. Source: Courtesy of Elizabeth Robbins, DVM.

Risk factors for the development of pyometra include prior hormonal therapy with estrogens or progestins [228], prior pregnancy termination [230, 231], having been in estrus within 12 weeks prior to presentation [229], and being nulliparous [226]. In addition, some breeds are thought to be overrepresented, including include the Rottweiler, Saint Bernard, Chow Chow, Golden Retriever, Miniature Schnauzer, Irish Terrier, Airedale Terrier, Cavalier King Charles Spaniel, Rough Collie, and Bernese Mountain Dog [229, 232, 233].

Pyometras are characterized by an accumulation of purulent material within the uterus, causing uterine enlargement, distension, and systemic malaise [229]. The experienced clinician should be able to appreciate the presence of the tubular uterus on abdominal palpation, and imaging via abdominal radiography or ultrasonography is helpful to confirm the diagnosis. The tubular uterus that is evident on imaging matches beautifully what is encountered during an ovariohysterectomy to manage the condition surgically (Figure 14.26).

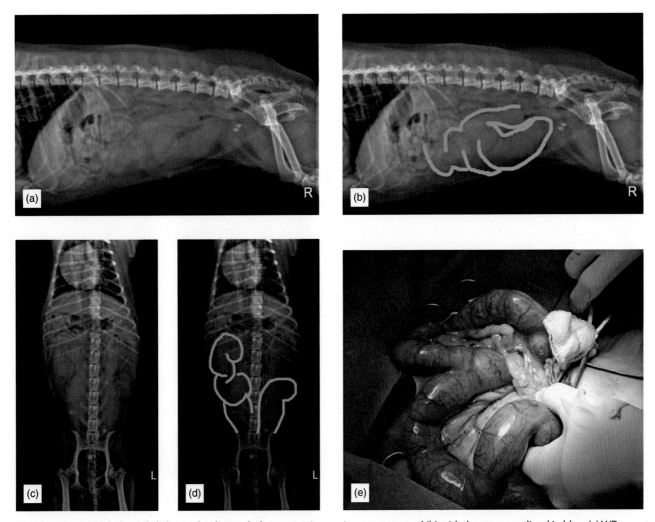

Figure 14.26 (a) Right lateral abdominal radiograph demonstrating canine pyometra and (b) with the uterus outlined in blue. (c) V/D radiograph demonstrating canine pyometra and (d) with the uterus outlined in blue. (e) Intra-operative depiction of pyometra.

There are two main types of pyometras, open and closed. In an open pyometra, the cervix remains open, allowing for the outflow of abnormal reproductive tract discharge. Because there is drainage of the purulent material, the patient tends to present for apparent vulvar discharge and is typically not as ill as is the patient with a closed pyometra.

In a closed pyometra, the cervix is closed, which results in retention of the abnormal uterine discharge. The uterus becomes palpably distended to the point that uterine rupture is possible. The clinician should take care to palpate gently when suspecting a pyometra to be present so as not to facilitate uterine rupture due to rough handling.

The physical examination of the female canine reproductive tract should also include a cursory evaluation of the external anatomy, the vulva. The astute clinician should take care to inspect the vulva for [218]:

- size;
- mucosal color;
- discharge;
- conformation.

The vulva is small during anestrus (Figure 14.27a), with its opening largely covered by the dorsal fold, a fold of skin that spans the space between the anus and vulva. The mucosa is pink and lacks sheen. There should be minimal to no vulvar discharge: if discharge is present, it may be mucoid. On average, anestrus lasts 3–4 months in the dog because most dogs come into heat every 6–7 months. However, there are breed-specific differences:

anestrus is prolonged in Collies, with a duration of 47 weeks [218, 234].

When the patient is in pro-estrus for an average of 9 days, the vulva begins to swell. Serosanguinous vulvar discharge is present. The discharge arises from the uterus and should not be malodorous [218, 234].

By the time the patient is in estrus, for an average of 9 days, the vulva has become quite pronounced such that its opening may be visible (Figure 14.27b). Despite its size, the vulva softens. The mucosa is paler than it was in anestrus, and tends to be edematous. This results in a classic sheen or glossiness to its appearance. Vulvar discharge is present. At the onset of estrus, vulvar discharge may appear to be increasingly hemorrhagic. As estrus progresses, vulvar discharge should fade from red to light pink or straw-colored. Most patients come into heat twice per year. Basenjis and Tibetan Mastiffs are the exception: they cycle only once per year [218, 234].

Early in diestrus, when pregnancy has been established, the patient may have a milky, odorless discharge. However, as diestrus progresses, vulvar discharge should cease [218, 234].

Unlike most other species, dogs that do not become pregnant continue through diestrus rather than abbreviating diestrus to return to proestrus and estrus [218, 234].

Postpartum discharge, colloquially referred to as lochia, is normal for approximately 3 weeks after delivery of pups. It is typically mucoid in texture and may be blood-tinged, green, or brown (Figure 14.28). It should not have an odor. If it does, or if it becomes more purulent, then metritis is possible.

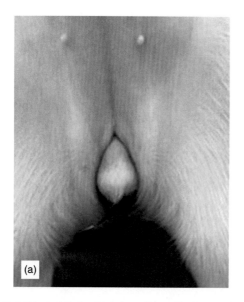 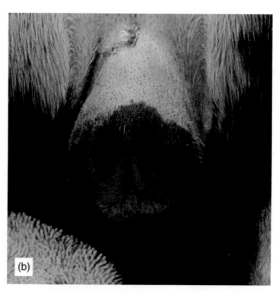

Figure 14.27 (a) Ventral abdominal view of the vulva in a patient that is in anestrus. Note that the vulva is small. (b) Ventral abdominal view of the vulva in a patient that is in estrus. The patient has been prepped for ovariohysterectomy. Note that the vulva is prominently swollen.

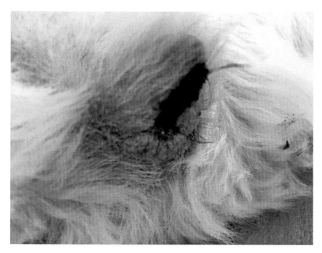

Figure 14.28 Close-up of vulva 2 days after the successful delivery of pups. Note the presence of lochia, which is normal.

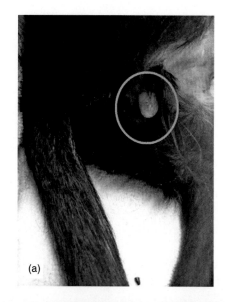

(a)

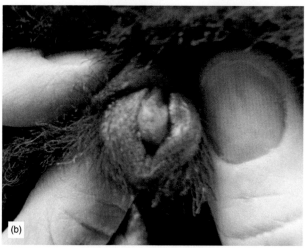

(b)

Figure 14.30 Clitoromegaly in a canine patient (a) that has been positioned in left lateral recumbency and (b) that is being viewed from behind.

In addition to evaluating the vulva for size, mucosal color, and discharge, the clinician should evaluate the vulvar conformation. Some dogs have hypoplastic, recessed, or "tucked up" vulvas (Figure 14.29). This conformation predisposes canine patients to perivulvar dermatitis and chronic and/or recurrent urinary tract infections. Some also present to the clinic for apparent urinary incontinence and/or vulvovaginitis. Clinical signs in these patients may be reduced by vulvoplasty. This cosmetic surgery is intended to reshape the vulva to make it less hidden, more open to the air, and therefore less prone to moist dermatitis, which initiates many of the problems for which patients present [235].

Other than a "tucked up" vulvar conformation, dogs may have a vulva that is misshapen and not considered normal. This can reflect an underlying intersex state, otherwise known as true hermaphrodism. These patients typically present for an apparent protruding vulvar mass that is in fact simply clitoromegaly (Figure 14.30) [151, 219, 236–238].

The internal vaginal examination of the bitch is beyond the scope of this book. Readers who are interested in vaginoscopy should consult appropriate resources in theriogenology.

14.10 Being Presented with a Female of Unknown Sexual Status

If, on initial presentation, the patient is acknowledged to be a stray and her sexual status is unknown, the clinician should ask for owner permission to shave the abdomen to look for a "spay scar." The presence of a "spay scar" increases the likelihood that the patient was spayed. The

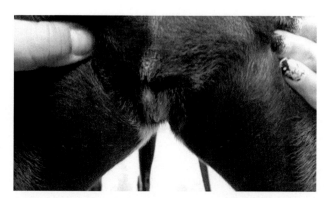

Figure 14.29 This patient's hypoplastic or recessed, "tucked up" vulvar conformation is obvious when the patient is viewed from behind.

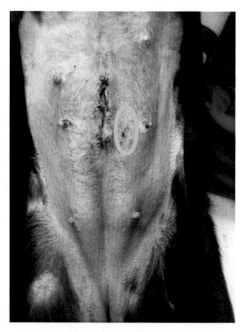

Figure 14.31 Tattoo identification along the ventrum to indicate that this patient has undergone ovariohysterectomy. The tattoo is placed at the time of surgery to signal that the patient has already been spayed.

presence of a "spay scar," however, is not a guarantee of sterilization: the patient could have been operated on at that location for something else, such as a cystotomy for urolithiasis.

The clinician should also take care to look for a tattoo that flanks the site where an ovariohysterectomy would have taken place (Figure 14.31) [239, 240].

14.11 Neonates

Puppies are born inside the amniotic sac, which the bitch bites through, in addition to the umbilical cord, to free the puppy and lick it, stimulating breathing [241].

Newborn puppies vary in birth weight depending upon the breed's anticipated size [242]:

- toy breeds: 100–400 g;
- medium breeds: 200–300 g;
- large breeds: 400–500 g;
- giant breeds: >700 g.

Because there is so much inter- and intrabreed variability, puppies should be considered as individuals with individual body weights measured on an accurate gram scale and recorded every 12–24 hours for the first 2 weeks of life. Within those 2 weeks, the birth weight of each pup should double [242].

For the first 2 weeks of life, puppies' heart rates routinely exceed 200 beats per minute, and their respiration is typically 15–35 breaths per minute [243–245]. They are not able to themoregulate reliably until they reach 4 weeks of age: their core temperature is initially 96–97 °F (35.5–36 °C) [36, 246].

Until 4 days of age, flexor tone predominates (Figure 14.32). This creates a comma shape that is characteristic of newborns. It also allows newborns to be flaccid and curled when they are scruffed by their mother [36, 246].

Eyelids do not separate and ear canals do not open until 5–14 days after birth, on average [36, 246] (Figure 14.33).

The menace and pupillary light reflexes are present by 10–21 days of age, and vision is normal by 4 weeks of age [36].

The neonate should have a strong rooting reflex and suckle response [36, 246], and the bitch should be monitored to make certain that she is allowing the puppies to nurse (Figure 14.34).

The abdomens should be enlarged post-nursing, and the puppies should be at rest (Figure 14.35). If puppies

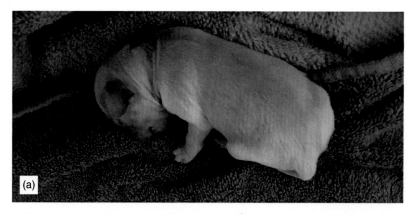
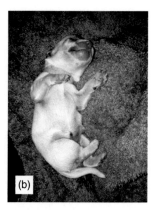

Figure 14.32 (a) Note how flexor tone predominates and the less than 1-week-old puppy tends to curl its body. (b) Note how predominant flexor tone is in this less than 1-week-old puppy. Source (a), (b): Courtesy of Nechama Bloom.

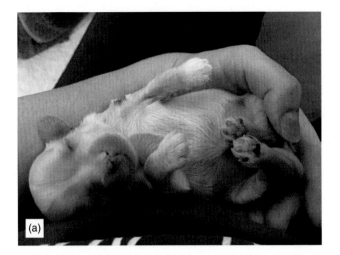

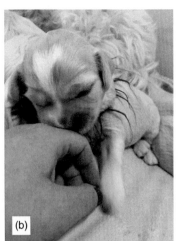

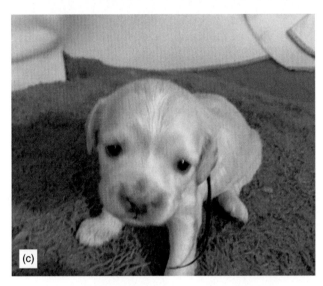

Figure 14.33 (a) Note how the upper and lower eyelids are closed in this 10-day-old puppy. The eyelids do not separate from one another until 5–14 days of age. This pup is right on schedule. (b) Note how the upper and lower eyelids are just beginning to separate in this 15-day-old puppy. (c) Note how the upper and lower eyelids are completely separated in this 18-day-old puppy. Source (a)–(c): Courtesy of Nechama Bloom.

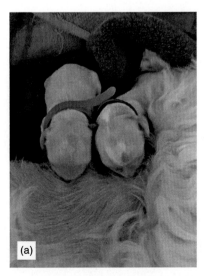

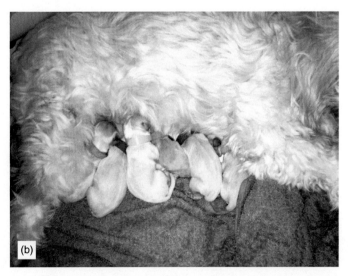

Figure 14.34 (a) Two 1-day-old puppies are nursing just hours after birth as the bitch continues to experience contractions to deliver the rest of the litter. (b) The bitch has completed delivery of the entire litter and is allowing all to nurse. Source (a), (b): Courtesy of Nechama Bloom.

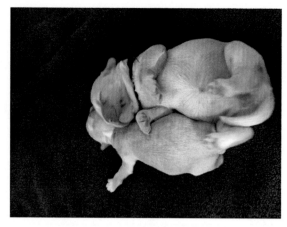

Figure 14.35 Two very content, sleeping, 7-day-old pups after nursing. Source: Courtesy of Nechama Bloom.

have swollen bellies but are restless, then further investigation is warranted to rule out impending illness.

As puppies age, their coat begins to take on its characteristic texture and appearance (Figure 14.36).

As puppies become ambulatory, their curiosity about their surroundings should peak. The puppy that is between 1 and 6 months of age should be examined at rest and at play. It should be engaged in the environment and react appropriately to environmental stimuli (Figure 14.37).

Gentle, positive handling at this age can facilitate the transformation of these puppies into well-socialized, tractable adults [242].

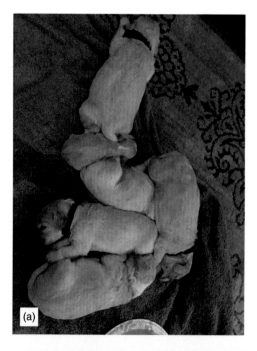

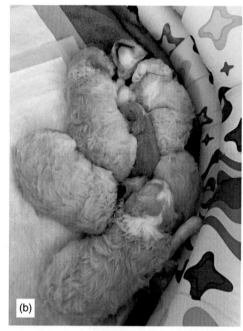

Figure 14.36 (a) 20-day-old pups with relatively straight coats. (b) By 27 days of age, the pups have developed curly coats. Source (a), (b): Courtesy of Nechama Bloom.

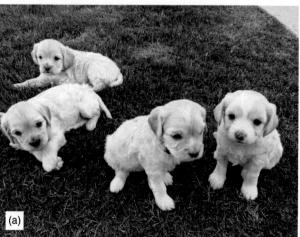

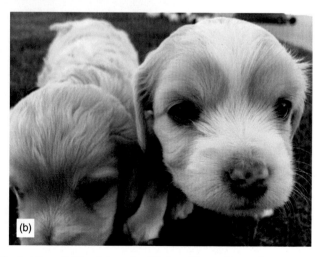

Figure 14.37 (a) 32-day-old pups exploring a grassy environment for the first time. (b) Two interactive 32-day-old pups have taken an active interest in the environment, including an interest in the photographer. Source (a), (b): Courtesy of Nechama Bloom.

References

1 Rothuizen, J., Schrauwen, E., Theyse, L.F.H., and Verhaert, L. (2009) Digestive tract, in *Medical History and Physical Examination in Companion Animals*, 2nd edn. (eds. A. Rijnberk and F.J. van Sluijs), Saunders Elsevier, St. Louis, pp. 86–100.

2 Leib, M.S. and Sartor, L.L. (2008) Esophageal foreign body obstruction caused by a dental chew treat in 31 dogs (2000–2006). *Journal of the American Veterinary Medical Association*, **232** (7), 1021–1025.

3 Michels, G.M., Jones, B.D., Huss, B.T., and Wagner-Mann, C. (1995) Endoscopic and surgical retrieval of fishhooks from the stomach and esophagus in dogs and cats: 75 cases (1977–1993). *Journal of the American Veterinary Medical Association*, **207** (9), 1194–1197.

4 Luthi, C. (1998) Esophageal foreign bodies in dogs: 51 cases (1992–1997). *European Journal of Comparative Gastroenterology*, **3**, 7–11.

5 Parker, N.R., Walter, P.A., and Gay, J. (1989) Diagnosis and surgical management of esophageal perforation. *Journal of the American Hospital Association*, **25** (5), 587–594.

6 Ryan, W.W. and Greene, R.W. (1975) The conservative management of esophageal foreign bodies and their complications: a review of 66 cases in dogs and cats. *Journal of the American Hospital Association*, **11**, 243–249.

7 Houlton, E.F., Herrtage, M.E., and Taylor, P.M. (1985) Thoracic oesophageal foreign bodies in the dog: a review of 90 cases. *Journal of Small Animal Practice*, **26**, 521–536.

8 Moore, A.H. (2001) Removal of oesophageal foreign bodies in dogs: use of the fluoroscopic method and outcome. *Journal of Small Animal Practice*, **42** (5), 227–230.

9 Spielman, B.L., Shaker, E.H., and Garvey, M.S. (1992) Esophageal foreign body in dogs – a retrospective study of 23 cases. *Journal of the American Hospital Association*, **28** (6), 570–574.

10 Sale, C.S.H. and Williams, J.M. (2006) Results of transthoracic esophagotomy retrieval of esophageal foreign body obstructions in dogs: 14 cases (2000–2004). *Journal of the American Hospital Association*, **42** (6), 450–456.

11 Pratt, C.L., Reineke, E.L., and Drobatz, K.J. (2014) Sewing needle foreign body ingestion in dogs and cats: 65 cases (2000–2012). *Journal of the American Veterinary Medical Association*, **245** (3), 302–308.

12 Rousseau, A., Prittie, J., Broussard, J.D. *et al.* (2007) Incidence and characterization of esophagitis following esophageal foreign body removal in dogs: 60 cases (1999–2003). *Journal of Veterinary Emergency and Critical Care*, **17** (2), 159–163.

13 Aronson, L.R., Brockman, D.J., and Brown, D.C. (2000) Gastrointestinal emergencies. *Veterinary Clinics of North America: Small Animal Practice*, **30** (3), 555–579, vi.

14 Thompson, H.C., Cortes, Y., Gannon, K. *et al.* (2012) Esophageal foreign bodies in dogs: 34 cases (2004–2009). *Journal of Veterinary Emergency and Critical Care*, **22** (2), 253–261.

15 Sellon, R.K. and Willard, M.D. (2003) Esophagitis and esophageal strictures. *Veterinary Clinics of North America: Small Animal Practice*, **33** (5), 945–967.

16 Washabau, R.J. (2003) Gastrointestinal motility disorders and gastrointestinal prokinetic therapy. *Veterinary Clinics of North America: Small Animal Practice*, **33** (5), 1007–1028, vi.

17 Holland, C.T., Satchell, P.M., and Farrow, B.R. (1996) Vagal esophagomotor nerve function and esophageal motor performance in dogs with congenital idiopathic megaesophagus. *American Journal of Veterinary Research*, **57** (6), 906–913.

18 Holland, C.T., Satchell, P.M., and Farrow, B.R. (2002) Selective vagal afferent dysfunction in dogs with congenital idiopathic megaoesophagus. *Autonomic Neuroscience: Basic & Clinical*, **99** (1), 18–23.

19 Gaynor, A.R., Shofer, F.S., and Washabau, R.J. (1997) Risk factors for acquired megaesophagus in dogs. *Journal of the American Veterinary Medical Association*, **211** (11), 1406–1412.

20 Shelton, G.D., Willard, M.D., Cardinet, G.H., 3rd, and Lindstrom, J. (1990) Acquired myasthenia gravis. Selective involvement of esophageal, pharyngeal, and facial muscles. *Journal of Veterinary Internal Medicine*, **4** (6), 281–284.

21 Shelton, G.D., Schule, A., and Kass, P.H. (1997) Risk factors for acquired myasthenia gravis in dogs: 1,154 cases (1991–1995). *Journal of the American Veterinary Medical Association*, **211** (11), 1428–1431.

22 Dye, T. (2003) The acute abdomen: a surgeon's approach to diagnosis and treatment. *Clinical Techniques in Small Animal Practice*, **18** (1), 53–65.

23 Saxon, W.D. (1994) The acute abdomen. *Veterinary Clinics of North America: Small Animal Practice*, **24** (6), 1207–1224.

24 Walters, P.C. (2000) Approach to the acute abdomen. *Clinical Techniques in Small Animal Practice*, **15** (2), 63–69.

25 Franks, J.N. and Howe, L.M. (2000) Evaluating and managing acute abdomen. *Veterinary Medicine*, **95** (1), 56.

26 Walters, J.M. (2003) Abdominal paracentesis and diagnostic peritoneal lavage. *Clinical Techniques in Small Animal Practice*, **18** (1), 32–38.

27 Swann, H., Hughes, D., and Drobatz, K.J. (1996) Use of abdominal fluid pH, pO2, [glucose] and [lactate] to differentiate bacterial peritonitis from nonbacterial causes of abdominal effusion in dogs and cats, in *Proceedings of the Fifth International Veterinary Emergency and Critical Care Society*, p. 884.

28 Fossum, T.W. (1997) Surgery of the abdominal cavity, in *Small Animal Surgery* (ed. T.W. Fossum), Mosby, St. Louis, pp. 179–199.

29 Crowe, D.T. (1984) Diagnostic abdominal paracentesis techniques – clinical evaluation in 129 dogs and cats. *Journal of the American Hospital Association*, **20** (2), 223–230.

30 Nyland, T.G. and Mattoon, J.S. (1995) Ultrasonography of the general abdomen, in *Veterinary Diagnostic Ultrasound* (eds. T.G. Nyland and J.S. Mattoon), Saunders, Philadelphia, pp. 43–51.

31 Smeak, D.D. (2012) Abdominal wall reconstruction and hernias, in *Veterinary Surgery: Small Animal*, 2nd edn. (eds. K.M. Tobias and S.A. Johnston), Saunders Elsevier, St. Louis, pp. 1353–1379.

32 Hermanson, J.W. and Evans, H.E. (1993) The muscular system, in *Miller's Anatomy of the Dog*, 3rd edn. (ed. H.E. Evans), Saunders Elsevier, Philadelphia, pp. 258–384.

33 Dyce, K.M., Sack, W.O., and Wensing, C.J.G. (1996) *Textbook of Veterinary Anatomy*, 2nd edn., Saunders Philadelphia.

34 Pratschke, K.M. (2014) Abdominal wall hernias and ruptures, in *Feline Soft Tissue and General Surgery* (eds. S.J. Langley-Hobbs, J.L. Demetriou, and J.F. Ladlow), Saunders Elsevier, St. Louis, pp. 269–280.

35 Read, R. (1985) Cranial abdominal hernias, in *Textbook of Small Animal Surgery* (ed. D.H. Slatter), Saunders Elsevier, Philadelphia, p. 853.

36 Hoskins, J.D. and Partington, B.P. (2001) Physical examination and diagnostic imaging procedures, in *Veterinary Pediatrics: Dogs and Cats from Birth to Six Months*, 3rd edn. (ed. J.D. Hoskins), Saunders Elsevier, Philadelphia, pp. 6–7.

37 Baker, T.W. and Davidson, A.P. (2011) Ultrasonogrpahy of the young patient, in *Small Animal Pediatrics: The First 12 Months of Life* (eds. M.E. Peterson and M.A. Kutzler), Saunders Elsevier, St. Louis, p. 197.

38 Ruble, R.P. and Hird, D.W. (1993) Congenital abnormalities in immature dogs from a pet store: 253 cases (1987–1988). *Journal of the American Veterinary Medical Association*, **202** (4), 633–636.

39 Rogers, W.A. and Ruebner, B.H. (1977) A retrospective study of probable glucocorticoid-induced hepatopathy in dogs. *Journal of the American Veterinary Medical Association*, **170** (6), 603–606.

40 Muller, P.B., Taboada, J., Hosgood, G. *et al.* (2000) Effects of long-term phenobarbital treatment on the liver in dogs. *Journal of Veterinary Internal Medicine*, **14** (2), 165–171.

41 Behrend, E.N., Kooistra, H.S., Nelson, R. *et al.* (2013) Diagnosis of spontaneous canine hyperadrenocorticism: 2012 ACVIM consensus statement (small animal). *Journal of Veterinary Internal Medicine*, **27** (6), 1292–1304.

42 Peterson, M.E., Nesbitt, G.H., and Schaer, M. (1981) Diagnosis and management of concurrent diabetes mellitus and hyperadrenocorticism in thirty dogs. *Journal of the American Veterinary Medical Association*, **178** (1), 66–69.

43 Meyer, H.P. and Rothuizen, J. (2013) The liver: history and physical examination, in *Canine and Feline Gastroenterology* (eds. R.J. Washabau and M.J. Day), Saunders Elsevier, St. Louis, pp. 856–863.

44 Walker, D., Abbondati, E., Cox, A.L. *et al.* (2016) Infectious canine hepatitis in red foxes (*Vulpes vulpes*) in wildlife rescue centres in the UK. *Veterinary Record*, **178** (17), 421.

45 Chapman, B.L., Hendrick, M.J., and Washabau, R.J. (1993) Granulomatous hepatitis in dogs: nine cases (1987–1990). *Journal of the American Veterinary Medical Association*, **203** (5), 680–684.

46 Fraga, E., Barreiro, J.D., Goicoa, A. *et al.* (2011) Abdominal ultrasonographic findings in dogs naturally infected with babesiosis. *Veterinary Radiology & Ultrasound*, **52** (3), 323–329.

47 Flatland, B., Moore, R.R., Wolf, C.M. *et al.* (2007) Liver aspirate from a Shar Pei dog. *Veterinary Clinical Pathology*, **36** (1), 105–108.

48 Loeven, K.O. (1994) Hepatic amyloidosis in two Chinese Shar Pei dogs. *Journal of the American Veterinary Medical Association*, **204** (8), 1212–1216.

49 Rifkin, J. and Miller, M.D. (2014) Copper-associated hepatitis in a Pembroke Welsh corgi. *Canadian Veterinary Journal/Revue Vétérinaire Canadienne*, **55** (6), 573–576.

50 Wouters, A.T., Casagrande, R.A., Wouters, F. *et al.* (2013) An outbreak of aflatoxin poisoning in dogs associated with aflatoxin B_1-contaminated maize products. *Journal of Veterinary Diagnostic Investigation*, **25** (2), 282–287.

51 Defarges, A. (2015) The physical examination. *Clinician's Brief*, September, 73–80.

52 Hobday, M.M., Pachtinger, G.E., Drobatz, K.J., and Syring, R.S. (2014) Linear versus non-linear gastrointestinal foreign bodies in 499 dogs: clinical presentation, management and short-term outcome. *Journal of Small Animal Practice*, **55** (11), 560–565.

53 Hayes, G. (2009) Gastrointestinal foreign bodies in dogs and cats: a retrospective study of 208 cases. *Journal of Small Animal Practice*, **50** (11), 576–583.

54 Gianella, P., Pfammatter, N.S., and Burgener, I.A. Oesophageal and gastric endoscopic foreign body removal: complications and follow-up of 102 dogs. *Journal of Small Animal Practice*, **50** (12), 649–654.

55 MacPhail, C. (2002) Gastrointestinal obstruction. *Clinical Techniques in Small Animal Practice*, **17** (4), 178–183.

56 Graham, J.P., Lord, P.F., and Harrison, J.M. (1998) Quantitative estimation of intestinal dilation as a predictor of obstruction in the dog. *Journal of Small Animal Practice*, **39** (11), 521–524.

57 Root, C.R., and Lord, P.F. (1971) Linear radiolucent gastrointestinal foreign bodies in cats and dogs – their radiographic appearance. *Veterinary Radiology & Ultrasound*, **12**, 45–52.

58 Tidwell, A.S. and Penninck, D.G. (1992) Ultrasonography of gastrointestinal foreign bodies. *Veterinary Radiology & Ultrasound*, **33** (3), 160–169.

59 Sharma, A., Thompson, M.S., Scrivani, P.V. *et al.* (2011) Comparison of radiography and ultrasonography for diagnosing small-intestinal

mechanical obstruction in vomiting dogs. *Veterinary Radiology & Ultrasound*, **52** (3), 248–255.

60 Tyrell, D. and Beck, C. (2006) Survey of the use of radiology vs. ultrasonography in the investigation of gastrointestinal foreign bodies in small animals. *Veterinary Radiology & Ultrasound*, **47**, 404–408.

61 Monnet, E. (2003) Gastric dilatation-volvulus syndrome in dogs. *Veterinary Clinics of North America: Small Animal Practice*, **33** (5), 987–1005, vi.

62 Sullivan, M. and Yool, D.A. (1998) Gastric disease in the dog and cat. *Veterinary Journal*, **156** (2), 91–106.

63 Glickman, L.T., Glickman, N.W., Perez, C.M. *et al.* (1994) Analysis of risk factors for gastric dilatation and dilatation-volvulus in dogs. *Journal of the American Veterinary Medical Association*, **204** (9), 1465–1471.

64 Schaible, R.H., Ziech, J., Glickman, N.W. *et al.* (1997) Predisposition to gastric dilatation-volvulus in relation to genetics of thoracic conformation in Irish setters. *Journal of the American Hospital Association*, **33** (5), 379–383.

65 Hosgood, G. (1994) Gastric dilatation-volvulus in dogs. *Journal of the American Veterinary Medical Association*, **204** (11), 1742–1747.

66 Glickman, L.T., Glickman, N.W., Schellenberg, D.B. *et al.* (2000) Non-dietary risk factors for gastric dilatation-volvulus in large and giant breed dogs. *Journal of the American Veterinary Medical Association*, **217** (10), 1492–1499.

67 Glickman, L.T., Glickman, N.W., Schellenberg, D.B. *et al.* (2000) Incidence of and breed-related risk factors for gastric dilatation-volvulus in dogs. *Journal of the American Veterinary Medical Association*, **216** (1), 40–45.

68 Millis, D.L., Nemzek, J., Riggs, C., and Walshaw, R. (1995) Gastric dilatation-volvulus after splenic torsion in two dogs. *Journal of the American Veterinary Medical Association*, **207** (3), 314–315.

69 Brourman, J.D., Schertel, E.R., Allen, D.A. *et al.* (1996) Factors associated with perioperative mortality in dogs with surgically managed gastric dilatation-volvulus: 137 cases (1988–1993). *Journal of the American Veterinary Medical Association*, **208** (11), 1855–1858.

70 Hall, J.A. (1989) Canine gastric dilatation-volvulus update. *Seminars in Veterinary Medicine and Surgery*, **4** (3), 188–193.

71 Wingfield, W.E., Cornelius, L.M., and Deyoung, D.W. (1974) Pathophysiology of the gastric dilation–torsion complex in the dog. *Journal of Small Animal Practice*, **15** (12), 735–739.

72 Orton, E.C. and Muir, W.W, 3rd. (1983) Hemodynamics during experimental gastric dilatation-volvulus in dogs. *American Journal of Veterinary Research*, **44** (8), 1512–1515.

73 Muir, W.W. (1982) Gastric dilatation-volvulus in the dog, with emphasis on cardiac arrhythmias. *Journal of the American Veterinary Medical Association*, **180** (7), 739–742.

74 Evans, H.E. and Christensen, G.C. (1979) *Miller's Anatomy of the Dog*, 2nd edn. Saunders, Philadelphia.

75 Bezuidenhout, A.J. (1993) The lymphatic system, in *Miller's Anatomy of the Dog*, 3rd edn. (ed. H.E. Evans), Saunders, Philadelphia, pp. 749–753.

76 Day, M.J., Lucke, V.M., and Pearson, H. (1995) A review of pathological diagnoses made from 87 canine splenic biopsies. *Journal of Small Animal Practice*, **36** (10), 426–433.

77 Eberle, N., von Babo, V., Nolte, I. *et al.* (2012) Splenic masses in dogs. Part 1. Epidemiologic, clinical characteristics as well as histopathologic diagnosis in 249 cases (2000–2011). *Tierarztliche Praxis, Ausgabe K, Kleintiere/Heimtiere*, **40** (4), 250–260 (in German).

78 Prymak, C., McKee, L.J., Goldschmidt, M.H., and Glickman, L.T. (1988) Epidemiologic, clinical, pathologic, and prognostic characteristics of splenic hemangiosarcoma and splenic hematoma in dogs – 217 cases (1985). *Journal of the American Veterinary Medical Association*, **193** (6), 706–712.

79 Wilson, D.V., Evans, A.T., Carpenter, R.E., and Mullineaux, D.R. (2004) The effect of four anesthetic protocols on splenic size in dogs. *Veterinary Anaesthesia and Analgesia*, **31** (2), 102–108.

80 Bajer, A., Mierzejewska, E.J., Rodo, A., and Welc-Faleciak, R. (2014) The risk of vector-borne infections in sled dogs associated with existing and new endemic areas in Poland. Part 2: Occurrence and control of babesiosis in a sled dog kennel during a 13-year-long period. *Veterinary Parasitology*, **202** (3–4), 234–420.

81 Cruz-Chan, J.V., Aguilar-Cetina, A.D., Villanueva-Lizama, L.E. *et al.* (2014) A canine model of experimental infection with *Leishmania (L.) mexicana. Parasites & Vectors*, **7**, 361.

82 Sofer, M., Michowitz, M., Mandelbaum, Y. *et al.* (1998) Percutaneous drainage of subcapsular splenic hematoma: an experimental model in dogs. *American Surgeon*, **64** (12), 1212–1214.

83 DeGroot, W., Giuffrida, M.A., Rubin, J. *et al.* (2016) Primary splenic torsion in dogs: 102 cases (1992–2014). *Journal of the American Veterinary Medical Association*, **248** (6), 661–668.

84 Saunders, H.M., Neath, P.J., and Brockman, D.J. (1998) B-mode and Doppler ultrasound imaging of the spleen with canine splenic torsion: a retrospective evaluation. *Veterinary Radiology & Ultrasound*, **39** (4), 349–353.

85 Neath, P.J., Brockman, D.J., and Saunders, H.M. (1997) Retrospective analysis of 19 cases of isolated torsion of the splenic pedicle in dogs. *Journal of Small Animal Practice*, **38** (9), 387–392.

86 Spangler, W.L. and Culbertson, M.R (1992). Prevalence, type, and importance of splenic diseases in dogs – 1,480 cases (1985–1989). *Journal of the American Veterinary Medical Association*, **200** (6), 829–834.

87 Cleveland, M.J. and Casale, S. (2016) Incidence of malignancy and outcomes for dogs undergoing splenectomy for incidentally detected nonruptured splenic nodules or masses: 105 cases (2009–2013). *Journal of the American Veterinary Medical Association*, **248** (11), 1267–1273.

88 Allett, B. and Hecht, S. (2016) Magnetic resonance imaging findings in the spine of six dogs diagnosed with lymphoma. *Veterinary Radiology & Ultrasound*, **57** (2), 154–161.

89 Eberhardt, F., Kohler, C., Krastel, D. *et al.* (2015) Sonographically detectable splenic disorders in dogs with malignant lymphoma. *Tierarztliche Praxis, Ausgabe K, Kleintiere/Heimtiere*, **43** (4), 215–220 (in German).

90 Evans, H.E. (1993) The digestive apparatus and abdomen, in *Miller's Anatomy of the Dog*, 3rd edn. (ed. H.E. Evans), Saunders, Philadelphia, pp. 385–461.

91 Axiak, S. and Hahn, K. (2013) Pancreas: neoplasia, in *Canine and Feline Gastroenterology* (eds. R.J. Washabau and M.J. Day), Saunders Elsevier, St. Louis, pp. 838–839.

92 Anderson, N.V. and Johnson, K.H. (1967) Pancreatic carcinoma in the dog. *Journal of the American Veterinary Medical Association*, **150** (3), 286–295.

93 Bennett, P.F., Hahn, K.A., Toal, R.L., and Legendre, A.M. (2001) Ultrasonographic and cytopathological diagnosis of exocrine pancreatic carcinoma in the dog and cat. *Journal of the American Hospital Association*, **37** (5), 466–473.

94 Brown, P.J., Mason, K.V., Merrett, D.J. *et al.* (1994) Multifocal necrotizing steatitis associated with pancreatic carcinoma in 3 dogs. *Journal of Small Animal Practice*, **35** (3), 129–132.

95 Steiner, J.M. (2003) Diagnosis of pancreatitis. *Veterinary Clinics of North America: Small Animal Practice*, **33** (5), 1181.

96 Hess, R.S., Saunders, H.M., Van Winkle, T.J. *et al.* (1998) Clinical, clinicopathologic, radiographic, and ultrasonographic abnormalities in dogs with fatal acute pancreatitis: 70 cases (1986–1995). *Journal of the American Veterinary Medical Association*, **213** (5), 665.

97 Saunders, H.M., Van Winkle, T.J., Drobatz, K. *et al.* (2002) Ultrasonographic findings in cats with clinical, gross pathologic, and histologic evidence of acute pancreatic necrosis: 20 cases (1994–2001). *Journal of the American Veterinary Medical Association*, **221** (12), 1724–1730.

98 Hall, E.J. (2013) Small intestine: diagnostic evaluation, in *Canine and Feline Gastroenterology* (eds. R.J. Washabau and M.J. Day), Saunders Elsevier, St. Louis, pp. 663–669.

99 Datz, C. (2011) Parasitic and protozoal diseases, in *Small Animal Pediatrics: The First 12 Months of Life* (eds. M.E. Peterson and M.A. Kutzler), Saunders Elsevier, St. Louis, pp. 154–160.

100 Rijnberk, A. and van Sluijs, F.S. (eds.) (2009) *Medical History and Physical Examination in Companion Animals*, 2nd edn., Saunders Elsevier, St. Louis.

101 Lappin, M.R. (2013) Small intestine: infection, in *Canine and Feline Gastroenterology* (eds. R.J. Washabau and M.J. Day), Saunders Elsevier, St. Louis, pp. 683–695.

102 German, A.J. (2013) Small intestine: inflammation, in *Canine and Feline Gastroenterology* (eds. R.J. Washabau and M.J. Day), Saunders Elsevier, St. Louis, pp. 669–678.

103 Allenspach, K., Wieland, B., Grone, A., and Gaschen, F. (2007) Chronic enteropathies in dogs: evaluation of risk factors for negative outcome. *Journal of Veterinary Internal Medicine*, **21** (4), 700–708.

104 Jergens, A.E., Moore, F.M., Haynes, J.S., and Miles, K.G. (1992) Idiopathic inflammatory bowel disease in dogs and cats: 84 cases (1987–1990). *Journal of the American Veterinary Medical Association*, **201** (10), 1603–1608.

105 German, A.J., Hall, E.J., and Day, M.J. (2003) Chronic intestinal inflammation and intestinal disease in dogs. *Journal of Veterinary Internal Medicine*, **17** (1), 8–20.

106 Jergens, A.E. (1999) Inflammatory bowel disease. Current perspectives. *Veterinary Clinics of North America: Small Animal Practice*, **29** (2), 501–521, vii.

107 Hall, E.J. and German, A.J. (2005) Diseases of the small intestine, in *Textbook of Veterinary Internal Medicine: Diseases of the Dog and Cat*, 6th edn. (eds. S.J. Ettinger and E.C. Feldman), Saunders Elsevier, St. Louis, pp. 1332–1378.

108 Craven, M., Simpson, J.W., Ridyard, A.E., and Chandler, M.L. (2004) Canine inflammatory bowel disease: retrospective analysis of diagnosis and outcome in 80 cases (1995–2002). *Journal of Small Animal Practice*, **45** (7), 336–342.

109 Littman, M.P., Dambach, D.M., Vaden, S.L., and Giger, U. (2000) Familial protein-losing enteropathy and protein-losing nephropathy in Soft Coated Wheaten Terriers: 222 cases (1983–1997). *Journal of Veterinary Internal Medicine*, **14** (1), 68–80.

110 Cave, N. (2013) Small intestine: obstruction, in *Canine and Feline Gastroenterology* (eds. R.J. Washabau and M.J. Day), Saunders Elsevier, St. Louis, pp. 699–706.

111 Boag, A.K., Coe, R.J., Martinez, T.A., and Hughes, D. (2005) Acid–base and electrolyte abnormalities in dogs with gastrointestinal foreign bodies. *Journal of Veterinary Internal Medicine*, **19** (6), 816–821.

112 Wilson, G.P. and Burt, J.K. (1974) Intussusception in the dog and cat: a review of 45 cases. *Journal of the American Veterinary Medical Association*, **164** (5), 515–518.

113 Lamb, C.R. and Mantis, P. (1998) Ultrasonographic features of intestinal intussusception in 10 dogs. *Journal of Small Animal Practice*, **39** (9), 437–441.

114 Patsikas, M.N., Jakovljevic, S., Moustardas, N. *et al.* (2003) Ultrasonographic signs of intestinal intussusception associated with acute enteritis or gastroenteritis in 19 young dogs. *Journal of the American Hospital Association*, **39** (1), 57–66.

115 Selting, K. (2007) Cancer of the gastrointestinal tract: Section G: Intestinal tumors, in *Withrow & MacEwen's Small Animal Clinical Oncology*, 4th edn. (ed. S.J. Withrow and D.M. Vail), Saunders Elsevier, St. Louis, pp. 491–503.

116 Couto, C.G., Rutgers, H.C., Sherding, R.G., and Rojko, J. (1989) Gastrointestinal lymphoma in 20 dogs. A retrospective study. *Journal of Veterinary Internal Medicine*, **3** (2), 73–78.

117 Miura, T., Maruyama, H., Sakai, M. *et al.* (2004) Endoscopic findings on alimentary lymphoma in 7 dogs. *Journal of Veterinary Medical Science*, **66** (5), 577–580.

118 Crawshaw, J., Berg, J., Sardinas, J.C. *et al.* (1998) Prognosis for dogs with nonlymphomatous, small intestinal tumors treated by surgical excision. *Journal of the American Hospital Association*, **34** (6), 451–456.

119 Paoloni, M.C., Penninck, D.G., and Moore, A.S. (2002) Ultrasonographic and clinicopathologic findings in 21 dogs with intestinal adenocarcinoma. *Veterinary Radiology & Ultrasound*, **43** (6), 562–567.

120 Birchard, S.J., Couto, C.G., and Johnson, S. (1986) Nonlymphoid intestinal neoplasia in 32 dogs and 14 cats. *Journal of the American Hospital Association*, **22** (4), 533–537.

121 Bergman, P.J. (2013) Small intestine: neoplasia, in *Canine and Feline Gastroenterology* (eds. R.J. Washabau and M.J. Day), Saunders Elsevier, St. Louis, pp. 710–714.

122 Dobson, J.M., Samuel, S., Milstein, H. *et al.* (2002) Canine neoplasia in the UK: estimates of incidence rates from a population of insured dogs. *Journal of Small Animal Practice*, **43** (6), 240–246.

123 Bastianello, S.S. (1983) A survey on neoplasia in domestic species over a 40-year period from 1935 to 1974 in the Republic of South Africa. 6. Tumours occurring in dogs. *Onderstepoort Journal of Veterinary Research*, **50** (3), 199–220.

124 Dorn, C.R., Taylor, D.O.N., Schneide, R. *et al.* (1968) Survey of animal neoplasms in Alameda and Contra Costa Counties California. 2. Cancer morbidity in dogs and cats from Alameda County. *Journal of the National Cancer Institute*, **40** (2), 307.

125 Cotchin, E. (1959) Some tumours of dogs and cats of comparative veterinary and human interest. *Veterinary Record*, **71**, 1040.

126 Cohen, M., Post, G.S., and Wright, J.C. (2003) Gastrointestinal leiomyosarcoma in 14 dogs. *Journal of Veterinary Internal Medicine*, **17** (1), 107–110.

127 Kapatkin, A.S., Mullen, H.S., Matthiesen, D.T., and Patnaik, A.K. (1992) Leiomyosarcoma in dogs: 44 cases (1983–1988). *Journal of the American Veterinary Medical Association*, **201** (7), 1077–1079.

128 Patnaik, A.K., Hurvitz, A.I., and Johnson, G.F. (1977) Canine gastrointestinal neoplasms. *Veterinary Pathology*, **14** (6), 547–555.

129 Myers, N.C. and Penninck, D.G. (1994) Ultrasonographic diagnosis of gastrointestinal smooth-muscle tumors in the dog. *Veterinary Radiology & Ultrasound*, **35** (5), 391–397.

130 Allenspach, K. (2013) Diagnosis of small intestinal disorders in dogs and cats. *Veterinary Clinics of North America: Small Animal Practice*, **43** (6), 1227–1240, v.

131 Marks, S.L. and Kather, E.J. (2003) Bacterial-associated diarrhea in the dog: a critical appraisal. *Veterinary Clinics of North America: Small Animal Practice*, **33** (5), 1029–1060.

132 Greene, C.E. (1998) Enteric bacterial infections, in *Infectious Diseases of the Dog and Cat* (ed. C.E. Greene), Saunders Elsevier, St. Louis, pp. 243–245.

133 Cave, N.J., Marks, S.L., Kass, P.H. *et al.* (2002) Evaluation of a routine diagnostic fecal panel for dogs with diarrhea. *Journal of the American Veterinary Medical Association*, **221** (1), 52–59.

134 Guilford, W.G. and Strombeck, D.R. (1996) Gastrointestinal tract infections, parasites, and toxicosis, in *Strombeck's Small Animal Gastroenterology*, 3rd edn. (eds. W.G. Guilford and S.A. Center), Saunders, Philadelphia, pp. 411–432.

135 Vail, D.M. (2007) Hematopoietic tumors: Section B: Feline lymphoma and leukemia, in *Withrow & MacEwen's Small Animal Clinical Oncology*, 4th edn. (ed. S.J. Withrow and D.M. Vail), Saunders Elsevier, St. Louis, pp. 733–752.

136 Zoran, D.L. (2013) Anorectum: infection, in *Canine and Feline Gastroenterology* (eds. R.J. Washabau and M.J. Day), Saunders Elsevier, St. Louis, pp. 784–785.

137 Harvey, C.E. (1974) Incidence and distribution of anal gland disease in the dog. *Journal of the American Hospital Association*, **10**, 573–576.

138 Hill, P.B., Lo, A., Eden, C.A. *et al.* (2006) Survey of the prevalence, diagnosis and treatment of dermatological conditions in small animals in general practice. *Veterinary Record*, **158** (16), 533–539.

139 Williams, J.M. (2005) *BSAVA Manual of Canine and Feline Gastroenterology*, 2nd edn., British Small Animal Veterinary Association; Gloucester, pp. 213–222.

140 van Duijkeren, E. (1995) Disease conditions of canine anal sacs. *Journal of Small Animal Practice*, **36** (1), 12–16.

141 Pappalardo, E., Martino, P.A., and Noli, C. (2002) Macroscopic, cytological and bacteriological evaluation of anal sac content in normal dogs and in dogs with selected dermatological diseases. *Veterinary Dermatology*, **13** (6), 315–322.

142 Lake, A.M., Scott, D.W., Miller, W.H., Jr., and Erb, H.N. (2004) Gross and cytological characteristics of normal canine anal-sac secretions. *Journal of Veterinary Medicine. A, Physiology, Pathology, Clinical Medicine*, **51** (5), 249–253.

143 Washabau, R.J. (2013) Anorectum: obstruction, in *Canine and Feline Gastroenterology* (eds. R.J. Washabau and M.J. Day), Saunders Elsevier, St. Louis, pp. 786–791.

144 Weir, E.C., Burtis, W.J., Morris, C.A. *et al.* (1988) Isolation of 16,000-dalton parathyroid hormone-like proteins from two animal tumors causing humoral hypercalcemia of malignancy. *Endocrinology*, **123** (6), 2744–2751.

145 Rosol, T.J., Nagode, L.A., Couto, C.G. *et al.* (1992) Parathyroid hormone (PTH)-related protein, PTH, and 1,25-dihydroxyvitamin D in dogs with cancer-associated hypercalcemia. *Endocrinology*, **131** (3), 1157–1164.

146 Burrows, C.F. and Ellison, G.V. (1993) Recto-anal disease, in *Textbook of Veterinary Internal Medicine: Diseases of the Dog and Cat*, 3rd edn. (eds. S.J. Ettinger and E.C. Feldman), Saunders, Philadelphia, pp. 1559–1575.

147 Matthiesen, D.T. and Marrietta, S.D. (1993) Diseases of anus and rectum, in *Textbook of Small Animal Surgery*, 2nd edn. (ed. D.H. Slatter), Saunders, Philadelphia, pp. 627–635.

148 Niebauer, G. (1993) Rectoanal disease, in *Disease Mechanisms in Small Animal Surgery* (ed. M.J. Bojrab), Lea & Febiger, Philadelphia, pp. 271–284.

149 Sjollema, B.E., Venker-van Haagen, A.J., van Sluijs, F.J. *et al.* (1993) Electromyography of the pelvic diaphragm and anal sphincter in dogs with perineal hernia. *American Journal of Veterinary Research*, **54** (1), 185–190.

150 Mann, F.A. (1993) Perineal herniation, in *Disease Mechanisms in Small Animal Surgery* (ed. M.J. Bojrab), Lea & Febiger, Philadelphia, pp. 92–97.

151 van Dongen, A.M. and L'Eplattenier, H.F. (2009) Kidneys and urinary tract, in *Medical History and Physical Examination in Companion Animals*, 2nd edn. (eds. A. Rijnberk and F.J. van Sluijs), Saunders Elsevier, St. Louis, pp. 101–107.

152 Hoey, S.E., Heder, B.L., Hetzel, S.J., and Waller, K.R. (2016) Use of computed tomography for measurement of kidneys in dogs without renal disease. *Journal of the American Veterinary Medical Association*, **248** (3), 282–287.

153 Finco, D.R., Stiles, N.S., Kneller, S.K. *et al.* (1971) Radiologic estimation of kidney size of the dog. *Journal of the American Veterinary Medical Association*, **159** (8), 995–1002.

154 Loback, M.A., Sullivan, M., and Mellor, D. (2012) Effect of breed, age, weight and gender on radiographic renal size in the dog. *Veterinary Radiology & Ultrasound*, **53**, 437–441.

155 Lee, R. and Leowijuk, C. (1982) Normal parameters in abdominal radiology of the dog and cat. *Journal of Small Animal Practice*, **23** (5), 251–269.

156 Debruyn, K., Paepe, D., Daminet, S. *et al.* (2013) Renal dimensions at ultrasonography in healthy Ragdoll cats with normal kidney morphology: correlation with age, gender and bodyweight. *Journal of Feline Medicine and Surgery*, **15** (12), 1046–1051.

157 Walter, P.A., Feeney, D.A., Johnston, G.R., and Fletcher, T.F. (1987) Feline renal ultrasonography – quantitative analyses of imaged anatomy. *American Journal of Veterinary Research*, **48** (4), 596–599.

158 Barr, F.J. (1990) Evaluation of ultrasound as a method of assessing renal size in the dog. *Journal of Small Animal Practice*, **31** (4), 174–179.

159 Jeffery, N.N., Douek, N., Guo, D.Y., and Patel, M.I. (2011) Discrepancy between radiological and pathological size of renal masses. *BMC Urology*, **11**, 2.

160 Barrera, R., Duque, J., Ruiz, P., and Zaragoza, C. (2009) Accuracy of ultrasonographic measurements of kidney dog for clinical use. *Revista Científica*, **19** (6), 576–583.

161 Barella, G., Lodi, M., Sabbadin, L.A., and Faverzani, S. (2012) A new method for ultrasonographic measurement of kidney size in healthy dogs. *Journal of Ultrasound*, **15** (3), 186–191.

162 Mareschal, A., d'Anjou, M.A., Moreau, M. *et al.* (2007) Ultrasonographic measurement of kidney-to-aorta ratio as a method of estimating renal size in dogs. *Veterinary Radiology & Ultrasound*, **48** (5), 434–438.

163 Laluha, P., Grest, P., Eichenberger, S. *et al.* (2006) Leiomyoma of a kidney in a dog: a rare diagnosis. *Schweizer Archiv für Tierheilkunde*, **148** (6), 303–307 (in German).

164 Gerber, B., Boretti, F.S., Kley, S. *et al.* (2005) Evaluation of clinical signs and causes of lower urinary tract disease in European cats. *Journal of Small Animal Practice*, **46** (12), 571–577.

165 Kruger, J.M., Osborne, C.A., Goyal, S.M. *et al.* (1991) Clinical evaluation of cats with lower urinary tract disease. *Journal of the American Veterinary Medical Association*, **199** (2), 211–216.

166 Fulkerson, C.M. and Knapp, D.W. (2015) Management of transitional cell carcinoma of the urinary bladder in dogs: a review. *Veterinary Journal*, **205** (2), 217–225.

167 Cain, D.T., Battersby, I., and Doyle, R. (2016) Response of dogs with urinary tract obstructions secondary to prostatic carcinomas to the alpha-1 antagonist prazosin. *Veterinary Record*, **178** (4), 96.

168 Bartges, J.W. and Callens, A.J. (2015) Urolithiasis. *Veterinary Clinics of North America: Small Animal Practice*, **45** (4), 747–768.

169 Burrow, R.D., Gregory, S.P., Giejda, A.A, and White, R.N. (2011) Penile amputation and scrotal urethrostomy in 18 dogs. *Veterinary Record*, **169** (25), 657.

170 Smeak, D.D. (2000) Urethrotomy and urethrostomy in the dog. *Clinical Techniques in Small Animal Practice*, **15** (1), 25–34.

171 Stiller, A.T., Lulich, J.P., and Furrow, E. (2014) Urethral plugs in dogs. *Journal of Veterinary Internal Medicine*, **28** (2), 324–330.

172 Houston, D.M., Moore, A.E., Favrin, M.G., and Hoff, B. (2003) Feline urethral plugs and bladder uroliths: a review of 5484 submissions 1998–2003. *Canadian Veterinary Journal/Revue Vétérinaire Canadienne*, **44** (12), 974–977.

173 Bartges, J.W., Kirk, C., and Lane, I.F. (2004) Update. Management of calcium oxalate uroliths in dogs and cats. *Veterinary Clinics of North America: Small Animal Practice*, **34** (4), 969–987, vii.

174 Johnston, G.R., Walter, P.A., and Feeney, D.A. (1986) Radiographic and ultrasonographic features of uroliths and other urinary-tract filling defects. *Veterinary Clinics of North America: Small Animal Practice*, **16** (2), 261–292.

175 Johnston, G.R., Feeney, D.A., and Osborne, C.A. (1979) Radiographic findings in urinary-tract infection. *Veterinary Clinics of North America: Small Animal Practice*, **9** (4), 749–774.

176 Park, R.D. and Wrigley, R.H. (2002) The urinary bladder, in *Textbook of Veterinary Diagnostic Radiology*, 4th edn. (ed. D.E. Thrall), Saunders, Philadelphia, pp. 571–592.

177 Feeney, D.A., Weichselbaum, R.C., Jessen, C.R., and Osborne, C.A. (1999) Imaging canine urocystoliths – detection and prediction of mineral content. *Veterinary Clinics of North America: Small Animal Practice*, **29** (1), 59.

178 Grauer, G.F. (2014) Ammonium urate urolithiasis. *Clinician's Brief*, December, 51–55.

179 Weichselbaum, R.C., Feeney, D.A., Jessen, C.R. *et al.* (1998) Evaluation of the morphologic characteristics and prevalence of canine urocystoliths from a regional urolith center. *American Journal of Veterinary Research*, **59** (4), 379–387.

180 Okafor, C.C., Pearl, D.L., Lefebvre, S.L. *et al.* (2013) Risk factors associated with struvite urolithiasis in dogs evaluated at general care veterinary hospitals in the United States. *Journal of the American Medical Association*, **243** (12), 1737–1745.

181 Seaman, R. and Bartges, J.W. (2001) Canine struvite urolithiasis. *Compendium: Continuing Education for Practicing Veterinarians*, **23** (5), 407.

182 Palma, D., Langston, C., Gisselman, K., and McCue, J. (2013) Canine struvite urolithiasis. *Compendium: Continuing Education for Practicing Veterinarians*, **35** (8), E1; quiz, E.

183 Osborne, C.A., Polzin, D.J., Abdullahi, S.U. *et al.* (1985) Struvite urolithiasis in animals and man: formation, detection, and dissolution. *Advances in Veterinary Science and Comparative Medicine*, **29**, 1–101.

184 Tarttelin, M.F. (1987) Feline struvite urolithiasis: factors affecting urine pH may be more important than magnesium levels in food. *Veterinary Record*, **121** (10), 227–230.

185 Rinkardt, N.E. and Houston, D.M. (2004) Dissolution of infection-induced struvite bladder stones by using a noncalculolytic diet and antibiotic therapy. *Canadian Veterinary Journal/Revue Vétérinaire Canadienne*, **45** (10), 838–840.

186 Houston, D.M., Rinkardt, N.E., and Hilton, J. (2004) Evaluation of the efficacy of a commercial diet in the dissolution of feline struvite bladder uroliths. *Veterinary Therapeutics: Research in Applied Veterinary Medicine*, **5** (3), 187–201.

187 Bartges, J. and Moyers, T. (2010) Evaluation of d,l-methionine and antimicrobial agents for dissolution of spontaneously-occurring infection-induced struvite urocystoliths in dogs, in *Proceedings of ACVIM Forum, Anaheim, CA*, p. 495.

188 Lekcharoensuk, C., Lulich, J.P., Osborne, C.A. *et al.* (2000) Patient and environmental factors associated with calcium oxalate urolithiasis in dogs. *Journal of the American Veterinary Medical Association*, **217** (4), 515–519.

189 Osborne, C.A., Lulich, J.P., Kruger, J.M. *et al.* (2009) Analysis of 451,891 canine uroliths, feline uroliths, and feline urethral plugs from 1981 to 2007: perspectives from the Minnesota Urolith Center. *Veterinary Clinics of North America: Small Animal Practice*, **39** (1), 183.

190 Osborne, C.A., Clinton, C.W., Bamman, L.K. *et al.* (1986) Prevalence of canine uroliths – Minnesota Urolith Center. *Veterinary Clinics of North America: Small Animal Practice*, **16** (1), 27–44.

191 Osborne, C.A., Lulich, J.P., Polzin, D.J. *et al.* (1999) Analysis of 77,000 canine uroliths – perspectives from the Minnesota Urolith Center. *Veterinary*

Clinics of North America: Small Animal Practice, **29** (1), 17.

192 Lulich, J.P., Osborne, C.A., and Bartges, J. (1999) Canine lower urinary tract disorders, in *Textbook of Veterinary Internal Medicine: Diseases of the Dog and Cat*, 5th edn. (eds. S.J. Ettinger and E.C. Feldman), Saunders, Philadelphia, pp. 1747–1783.

193 Bartges, J.W., Osborne, C.A., Lulich, J.P. *et al.* (1994) Prevalence of cystine and urate uroliths in bulldogs and urate uroliths in dalmatians. *Journal of the American Veterinary Medical Association*, **204** (12), 1914–1918.

194 de Gier, J. and van Sluijs, F.J. (2009) Male reproductive tract, in *Medical History and Physical Examination in Companion Animals*, 2nd edn. (eds. A. Rijnberk and F.J. van Sluijs), Saunders Elsevier, St. Louis, pp. 117–122.

195 Foster, R.A. (2012) Common lesions in the male reproductive tract of cats and dogs. *Veterinary Clinics of North America: Small Animal Practice*, **42** (3), 527–545, vii.

196 Krawiec, D.R. (1994) Canine prostatic disease. *Journal of the American Veterinary Medical Association*, **204**, 1561–1564.

197 Fan, T.M. and de Lorimier, L.-P. (2007) Tumors of the male reproductive system, in *Withrow & MacEwen's Small Animal Clinical Oncology*, 4th edn. (ed. S.J. Withrow and D.M. Vail), Saunders Elsevier, St. Louis, pp. 637–648.

198 Bell, F.W., Klausner, J.S., Hayden, D.W. *et al.* (1991) Clinical and pathologic features of prostatic adenocarcinoma in sexually intact and castrated dogs: 31 cases (1970–1987). *Journal of the American Veterinary Medical Association*, **199** (11), 1623–1630.

199 Teske, E., Naan, E.C., van Dijk, E.M. *et al.* (2002) Canine prostate carcinoma: epidemiological evidence of an increased risk in castrated dogs. *Molecular and Cellular Endocrinology*, **197** (1–2), 251–255.

200 Sorenmo, K.U., Goldschmidt, M., Shofer, F. *et al.* (2003) Immunohistochemical characterization of canine prostatic carcinoma and correlation with castration status and castration time. *Veterinary and Comparative Oncology*, **1** (1), 48–56.

201 Johnston, S.D., Root Kustritz, M.V., and Olson, P.N.S. (2001) *Canine and Feline Theriogenology*, Saunders, Philadelphia.

202 Keenan, L.R.J. (1998) The infertile male, in *Manual of Small Animal Reproduction and Neonatology* (ed. G. Simpson), British Small Animal Veterinary Association, Cheltenham, pp. 83–93.

203 Hayes, H.M., Jr. and Wilson, G.P. (1986) Hospital incidence of hypospadias in dogs in North America. *Veterinary Record*, **118** (22), 605–607.

204 Christiansen, I. (1984) *Reproduction in the Dog and Cat*, Bailliere Tindall, London.

205 Kutzler, M.A. (2011) The reproductive tract, in *Small Animal Pediatrics: The First 12 Months of Life* (eds. M.E. Peterson and M.A. Kutzler), Saunders Elsevier, St. Louis, pp. 405–417.

206 Christensen, B.W. (2012) Disorders of sexual development in dogs and cats. *Veterinary Clinics of North America: Small Animal Practice*, **42** (3), 515–526, vi.

207 Peter, A.T. (2001) The reproductive system, in *Veterinary Pediatrics: Dogs and Cats from Birth to Six Months*, 3rd edn. (ed. J.D. Hoskins), Saunders Elsevier, Philadelphia, pp. 463–75.

208 Rhoades, J.D. and Foley, C.W. (1977) Cryptorchidism and intersexuality. *Veterinary Clinics of North America: Small Animal Practice*, **7** (4), 789–794.

209 Baumans, V., Dijkstra, G., and Wensing, C.J. (1981) Testicular descent in the dog. *Anatomia, Histologia, Embryologia*, **10** (2), 97–110.

210 Meyers-Wallen, V.N. (2012) Gonadal and sex differentiation abnormalities of dogs and cats. *Sexual Development*, **6** (1–3), 46–60.

211 Yates, D., Hayes, G., Heffernan, M., and Beynon, R. (2003) Incidence of cryptorchidism in dogs and cats. *Veterinary Record*, **152** (16), 502–504.

212 Romagnoli, S.E. (1991) Canine cryptorchidism. *Veterinary Clinics of North America: Small Animal Practice*, **21** (3), 533–544.

213 Reif, J.S. and Brodey, R.S. (1969) The relationship between cryptorchidism and canine testicular neoplasia. *Journal of the American Veterinary Medical Association*, **155** (12), 2005–2010.

214 Kutzler, M.A. (2011) The reproductive tract, in *Small Animal Pediatrics: The First 12 Months of Life* (eds. M.E. Peterson and M.A. Kutzler), Saunders Elsevier, St. Louis, pp. 405–417.

215 Pearson, H., and Kelly, D.F. (1975) Testicular torsion in the dog: a review of 13 cases. *Veterinary Record*, **97** (11), 200–204.

216 Hayes, H.M., Wilson, G.P., and Pendergrass, T.W. (1985) Canine cryptorchidism and subsequent testicular neoplasia: case control study with epidemiologic update. *Teratology*, **32**, 51–56.

217 Pendergrass, T.W., and Hayes, H.M. (1975) Cryptorchidism and related defects in dogs: epidemiologic comparisons with man. *Teratology*, **12**, 51–56.

218 Schaefers-Okkens, A.C. and Kooistra, H.S. (2009) Female reproductive tract, in *Medical History and Physical Examination in Companion Animals*, 2nd edn. (eds. A. Rijnberk and F.J. van Sluijs), Saunders Elsevier, St. Louis, pp. 108–116.

219 Ortega-Pacheco, A., Gutierrez-Blanco, E., and Jimenez-Coello, M. (2012) Common lesions in the female reproductive tract of dogs and cats. *Veterinary Clinics of North America: Small Animal Practice*, **42** (3), 547–559, vii.

220 Little, S.E. (2012). Female reproduction, in *The Cat: Clinical Medicine and Management* (ed. S.E. Little), Saunders Elsevier, St. Louis, pp. 1195–1227.

221 Concannon, P., Whaley, S., Lein, D., and Wissler, R. (1983) Canine gestation length: variation related to time of mating and fertile life of sperm. *American Journal of Veterinary Research*, **44** (10), 1819–1821.

222 Smith, F.O. (2011) Prenatal care of the bitch and queen, in *Small Animal Pediatrics: The First 12 Months of Life* (eds. M.E. Peterson and M.A. Kutzler), Saunders Elsevier, St. Louis, pp. 1–10.

223 Johnston, S.D., Root Kustritz, M.V., and Olson, P.S. (2001) Disorders of the canine uterus and uterine tubes (oviducts), in *Canine and Feline Theriogenology*, 1st edn., Saunders, Philadelphia, pp. 206–224.

224 Feldman, E.C. and Nelson, R.W. (2004) Cystic endometrial hyperplasia/pyometra complex, in *Canine and Feline Endocrinology and Reproduction*, 3rd edn., Saunders, St. Louis, pp. 852–867.

225 Hardy, R.M. and Osborne, C.A. (1974) Canine pyometra: pathogenesis, physiology, diagnosis and treatment of uterine and extra-uterine lesions. *Journal of the American Hospital Association*, **10**, 245–268.

226 Dow, C. (1957) The cystic hyperplasia–pyometra complex in the bitch. *Veterinary Record*, **69**, 1409–1415.

227 Ewald, B.H. (1961) A survey of the cystic hyperplasia–pyometra complex in the bitch. *Small Animal Clinician*, **1**, 383–386.

228 Wheaton, L.G., Johnson, A.L., Parker, A.J., and Kneller, S.K. (1989) Results and complications of surgical treatment of pyometra – a review of 80 cases. *Journal of the American Hospital Association*, **25** (5), 563–568.

229 Pretzer, S.D. (2008) Clinical presentation of canine pyometra and mucometra: a review. *Theriogenology*, **70** (3), 359–363.

230 Bowen, R.A., Behrendt, M.D., Wheeler, S.L. *et al.* (1985) Efficacy and toxicity of estrogens commonly used to terminate canine pregnancy. *Journal of the American Veterinary Medical Association*, **186** (8), 783–788.

231 Sutton, D.J., Geary, M.R., and Bergman, J.G. (1997) Prevention of pregnancy in bitches following unwanted mating: a clinical trial using low dose oestradiol benzoate. *Journal of Reproduction and Fertility, Supplement*, **51**, 239–243.

232 Krook, L., Larsson, S., and Rooney, J.R. (1960) The interrelationship of diabetes mellitus, obesity, and pyometra in the dog. *American Journal of Veterinary Research*, **21**, 120–127.

233 Smith, F.O. (2006) Canine pyometra. *Theriogenology*, **66** (3), 610–612.

234 Root Kustritz, M.V. (2010) *Clinical Canine and Feline Reproduction: Evidence-Based Answers*, Wiley-Blackwell, Ames, IA.

235 Hammel, S.P., and Bjorling, D.E. (2002) Results of vulvoplasty for treatment of recessed vulva in dogs. *Journal of the American Hospital Association*, **38** (1), 79–83.

236 Groppetti, D., Genualdo, V., Bosi, G. *et al.* (2012) XX SRY-negative true hermaphrodism in two dogs: clinical, morphological, genetic and cytogenetic studies. *Sexual Development*, **6** (1–3), 135–142.

237 Wernham, B.G. and Jerram, R.M. (2006) Male pseudohermaphroditism in a Labrador Retriever, and

a review of mammalian sexual differentiation. *New Zealand Veterinary Journal*, **54** (5), 248–252.

238 Silversides, D.W., Benoit, J.M., Collard, F., and Gilson, C. (2011) Disorder of sex development (XX male, SRY negative) in a French bulldog. *Canadian Veterinary Journal/Revue Vétérinaire Canadienne*, **52** (6), 670–672.

239 Kahler, S.C. (1995) Tattoo identification eliminates possibility of initiating repeat spay/neuter surgery. *Journal of the American Veterinary Medical Association*, **207** (9), 1149, 1154.

240 Davis, F.L., Jr. (1981) Tattoo identification of spayed or neutered dogs and cats. *Journal of the American Veterinary Medical Association*, **179** (12), 1421–1422.

241 Rickard, V. (2011) Birth and the first 24 hours, in *Small Animal Pediatrics: The First 12 Months of Life* (eds. M.E. Peterson and M.A. Kutzler), Saunders Elsevier, St. Louis, pp. 11–19.

242 Hoskins, J.D. (1995) Physical examination and diagnostic imaging procedures: the physical examination, in *Veterinary Pediatrics: Dogs and Cats from Birth to Six Months*, 2nd edn. (ed. J.D. Hoskins), Saunders, Philadelphia, pp. 1–7.

243 Hoskins, J.D., and Partington, B.P. (2001) Physical examination and diagnostic imaging procedures, in *Veterinary Pediatrics: Dogs and Cats from Birth to Six Months*, 3rd edn. (ed. J.D. Hoskins), Saunders Elsevier, Philadelphia, pp. 1–21.

244 Mosier, J.E. (1978) The puppy from birth to six weeks. *Veterinary Clinics of North America: Small Animal Practice*, **8** (1), 79–100.

245 Small, E. (1980) Pediatrics, in *Current Veterinary Therapy*, vol. VII (ed. R.W. Kirk), Saunders, Philadelphia, p. 77.

246 Root Kustritz, M.V. (2011) History and physical examination of the neonate, in *Small Animal Pediatrics: The First 12 Months of Life* (eds. M.E. Peterson and M.A. Kutzler), Saunders Elsevier, St. Louis, pp. 20–27.

15

Examining the Musculoskeletal System of the Dog

15.1 Muscle Condition Score (MCS)

Obesity within the companion animal population in the United States is on the rise [1, 2], affecting up to 50% of the nation's pets [3–6] and between 22 and 40% of pets worldwide [7]. As was discussed at length in Section 10.2, obesity is a risk factor for a multitude of systemic maladies [1, 8–14] and shortens lifespan [13, 15].

The concept of body condition score (BCS) emerged as a starting point for the veterinary team to discuss weight management and lifestyle concerns with the client. Because BCS is correlated with body weight, patients with an elevated BCS could be identified as overweight or obese, and could be enrolled in a clinic weight loss program, depending upon client buy-in and compliance [16].

Currently, most veterinary practices routinely assess BCS using either a five- or nine-point scale [17, 18]. Both scales assess BCS along a sliding scale, in which the extremes reflect emaciation and morbid obesity. When used to assess patients with <45% body fat, these scales have been validated [18, 19]. Unfortunately, as the percentage of body fat in veterinary patients exceeds 45%, both the five- and nine-point scales fall short of accurately predicting body fat. This is of concern given the upward trends in pet obesity worldwide [7, 10, 20].

Another significant shortcoming in assessing BCS is that it does not allow the clinician to capture patients that have lost appreciable lean body mass. For example, it is not uncommon for geriatric patients to be both obese and sarcopenic. These patients are at risk of being underscored for BCS by the inexperienced clinician, who may erroneously factor muscle mass into the BCS even though BCS is strictly an assessment of body fat.

Underweight patients are also at risk of the veterinary team failing to identify loss of lean body mass [21]. Weight loss in lean patients may be documented as loss of body fat alone when in fact lean body mass has been reduced.

When lean body mass is lost, it may be age-related (sarcopenia) or disease-related (cachexia) [22]. In either case, it is important for the veterinary team to capture that loss: loss of lean body mass has been linked to higher morbidity and mortality in people [22–25] and also decreased survival in veterinary patients [26–28].

In order to capture lean body mass, a separate scoring system is needed: in addition to receiving a BCS, each patient should also receive a muscle mass score (MMS) or muscle condition score (MCS) [16].

As with BCS, the determination of MCS requires gross observation and palpation. In particular, thick-coated patients are most at risk of being overscored without palpation. The plushness of their coats can mask mild to moderate muscle atrophy that can only be appreciated with a hands-on approach (Figure 15.1) [16].

The easiest areas on the body on which to appreciate muscle mass and recognize muscle wasting are the bony prominences over which there are rarely fat stores to complicate a determination of muscle mass as being adequate or inadequate [16]. The prominence of the temporal bones, scapulae, transverse processes of the lumbar vertebrae, and wings of the ilia are the most common locations on the body that factor into a determination of MCS [16, 29–32] (Figure 15.2).

Based upon muscle mass assessment at these locations, dogs are ranked on a four-point scale [16, 33]. Depending upon the study consulted, clinicians may arrange their numerical scoring differently. For example, a 2012 canine study assigned a score of "0" to a patient without muscle wasting and a "3" to a patient with severe muscle wasting [34]. By contrast, a 2011 feline study assigned a score of "3" to a well-muscled, "normal" individual compared with a "0," which reflected severe muscle wasting [21].

The author prefers the latter approach and uses the following numerical scale for MCS in the dog:

- MCS of 3 equates to normal muscle mass. There is no muscle wasting.
- MCS of 2 equates to mild wasting of muscle mass.
- MCS of 1 equates to moderate wasting of muscle mass.
- MCS of 0 equates to severe wasting of muscle mass.

It is less important to adopt the author's method and more important that each practice strives for consistency so that an assessment of MCS is practical, user-friendly, and universally understood by every member of the veterinary team.

In addition to numerically providing each patient with a MCS, the clinician should note whether muscle wasting

Performing the Small Animal Physical Examination, First Edition. Ryane E. Englar.
© 2017 John Wiley & Sons, Inc. Published 2017 by John Wiley & Sons, Inc.

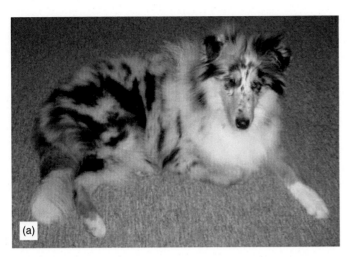
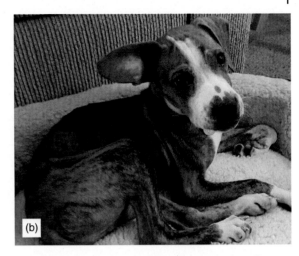

Figure 15.1 (a) MCS and BCS will be difficult to determine based upon observation of this plush-coated merle Collie. Palpation is required to be accurate in one's determination of both scores. Source: Courtesy of B. Santos. (b) MCS and BCS will be easier to determine based upon observation of this short-coated dog. However, palpation should still be employed to confirm both scores. Source: Courtesy of Analucia P. Aliaga.

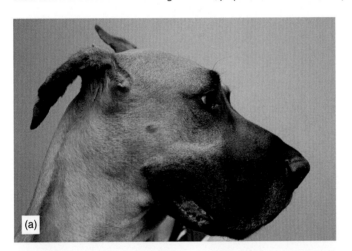
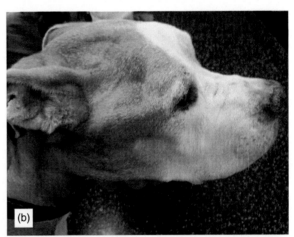

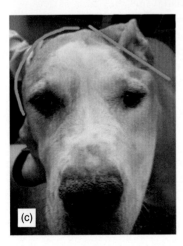
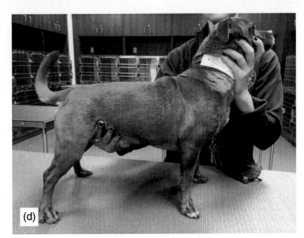
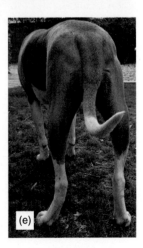

Figure 15.2 (a) The temporal musculature of this Great Dane appears to be normal based upon gross visual examination. Source: Courtesy of the Media Resources Department at Midwestern University. (b) In contrast to the patient in (a), there is marked temporal muscle atrophy of this canine patient, when viewed in profile. Source: Courtesy of Daniel Foy, MS, DVM, DACVIM, DACVECC. (c) When the same patient as in (b) is viewed from the front, the astute clinician will note the marked asymmetry of the temporal muscles on comparing the left and right sides of the cranium. Source: Courtesy of Daniel Foy, MS, DVM, DACVIM, DACVECC. (d) Appreciating normal whole-body musculature in a canine patient that is being viewed in profile. (e) Appreciating normal caudal thigh musculature in a canine patient that is being viewed from behind. Source: Courtesy of Kiefer Hazard. (Continued)

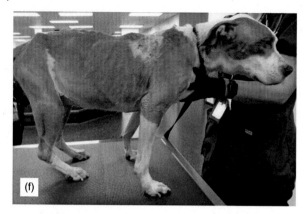

Figure 15.2 (*Continued*)
(f) Compared with the patients in (d) and (e), this patient is emaciated with both a low BCS and low MCS. Note that the temporal bones, scapulae, transverse processes of the lumbar vertebrae, and wings of the ilia are abnormally prominent owing to muscle wasting secondary to neglect.

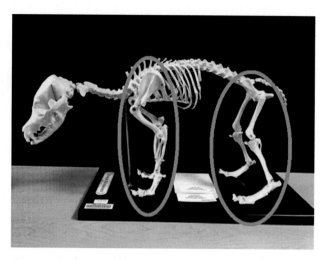

Figure 15.3 The dog skeleton when viewed in profile. The appendicular skeleton is highlighted in blue, to include both the forelimbs and hind limbs.

is focal or generalized, and symmetrical or asymmetric. These details can provide the astute clinician with clues as to the underlying cause of the wasting. For example, a dog with a prior orthopedic injury to the right hind limb may have residual focal muscle wasting of the caudal thigh from disuse; a dog with osteoarthritis of both hind limbs may have bilaterally symmetrical caudal thigh muscle atrophy due to decreased range of motion and mobility; and a dog with a prior amputation of the left forearm is likely to have focal muscle wasting of the muscles that would have been important components of the thoracic girdle.

Because loss of muscle mass is associated with adverse outcomes in human medicine, early recognition of muscle wasting is emphasized so as to allow for earlier medical interventions that may expand the patient's quantity and quality of life [16, 22, 23, 25].

15.2 The Skeleton as a Whole

Recall from Section 7.2 that there is an axial and an appendicular skeleton, and that the latter connects to the former by means of the thoracic and pelvic girdles [35] (Figure 15.3).

Both aspects of the skeleton should be assessed in each patient as part of a wellness examination. This is important in new patients to establish a baseline. However, examining the skeleton is particularly critical in new puppy visits in which the clinician may be asked to provide a health certificate or some statement to suggest that the puppy is fit for sale [35].

15.2.1 Key Components of the Axial Skeleton to Appreciate on Physical Examination

An examination of the axial skeleton should assess the cranium and facial bones.

Recall from Section 7.2.1 that there is a normal prenatal gap between the frontal and parietal bones, the fontanelle [36, 37]. This structure should close before birth or shortly thereafter [36–38]. Failure of the fontanelle to close before birth is a common occurrence in toy breeds of dogs.

When dogs present with this condition, the fontanelle is said to be open or persistent. The Chihuahua has breed-specific terminology: an open fontanelle in the Chihuahua is referred to as a molera. The molera is written into the American Kennel Club's breed standard as optional for Chihuahuas [39].

Puppies with open fontanelles may be at increased risk of sustained cerebral trauma. Puppies with open fontanelles also have a higher risk of concurrent congenital hydrocephalus [40]. It is estimated that one-third of dogs with open fontanelles have ventriculomegaly with concurrent neurological signs and one-third of dogs with open fontanelles have ventriculomegaly without concurrent neurological signs [41, 42]. Ventriculomegaly can be diagnosed via ultrasound of the brain that is performed through the open fontanelle [43–47]. Compared with the paired slit-like anechoic ventricles of a normal puppy, enlarged ventricles are wider and may actually appear to converge [46].

However, not all puppies with open fontanelles have hydrocephalus, and many are neurologically normal. Therefore, an open fontanelle is not diagnostic for hydrocephalus [41, 42, 48]. That being said, the presence or absence of an open fontanelle should be confirmed at every new puppy wellness examination.

In addition to feeling for an open fontanelle, the structure of the facial bones should be appreciated for symmetry and breed-specific traits. Recall from Section 11.1 that the brachycephalic breeds such as the English Bulldog and French Bulldog are morphologically distinct, with higher cephalic indices, shallow orbits, and shortened brain cases. This combination results in muzzles that have a "pushed in" appearance [49–52] (Figure 15.4).

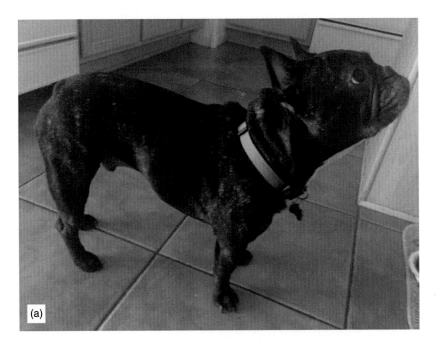
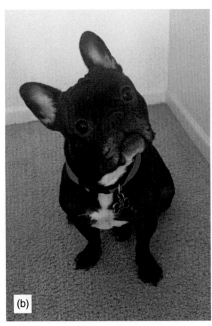

Figure 15.4 (a) Profile view and (b) head-on view of a brachycephalic dog that has the classic "pushed in" appearance to its muzzle due to distorted facial bone structure. Source (a), (b): Courtesy of Cailin McElhenny.

The experienced clinician should also note the posture and carriage of the neck. Any reluctance to move the neck in one or more locations should be noted as the details pertaining to this hesitancy may affect how the clinician prioritizes the list of differential diagnoses.

A dog is said to be exhibiting ventroflexion of the neck when the chin is tucked in nearer to the chest in a way that gives the illusion that the dog is bowing its head. Cervical ventroflexion may be a fear response: the dog hunches as if in an attempt to disappear [53]. It may also occur secondary to generalized muscle weakness as in the cat, although this occurs with less frequency in the dog [54]. In the canine patient, cervical ventroflexion is more often the result of neck guarding secondary to pain, as from cervical intervertebral disc disease (IVDD) [55–59].

On the other hand, a dog may be reluctant to ventroflex the neck in particular disease states in which such directional movement causes pain. For example, dogs with atlantoaxial subluxation, syringomyelia, or even an atlantoaxial epidural abscess may be reluctant to ventroflex at the neck and may prefer to hold their head and neck parallel to the spine [55, 56, 60–62].

A dog may also have structural, albeit rare, congenital cervical kyphosis that causes a "hunchback" or "camel hump" appearance of the neck. In this condition, the patient is not consciously holding its head and neck at a certain height; the patient is structurally built with anatomic deviation from the norm. To date, this condition has only been reported in sighthounds [63, 64].

More often, these skeletal changes are subtle and identified only through radiography. However, sometimes it is possible to appreciate kyphosis, lordosis, or scoliosis on physical examination alone. These may indicate congenital or acquired spinal deformities as from automobile trauma. They may also increase the patient's risk of developing disc compression: the abnormal architecture of the vertebral column may predispose the patient to pinching of the spinal cord with resultant neuropathy.

15.2.2 Key Components of the Appendicular Skeleton to Appreciate on Physical Examination

An examination of the appendicular skeleton should include the following characteristics in addition to palpation of the forelimbs and hind limbs:

- skeletal conformation;
- weight-bearing status;
- gait.

Skeletal conformation refers to how body parts are proportioned in relation to one another, and how the skeleton as a foundation impacts the supporting architecture of muscles and connective tissue. Skeletal conformation of the canine patient may be impacted by disorders of growth and development. For example, osteochondrodysplasia is an inherited condition of abnormal growth of the bone and cartilage. Most notably, this results in long bone deformities and apparent dwarfism. Osteochondrodysplasia has been reported in the Great Pyrenees [65], Alaskan Malamutes [66–68], Samoyeds [69, 70], Scottish Deerhounds [71], Labrador Retrievers [72], Irish Setters [73], Miniature Poodle [74], and Norwegian Elkhounds [75].

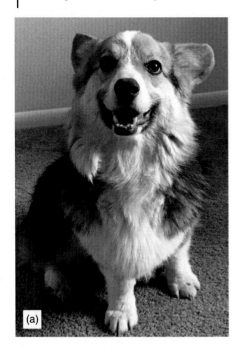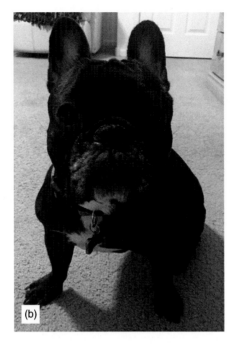

Figure 15.5 (a) Corgi with breed-specific chondrodystrophic limbs. Source: Courtesy of Cora R. Zenko. (b) French Bulldog with breed-specific chondrodystrophic limbs. Source: Courtesy of Cailin McElhenny.

One specific type of osteochondrodysplasia is achondroplasia. Achondroplasia also results in dwarfism characterized by foreshortened limbs. However, it is written into the breed standard, meaning that it is considered to be the norm in affected breeds [76, 77]. For example, breeds that are known for achondroplasia include Dachshunds and Pembroke Welsh Corgis. Sometimes these breeds are referred to as being chondrodystrophic, meaning that their cartilage is malformed (Figure 15.5).

Dwarfism may also be secondary to underlying endocrinopathies such as central hypothyroidism, which has been reported in Miniature and Giant Schnauzers. These patients tend to present with disproportionate dwarfism and macroglossia [78, 79].

In addition to whole-body conformation, individual limbs should be evaluated for skeletal deviations from the norm. Varus deformities are characterized as having a deviation in one or more limbs toward the median line, in the sagittal plane. For example, a patient that presents with carpal varus will have a limb distal to the "wrist" that angles toward the median line. In contrast, a patient with carpal valgus will have an angular limb deformity in which the limb distal to the "wrist" angles away from the median line. In the author's experience, valgus deformities are more commonly seen in dogs than carpal varus (Figure 15.6) [80–83].

Varus and valgus deformities may be a consequence of carpal laxity syndrome, a condition that is characterized by an excessively abnormal range of motion at the carpus (Figure 15.7). This condition is more typically seen in rapidly growing, medium- to large-sized breeds between the ages of 6 weeks and 7 months. Males are overrepresented, as are Doberman Pinschers and Shar Peis [80, 84, 85].

Abnormal laxity of joints is not limited to forelimbs. Dogs may also present for abnormal hind end laxity, including the following:

- Coxofemoral joint laxity [86, 87], which has been linked to canine hip dysplasia [88].
- Intertarsal laxity (Figure 15.8) [89], which may be secondary to trauma or age-related degeneration, which occurs with greater frequency in the Collie or Shetland Sheepdog breeds [90, 91].

In addition to evaluating for limb deformities, the clinician should note if the patient is weight bearing and, if so, if there are any stipulations to record. For example, a patient may be apparently weight bearing at rest but not at a walk, or at a walk but not at a trot.

In general, lameness examinations tend to be less of a challenge in dogs than in cats: it is much easier to trot a dog than a cat, especially if the clinician is able to engage the client in the process. The canine patient is also typically more willing to walk and/or trot side-by-side its owner than if only technical staff are involved. In the author's experience, the canine patient can often be tricked into a hefty gait by pointing the client in the direction of the clinic's exit, with the dog on a leash. Timid dogs that are treat motivated may be coaxed into a walk by having the owner continuously offer treats.

Owners may also be encouraged to volunteer audiovisual footage taken with their own video-recording devices to document abnormal gaits witnessed in the home environment.

If the patient is visibly lame, the clinician should attempt to answer the following questions [35, 92]:

- Is the lameness a new finding or a recurrent concern?

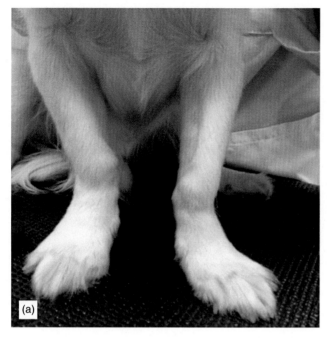

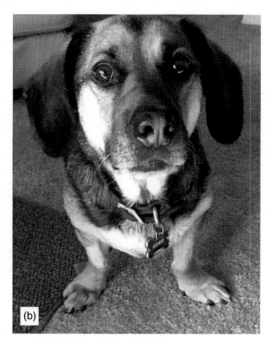

Figure 15.6 (a) Bilateral carpal valgus. (b) A second example of bilateral carpal valgus. Source: Courtesy of Jessica Herrod.

- Was there a known inciting factor that triggered the lameness?
- Is the patient partially bearing weight or not bearing any weight at all? A patient that is non-weight bearing may hold up the affected limb(s). The patient may also reproducibly lean against the examination room wall to take pressure off of the affected limb(s).
- Is the lameness persistent or does it come and go?
- Does the patient exhibit shifting leg lameness? That is, does the lameness originate in one limb only to "jump" to another during the course of the examination?
- Does the patient exhibit difficulty or discomfort when standing up or sitting down?

- Is the patient's lameness worse after inactivity or is it worse after activity, such as faster gaits or stepping up and down, on and off a curb?
- Does the lameness progressively worsen with continued movement?

Grading the lameness is helpful in outlining progression of disease [35, 93, 94]. That being said, there is not one universal, standard scoring system for lameness. The author's clinic has decided upon the following scoring system:

- Grade 1: Shifts weight off affected leg when at rest or standing, but does not exhibit lameness at a walk or a trot.
- Grade 2: Mild lameness at a trot, none at a walk.
- Grade 3: Mild to moderate lameness at a walk and a trot.

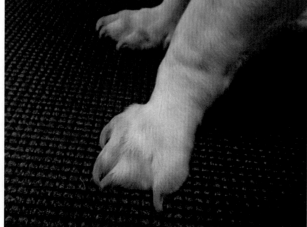

Figure 15.7 Right carpal laxity. Source: Courtesy of Elizabeth Robbins, DVM.

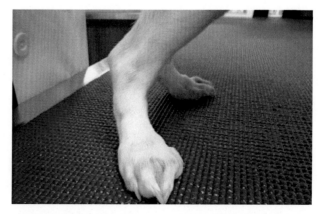

Figure 15.8 Right tarsal laxity. Source: Courtesy of Elizabeth Robbins, DVM.

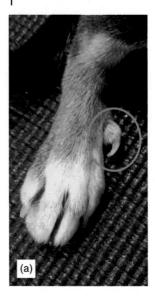 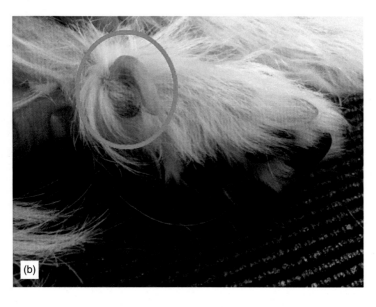

Figure 15.9 Rear dewclaw associated with (a) the right and (b) left hind paw.

- Grade 4: Carries limb when trotting, although may place leg when standing.
- Grade 5: Non-weight bearing.

It is less important to adopt the author's method and more important that each practice strives for consistency so that an assessment of lameness is practical, user-friendly, and universally understood by every member of the veterinary team.

15.2.3 Additional Components of the Skeleton to Appreciate on Physical Examination

Prior to examining the forelimbs and hind limbs in depth, the astute clinician should note the presence of any other dysostoses, congenital developmental disorders of bone. One of the more common dysostoses that is seen in canine patients is the presence of rear dewclaws: rather than having four digits on the hind paw, they have five. In other words, these patients have a first digit on their rear paw(s) in the same way they are expected to have five digits per forepaw (Figure 15.9).

Rear dewclaws are often bilateral, but are not required to be so. When they occur, rear dewclaws may be loose in their attachment or bony. Whether or not each rear dewclaw has both the first and second phalanges varies. Certain breeds are expected to have rear dewclaws based upon their breed standard. For example, double rear dewclaws are an expectation for the Great Pyrenees and Briards. Rear dewclaws are heritable [95, 96].

When rear dewclaws are present at birth and not desired – for example, rear dewclaw removal is required as per the breed standard for the Bernese Mountain Dog [97] – they should be removed between 3 and 5 days of age. This is often paired with tail docking in breeds for which elective caudectomy is indicated [96].

Rear dewclaw removal is thought to be an effective way to reduce the risk of hunting-associated trauma: working

dogs that earn their keep by racing through the brush may be at increased risk of injury to this extra dangly appendage [96].

In the event that rear dewclaws are retained, regular nail trimming is an important part of routine care for these patients. These claws are at increased risk of overgrowing, potentially to the extent that they drive into digital pads.

15.3 The Appendicular Skeleton: The Forelimb

The appendicular skeleton should be examined in every dog as part of a comprehensive physical examination. However, it is especially important that the clinician take a detail-oriented approach to the patient's extremities when its presenting complaint is limb-related.

Of the differentials that are possible for forelimb lameness, the following represent the most common broad categories [98–103] (Figure 15.10):

- Developmental, such as an angular limb deformity, osteochondrosis [104], and elbow dysplasia [105].
- Nutrition, including nutritional secondary hyperparathyroidism [106–111].
- Traumatic, such as a fracture [112] or digital paw pad laceration [113].
- Degenerative, such as osteoarthritis [105].
- Immune-mediated [114–116].
- Infectious:
  - Bacterial, such as Lyme disease [117, 118] or rickettsial diseases [119, 120].
  - Fungal, as from coccidioidomycosis, the causative agent of valley fever [121, 122].
- Primary neoplastic, such as osteosarcoma [123, 124] and digital squamous cell carcinoma [125].
- Metastatic disease, as from canine prostatic adenocarcinoma [126].

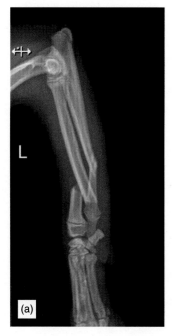 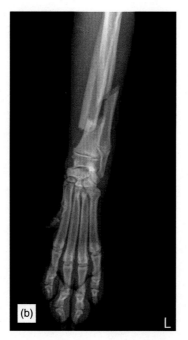 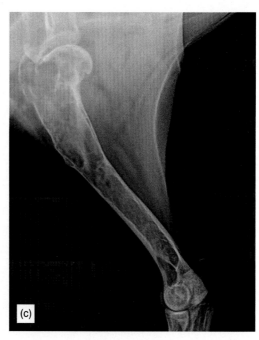

Figure 15.10 (a) Lateral radiographic view of the left antebrachium, demonstrating fractures of the radius and ulna. Source: Courtesy of Stephanie Shaver, DVM, DACVS-SA and Analucia P. Aliaga. (b) Orthogonal view of the left antebrachium depicted in (a), demonstrating fractures of the radius and ulna. Source: Courtesy of Stephanie Shaver, DVM, DACVS-SA and Analucia P. Aliaga. (c) Radiographic depiction of an aggressive bony lesion of the proximal humerus, secondary to fungal osteomyelitis.

- Palmar surface discomfort, as from interdigital cysts [127] or interdigital dermatitis.
- Other.

There are so many differential diagnoses for forelimb lameness in the dog that history and physical examination play important roles in prioritizing which diagnoses to pursue with follow-up diagnostic testing. In the author's experience, students are apt to want to leap to the diagnosis when in fact there is an important preceding step: localization of the lameness, that is, identifying the source of the lameness prior to identifying the cause.

Before the cause of the lameness can be identified, the clinician must be open to hearing what, if anything, the client has noticed at home. Subtleties in what the owner has picked up on with regard to the lameness can be exceptionally helpful, especially when a patient is adrenalized in the clinic and less likely to demonstrate the lameness [128]:

- When there is a unilateral forelimb lameness, the owner may report that the dog has a head bob when bearing weight on the painful limb.
- When there is bilateral forelimb lameness, the owner may report that the dog abbreviates its stride by taking short, choppy steps.

After taking a thorough history, the clinician may proceed to palpation, which assesses for:

- Symmetry between the forelimbs in terms of bone contour: is there continuity of bone or are there palpable (closed) or visible (open) fractures?
- Symmetry between the forelimbs in terms of muscle mass.
- Symmetry between the forelimbs in terms of joints: is there joint swelling, heat, or effusion?

There is not one "right" way to palpate the forelimbs. In what order to palpate is a matter of clinician preference. Some clinicians prefer to start distal and work their way up proximally, from the digits to the scapulae [92]; others work preferentially in reverse. The author tends to perform palpation from distal to proximal because, in her experience, dogs tend not to dislike toe touching as intensely as cats. On the rare occasion that a client points out a patient's aversion to toe touching, the author reverses the order and palpates from proximal to distal.

The order of the orthopedic examination matters less than it does that the clinician is systematic in approach and includes all of the following structures:

- The thoracic girdle, which includes the scapulae and the clavicles [129, 130].
- The humerus, which comprises the brachium or arm [129, 130].
- The radius and ulna, which compose the antebrachium or forearm [129, 130].
- The carpus or wrist [129, 130].
- The metacarpals.
- The phalanges.

Each of these regions should be palpated superficially, followed by deep palpation and any associated range of motion manipulations through joints. It is common to begin this portion of the examination with the patient standing. However, by the time that range of motion manipulations are required, it is easiest to transition the patient into lateral recumbency. If one forelimb is known to be sensitive, then the author tends to examine that forelimb last [92].

When examining the thoracic girdle, only the scapulae are palpable. The clavicles are only apparent radiographically [35, 129]. The scapulae palpate as large, flat bones of the shoulder. Their outline has been described by Evans in 1993 (p. 182) as forming "an imperfect triangle having two surfaces, three borders, and three angles" [129].

The lateral surface of each scapula is divided by the spine of the scapula, which is prominent and palpable on a dog of ideal BCS. The supraspinous fossa containing the supraspinatus muscle is dorsal to the spine of the scapula and the infraspinous fossa, containing the infraspinatus muscle, sits ventrally. These two muscles are palpable. They should be symmetrical when comparing left and right forelimbs, and both should be non-painful on manipulation [35, 129].

The acromion is the widest portion of the distal spine of the scapula. The acromion should be palpable as an important landmark from which muscles such as the deltoid originate [35, 129] (Figure 15.11).

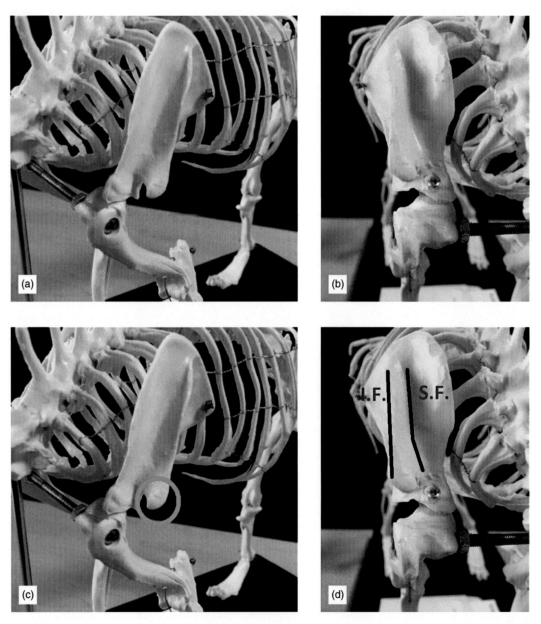

Figure 15.11 (a) Three-quarter view of the left scapula from plastic model of the dog skeleton. (b) Head-on view of the right scapula from plastic model of the dog skeleton. (c) Three-quarter view of the left scapula from plastic model of the dog skeleton, with the acromion circled in blue. (d) Head-on view of the right scapula from plastic model of the dog skeleton, with key structures identified. The spine of the scapula is outlined with black lines. The supraspinous fossa is labeled S.F. and the infraspinous fossa I.F.

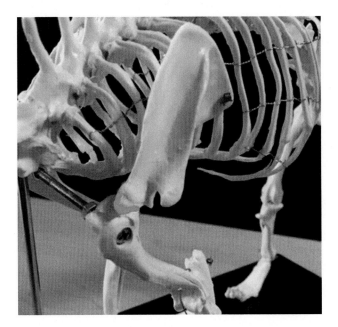

Figure 15.12 Three-quarter view of the left scapula from plastic model of the dog skeleton, with the supraglenoid tubercle outlined in blue.

Another important landmark of each scapula is the supraglenoid tubercle, from which the biceps brachii tendon originates [129] (Figure 15.12).

The shoulder joint is formed by the articulation of the scapula and the proximal humerus. The greater tubercle of the proximal humerus, which is palpable, is where the supraspinatus muscle inserts [129] (Figure 15.13).

The shoulder joint should be assessed for swelling, palpable heat that could indicate active inflammation, crepitus, pain, and tolerance of range of motion. In a German Shepherd Dog, the shoulder joint can be maintained at 47° in flexion and 159° in extension, and in a Labrador Retriever, the shoulder joint can be maintained at 57° in flexion and 165° in extension, as measured via goniometry [131].

The body of the humerus should be palpated for angular limb deformities, swelling, asymmetry between the left and right forelimb, and pain [35].

The medial and lateral epicondyles are palpable at the distal humerus [129] (Figure 15.14).

Recall that in the dog, unlike the cat, there is not a supracondylar foramen on the medial aspect of the distal humerus, through which the median nerve and brachial artery pass [132]. The distal humerus of the dog is also distinct from that of the cat because dogs, unlike cats, have an opening at the olecranon fossa. Although this structure is not palpable in the live dog, it is important to note because the radiographic appearance of the distal humerus in the dog will differ from that of the cat [132].

Distally, the radius and ulna articulate with the humerus to form the elbow joint (Figure 15.15). The elbow joint is a common site of osteoarthritis in the dog [133, 134]. Developmentally, the elbow may also become dysplastic.

Elbow dysplasia is a heritable condition that includes one or more of the following defects [135]:

- fragmented medial coronoid process (FCP);
- osteochondrosis of the humerus;
- ununited anconeal process (UAP);
- articular cartilage injury;
- incongruity of the elbow joint.

There is overlap, for example, between UAP and elbow joint incongruity, specifically when the latter is caused by a foreshortened ulna. When the ulna is abbreviated in length, the humeral condyle is strapped for space between the anconeal process and the radius. The pressure that it takes to squeeze the humeral condyle into that tight fit is directed onto the anconeal process, which can lead to UAP or even a fracture of the anconeal process [136, 137].

There is also overlap between FCP and elbow joint incongruity, specifically when the latter is caused by a foreshortened radius. When the radius is abbreviated in length, the medial aspect of the humeral condyle and the medial coronoid process are placed under increased

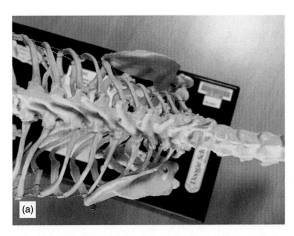
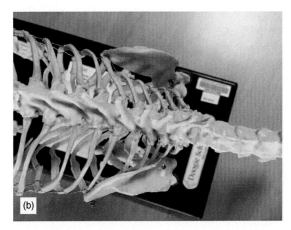

Figure 15.13 (a) Aerial view of the thoracic girdle of the dog skeleton and (b) with the greater tubercle of each humerus outlined in red.

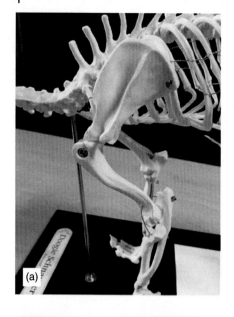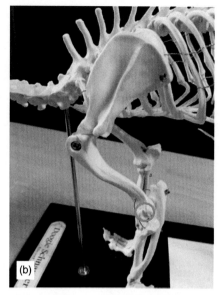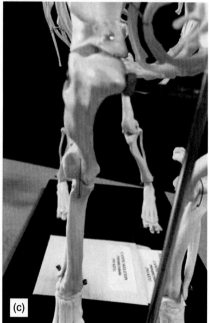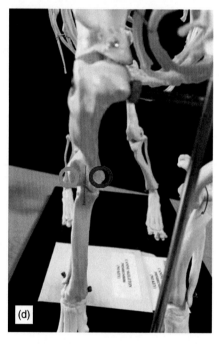

Figure 15.14 (a) Lateral view of the left humerus from plastic model of the dog skeleton and (b) with the lateral epicondyle of the humerus outlined in a blue circle. (c) Head-on view of the right humerus from plastic model of the dog skeleton and (d) with the lateral epicondyle outlined in a blue circle and the medial epicondyle in a red circle.

pressure. The pressure may be great enough to result in fracture of the coronoid process [136, 138, 139].

Labrador Retrievers are overrepresented in the United Kingdom with an incidence of 17% [140, 141]; Bernese Mountain Dogs are overrepresented in The Netherlands with an incidence of 70% [142]. Other breeds that have been reported in the medical literature worldwide include the Rottweiler, Golden Retriever, and German Shepherd Dog [138]. Different breeds may share different inheritance patterns, and each defect may be inherited independently [135, 143–146]. An early age of onset is typical for elbow dysplasia [135], which is more likely to occur in males than females [147].

Although a literature review and a discussion on the comprehensive diagnostic work-up for elbow dysplasia are beyond the scope of this text, the author considers it important that the veterinary student be aware of conditions that may affect the elbow. If elbow pain or forelimb lameness is present, it is imperative for the well-being of the patient that the clinician be cognizant of what may require subsequent evaluation and why.

The elbow should be assessed for swelling, palpable heat that could indicate active inflammation, crepitus, pain, and tolerance of range of motion. In a German Shepherd Dog, the elbow joint can be maintained at 25° in flexion and 155° in extension, and in a Labrador Retriever, the

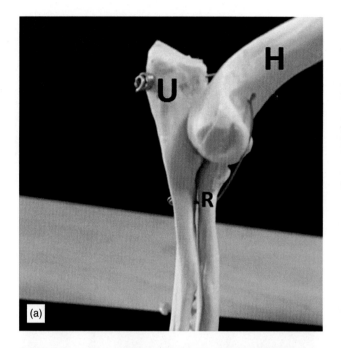

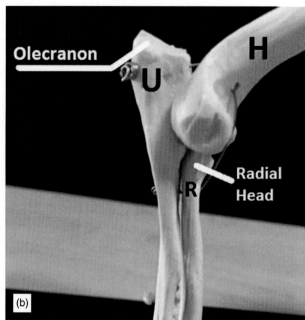

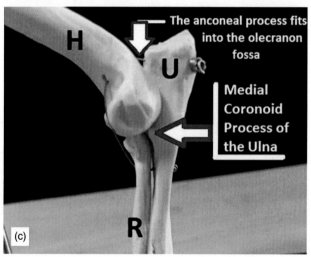

Figure 15.15 (a) Lateral aspect of the right elbow joint from plastic model of the dog skeleton and (b) with the olecranon of the ulna and the radial head indicated. (c) Medial aspect of the right elbow joint from plastic model of the dog skeleton, with the medial coronoid process of the ulna and the region of the anconeal process indicated. In each image, the key landmarks are labeled as follows: U = ulna; R = radius; H = humerus.

shoulder joint can be maintained at 36° in flexion and 165° in extension, as measured via goniometry [131].

Moving distally to the antebrachium, the radius is the primary weight bearer. It is shorter than the ulna, which serves primarily as a means of muscle attachment. Proximally, its caudal surface articulates with the ulna; distally, its lateral border articulates with the ulna. Distally, the radius also articulates with the carpus to form the radiocarpal joint [129].

On palpation of the proximal antebrachium, it is possible to appreciate the radial head laterally and the caudally-directed protrusion of the ulna, the olecranon. The olecranon plays an important role as a lever for the extensor muscles of the elbow [129].

The radius and ulna crisscross such that on palpation of the distal antebrachium, the radius is now the more medial of the two bones. The styloid process of the distal ulna is palpable laterally, where it articulates with the accessory carpal bone [129] (Figure 15.16).

The carpus includes seven bones arranged in two rows (Figure 15.17). The distal row of carpal bones articulates with five metacarpal bones. The second through fifth metacarpal bones each bear three phalanges to form the second through fifth digits; the first metacarpal bone, located medially, bears only two phalanges [129] (Figure 15.18).

Given the size of a dog's forepaw, it is very difficult to identify the individual carpal bones through palpation alone, with the exception of the accessory carpal bone. Therefore, the clinician's goal in examining the carpus is less to identify individual bones and more to identify any abnormalities such as swelling, heat, crepitus, pain, and asymmetry between the left and right forepaws.

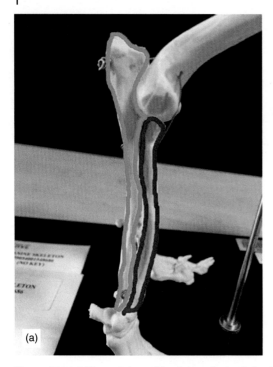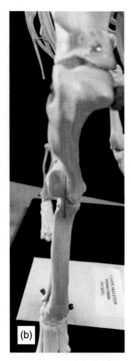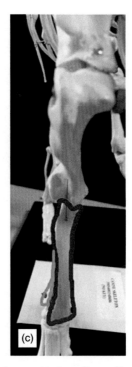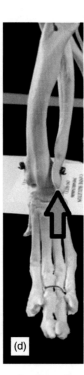

Figure 15.16 (a) Lateral view of the right radius and ulna from plastic model of the dog skeleton, with the radius outlined in red and the ulna in blue. (b) Head-on view of the right radius and ulna from plastic model of the dog skeleton and (c) with the radius outlined in red and the ulna in blue. Note how the distal radius is medial to the distal ulna. (d) Head-on view of the left radius and ulna from plastic model of the dog skeleton, with the styloid process of the distal ulna identified by the blue arrow. Again, note how the distal ulna is lateral to the distal radius.

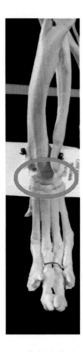

Figure 15.17 Head-on view of the left carpus from a plastic model of the dog skeleton. The left carpus is circled in blue.

The carpus should also be put through range of motion exercises. In a German Shepherd Dog, the carpus can be maintained at 34° in flexion and 198° in extension, and in a Labrador Retriever, the carpus can be maintained at 32° in flexion and 196° in extension, as measured via goniometry [131].

The individual metacarpal bones can be palpated as can the digits, taking care to manipulate them in such a way as to test for the ability to extend and retract the associated claws. However, size is a huge limitation when it comes to examination of the forepaw. Fractures of carpal and metacarpal bones and phalanges can be missed when evaluated based on the physical examination alone [92]. Radiographs provide confirmation regarding the presence or absence of fractures and should be encouraged any time pain, swelling, or lameness is localized to the distal forelimb.

15.4 The Appendicular Skeleton: The Hind Limb

As noted in Section 15.3, the appendicular skeleton should be examined in every dog as part of a comprehensive physical examination. However, it is especially important that the clinician takes a detail-oriented

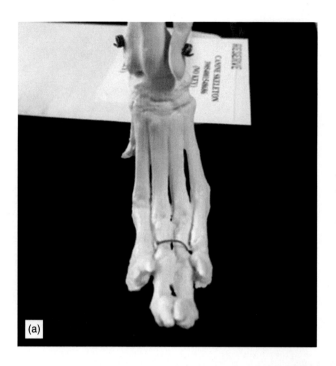
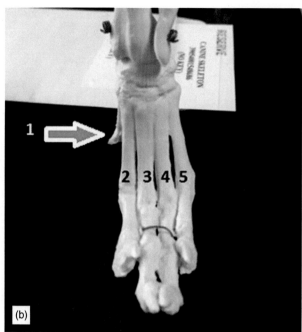
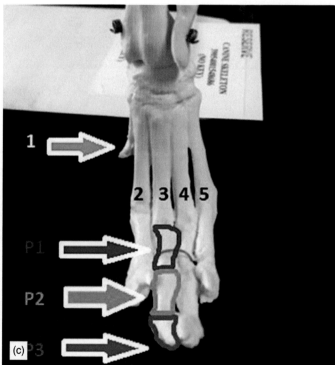
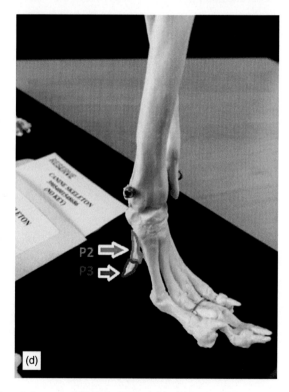

Figure 15.18 (a) Aerial view of the left forepaw from a plastic model of the dog skeleton and (b) with the metacarpal bones labeled 1–5. The most medial metacarpal bone is considered 1 and the most lateral metacarpal bone is considered 5. (c) Aerial view of the left forepaw from a plastic model of the dog skeleton with the metacarpal bones labeled 1–5 and the phalanges labeled as P1 (blue), P2 (orange), and P3 (purple). Note that P1 is the most proximal and P3 is the most distal phalanx. (d) Aerial view of the left forepaw from a plastic model of the dog skeleton, with only metacarpal 1 labeled. Note that there are only two phalanges arising distal to the first metacarpal bone: these are P2 and P3.

approach to the patient's extremities when its presenting complaint is limb-related.

Of the differentials that are possible for hind limb lameness, the following represent the most common broad categories:

- Developmental, such as hip dysplasia [148–150].
- Nutrition, including nutritional secondary hyperparathyroidism [106–111].
- Traumatic, such as a fracture [112] or digital paw pad laceration [113].
- Degenerative, such as osteoarthritis [105].
- Immune-mediated [114–116].
- Infectious:
  - Bacterial, such as Lyme disease [117, 118] or rickettsial diseases [119, 120].
  - Fungal, as from coccidioidomycosis, the causative agent of valley fever [121, 122].
- Primary neoplastic, such as osteosarcoma [123, 124] and digital squamous cell carcinoma [125].
- Metastatic disease, as from canine prostatic adenocarcinoma [126].
- Plantar surface discomfort, as from interdigital cysts [127] or interdigital dermatitis.
- Other.

Note that there is much overlap between these broad categories for hind limb lameness and those for forelimb lameness.

Before the cause of the lameness can be identified, the clinician must be open to hearing what, if anything, the client has noticed at home. Subtleties in what the owner has picked up on with regard to the lameness can be exceptionally helpful, especially when a patient is adrenalized in the clinic and less likely to demonstrate the lameness [128]:

- When there is a unilateral hind limb lameness, the owner may report that the dog has a hip hike: the hip of the affected leg elevates when bearing weight on the painful limb.
- When there is bilateral hind limb lameness, the owner may report that the dog abbreviates its stride by taking short, choppy steps.

After taking a thorough history, the clinician may proceed to palpation, which assesses for:

- Symmetry between the hind limbs in terms of bone contour: is there continuity of bone or are there palpable (closed) or visible (open) fractures?
- Symmetry between the hind limbs in terms of muscle mass.
- Symmetry between the hind limbs in terms of joints: is there joint swelling, heat, or effusion?

Just as there is not one right way to palpate the forelimbs, so there is not one right way to palpate the hind limbs. In what order to palpate is a matter of clinician preference. Some clinicians prefer to start distal and work their way up proximally, from the digits to the pelvis [92]; others work preferentially in reverse. The author tends to perform palpation from distal to proximal because, in her experience, dogs tend not to dislike toe touching as intensely as cats. On the rare occasion that a client points out a patient's aversion to toe touching, the author reverses the order and palpates from proximal to distal.

The order of the orthopedic examination matters less than it does that the clinician is systematic in approach and includes all of the following structures:

- The pelvic girdle, which includes the ilium, ischium, pubis, and acetabulum [129, 130].
- The femur, which comprises the thigh [129, 130].
- The tibia and fibula, which compose the lower leg [129, 130].
- The tarsus or ankle [129, 130].
- The metatarsals.
- The phalanges.

As with the forelimbs, each of these hind limb regions should be palpated superficially, followed by deep palpation and any associated range of motion manipulations through joints. It is common to begin this portion of the examination with the patient standing. However, by the time that range of motion manipulations are required, it is easiest to transition the patient into lateral recumbency. If one hind limb is known to be sensitive, then the author tends to examine that hind limb last [92].

When examining the pelvic girdle, the wings of the ilia and the ischiatic tuberosity are palpable [35, 129] (Figure 15.19).

Pelvic trauma is common in dogs owing to their tendency to be involved in vehicular accidents [151]. When hit-by-car injuries are sustained, dogs often fracture their pelvis. In fact, pelvic fractures represent one-fifth to one-fourth of all diagnosed fractures in the dog [152, 153].

Canine patients tend to lack the massive hemorrhage that is consistent with pelvic fractures in people and that accounts for a mortality rate of up to 50% [154, 155]. Uroabdomen is also uncommonly seen in dogs with pelvic fractures [156–161]. However, because the pelvis is a box and a fracture in one location of the box typically results in subsequent fractures of the box elsewhere, intra-abdominal damage to organs, tissues, and other vital structures such as nerves is possible [151]. For example, nerve damage that is associated with sacral fractures may result in hind limb dysfunction, urinary retention, and/or urinary and fecal incontinence; pelvic floor fractures may result in constipation or obstipation [151, 162, 163].

Ilial fractures are reported most often when it comes to pelvic trauma. Acetabular fractures also occur with

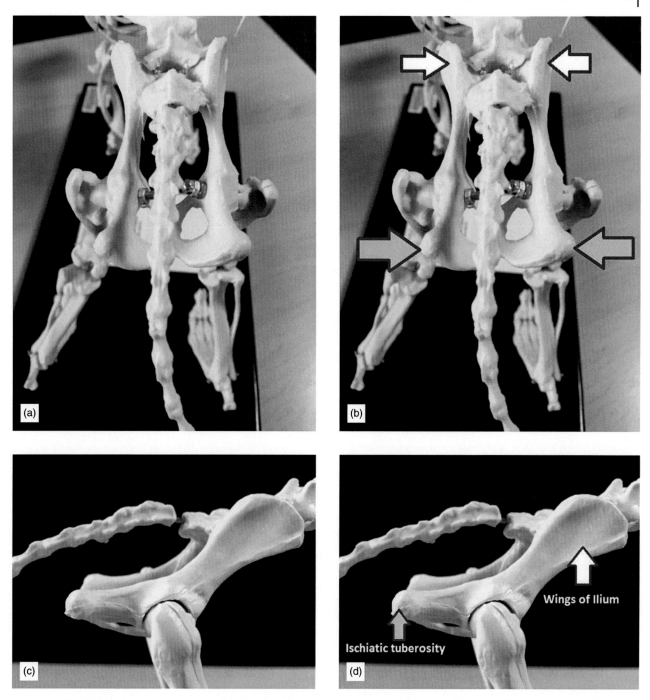

Figure 15.19 (a) End-on-view of a plastic model of a dog skeleton. The emphasis is on the pelvis. (b) As (a), with the wings of the ilia identified by white arrows and the ischiatic tuberosities by pink arrows. (c) Lateral view of a plastic model of a dog skeleton. The emphasis is on the pelvis. (d) As (c), with the wing of the right ilium identified by a white arrow and the ischiatic tuberosity by a pink arrow.

frequency; however, this location carries a more guarded prognosis because the acetabulum is a structure that is vital to the integrity of the coxofemoral joint [151, 152].

Pelvic fractures may occur with or without coxofemoral luxations. When luxation of the coxofemoral joint occurs in dogs, 90% of the time it occurs in a cranio-dorsal direction [164, 165].

Radiographs are diagnostic for coxofemoral luxation. See Figure 7.22 for an example of cranio-dorsal coxofemoral luxation in a cat. The author does not have an equivalent radiograph for a dog, but they are comparable in terms of appearance.

The astute clinician is able to diagnose cranio-dorsal coxofemoral luxation based upon abnormal physical

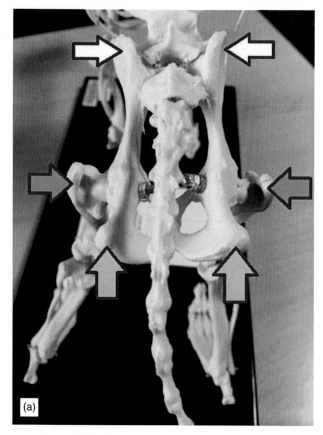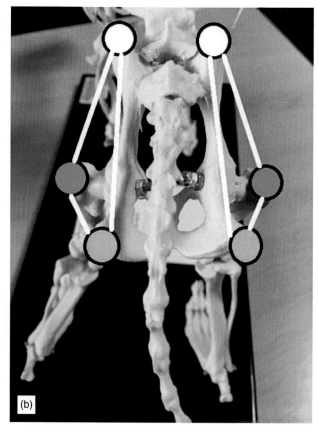

Figure 15.20 (a) End-on-view of a plastic model of a dog skeleton. The emphasis is on the pelvis. The wings of the ilia are identified by white arrows, the ischiatic tuberosities by pink arrows, and the greater trochanters by blue arrows. (b) Note the imaginary triangle that is formed by the wings of the ilia (identified by white circles), the ischiatic tuberosities (identified by pink circles), and the greater trochanters (identified by blue circles).

examination findings alone. In a normal dog, the wings of the ilia, ischiatic tuberosities, and greater trochanters should form a triangle that is symmetrical on both the left and right sides (Figure 15.20).

When there is a cranio-dorsal coxofemoral luxation, the greater trochanter on the affected side pathologically migrates in a cranio-dorsal direction, causing a disruption in this triangle. This can be appreciated on radiographic examination – see Figure 7.24 [35].

Another way to assess for cranio-dorsal coxofemoral luxation is for the clinician to place his thumb between the greater trochanter and the ischiatic tuberosity. Simultaneously, the clinician applies pressure to lift both hind limbs gently up and extend them caudally. Leg length is compared by assessing the location of the right and left calcanei. In cases involving cranio-dorsal coxofemoral luxation, the affected side will appear to have the shorter leg because the femur has been moved in a cranio-dorsal direction from its original seat within the acetabulum [35].

In addition to pelvic trauma, congenital pelvic deformities are possible. Hip dysplasia is a heritable condition of primarily large- and giant-breed dogs that is characterized by abnormal, inadequate coverage of the femoral head by the acetabulum [148, 166, 167]. Hip laxity is a significant risk factor for the develop of hip dysplasia [168], as is the breed of dog. German Shepherd Dogs and Labrador Retrievers are overrepresented; however, selective breeding in under five generations has proven effective at diminishing the percentage of affected patients in both breeds [169].

Although the prevalence is relatively low at 3.52%, the incidence of canine hip dysplasia is increasing [170]. Part of the concern surrounding canine hip dysplasia is that even though strides have been made to understand better the polygenetic nature of the disease, environmental factors that predispose the patient may be well outside the clinician's control. For example, increased birth weight and increased litter size are risk factors that cannot be controlled [170].

For other risk factors, the veterinary team may have some degree of influence, yet ultimately it is up to the client and the mutual lifestyle that is shared by the client and patient. For example, elevated body condition scoring increases the incidence of disease; however, the client may be non-compliant when it comes to weight management even if the veterinary team has attempted to intervene. Similarly, rapid growth and development may hasten the onset of disease. Yet clients may choose against purchasing breed-specific (i.e. large-breed) puppy formula that balances the calcium to phosphorus ratio in such a way as to encourage slow growth. Clients may also elect to free feed rather than meal feed, increasing the chance of obesity [171, 172], which may in turn increase the risk for hip dysplasia [170].

Patients may present for routine screening for hip dysplasia because they are intended to be breeding stock, or patients may present for routine screening because of a familial history of disease. Alternatively, patients may present for clinical lameness, apparent stiffness, and/or difficulty with stairs [170].

One or both limbs may be affected. Immature patients may present with an altered gait. Clients and students alike often make reference to a classic "bunny-hopping" gait that may bear a striking resemblance to the gait that is appreciated following cranial cruciate ligament rupture [170].

A dog of the appropriate signalment with a presenting complaint that is supportive of the diagnosis of canine hip dysplasia should be considered potentially dysplastic until proven wrong.

Any patient with hind limb lameness, particular a young, large- to giant-breed dog, should have both coxofemoral joints assessed for swelling, palpable heat, crepitus, pain, and range of motion. Although dogs are not able to extend their hips as far as cats can, they still have decent range of motion at the coxofemoral joint. In a German Shepherd Dog, the hip can be maintained at 44° in flexion and 155° in extension, and in a Labrador Retriever, the hip can be maintained at 50° in flexion and 162° in extension, as measured via goniometry [131, 132, 173].

Dogs with hip dysplasia may resent hip manipulation, particularly full hip extension and abduction, in such a way as to resist the clinician's attempts to elicit full range of motion [170, 174].

Dogs that are suspicious for hip dysplasia should be subjected to the Ortolani test, which may require sedation. The Ortolani test is a maneuver that assesses the patient for hip laxity. With the patient in dorsal or lateral recumbency, the stifle and hip are held at 90° of flexion. One hand of the clinician is held at the level of the stifle; the opposite hand is placed over the hip, taking care to have the thumb seated over the greater trochanter. Using the hand on the stifle, the clinician applies a compressive force along the femur; using the opposite hand, the clinician applies a countercompressive force over the hip. No hip laxity should be felt in a non-dysplastic, normal dog at this point; however, if there is any degree of laxity, the thumb over the greater trochanter will feel the femoral head subluxate. Next, while maintaining the compressive

force along the femur, the stifle is abducted. In a dog with a positive Ortolani test, the clinician will feel a "click" or a "pop" as the femoral head reduces back into the acetabulum, suggesting that there is inadequate coverage of the femoral head [174, 175].

A positive Ortolani sign increases suspicion that the patient has hip dysplasia. However, radiographs are diagnostic for the condition. In an attempt to reduce perceived subjectivity of scoring of hips for hip dysplasia, several standardized approaches have been developed. These include the following [176]:

- The Orthopedic Foundation for Animals (OFA) approach: a ventrodorsal view is examined with the hips in full extension [170].
- The PennHIP technique [177]: in addition to the hip-extended view, there are distraction and compression views to increase patient data. The theory is that the hip-extended views may mask subtle hip dysplasia because the joint capsule is taut when the hips are hyperextended. The additional two views provide extra details regarding how well the femoral heads are seated within the acetabulum.
- The Norberg angle [178, 179]: this modality has historically been employed more in Europe than in the United States. It involves drawing a line connecting the centers of both femoral heads and a line drawn between the craniodorsal rim and the femoral head of the same side. Where the two lines intersect, they create an angle. The greater the angle, the lower is the risk for hip laxity.

Radiographic interpretation of hip dysplasia is beyond the scope of this text; however, the author finds it important that the veterinary student be aware of hip dysplasia as a condition and recognizes that there are various ways by which a diagnosis can be confirmed.

The student clinician should also recognize that radiographic signs do not always correlate with the severity of clinical disease. Mild changes on radiographs may be present in a dog that is clinical for advanced disease. By contrast, severe changes on radiographs may be found in a dog that presents with only subtle signs of disease.

In addition to the acetabulum of the hip, recall that the proximal femur is a key component of the coxofemoral joint. The femoral head, a hemispherical projection, articulates with the acetabulum of the pelvis. Hyaline cartilage lines the articulating surface of the femoral head with the exception of the fovea capitis, a depression along the medial aspect of the proximal epiphysis. The fovea capitis is the site of attachment of the ligament of the head of the femur, which anchors the femur to the ventral acetabulum. The femoral neck supports the head and joins it to the proximal femoral epiphysis [129, 130, 180].

Recall from Section 7.4 that the proximal femur is exposed to large amounts of tensile and compressive forces during everyday activity. The leaves of the trabeculae of the proximal femur are arranged to withstand these forces. Additional reinforcement is provided by the linea transversa, a ridge extending from the base of the femoral head to the greater trochanter. Together, the trabeculae and linea transversa counteract bending forces to stabilize the trabeculae and linea transversa counteract bending forces to stabilize the proximal femur and coxofemoral joint [129, 130, 180].

The greater trochanter further stabilizes the skeleton by serving as an attachment site for the middle gluteal, deep gluteal, and piriformis muscles. These muscles initiate hip extension, abduction, and medial rotation of the pelvic limb. [129, 130, 180, 181].

The trochanteric fossa is a depression that is located medial to the greater trochanter and is the point of attachment for the internal and external obturator and gemelli muscles to achieve lateral rotation of the hip. Distal and caudomedial to the femoral neck is the lesser trochanter. Here, the iliopsoas muscle attaches to enable flexion of the hip [129, 130, 180, 181] (Figure 15.21).

The greater trochanter should be palpable on physical examination of the dog compared with the remainder of the proximal femur, which is less easily accessed.

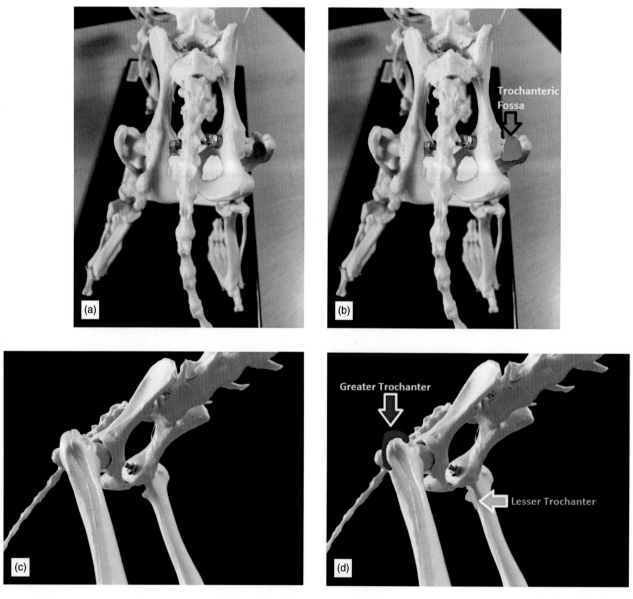

Figure 15.21 (a) Overhead view of a plastic model of a dog skeleton. The emphasis is on the femur. (b) As (a), with the trochanteric fossa outlined in orange. (c) Alternative view of the pelvis and proximal femur of a dog skeleton. (d) As (c), with the lesser trochanter outlined in pink and the greater trochanter in blue.

Proximal femoral fractures are possible in the dog: avulsion fracture of the lesser trochanter [182] and proximal femoral physeal fractures [183] have been reported. However, when femoral fractures occur in dogs, they are more likely to impact the distal growth plate [184]. Therefore, the entire length of the femur, not just the proximal femur, should be assessed in any dog, particularly one that is presenting for hind limb lameness. As with all other long bones, the body of the femur should be palpated for swelling, pain, and asymmetry between the left and right femurs.

The medial and lateral epicondyles are palpable at the distal femur [129, 130]. The femoral trochlea, located at the cranial surface of the distal femur, between the medial and lateral epicondyles of the femur, is not palpable on physical examination. However, the patella or knee cap articulates with this smooth surface [129] (Figure 15.22).

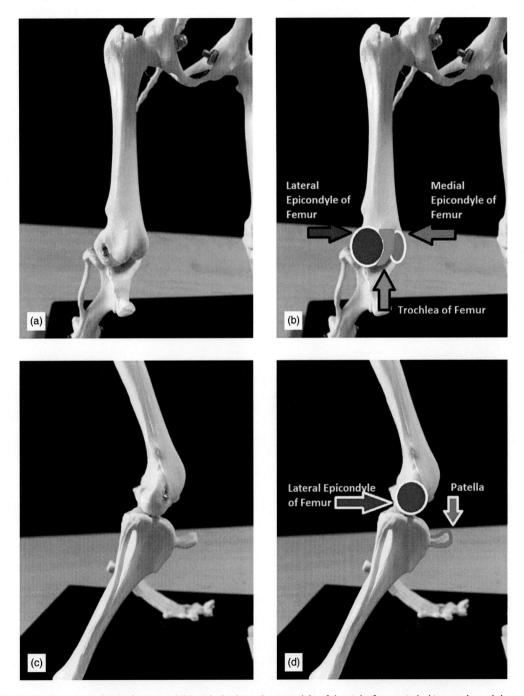

Figure 15.22 (a) Head-on view of right femur and (b) with the lateral epicondyle of the right femur circled in purple and the medial epicondyle of the right femur circled in orange. The trochlea of the femur is drawn in, in blue. (c) Lateral view of right femur and (d) with the lateral epicondyle of the right femur circled in purple and the patella outlined in orange.

The patella is palpable in dogs as an ossification within the tendon of insertion of the quadriceps femoris muscle, which extends the stifle [129]. To locate the patella, it may be easiest for the clinician first to identify the tibial crest, a prominence at the cranial aspect of the proximal tibia. Proximal to the tibial crest is the tibial tuberosity. The patellar tendon runs from the tibial tuberosity to the patella. So, by tracking the patellar tendon proximally from the tibial tuberosity, the clinician should reach the patella (Figure 15.23).

The patella's ability to luxate should be tested on physical examination. Patellar luxation is a common orthopedic malady of dogs [185–188]. Dogs are not typically born with one or both patellae luxated. More typically, during growth and development, the patella begins to shift outside its normal anatomic boundary. Rather than being seated at all times within the patellar groove, it may slip in and out of position, due in part to an abnormally shallow patellar groove. As the grade of luxation progresses, the patella spends increasingly less time in the correct position [185].

Different clinicians may reference different grading systems. The author uses the following system to capture grades of patellar luxations in the dog [189]:

- Grade 1: The patella is seated in its correct anatomic position within the patellar groove and does not typically luxate spontaneously, although it can be manually luxated. When it is manually luxated by the clinician and the clinician's pressure is released, the patella returns to its normal anatomic position. There is no impact on flexion and extension of the stifle.

- Grade 2: The patella is typically seated in its correct anatomic position within the patellar groove, but it may luxate spontaneously with flexion of the stifle joint. It may also be manually luxated. Once out of position, the patella may stay luxated until the patient extends at the stifle joint or until the clinician manually reduces the patella.

- Grade 3: The patella is typically out of position, yet can be manually replaced to its normal anatomic location when the patient extends at the stifle.

- Grade 4: The patella is always out of position and cannot be reduced: there is no ability to manually replace it within the patellar groove.

Over time, patellar luxation destabilizes the stifle joint by eroding the joint surfaces. This may incite joint-associated pain with resultant lameness and the development of osteoarthritis [185, 190].

Patellar luxation may be medial (MPL) or lateral (LPL), unilateral or bilateral [188, 189, 191–193]. A large-scale epidemiological study in England that reviewed the electronic medical records of 210,824 dogs spanning 119 primary-care clinics found the prevalence to be 1.30% [185].

MPLs occur most commonly in toy and small-breed dogs [188, 194]. Pomeranians, Yorkshire Terriers, and Chihuahuas are overrepresented [185, 195]. However, large and giant breeds with MPL have also been reported [191, 192]. Patients with MPL often have concurrent anatomic anomalies. In addition to having a shallower than normal patellar groove, they may have medial displacement of the quadriceps muscle group.

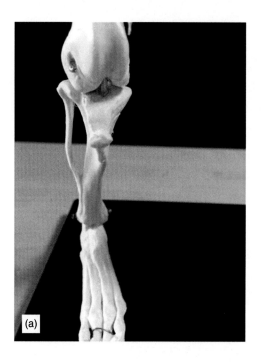 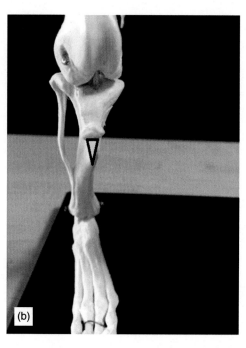

Figure 15.23 (a) Head-on view of the canine hind limb with emphasis on the cranial aspect of the tibia and (b) with the tibial crest outlined as a blue triangle.

As a result, the medial aspect of the distal femoral physis is put under enough pressure to retard growth. At the same time, there is no simultaneous pressure on the lateral aspect of the distal femoral physis such that growth continues normally at this location. The net result is that the distal femur becomes bowed laterally. In mild cases, this may only be apparent on radiographic examination, however, in moderate to severe cases, it is grossly visible [189].

When LPLs occur, they are more commonly seen in large and giant breeds [189]. However, MPLs occur with greater frequency than LPLs in large- and giant-breed dogs: in a retrospective study evaluating 124 cases of patellar luxation in dogs, 83% of large-breed dogs had a diagnosed MPL compared with 17% with LPL [192]. Toy and small breeds with LPL have also been reported, albeit rarely: in the aforementioned study, only 2% of small-breed dogs were diagnosed with LPL compared with 98% with MPL [192].

LPL is thought to be due to abnormal, excessive rotation externally of the proximal femur. The resultant shift in the pull of the quadriceps muscle group laterally forces the patella lateral to the patellar groove [189].

In addition to localizing the patella and identifying whether or not patellar luxation is present, the stifle joint should be assessed for swelling, palpable heat that could indicate active inflammation, crepitus, pain, and tolerance of range of motion. In a German Shepherd Dog, the stifle joint can be maintained at 33° in flexion and 153° in extension, and in a Labrador Retriever, the stifle joint can be maintained at 42° in flexion and 162° in extension, as measured via goniometry [131].

See Section 7.4 to review the anatomy of the stifle joint, in particular the medial and lateral collateral ligaments and the cranial and caudal cruciate ligaments [196]. In particular, cranial cruciate ligament disease (CCLD), otherwise referred to as rupture of the cranial cruciate ligament (CCLR), is a common source of hind limb lameness in the dog [197–199]. CCLR is thought to result from progressive degeneration of the CCL, although acute rupture of the CCL may occur secondary to trauma [198].

Large-breed dogs are overrepresented in the medical literature, in particular the Newfoundland, Rottweiler, Labrador Retriever, Staffordshire Bull Terrier, and Boxer. Also overrepresented are the West Highland White Terrier and the Yorkshire Terrier. The Cocker Spaniel appears to be a "safer" breed, that is, the breed's risk of developing CCLR is lower [185, 197, 200–202].

Unilateral or bilateral CCLR is possible. When CCLR occurs in a breed that is predisposed, bilateral occurrence is more typical, with the second pelvic limb succumbing to CCLD within 1 year of the first [201].

A large-scale epidemiological study in England that reviewed the electronic medical records of 171,522 dogs spanning 97 primary-care clinics found the prevalence to be 0.56%. Overweight dogs and spayed females may be at increased risk [197, 198, 203–205], and dogs belonging to a breed that is predisposed are at risk of developing CCLR at a younger age [206].

Over time, CCLR destabilizes the stifle joint by eroding the joint surfaces. This may incite joint-associated pain with resultant lameness and the development of osteoarthritis. Meniscal damage is common. In particular, the medial meniscus tends to become frayed [207]. In addition, the proximal patella, patellar groove, and mediodorsal tibia tend to develop osteophytes that can be appreciated on radiographic examination of the stifle [207, 208].

Canine patients may present for acute lameness, as occurs from an acute CCLR, or a prolonged history of intermittent lameness, as occurs from either a partial tear or chronic injury to the CCL. Patients with acute CCLR tend to be non- or minimally weight bearing, as evident by toe touching in the examination room. Patients with chronic CCL injury may have increased difficulty changing position from standing to being seated and vice versa. They may tuck the affected leg out to the side. They may become exercise intolerant with lameness that worsens after activity, and their lameness may be accentuated when ambulating after long periods of rest. Owners may report and clinicians may observe a classic "bunny-hopping" gait [207].

On physical examination, patients with CCLR may present with stifle effusion and overt aversion to stifle manipulation by the attending clinician. Sedation may be required to eliminate tension in the patient's muscles that may challenge the clinician's ability to assess the stifle and put it through range of motion effectively. When the stifle is flexed and extended, there may or may not be a "click." When present, this "click" has historically been considered indicative of meniscal tearing. However, this is an inconsistent finding at best [132, 207, 209].

When cranial cruciate ligament injury is suspected, it can be confirmed by the cranial drawer or tibial thrust tests [132, 207, 210, 211]. The cranial drawer test is performed with the patient in lateral recumbency. If the patient's right stifle is suspected of cranial cruciate ligament injury, then the patient should be placed gently in left lateral recumbency so that the right hind limb is available for manipulation. In this example, the tip of the clinician's left index finger will be placed over the patella and his thumb will be placed over the femoral fabella. This serves to anchor the femur. The clinician then lays his right index finger over the tibial crest and plants his right thumb behind the head of the fibula. This stabilizes the proximal tibia. Holding the femur

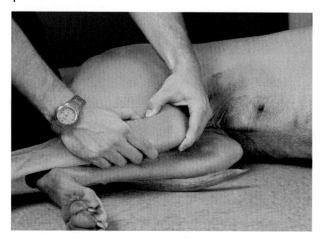

Figure 15.24 Testing for cranial drawer in this canine patient's right stifle. Source: Courtesy of the Media Resources Department at Midwestern University.

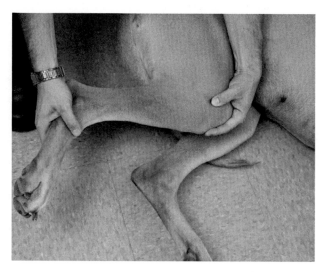

Figure 15.25 Testing for tibial thrust in this canine patient's right stifle. Source: Courtesy of the Media Resources Department at Midwestern University.

steady, the clinician then applies cranially directed force to the tibia with his right hand to attempt cranial translocation of the tibia. If this occurs, then the stifle has been pathologically hyperextended. The patient is said to be positive for cranial drawer, which confirms injury to the cranial cruciate ligament [35, 196, 207] (Figure 15.24).

The tibial thrust test is also typically performed with the patient in lateral recumbency. The premise of this test is that when the tarsus is flexed while the stifle is extended, an intact cranial cruciate ligament should prevent hyperextension of the stifle. As before, if the patient's right stifle is suspected of cranial cruciate ligament injury, then the patient should be placed gently in left lateral recumbency so that the right hind limb is available for manipulation. The clinician gently lays his left index finger over the patient's patella and tibial crest. He uses the placement of this forefinger to sense for abnormal cranial movement of the tibia as his right hand grasps the right metatarsal region and directs the tarsus into flexion. If cranial cruciate ligament injury is present, then forward motion of the tibia will be appreciated [35, 207, 211] (Figure 15.25).

The clinician should also assess for the stability of the medial and lateral collateral ligaments. To assess for medial collateral ligament stability, the patient is again placed in lateral recumbency with the limb of interest up and available for manipulation. The limb of interest is held in extension. The clinician grasps the limb's distal femur in one hand and the proximal tibia in the other. With the hand that is on the proximal tibia, the clinician attempts to abduct the tibia relative to the femur. If the medial collateral ligament is intact, the clinician should not feel displacement of the tibia [35, 212, 213].

To assess for lateral collateral ligament stability, the patient remains in lateral recumbency, with the "up" limb held in extension. The clinician grasps the limb's distal femur in one hand and the proximal tibia in the other. With the hand that is on the proximal tibia, the clinician attempts to adduct the tibia relative to the femur. If the lateral collateral ligament is intact, the clinician should not feel the lateral joint space open up [35, 212, 213].

In addition to the stifle, the clinician should consider the crus and recall from Section 7.4 that this region of the body consists of the more cranially positioned tibia and the narrow fibula. The tibia bears the bulk of the weight for the crus; the function of the laterally located fibula is to serve as a site for muscle attachment [129]. The proximal tibia is flat to allow for articulation with the femur. The medial and lateral tibial condyles are separated from the medial and lateral femoral condyles only by the medial and lateral menisci, which are incomplete, biconcave discs [129].

Between the tibial condyles and caudally located is the popliteal notch. Recall that this is an attachment site for the caudal cruciate ligament [196, 214].

Distally, the tibia ends as the medial malleolus. Caudal to the medial malleolus are distinct notches and sulci that provide attachment sites for tarsal flexors [129].

Proximally, the head of the fibula articulates with the caudolateral aspect of the lateral tibial condyle. Distally, it ends as the lateral malleolus. Along the medial aspect of the lateral malleolus there is an articulating surface that allows for the intimate connection involving the trochlea of the tibial tarsal bone or talus [129].

Although the tarsus is like the carpus in that they both consist of seven bones, there are two key differences.

Figure 15.26 (a) Profile view of the right crus and tarsus and (b) with emphasis on the tuber calcanei, which is circled in blue.

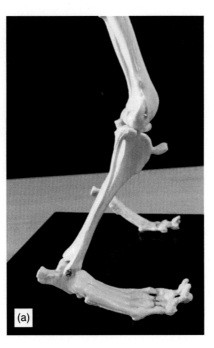
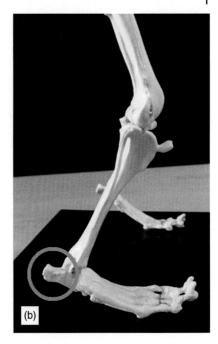

First, both the tibia and fibula articulate only with the tibial tarsal bone, whereas the radius and ulna have a broader connection to the carpus. Second, the tarsus is three times longer than the carpus. Third, the tarsus contains an extremely varied set of tarsal bones based upon size and shape. The largest, longest bone of the tarsus is the calcaneus. Proximally, the calcaneus forms a prominent level, the tuber calcanei, upon which the calcanean tendon inserts (Figure 15.26). Distally, it forms a stable joint with the tibial tarsal bone [129].

The distal row of tarsal bones articulates with four metatarsal bones that are identified as being the second through fifth. The second metatarsal bone is the most medially located [129]. Each metatarsal bone bears three phalanges to form the second through fifth digits [129] (15.27).

Given the size of a dog's hind paw, it is very difficult to identify the individual tarsal bones through palpation alone, with the exception of the calcaneus. Therefore, the clinician's goal in examining the tarsus is less to identify individual bones and more to identify any abnormalities such as swelling, heat, crepitus, asymmetry between the left and right forepaw, and pain.

The clinician should also assess tarsal range of motion. In a German Shepherd Dog, the tarsal joint can be maintained at 30° in flexion and 149° in extension, and in a Labrador Retriever, the tarsal joint can be maintained at 39° in flexion and 164° in extension, as measured via goniometry [131].

In addition, the clinician should assess the stability of the medial and lateral tarsal collateral ligaments,

each of which is composed of two bands, a short and a long. To assess for instability of each band, the tarsus should be tested for displacement in flexion (damage to the short band will result in instability) and also in extension (damage to the long band will result in instability).

The individual metatarsal bones can be palpated as can the digits. However, as was the case in the cat, size remains a limitation when it comes to the examination of the hind paw. Fractures of tarsal and metatarsal bones and phalanges can easily be missed when evaluated based on the physical examination alone [92]. Radiographs should be prioritized any time pain, swelling, or lameness is localized to the distal hind limb.

In general, the orthopedic examination is less challenging in the dog than in the cat because overall canine patients tend to be more tractable when it comes to limb manipulation and gait analysis. Yet many of the orthopedic manipulations may seem unnatural to the student clinician who is performing them for the very first time. Students should consider practicing orthopedic maneuvers on any anesthetized patient just as was advised for honing in on abdominal palpation skills. The anesthetized patient lacks tension and therefore it will be easier for the inexperienced clinician to develop confidence that what they are feeling is in fact truly present. The more student clinicians practice, the more likely they will pick up on subtle changes that can facilitate diagnostic, medical, and/or surgical management.

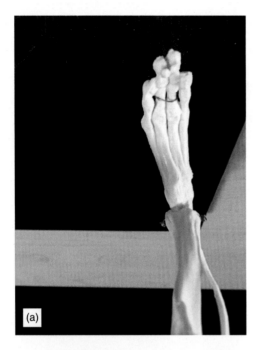

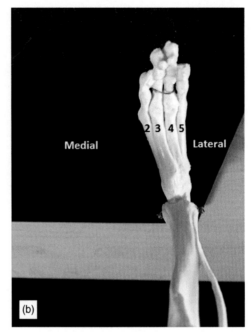

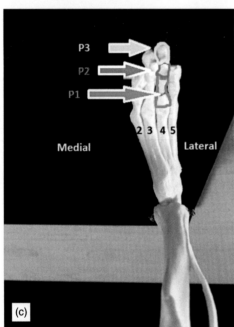

Figure 15.27 (a) Skeletal model of the right distal hind limb of the dog, (b) with the metatarsal bones labeled 2–5 (the most medial metacarpal bone is considered 2 and the most lateral metacarpal bone is considered 5), and (c) with the metatarsal bones labeled 2–5 and the phalanges labeled P1, P2, and P3, where P1 is the most proximal and P3 is the most distal phalanx.

References

1 German, A.J. (2006) The growing problem of obesity in dogs and cats. *Journal of Nutrition*, **136** (7 Suppl.), 1940S–1946S.

2 Churchill, J. and Ward, E. (2016) Communicating with pet owners about obesity: roles of the veterinary health care team. *Veterinary Clinics of North America: Small Animal Practice*, **46** (5), 899–911.

3 Brooks, D., Churchill, J., Fein, K. *et al.* (2014) 2014 AAHA weight management guidelines for dogs and cats. *Journal of the American Animal Hospital Association*, **50** (1), 1–11.

4 Colliard, L., Paragon, B.M., Lemuet, B. *et al.* (2009) Prevalence and risk factors of obesity in an urban population of healthy cats. *Journal of Feline Medicine and Surgery*, **11** (2), 135–140.

5 Pibot, P., Biourge, V., and Elliot, D. (2006) *Encyclopedia of Canine Clinical Nutrition*, Royal Canin, Almargues.

6 Lund, E.M., Armstrong, P.J., and Kirk, C.A. (2005) Prevalence and risk factors for obesity in adult cats from private US veterinary practices. *International Journal of Applied Research in Veterinary Medicine*, **3** (2), 88–96.

7 McGreevy, P.D., Thomson, P.C., Pride, C. *et al.* (2005) Prevalence of obesity in dogs examined by Australian veterinary practices and the risk factors involved. *Veterinary Record*, **156** (22), 695.

8 White, G.A., Hobson-West, P., Cobb, K. *et al.* (2011) Canine obesity: is there a difference between veterinarian and owner perception? *Journal of Small Animal Practice*, **52** (12), 622–626.

9 German, A.J. (2010) Obesity in companion animals. *Companion Animal Practice*, 32, 42–50.

10 Lund, E.M., Armstrong, P.J., Kirk, C.A., and Klausner, J.S. (2006) Prevalence and risk factors for obesity in adult dogs from private U.S. veterinary practices. *International Journal of Applied Research in Veterinary Medicine*, **4**, 177–186.

11 Markwell, P.J., Vanerk, W., Parkin, G.D. *et al.* (1990) Obesity in the dog. *Journal of Small Animal Practice*, **31** (10), 533–537.

12 Weeth, L.P., Fascetti, A.J., Kass, P.H. *et al.* (2007) Prevalence of obese dogs in a population of dogs with cancer. *American Journal of Veterinary Research*, **68** (4), 389–398.

13 Kealy, R.D., Lawler, D.F., Ballam, J.M. *et al.* (2002) Effects of diet restriction on life span and age-related changes in dogs. *Journal of the American Veterinary Medical Association*, **220**, 1315–1320.

14 Mattheeuws, D., Rottiers, R., Kaneko, J.J., and Vermeulen, A. (1984) Diabetes mellitus in dogs: relationship of obesity to glucose tolerance and insulin response. *American Journal of Veterinary Research*, **45** (1), 98–103.

15 Lawler, D.F., Larson, B.T., Ballam, J.M. *et al.* (2008) Diet restriction and ageing in the dog: major observations over two decades. *British Journal of Nutrition*, **99** (4), 793–805.

16 Baldwin, K., Bartges, J., Buffington, T. *et al.* (2010) AAHA nutritional assessment guidelines for dogs and cats. *Journal of the American Animal Hospital Association*, **46** (4), 285–296.

17 Laflamme, D. (1997) Development and validation of a body condition score system for dogs. *Canine Practice*, **22** (4), 10–15.

18 Toll, P.W., Yamka, R.M., Schoenherr, W.D. *et al.* (2010) Obesity, in *Small Animal Clinical Nutrition* (eds. M.S. Hand, C.D. Thatcher, R.L. Remillard, *et al.*), Mark Morris Institute, Topeka, KS, pp. 501–542.

19 Witzel, A.L., Kirk, C.A., Henry, G.A. *et al.* (2014) Use of a novel morphometric method and body fat index system for estimation of body composition in overweight and obese dogs. *Journal of the American Veterinary Medical Association*, **244** (11), 1279–1284.

20 Courcier, E.A., Thomson, R.M., Mellor, D.J., and Yam, P.S. (2010) An epidemiological study of environmental factors associated with canine obesity. *Journal of Small Animal Practice*, **51** (7), 362–367.

21 Michel, K.E., Anderson, W., Cupp, C., and Laflamme, D.P. (2011) Correlation of a feline muscle mass score with body composition determined by dual-energy X-ray absorptiometry. *British Journal of Nutrition*, **106** (Suppl. 1), S57–S59.

22 Freeman, L.M. (2012) Cachexia and sarcopenia: emerging syndromes of importance in dogs and cats. *Journal of Veterinary Internal Medicine*, **26** (1), 3–17.

23 Anker, S.D., Ponikowski, P., Varney, S. *et al.* (1997) Wasting as independent risk factor for mortality in chronic heart failure. *Lancet*, **349** (9058), 1050–1053.

24 Anker, S.D., Negassa, A., Coats, A.J. *et al.* (2003) Prognostic importance of weight loss in chronic heart failure and the effect of treatment with angiotensin-converting-enzyme inhibitors: an observational study. *Lancet*, **361** (9363), 1077–1083.

25 Freeman, L.M. and Roubenoff, R. (1994) The nutrition implications of cardiac cachexia. *Nutrition Reviews*, **52** (10), 340–347.

26 Baez, J.L., Michel, K.E., Sorenmo, K., and Shofer, FS. (2007) A prospective investigation of the prevalence and prognostic significance of weight loss and changes in body condition in feline cancer patients. *Journal of Feline Medicine and Surgery*, **9** (5), 411–417.

27 Scarlett, J.M. and Donoghue, S. (1998) Associations between body condition and disease in cats. *Journal of the American Veterinary Medical Association*, **212** (11), 1725–1731.

28 Doria-Rose, V.P. and Scarlett, J.M. (2000) Mortality rates and causes of death among emaciated cats. *Journal of the American Veterinary Medical Association*, **216** (3), 347–351.

29 Thayer, V. (2012) Deciphering the cat: the medical history of physical examination, in *The Cat: Clinical Medicine and Management* (ed. S.E. Little), Saunders Elsevier, St. Louis, pp. 36–39.

30 Bartges, J., Raditic, D., Kirk, C. *et al.* (2012) Nutritional management of diseases, in *The Cat: Clinical Medicine and Management* (ed. S.E. Little), Saunders Elsevier, St. Louis, p. 261.

31 Little, S.E. (2012) Managing the senior cat, in *The Cat: Clinical Medicine and Management* (ed. S.E. Little), Saunders Elsevier, St. Louis, p. 1169.

32 Chandler, M. (2014) Nutrition for the surgical patient, in *Feline Soft Tissue and General Surgery* (eds. S.J. Langley-Hobbs, J.L. Demetriou, and J.F. Ladlow), Saunders Elsevier, St. Louis, pp. 55–58.

33 WSAVA Nutritional Assessment Guidelines Task Force Members, Freeman, L., Becvarova, I., Cave, N. *et al.* (2011) WSAVA Nutritional Assessment Guidelines. *Journal of Small Animal Practice*, **52** (7), 385–396.

34 Hutchinson, D., Sutherland-Smith, J., Watson, A.L., and Freeman, L.M. (2012) Assessment of methods of evaluating sarcopenia in old dogs. *American Journal of Veterinary Research*, **73** (11), 1794–1800.

35 Hazewinkel, H.A.W., Meij, B.P., Theyse, L.F.H., and van Rijssen, B. (2009) Locomotor system, in *Medical History and Physical Examination in Companion Animals*, 2nd edn. (eds. A. Rijnberk and F.J. van Sluijs), Saunders Elsevier, St. Louis, pp. 135–159.

36 Dyce, K.M., Sack, W.O., and Wensing, C.J.G. (1996) Some basic facts and concepts, in *Textbook of Veterinary Anatomy*, 2nd edn. (eds. K.M. Dyce, W.O. Sack, and C.J.G. Wensing), Saunders, Philadelphia.

37 Evans, H.E. (1993) Prenatal development, in *Miller's Anatomy of the Dog*, 3rd edn. (ed. H.E. Evans), Saunders Elsevier, Philadelphia.

38 Stades, F.C. and Stokhof, A.A. (2009) Health certification, in *Medical History and Physical Examination in Companion Animals*, 2nd edn. (eds. A. Rijnberk and F.J. van Sluijs), Saunders Elsevier, St. Louis, pp. 245–246.

39 American Kennel Club (2008) *Official Standard of the Chihuahua*, http://images.akc.org/pdf/breeds/standards/Chihuahua.pdf?_ga=1.215017687.1321975590.1442621488 (accessed 27 June 2016).

40 Przyborowska, P., Adamiak, Z., Jaskolska, M., and Zhalniarovich, Y. (2013) Hydrocephalus in dogs: a review. *Veterinarni Medicina*, **58** (2), 73–80.

41 Root Kustriz, M.V. (2011) History and physical examination of the weanling and adolescent, in *Small Animal Pediatrics: The First 12 Months of Life* (eds. M.E. Peterson and M.A. Kutzler), Saunders Elsevier, St. Louis, pp. 28–33.

42 Root Kustriz, M.V. (2011) History and physical examination of the neonate, in *Small Animal Pediatrics: The First 12 Months of Life* (eds. M.E. Peterson and M.A. Kutzler), Saunders Elsevier, St. Louis, pp. 20–27.

43 Brown, J.A., Rachlin, J., Rubin, J.M., and Wollmann, R.L. (1984) Ultrasound evaluation of experimental hydrocephalus in dogs. *Surgical Neurology*, **22** (3), 273–276.

44 Esteve-Ratsch, B., Kneissl, S., and Gabler, C. (2001) Comparative evaluation of the ventricles in the Yorkshire Terrier and the German Shepherd dog using low-field MRI. *Veterinary Radiology & Ultrasound*, **42** (5), 410–413.

45 Adamiak, Z., Jaskolska, M., and Pomianowski, A. (2012) Low-field magnetic resonance imaging of canine hydrocephalus. *Pakistan Veterinary Journal*, **32** (1), 128–130.

46 Thomas, W.B. (2010) Hydrocephalus in dogs and cats. *Veterinary Clinics of North America: Small Animal Practice*, **40** (1), 143.

47 Partington, B.P. (1995) Physical examination and diagnostic imaging procedures: diagnostic imaging techniques, in *Veterinary Pediatrics: Dogs and Cats from Birth to Six Months*, 2nd edn. (ed. J.D. Hoskins), Saunders, Philadelphia, pp. 7–21.

48 Hoskins, J.D. and Shelton, G.D. (2001) The nervous and neuromuscular systems, in *Veterinary Pediatrics: Dogs and Cats from Birth to Six Months*, 3rd edn. (ed. J.D. Hoskins), Saunders Elsevier, Philadelphia, pp. 425–62.

49 Haworth, K.E., Islam, I., Breen, M. *et al.* (2001) Canine TCOF1; cloning, chromosome assignment and genetic analysis in dogs with different head types. *Mammalian Genome*, **12** (8), 622–629.

50 Wayne, R.K. (1986) Cranial morphology of domestic and wild canids – the influence of development on morphological change. *Evolution*, **40** (2), 243–261.

51 Young, A. and Bannasch, D. (2006) Morphological variation in the dog, in *The Dog and its Genome* (eds. E.A. Ostrander, U. Giger, and K. Lindblad-Toh), Cold Spring Harbor Laboratory Press, Cold Spring Harbor, NY, pp. 47–65.

52 Schoenebeck, J.J. and Ostrander, E.A. (2013) The genetics of canine skull shape variation. *Genetics*, **193** (2), 317–325.

53 Overall, K.L. (1997) Normal canine behavior, in *Clinical Behavioral Medicine for Small Animals* (ed. K.L. Overall), Mosby, St. Louis, pp. 9–44.

54 Grevel, V., Opitz, M., Steeb, C., and Skrodzki, M. (1993) Myopathy due to potassium deficiency in eight cats and a dog. *Berliner und Münchener Tierärztliche Wochenschrift*, **106** (1), 20–26 (in German).

55 Rusbridge, C. (2005) Neurological diseases of the Cavalier King Charles spaniel. *Journal of Small Animal Practice*, **46** (6), 265–272.

56 Ryan, T.M., Platt, S.R., Llabres-Diaz, F.J. *et al.* (2008) Detection of spinal cord compression in dogs with cervical intervertebral disc disease by magnetic resonance imaging. *Veterinary Record*, **163** (1), 11–15.

57 Brisson, B.A. (2010) Intervertebral disc disease in dogs. *Veterinary Clinics of North America: Small Animal Practice*, **40** (5), 829.

58 Denny, H.R. (1978) The surgical treatment of cervical disc protrusions in the dog: a review of 40 cases. *Journal of Small Animal Practice*, **19** (5), 251–257.

59 Morgan, P.W., Parent, J., and Holmberg, D.L. (1993) Cervical pain secondary to intervertebral disc disease in dogs – radiographic findings and surgical implications. *Progress in Veterinary Neurology*, **4** (3), 76–80.

60 Loughin, C.A. and Marino, D.J. (2016) Atlantooccipital overlap and other craniocervical junction abnormalities in dogs. *Veterinary Clinics of North America: Small Animal Practice*, **46** (2), 243.

61 Freeman, A.C., Platt, S.R., Kent, M. *et al.* (2014) Chiari-like malformation and syringomyelia in American Brussels Griffon dogs. *Journal of Veterinary Internal Medicine*, **28** (5), 1551–1559.

62 Linon, E., Geissbuhler, U., Karli, P., and Forterre, F. (2014) Atlantoaxial epidural abscess secondary to grass awn migration in a dog. *Veterinary and Comparative Orthopaedics and Traumatology*, **27** (2), 155–158.

63 Forterre, F., Casoni, D., Tomek, A. *et al.* (2015) Congenital cervical kyphosis in two young sighthounds. *Veterinary and Comparative Orthopaedics and Traumatology*, **28** (1), 73–78.

64 Parker, A.J., Park, R.D., and Stowater, J.L. (1973) Cervical kyphosis in an Afghan Hound. *Journal of the American Veterinary Medical Association*, **162** (11), 953–955.

65 Bingel, S.A. and Sande, R.D. (1994) Chondrodysplasia in five Great Pyrenees. *Journal of the American Veterinary Medical Association*, **205** (6), 845–848.

66 Bingel, S.A., Sande, R.D., and Wight, T.N. (1985) Chondrodysplasia in the Alaskan Malamute – characterization of proteoglycans dissociatively extracted from dwarf growth plates. *Laboratory Investigation*, **53** (4), 479–485.

67 Bingel, S.A., Sande, R.D., and Newbrey, J. (1983) Dwarfism in the Alaskan Malamute – ultrastructural features of dwarf growth plate chondrocytes. *Calcified Tissue International*, **35** (2), 216–224.

68 Fletch, S.M., Smart, M.E., Pennock, P.W., and Subden, R.E. (1973) Clinical and pathologic features of chondrodysplasia (dwarfism) in the Alaskan Malamute. *Journal of the American Veterinary Medical Association*, **162** (5), 357–361.

69 Meyers, V.N., Jezyk, P.F., Aguirre, G.D., and Patterson, D.F. (1983) Short-limbed dwarfism and ocular defects in the Samoyed dog. *Journal of the American Veterinary Medical Association*, **183** (9), 975–979.

70 Aroch, I., Ofri, R., and Aizenberg, I. (1996) Haematological, ocular and skeletal abnormalities in a Samoyed family. *Journal of Small Animal Practice*, **37** (7), 333–339.

71 Breur, G.J., Zerbe, C.A., Slocombe, R.F. *et al.* (1989) Clinical, radiographic, pathologic, and genetic features of osteochondrodysplasia in Scottish deerhounds. *Journal of the American Veterinary Medical Association*, **195** (5), 606–612.

72 Frischknecht, M., Niehof-Oellers, H., Jagannathan, V. *et al.* (2013) A *COL11A2* mutation in Labrador Retrievers with mild disproportionate dwarfism. *PLoS One*, **8** (3), e60149.

73 Hanssen, I., Falck, G., Grammeltvedt, A.T. *et al.* (1998) Hypochondroplastic dwarfism in the Irish setter. *Journal of Small Animal Practice*, **39** (1), 10–44.

74 Neff, M.W., Beck, J.S., Koeman, J.M. *et al.* (2012) Partial deletion of the sulfate transporter *SLC13A1* is associated with an osteochondrodysplasia in the Miniature Poodle breed. *PLoS One*, **7** (12), e51917.

75 Kyostila, K., Lappalainen, A.K., and Lohi, H. (2013) Canine chondrodysplasia caused by a truncating mutation in collagen-binding integrin alpha subunit 10. *PLoS One*, **8** (9), e75621.

76 American Kennel Club (2007) *Official Standard of the Dachshund*, http://images.akc.org/pdf/breeds/standards/Dachshund.pdf?_ga=1.220350552 .1321975590.1442621488 (accessed 19 January 2017).

77 American Kennel Club (1993) *Official Standard of the Pembroke Welsh Corgi*, http://images.akc.org/pdf/breeds/standards/PembrokeWelshCorgi.pdf?_ga =1.246130884.1321975590.1442621488 (accessed 19 January 2017).

78 Voorbij, A.M., Leegwater, P.A., Buijtels, J.J. *et al.* (2016) Central hypothyroidism in Miniature Schnauzers. *Journal of Veterinary Internal Medicine*, **30** (1), 85–91.

79 Greco, D.S., Feldman, E.C., Peterson, M.E. *et al.* (1991) Congenital hypothyroid dwarfism in a family of Giant Schnauzers. *Journal of Veterinary Internal Medicine*, **5** (2), 57–65.

80 Harasen, G. (2010) Canine carpal conundrums. *Canadian Veterinary Journal/Revue Vétérinaire Canadienne*, **51** (8), 909–910.

81 Comerford, E.J., Doran, I.C., and Owen, M.R. (2006) Carpal derangement and associated carpal valgus in a dog. *Veterinary and Comparative Orthopaedics and Traumatology*, **19** (2), 113–116.

82 Sereda, C.W., Lewis, D.D., Radasch, R.M. *et al.* (2009) Descriptive report of antebrachial growth deformity correction in 17 dogs from 1999 to 2007, using hybrid linear-circular external fixator constructs. *Canadian Veterinary Journal/Revue Vétérinaire Canadienne*, **50** (7), 723–732.

83 Langley-Hobbs, S.J., Hamilton, M.H., and Pratt, J.N.J. (2007) Radiographic and clinical features of carpal varus associated with chronic sprain of the lateral collateral ligament complex in 10 dogs. *Veterinary and Comparative Orthopaedics and Traumatology*, **20** (4), 324–330.

84 Cetinkaya, M.A., Yardimci, C., and Saglam, M. (2007) Carpal laxity syndrome in forty-three puppies. *Veterinary and Comparative Orthopaedics and Traumatology*, **20** (2), 126–130.

85 Shires, P.K., Hulse, D.A., and Kearney, M.T. (1985) Carpal hyperextension in two-month-old pups. *Journal of the American Veterinary Medical Association*, **186** (1), 49–52.

86 Lopez, M.J., Quinn, M.M., and Markel, M.D. (2006) Evaluation of gait kinetics in puppies with coxofemoral joint laxity. *American Journal of Veterinary Research*, **67** (2), 236–241.

87 Lopez, M.J., Quinn, M.M., and Markel, M.D. (2006) Associations between canine juvenile weight gain and coxofemoral joint laxity at 16 weeks of age. *Veterinary Surgery*, **35** (3), 214–218.

88 Madsen, J.S. (1997) The joint capsule and joint laxity in dogs with hip dysplasia. *Journal of the American Veterinary Medical Association*, **210** (10), 1463.

89 Harasen, G. (2002) Arthrodesis – Part II: The tarsus. *Canadian Veterinary Journal/Revue Vétérinaire Canadienne*, **43** (10), 806–808.

90 Johnson, K.A. (1995) Arthrodesis, in *Small Animal Orthopedics* (ed. M.L. Olmstead), Mosby, St. Louis, pp. 527–529.

91 Piermattei, D.L., Flo, G.L., and Brinker, W.O. (1997) *Brinker, Piermattei, and Flo's Handbook of Small Animal Orthopedics and Fracture Repair*, 3rd edn., Saunders, Philadelphia, pp. 642–652.

92 Voss, K. and Steffen, F. (2009) Patient assessment, in *Feline Orthopedic Surgery and Musculoskeletal Disease* (eds. P.M. Montavon, K. Voss, and S.J. Langley-Hobbs), Saunders Elsevier, St. Louis, pp. 3–20.

93 Arnoczky, S.P. and Tarvin, G.B. (1981) Physical examination of the musculoskeletal system. *Veterinary Clinics of North America: Small Animal Practice*, **11** (3), 575–593.

94 Piermattei, D.L., Flo, G.L., and DeCamp, C.E. (2006) *Piermattei and Flo's Handbook of Small Animal*

Orthopedics and Fracture Repair, 4th edn., Saunders, Philadelphia.

95 Park, K., Kang, J., Park, S. *et al.* (2004) Linkage of the locus for canine dewclaw to chromosome 16. *Genomics*, **83** (2), 216–224.

96 MacPhail, C.M. (2013) Surgery of the integumentary system, in *Small Animal Surgery*, 4th edn. (ed. T.W. Fossum), Mosby Elsevier, St. Louis, pp. 190–288.

97 American Kennel Club (1990) *Official Standard of the Bernese Mountain Dog*, http://images.akc.org/pdf/breeds/standards/BerneseMountainDog.pdf?_ga=1.146007796.1321975590.1442621488 (accessed 27 June 2016).

98 Kunkel, K.A. and Rochat, M.C. (2008) A review of lameness attributable to the shoulder in the dog. Part one. *Journal of the American Animal Hospital Association*, **44** (4), 156–162.

99 Kunkel, K.A. and Rochat, M.C. (2008) A review of lameness attributable to the shoulder in the dog. Part two. *Journal of the American Animal Hospital Association*, **44** (4), 163–170.

100 Cook, J.L. (2001) Forelimb lameness in the young patient. *Veterinary Clinics of North America: Small Animal Practice*, **31** (1), 55.

101 Schulz, K.S. (2001) Forelimb lameness in the adult patient. *Veterinary Clinics of North America: Small Animal Practice*, **31** (1), 85.

102 Renberg, W.C. (2001) Evaluation of the lame patient. *Veterinary Clinics of North America: Small Animal Practice*, **31** (1), 1

103 Rochat, M.C. (2005) Emerging causes of canine lameness. *Veterinary Clinics of North America: Small Animal Practice*, **35** (5), 1233–1239, vii.

104 Lande, R., Reese, S.L., Cuddy, L.C. *et al.* (2014) Prevalence of computed tomographic subchondral bone lesions in the scapulohumeral joint of 32 immature dogs with thoracic limb lameness. *Veterinary Radiology & Ultrasound*, **55** (1), 23–28.

105 Kunst, C.M., Pease, A.P., Nelson, N.C. *et al.* (2014) Computed tomographic identification of dysplasia and progression of osteoarthritis in dog elbows previously assigned OFA grades 0 and 1. *Veterinary Radiology & Ultrasound*, **55** (5), 511–520.

106 Stogdale, L. (1979) Foreleg lameness in rapidly growing-dogs. *Journal of the South African Veterinary Association*, **50** (3), 193–200.

107 Bennett, D. (1976) Nutrition and bone disease in the dog and cat. *Veterinary Record*, **98** (16), 313–321.

108 Krook, L. and Whalen, J.P. (2010) Nutritional secondary hyperparathyroidism in the animal kingdom: report of two cases. *Clinical Imaging*, **34** (6), 458–461.

109 de Fornel-Thibaud, P., Blanchard, G., Escoffier-Chateau, L. *et al.* (2007) Unusual case of osteopenia associated with nutritional calcium and vitamin D deficiency in an adult dog. *Journal of the American Animal Hospital Association*, **43** (1), 52–60.

110 Taylor, M.B., Geiger, D.A., Saker, K.E., and Larson, M.M. (2009) Diffuse osteopenia and myelopathy in a puppy fed a diet composed of an organic premix and raw ground beef. *Journal of the American Veterinary Medical Association*, **234** (8), 1041–1048.

111 Lourens, D.C. (1980) Nutritional or secondary hyperparathyroidism in a German Shepherd litter. *Journal of the South African Veterinary Association*, **51** (2), 121–123 (in Afrikaans).

112 Nortje, J., Bruce, W.J., and Worth, A.J. (2015) Surgical repair of humeral condylar fractures in New Zealand working farm dogs – long-term outcome and owner satisfaction. *New Zealand Veterinary Journal*, **63** (2), 110–116.

113 Duffy, A.L. and Hackett, T.B. (2010) Canine pedal injury resulting from metal landscape edging. *Journal of Veterinary Emergency and Critical Care*, **20** (5), 533–536.

114 Foster, J.D., Sample, S., Kohler, R. *et al.* (2014) Serum biomarkers of clinical and cytologic response in dogs with idiopathic immune-mediated polyarthropathy. *Journal of Veterinary Internal Medicine*, **28** (3), 905–911.

115 Johnson, K.C. and Mackin, A. (2012) Canine immune-mediated polyarthritis. Part 1: Pathophysiology. *Journal of the American Animal Hospital Association*, **48** (1), 12–17.

116 Johnson, K.C. and Mackin, A. (2012) Canine immune-mediated polyarthritis. Part 2: Diagnosis and treatment. *Journal of the American Animal Hospital Association*, **48** (2), 71–82.

117 Chomel, B. (2015) Lyme disease. *Revue Scientifique et Technique*, **34** (2), 569–576.

118 Krupka, I. and Straubinger, R.K. (2010) Lyme borreliosis in dogs and cats: background, diagnosis, treatment and prevention of infections with *Borrelia burgdorferi sensu stricto*. *Veterinary Clinics of North America: Small Animal Practice*, **40** (6), 1103.

119 Solano-Gallego, L., Capri, A., Pennisi, M.G. *et al.* (2015) Acute febrile illness is associated with *Rickettsia* spp infection in dogs. *Parasites & Vectors*, **8**, 216.

120 Mazepa, A.W., Kidd, L.B., Young, K.M., and Trepanier, L.A. (2010) Clinical presentation of 26 *Anaplasma phagocytophilum*-seropositive dogs residing in an endemic area. *Journal of the American Animal Hospital Association*, **46** (6), 405–412.

121 Graupmann-Kuzma, A., Valentine, B.A., Shubitz, L.F. *et al.* (2008) Coccidioidomycosis in dogs and cats: a review. *Journal of the American Animal Hospital Association*, **44** (5), 226–235.

122 Johnson, L.R., Herrgesell, E.J., Davidson, A.P., and Pappagianis, D. (2003) Clinical, clinicopathologic, and radiographic findings in dogs with coccidioidomycosis: 24 cases (1995–2000). *Journal of the American Veterinary Medical Association*, **222** (4), 461–466.

123 Sivacolundhu, R.K., Runge, J.J., Donovan, T.A. *et al.* (2013) Ulnar osteosarcoma in dogs: 30 cases (1992–2008). *Journal of the American Veterinary Medical Association*, **243** (1), 96–101.

124 Gasch, E.G., Rivier, P., and Bardet, J.F. (2013) Free proximal cortical ulnar autograft for the treatment of distal radial osteosarcoma in a dog. *Canadian Veterinary Journal/Revue Vétérinaire Canadienne*, **54** (2), 162–166.

125 Henry, C.J., Brewer, W.G., Whitley, E.M. *et al.* (2005) Canine digital tumors: a Veterinary Cooperative Oncology Group retrospective study of 64 dogs. *Journal of Veterinary Internal Medicine*, **19** (5), 720–724.

126 Shafiee, R., Shariat, A., Khalili, S. *et al.* (2015) Diagnostic investigations of canine prostatitis incidence together with benign prostate hyperplasia, prostate malignancies, and biochemical recurrence in high-risk prostate cancer as a model for human study. *Tumour Biology*, **36** (4), 2437–2445.

127 Duclos, D.D., Hargis, A.M., and Hanley, P.W. (2008) Pathogenesis of canine interdigital palmar and plantar comedones and follicular cysts, and their response to laser surgery. *Veterinary Dermatology*, **19** (3), 134–141.

128 Fox, D.B. (2007) Orthopedic examination of the forelimb in the dog. *Clinician's Brief, June*, 19–22.

129 Evans, H.E. (1993) The skeleton, in *Miller's Anatomy of the Dog*, 3rd edn. (ed. H.E. Evans), Saunders Elsevier, Philadelphia, pp. 122–218.

130 Gilbert, S.G. (1989) *Pictorial Anatomy of the Cat*, University of Washington Press, Seattle.

131 Thomas, T.M., Marcellin-Little, D.J., Roe, S.C. *et al.* (2006) Comparison of measurements obtained by use of an electrogoniometer and a universal plastic goniometer for the assessment of joint motion in dogs. *American Journal of Veterinary Research*, **67** (12), 1974–1979.

132 Grierson, J. (2012) Hips, elbows and stifles: common joint diseases in the cat. *Journal of Feline Medicine and Surgery*, **14** (1), 23–30.

133 Clements, D.N., Fitzpatrick, N., Carter, S.D., and Day, P.J.R. (2009) Cartilage gene expression correlates with radiographic severity of canine elbow osteoarthritis. *Veterinary Journal*, **179** (2), 211–218.

134 Morgan, J.P., Wind, A., and Davidson, A.P. (1999) Bone dysplasias in the Labrador retriever: a radiographic study. *Journal of the American Animal Hospital Association*, **35** (4), 332–340.

135 Michelsen, J. (2013) Canine elbow dysplasia: aetiopathogenesis and current treatment recommendations. *Veterinary Journal*, **196** (1), 12–19.

136 Samoy, Y., Van Ryssen, B., Gielen, I. *et al.* (2006) Review of the literature – elbow incongruity in the dog. *Veterinary and Comparative Orthopaedics and Traumatology*, **19** (1), 1–8.

137 Van Sickle, D.C. (1966) A comparative study of the postnatal elbow development of the Greyhound and the German Shepherd dog. *Journal of the American Veterinary Medical Association*, **147**, 1650.

138 Kirberger, R.M. and Fourie, S.L. (1998) Elbow dysplasia in the dog: pathophysiology, diagnosis and control. *Journal of the South African Veterinary Association*, **69** (2), 43–54.

139 Olson, N.C., Brinker, W.O., Carrig, C.B., and Tvedten, H.W. (1981) Asynchronous growth of the canine radius and ulna – surgical correction following experimental premature closure of the distal radial physis. *Veterinary Surgery*, **10** (3), 125–131.

140 Morgan, J.P., Wind, A., and Davidson, A.P. (1999) Bone dysplasias in the Labrador retriever: a radiographic study. *Journal of the American Animal Hospital Association*, **35** (4), 332–340.

141 Morgan, J., Wind, A., and Davidson, A.P. (2000) Elbow dysplasia, in *Hereditary Bone and Joint Diseases in the Dog*, Schültersche, Hannover, pp. 41–94.

142 Hazewinkel, H.A.W., Meij, B.P., Nap, R.C., and Dijkshoorn, N.E. (1995) Radiographic views for elbow dysplasia screening in Bernese Mountain Dogs, in *Proceedings of the 7th International Elbow Working Group Meeting*, Konstanz, Germany, pp. 32–37.

143 Clements, D.N. (2006) Gene expression in normal and diseased elbows, in *Proceedings of the Autumn Meeting of the British Veterinary Orthopaedic Association, Chester*, pp. 6–7.

144 Grondalen, J. and Lingaas, F. (1991) Arthrosis in the elbow joint of young rapidly growing dogs – a genetic investigation. *Journal of Small Animal Practice*, **32** (9), 460–464.

145 Lewis, T.W., Ilska, J.J., Blott, S.C., and Woolliams, J.A. (2011) Genetic evaluation of elbow scores and the relationship with hip scores in UK Labrador retrievers. *Veterinary Journal*, **189** (2), 227–233.

146 Maki, K., Janss, L.L.G., Groen, A.F. *et al.* (2004) An indication of major genes affecting hip and elbow dysplasia in four Finnish dog populations. *Heredity*, **92** (5), 402–408.

147 Meyer-Lindenberg, A., Fehr, M., and Nolte, I. (2006) Co-existence of UAP and FCP of the ulna in the dog. *Journal of Small Animal Practice*, **47**, 61–65.

148 Ginja, M.M., Silvestre, A.M., Gonzalo-Orden, J.M., and Ferreira, A.J. (2010) Diagnosis, genetic control and preventive management of canine hip dysplasia: a review. *Veterinary Journal*, **184** (3), 269–276.

149 Wilson, B., Nicholas, F.W., and Thomson, P.C. (2011) Selection against canine hip dysplasia: success or failure? *Veterinary Journal*, **189** (2), 160–168.

150 Woolliams, J.A., Lewis, T.W., and Blott, S.C. (2011) Canine hip and elbow dysplasia in UK Labrador retrievers. *Veterinary Journal*, **189** (2), 169–176.

151 Stieger-Vanegas, S.M., Senthirajah, S.K., Nemanic, S. *et al.* (2015) Evaluation of the diagnostic accuracy of four-view radiography and conventional computed tomography analysing sacral and pelvic fractures in dogs. *Veterinary and Comparative Orthopaedics and Traumatology*, **28** (3), 155–163.

152 Harasen, G. (2007) Pelvic fractures. *Canadian Veterinary Journal/Revue Vétérinaire Canadienne*, **48** (4), 427–428.

153 Draffan, D., Clements, D., Farrell, M. *et al.* (2009) The role of computed tomography in the classification and management of pelvic fractures. *Veterinary and Comparative Orthopaedics and Traumatology*, **22** (3), 190–197.

154 Burkhardt, M., Nienaber, U., Pizanis, A. *et al.* (2012) Acute management and outcome of multiple trauma patients with pelvic disruptions. *Critical Care*, **16** (4), R163.

155 Meeson, R. and Corr, S. (2011) Management of pelvic trauma: neurological damage, urinary tract disruption

and pelvic fractures. *Journal of Feline Medicine and Surgery*, **13** (5), 347–361.

156 Hoffberg, J.E., Koenigshof, A.M., and Guiot, L.P. (2016) Retrospective evaluation of concurrent intra-abdominal injuries in dogs with traumatic pelvic fractures: 83 cases (2008–2013). *Journal of Veterinary Emergency and Critical Care*, **26** (2), 288–294.

157 Boysen, S.R., Rozanski, E.A., Tidwell, A.S. *et al.* (2004) Evaluation of a focused assessment with sonography for trauma protocol to detect free abdominal fluid in dogs involved in motor vehicle accidents. *Journal of the American Veterinary Medical Association*, **225** (8), 1198–1204.

158 Simpson, S.A., Syring, R., and Otto, C.M. (2009) Severe blunt trauma in dogs: 235 cases (1997–2003). *Journal of Veterinary Emergency and Critical Care*, **19** (6), 588–602.

159 Streeter, E.M., Rozanski, E.A., Laforcade-Buress, A. *et al.* (2009) Evaluation of vehicular trauma in dogs: 239 cases (January–December 2001). *Journal of the American Veterinary Medical Association*, **235** (4), 405–408.

160 Stafford, J.R. and Bartges, J.W. (2013) A clinical review of pathophysiology, diagnosis, and treatment of uroabdomen in the dog and cat. *Journal of Veterinary Emergency and Critical Care*, **23** (2), 216–229.

161 Kolata, R.J. and Johnston, D.E. (1975) Motor vehicle accidents in urban dogs: a study of 600 cases. *Journal of the American Veterinary Medical Association*, **167** (10), 938–941.

162 Lee, K., Heng, H.G., Jeong, J. *et al.* (2012) Feasibility of computed tomography in awake dogs with traumatic pelvic fracture. *Veterinary Radiology & Ultrasound*, **53** (4), 412–416.

163 Anderson, A. and Coughlan, A.R. (1997) Sacral fractures in dogs and cats: a classification scheme and review of 51 cases. *Journal of Small Animal Practice*, **38** (9), 404–409.

164 Fry, P.D. (1974) Observations on the surgical treatment of hip dislocation in the dog and cat. *Journal of Small Animal Practice*, **15** (11), 661–670.

165 Christopher, S.A. (2011) What is your diagnosis? *Journal of the American Veterinary Medical Association*, **239** (3), 301–302.

166 Maki, K., Janss, L.L., Groen, A.F. *et al.* (2004) An indication of major genes affecting hip and elbow dysplasia in four Finnish dog populations. *Heredity*, 92 (5), 402–408.

167 Janutta, V. and Distl, O. (2006) Inheritance of canine hip dysplasia: review of estimation methods and of heritability estimates and prospects on further developments. *DTW. Deutsche Tierärztliche Wochenschrift*, **113** (1), 6–12.

168 Smith, G.K., Popovitch, C.A., Gregor, T.P., and Shofer, F.S. (1995) Evaluation of risk factors for degenerative joint disease associated with hip dysplasia in dogs. *Journal of the American Veterinary Medical Association*, **206** (5), 642–647.

169 Leighton, E.A. (1997) Genetics of canine hip dysplasia. *Journal of the American Veterinary Medical Association*, **210** (10), 1474–1479.

170 Baltzer, W. (2001) Canine hip dysplasia: Part 1. *Clinician's Brief*, October, 23–26.

171 Marshall, W., Bockstahler, B., Hulse, D., and Carmichael, S. (2009) A review of osteoarthritis and obesity: current understanding of the relationship and benefit of obesity treatment and prevention in the dog. *Veterinary and Comparative Orthopaedics and Traumatology*, **22** (5), 339–345.

172 Budsberg, S.C. and Bartges, J.W. (2006) Nutrition and osteoarthritis in dogs: does it help? *Veterinary Clinics of North America: Small Animal Practice*, **36** (6), 1307–1323, vii.

173 Chandler, J.C. and Beale, B.S. (2002) Feline orthopedics. *Clinical Techniques in Small Animal Practice*, **17** (4), 190–203.

174 Innes, J. (2007) Palpating for the Ortolani sign when diagnosing hip dysplasia. *Clinician's Brief*, January, 71–72.

175 Fox, D.B. (2007) Orthopedic examination of the rear limb in the dog. *Clinician's Brief*, July, 63–66.

176 Lust, G., Todhunter, R.J., Erb, H.N. *et al.* (2001) Comparison of three radiographic methods for diagnosis of hip dysplasia in eight-month-old dogs. *Journal of the American Veterinary Medical Association*, **219** (9), 1242–1246.

177 Smith, G.K. (1997) Advances in diagnosing canine hip dysplasia. *Journal of the American Veterinary Medical Association*, **210** (10), 1451–1457.

178 Farese, J.P., Todhunter, R.J., Lust, G. *et al.* (1998) Dorsolateral subluxation of hip joints in dogs measured in a weight-bearing position with radiography and computed tomography. *Veterinary Surgery*, **27** (5), 393–405.

179 Comhaire, F.H. and Schoonjans, F.A. (2011) Canine hip dyslasia: the significance of the Norberg angle for healthy breeding. *Journal of Small Animal Practice*, **52** (10), 536–542.

180 Guiot, L.P., Demianiuk, R.M., and Dejardin, L.M. (2012) Fractures of the femur, in *Veterinary Surgery: Small Animal*, vol. 1 (eds. K.M. Tobias and S.A. Johnston), Saunders Elsevier, St. Louis, pp. 865–905.

181 Sebastiani, A.M. and Fishbeck, D.W. (1998) *Mammalian Anatomy: the Cat*, Morton, Englewood, CO.

182 Vidoni, B., Henninger, W., Lorinson, D., and Mayrhofer, E. (2005) Traumatic avulsion fracture of the lesser trochanter in a dog. *Veterinary and Comparative Orthopaedics and Traumatology*, **18** (2), 105–109.

183 Guerrero, T.G., Koch, D., and Montavon, P.M. (2005) Fixation of a proximal femoral physeal fracture in a dog using a ventral approach and two Kirschner wires. *Veterinary and Comparative Orthopaedics and Traumatology*, **18** (2), 110–114.

184 Engel, E. and Kneissl, S. (2014) Salter–Harris fractures in dogs and cats considering problems in radiological reports – a retrospective analysis of 245 cases between 1991 and 2012. *Berliner und Münchener Tierärztliche Wochenschrift*, **127** (1–2), 77–83 (in German).

185 O'Neill, D.G., Meeson, R.L., Sheridan, A. *et al.* (2016) The epidemiology of patellar luxation in dogs attending primary-care veterinary practices in England. *Canine Genetics and Epidemiology*, **3**, 4.

186 Knight, G.C. (1963) Abnormalities and defects in pedigree dogs – III. Tibio-femoral joint deformity and patellar luxation. *Journal of Small Animal Practice*, **4** (6), 463–464.

187 Ness, M.G., Abercromby, R.H., May, C. *et al.* (1996) A survey of orthopaedic conditions in small animal veterinary practice in Britain. *Veterinary and Comparative Orthopaedics and Traumatology*, **9** (2), 43–52.

188 Roush, J.K. (1993) Canine patellar luxation. *Veterinary Clinics of North America: Small Animal Practice*, **23** (4), 855–868.

189 Schulz, K. (2007) Diseases of the joints: medial patellar luxation, in *Small Animal Surgery*, 3rd edn. (ed. T.W. Fossum), Mosby Elsevier, St. Louis, pp. 1289–1296.

190 Dokic, Z., Lorinson, D., Weigel, J.P., and Vezzoni, A. (2015) Patellar groove replacement in patellar luxation with severe femoro-patellar osteoarthritis. *Veterinary and Comparative Orthopaedics and Traumatology*, **28** (2), 124–130.

191 Remedios, A.M., Basher, A.W., Runyon, C.L., and Fries, C.L. (1992) Medial patellar luxation in 16 large dogs. A retrospective study. *Veterinary Surgery*, **21** (1), 5–9.

192 Hayes, A.G., Boudrieau, R.J., and Hungerford, L.L. (1994) Frequency and distribution of medial and lateral patellar luxation in dogs: 124 cases (1982–1992). *Journal of the American Veterinary Medical Association*, **205** (5), 716–720.

193 Gibbons, S.E., Macias, C., Tonzing, M.A. *et al.* (2006) Patellar luxation in 70 large breed dogs. *Journal of Small Animal Practice*, **47** (1), 3–9.

194 LaFond, E., Breur, G.J., and Austin, C.C. (2002) Breed susceptibility for developmental orthopedic diseases in dogs. *Journal of the American Animal Hospital Association*, **38** (5), 467–477.

195 Priester, W.A. (1972) Sex, size, and breed as risk factors in canine patellar dislocation. *Journal of the American Veterinary Medical Association*, **160** (5), 740.

196 Palmer, R.H. (2005) *Diagnosing Cranial Cruciate Ligament Pathology*, http://veterinarymedicine. dvm360.com/diagnosing-cranial-cruciate-ligament-pathology (accessed 2 May 2016).

197 Taylor-Brown, F.E., Meeson, R.L., Brodbelt, D.C. *et al.* (2015) Epidemiology of cranial cruciate ligament disease diagnosis in dogs attending primary-care veterinary practices in England. *Veterinary Surgery*, **44** (6), 777–783.

198 Comerford, E.J., Smith, K., and Hayashi, K. (2011) Update on the aetiopathogenesis of canine cranial cruciate ligament disease. *Veterinary and Comparative Orthopaedics and Traumatology*, **24** (2), 91–98.

199 Molsa, S.H., Hyytiainen, H.K., Hielm-Bjorkman, A.K., and Laitinen-Vapaavuori, O.M. (2014) Long-term functional outcome after surgical repair of cranial cruciate ligament disease in dogs. *BMC Veterinary Research*, **10**, 266.

200 Witsberger, T.H., Villamil, J.A., Schultz, L.G. *et al.* (2008) Prevalence of and risk factors for hip dysplasia and cranial cruciate ligament deficiency in dogs. *Journal of the American Veterinary Medical Association*, **232** (12), 1818–1824.

201 Buote, N., Fusco, J., and Radasch, R. (2009) Age, tibial plateau angle, sex, and weight as risk factors for contralateral rupture of the cranial cruciate ligament in Labradors. *Veterinary Surgery*, **38** (4), 481–489.

202 Macias, C., McKee, W.M., and May, C. (2002) Caudal proximal tibial deformity and cranial cruciate ligament rupture in small-breed dogs. *Journal of Small Animal Practice*, **43** (10), 433–438.

203 Doverspike, M., Vasseur, P.B., Harb, M.F., and Walls, C.M. (1993) Contralateral cranial cruciate ligament rupture – incidence in 114 dogs. *Journal of the American Animal Hospital Association*, **29** (2), 167–170.

204 Powers, M.Y., Martinez, S.A., Lincoln, J.D. *et al.* (2005) Prevalence of cranial cruciate ligament rupture in a population of dogs with lameness previously attributed to hip dysplasia: 369 cases (1994–2003). *Journal of the American Veterinary Medical Association*, **227** (7), 1109–1111.

205 Slauterbeck, J.R., Pankratz, K., Xu, K.T. *et al.* (2004) Canine ovariohysterectomy and orchiectomy increases the prevalence of ACL injury. *Clinical Orthopaedics and Related Research*, **429**, 301–305.

206 Duval, J.M., Budsberg, S.C., Flo, G.L., and Sammarco, J.L. (1999) Breed, sex, and body weight as risk factors for rupture of the cranial cruciate ligament in young dogs. *Journal of the American Veterinary Medical Association*, **215** (6), 811–814.

207 Schulz, K. (2007) Diseases of the joints: cranial cruciate ligament rupture, in *Small Animal Surgery*, 3rd edn. (ed. T.W. Fossum), Mosby Elsevier, St. Louis, pp. 1254–1275.

208 Voss, K., Langley-Hobbs, S.J., and Montavon, P.M. (2009) Stifle joint, in *Feline Orthopedic Surgery and Musculoskeletal Disease* (eds. P.M. Montavon, K. Voss, and S.J. Langley-Hobbs), Saunders Elsevier, St. Louis, pp. 475–490.

209 Scott, H. and McLaughlin, R. (2006) *Feline Orthopedics*, Manson Publishing, London.

210 Thomson, M. (2006) The cat with lameness, in *Problem-Based Feline Medicine* (ed. J. Rand), Saunders Elsevier, Edinburgh, pp. 976–991.

211 Henderson, R.A. and Milton, J.L. (1978) Tibial compression mechanism – diagnostic aid in stifle injuries. *Journal of the American Animal Hospital Association*, **14** (4), 474–479.

212 Schulz, K. (2007) Diseases of the joints: collateral ligament injury, in in *Small Animal Surgery*, 3rd edn. (ed. T.W. Fossum), Mosby Elsevier, St. Louis, pp. 1280–1283.

213 Millis, D.L. and Mankin, J. (2014) Orthopedic and neurologic evaluation, in *Canine Rehabilitation and Physical Therapy*, 2nd edn. (eds. D.L. Millis, D. Levine, and R.A. Taylor), Saunders Elsevier, St. Louis, pp. 180–192.

214 Evans, H.E. (1993) Arthrology, in *Miller's Anatomy of the Dog*, 3rd edn. (ed. H.E. Evans), Saunders Elsevier, Philadelphia, pp. 219–257.

16

Evaluating the Nervous System of the Dog

16.1 Assessing Behavior and Mental Status

Neurologic dysfunction is not always restricted to loco-motion and gait. At its most subtle, neurologic dysfunction can involve abnormal behavior that is sporadic or owner-reported based upon observations witnessed within the home environment [1–4].

Owners may report that the patient is sleeping more or is less responsive to its environment. This is often assumed to be age-related. Clients may subscribe to the belief that the patient is "slowing down" and that reduced activity represents the patient's "new normal" when in fact the patient's mentation may be compromised [4].

Owners may report a decreased appetite that turns out not to be gastrointestinal-related. Rather, the history of inappetence and clarification as to what the owner is observing directly at home may lead the clinician down the path to suspect the onset of cervical pain: it may be that the patient is unable or unwilling to lower its neck to reach the food bowl [4].

Owners may present the patient for presumptive otitis externa as a result of head-shaking, scratching at the ear, and facial rubbing that in fact may reflect underlying neuropathic pain as from Chiari-like malformation and syringomyelia in King Charles Cavalier Spaniels [5–8].

Owners may make note of odd, isolated episodes of licking and biting at the air as if at an imaginary object that is suggestive of fly-catching syndrome [9–11], an idiopathic neurologic-based disorder that may be epilepsy based [11], obsessive–compulsive [12], or dyskinetic, as from an extrapyramidal lesion [9].

Owners may report a sudden behavioral change, typically representative of extremes: either full-out aggression or a complete retreat from all household activity. This may be the first sign of intracranial neoplasia within the frontal lobe [13].

Historical data can be especially telling [13, 14] with regard to progression of underlying disease, and the client should be questioned in terms of:

- description of the behavior;
- onset;
- duration;
- frequency;
- time of day;
- apparent connection to other activities.

Owners should be encouraged to provide audiovisual recordings as able, especially when the observed behaviors are infrequent and unlikely to be present on physical examination.

After taking a thorough history, the clinician should make initial observations regarding the patient and its interactions within the examination room prior to physically examining the dog. Although the clinician may not witness some or all of the behaviors that were described by the client, the clinician may identify additional findings to augment or clarify the client's concerns [4, 15].

The clinician should determine if the patient is conscious [2, 15]. A conscious patient is said to be awake and aware of its surroundings [1, 14]. Note that the patient's response to the environment may vary, yet it may still be considered conscious. For instance, three very different patients may be hypervigilant, attentive, and quietly aware, yet all three states are compatible with consciousness (Figure 16.1).

It is important to recognize that an alert dog does not necessarily have to be interactive. An alert dog can be introverted and doing its best to avoid eye contact and being engaged with others in the same confined space. For example, a dog that is cowering under the chair of an examination room, pressing itself into the wall, is alert.

To help decide whether or not a dog is alert, the clinician should determine if it is responding appropriately to environmental stimuli. For instance, it would be abnormal for an anxious adult dog in a high-stress environment such as an examination room to sleep.

Consciousness is not all-or-nothing [1, 2, 14]: there is a sliding scale to qualify reductions in consciousness. In order of increasing severity, patients may be described as follows [2, 15]:

- depressed;
- obtunded;
- stuporous;
- comatose.

Performing the Small Animal Physical Examination, First Edition. Ryane E. Englar.
© 2017 John Wiley & Sons, Inc. Published 2017 by John Wiley & Sons, Inc.

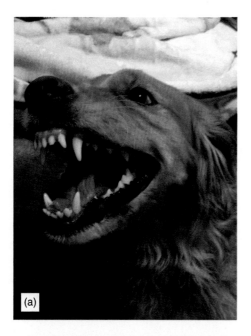

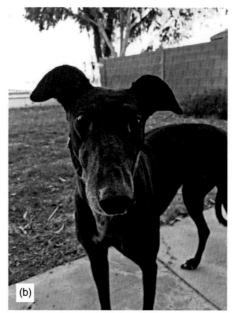

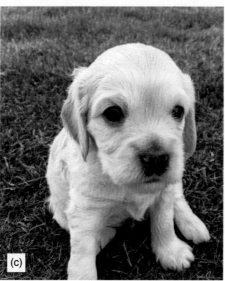

Figure 16.1 (a) Hypervigilant patient that is overstimulated to the point of reacting with aggression. Source: Courtesy of Christiana and Kaylee Otterson. (b) Attentive, alert patient in its home environment. Source: Courtesy of Meghan Teixeira and Matt Stait. (c) Quietly aware, yet conscious patient. Source: Courtesy of Nechama Bloom.

Review Section 8.1 to be able to differentiate between the levels of consciousness that are outlined here.

16.2 Assessing Posture

Posture should be taken into consideration relative to the age of the patient. At birth, puppies are able to lift their head; however, they are unable to maintain themselves in an upright posture until roughly 2 weeks of age [16, 17] (Figure 16.2).

Flexor tone predominates for the first few days of life, creating the classic comma shape that is characteristic of newborns [18, 19] (Figure 16.3).

Extensor dominance emerges by the time a puppy is 4–5 days old, and lasts for a little under a month. At that point, the puppy will no longer tolerate being held in suspension [16, 20].

By 1 month of age, the puppy's posture should mirror an adult's: the head and neck are held upright, with right- and left-sided symmetry, and the trunk should be held evenly without a unilateral tilt [1, 14]. Thereafter, when the patient is standing, the weight distribution between limbs should be roughly equal [1, 14]. The patient should also be bilaterally symmetrical in terms of posture.

Asymmetry may be subtle, but clinically important. The astute clinician should identify and note the presence of

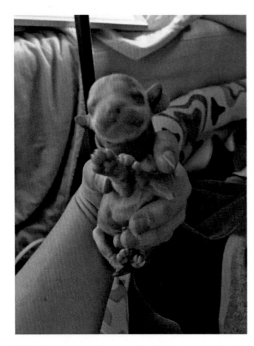

Figure 16.2 This 1-day-old puppy is able to raise its head. Source: Courtesy of Nechama Bloom.

a head tilt, the direction of the head tilt, and whether or not there is concurrent facial asymmetry.

In a dog, a head tilt could be caused by a large number of differentials:

- Severe otitis externa [21].
- Inflammatory middle ear disease [21, 22].

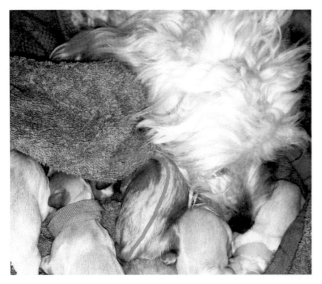

Figure 16.3 Note the predominant flexor tone of this 1-day-old puppy, which creates the classic comma shape that has been drawn in with blue to depict the curl of the spine. Source: Courtesy of Nechama Bloom.

- Ischemic injury as from a cerebrovascular accident or stroke [23–25].
- Vestibular disease [26–30]:
  - Peripheral
  - Central.
- Disorders of development and growth [31]:
  - Occipitoatlantoaxial malformations (OAAMs).
- Infectious disease:
  - Bacterial
    o Listeriosis [32]
    o Rickettsial bacteria such as *Ehrlichia* [33]
    o Streptococcal meningoencephalitis [34].
  - Fungal [35].
  - Viral
    o Rabies [36]
    o Pseudorabies, a type of herpesvirus [37].
- Granulomatous meningoencephalitis, a type of inflammatory disease of the central nervous system [38, 39].
- Endocrinopathy:
  - Hypothyroidism [40].
- Trauma, such as being hit by a car [41].
- Neoplasia, such as trigeminal nerve tumors [42, 43] and brain tumors [44, 45].

Note that not all of these differentials are diseases of the nervous system. Some are and some are not, and differentiating between them can be challenging. However, some basic tips may help to lump "like" differentials and rule out others.

For instance, when head tilts are related to underlying vestibular disease, the patient may present with concurrent ataxia or nystagmus. In classic, unilateral vestibular disease, the head tilt is ipsilateral to the lesion. However, if vestibular disease is bilateral, the head tilt may be extinguished [46].

Furthermore, in patients with both a head tilt and circling behavior, vestibular disease is less likely and thalamic and cerebral diseases must be prioritized [14, 46].

For these reasons, a thorough neurologic examination is key to ruling in probable diagnoses, by picking up on additional clues that, when paired with a head tilt, may explain the presentation of the patient.

A head tilt is not the only abnormality in posture that may be present on physical examination. Neck posture could deviate from the norm. See Section 15.2.1 to review musculoskeletal reasons that could affect neck posture. Cervical ventroflexion, in particular, was discussed. Additional non-neurologic causes for the cervical region to appear misshapen are congenital malformations or acquired orthopedic disease. For instance, abnormal shaping of the vertebral column can lead to [1]

- scoliosis, sideways deviation in the spinal column;
- kyphosis, a dorsal deviation in the spinal column;
- lordosis, a ventral deviation in the spinal column.

By contrast, when neck posture abnormalities are due to neurologic dysfunction, the neck is often twisted rather than simply deviated in a state referred to as torticollis [14].

Alternatively, patients may have a normal head and neck posture, yet position one or more limbs in space abnormally. In these cases, a more thorough investigation of the affected limb is required by means of palpation and postural reflexes to assist with lesion localization [13].

Abnormal postures are not isolated to weight-bearing, standing patients. Patients that are recumbent are also subject to changes in posture that are easily recognized and, when present, denote serious neurologic dysfunction [14, 15]. Recall from Section 8.2 that [14, 15]:

- Extension of all limbs in recumbency, with or without opisthotonus, head and neck dorsiflexion, is characteristic of a brain stem lesion, and is referred to as decerebrate rigidity.
- Thoracic limb extension with hip flexion and opisthotonus is characteristic of acute cerebellar injury and is referred to as decerebellate rigidity.
- Thoracic limb extension with bilateral pelvic limb paralysis is characteristic of thoracolumbar spinal segment injury and is referred to as the Schiff–Sherrington posture.

16.3 Assessing Coordination and Gait

Review the discussion in Section 8.3 regarding what is necessary for a patient to generate a gait. As described there, a normal gait should be smooth, strong, and even. Forelimb stride should be roughly equivalent to hind limb stride. Foot placement should be solid, without hesitation, and crisp, meaning that each foot strikes the ground and comes up off the ground without the dorsal surface of the paw knuckling [14].

Subtle gait changes are most easily detected when the patient makes tight turns or sudden movements [13, 14]. This is much easier to reproduce in dogs than cats because directional movement in the dog can be heavily guided by the handler who is holding the leash.

When gait changes are noted, the clinician should record the following:

- The limb(s) involved.
- Whether or not there is a component of weakness [13, 15] (see Section 8.3 to review associated terms):
  - If so, does the weakness stem from the lower motor neuron (LMN), meaning that the patient has difficulty supporting weight?
  - Or does the weakness stem from the upper motor neuron (UMN), meaning that the patient can support weight, but has a delay in the swing phase of the gait?

- Whether the perceived weakness is linked to exertion [13].
- Whether or not there is a component of paralysis [13, 15] (see Section 8.3. to review associated terms).
- The quality of the gait.

The clinician should ask whether the gait appears to be coordinated. Gait incoordination that is not attributed to weakness is referred to as ataxia [2, 14]. Recall from Section 8.3 that there are three main categories of ataxia [14, 15]:

1) cerebellar ataxia;
2) vestibular ataxia;
3) proprioceptive or sensory ataxia.

Cerebellar ataxia stems from underlying cerebellar disease that results in an abnormal rate, range, or force of movement. A classic example of cerebellar ataxia is the "toy soldier" gait, where the patient has a very stilted, high-stepping, over-reaching gait, each step of which may also demonstrate exaggerated flexion [13].

Vestibular ataxia reflects a true lack of balance. This may be due to peripheral vestibular disease, as in medical conditions that involve the tympanic bulla, or central vestibular disease, as occurs when lesions arise at the cerebello-ponto-medullary angle [46].

When unilateral vestibular disease is present, the patient will lean, drift, or fall toward one side. This may be overt or subtle. The patient may simply try to lean against the examination room wall as it walks to "hold itself up." A head tilt may or may not be present [14, 46]. When vestibular disease is bilateral, the patient tends to be reluctant to move and classically presents with wide, side-to-side swaying of the head and neck [14, 46].

Proprioceptive or sensory ataxia occurs when there is a lesion in the peripheral nerve, dorsal root, spinal cord, or brain stem. This adversely affects the patient's ability to sense where its limbs are positioned in space. As a result, the patient appears to be clumsy and exceptionally uncoordinated. Clients may say that their dog appears to be intoxicated. Dogs with this type of ataxia will typically try to stand with a wide base to attempt stability. They also often exhibit knuckling with or without concurrent paresis [14, 46].

16.4 Assessing Postural Reactions

Postural reactions supplement gait analysis by confirming that the patient knows where its head and neck, body, and feet are relative to each other in space. In order for the dog to have a spatial sense of its own anatomy relative to its environment, all components of the nervous system must be intact and functionally communicating with one another. When there is dysfunction in one or more parts of the pathway, there will be deficits in one or more postural responses [2, 14].

Deficits in postural reactions may be more apparent to the veterinary student than the subtleties of gait analysis, which is why they are mentioned here [2, 14].

The most common postural reactions that are assessed in dogs are the same in cats [1, 2, 13–15]:

- proprioceptive positioning;
- placing response;
- hopping;
- hemi-walking;
- wheel-barrowing.

Although repetitive, the author feels that it is important to review postural reactions in depth because of the value of the information that they can provide.

Proprioceptive positioning is sometimes referred to as position sense [13] or the knuckling-over reflex [1]. This test requires the clinician to evaluate each foot. With the patient standing and supported, the clinician methodically grasps each paw, one at a time, and positions it such that the dorsal surface comes into contact with the ground. [1, 13–15, 47]:

- The front paws are most easily accessed from their respective side. For example, the left front paw is most accessible from the left side whereas the right front paw is most accessible from the right.
- The hind paws are most easily accessed when the veterinarian stands behind the patient with the patient facing away from the veterinarian.

Supporting the patient throughout the examination is essential. A patient may have normal proprioception but "fail" this test because of weakness. Supporting the patient eliminates the risk that weakness will yield inaccurate test results.

A patient with normal proprioception will "recognize" that the dorsum of the paw is not an appropriate anatomic position to maintain and will quickly right its paw so that the palmar or plantar aspect makes contact with the floor instead as is the normal posture of a standing dog [13, 15]. A patient with normal proprioception may even anticipate the clinician's attempt to place its paw in a way that does not anatomically feel right. The patient may even refuse to allow the paw to be misplaced on the floor [1, 13, 15]. By contrast, a patient that has one or more lesions along the reflex arc will not attempt to right the wrong, and will remain standing as is, trying to bear weight abnormally on the dorsal surface of the affected paw (Figure 16.4) [13, 15].

Knuckling is not pathognomonic for any one disease. Knuckling has been reported in the veterinary medical literature for a number of differentials, including the following:

- Vertebral canal compression, with associated compression of the spine, as from:
  - intervertebral disc disease (IVDD) [48, 49]

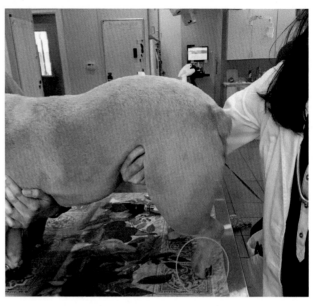

Figure 16.4 This patient is demonstrating abnormal knuckling of the left pelvic limb. Source: Courtesy of Shirley Yang, DVM.

  - cyst [50–52]
  - tumor [53].
- Infectious disease, such as canine distemper [54, 55].
- Prototheosis [56].
- Ischemic injury as from a cerebrovascular accident [23–25] or infarct [57].
- Fibrocartilaginous embolism [58].
- Degeneration:
  - of the axons [59]
  - of the articular facets [60].
- Neuroaxonal dystrophy [61], characterized by swelling of the axons.

Of these differentials, IVDD is commonplace in veterinary medicine as a surgical neurologic disease [62, 63]. IVDD involves one or more of the discs that sit between each vertebral body. Normal discs can be likened to a jelly donut: they have a gelatinous core called the nucleus pulposus, surrounded by a fibrous outer ring, the annulus fibrosus [63, 64]. The annulus fibrosus is on average twice as thick ventrally as dorsally such that the nucleus pulposus is not truly centered with the disc. Rather, the nucleus pulposus is eccentrically located. This may explain its tendency to herniate dorsally, toward the vertebral canal. The end result is disc extrusion, referred to as Hansen Type 1 IVDD [63–65].

As dogs age, their discs naturally degenerate [63, 66, 67]. Their water content decreases and, with it, some of their ability to withstand pressure [68, 69]. Disc degeneration progresses along the entire length of the spine, and occurs sooner in life in dogs that are chondrodystrophic: by 1 year of age, dogs such as Dachshunds will have easily lost three-quarters of their gelatinous nucleus pulposus [67–72].

The width of each disc varies depending upon their location along the spine. The narrowest discs occur between C2–C3 and L4–L5 [63, 73]. The widest discs occur between C4–C5, C5–C6, and L2–L3 [63, 73]. In general, cervical and lumbar discs are wider than thoracic discs [64, 67], and Dachshunds tend to have the widest discs of any breed [73].

Dachshunds also tend to have discs that calcify as they age. Depending upon the study, up to 90% of Dachshunds may develop such mineralization with an average of 2.3 calcified discs per dog [67, 69, 74, 75]. In particular, discs between T10–T13 are most likely to calcify and image radiographically [63, 74–77].

In addition to a change in the composition of the nucleus pulposus due to aging, the annulus fibrosus can also undergo degeneration. This tends to occur focally, as opposed to the entire length of the spine. Mineralization rarely occurs, and older, non-chondrodystrophic dogs are most at risk. The concern in these patients is that this type of degeneration causes the nucleus pulposus to push against the weakened annulus fibrosus. The end result is disc protrusion, referred to as Hansen Type 2 IVDD [63, 67, 69].

Small- to medium-sized dogs appear to be at an increased risk of developing IVDD, especially those that are chondrodystrophic [63, 78]. For example, the risk that a Dachshund carries for the development of IVDD is 12.6 times greater than in other breeds [78]. Of all cases of acute IVDD in dogs, Dachshunds represent 45–73% [67, 79–82], and 62% of certain lineages are expected to develop IVDD at some point in their lifetime [80, 81]. The Pekingese, Beagle, and Cocker Spaniel are also predisposed [78], and when IVDD occurs in the Beagle, it is 10 times more likely to target the cervical region than the thoracolumbar region [79]. Similarly, the cervical region is more likely to be implicated in cases of IVDD in the aged population than in the young [79].

It used to be thought, based upon postmortem evaluation, that Hansen Type 1 IVDD occurred primarily in chondrodystrophic breeds and Hansen Type 2 IVDD primarily in non-chondrodystrophic dogs and/or large breeds [67, 69]. Although it is true that chondrodystrophic breeds are less likely to develop Hansen Type 2 IVDD [69, 83, 84], large-breed dogs may develop both Hansen Type 1 and Type 2 IVDD. German Shepherds are predisposed to both presentations [85, 86]. In addition, among the large-breed dogs, Hansen Type 1 also occurs with greater frequency in Doberman Pinschers, Rottweilers, Dalmatians, and Labrador Retrievers [85–87].

Cervical disc disease represents up to one-quarter of all case presentations for IVDD [78, 79, 88]. Patients frequently present for neck-guarding with and without neurologic deficits, including knuckling [89–93]. Hansen Type 1 IVDD is more often implicated in this region of the spine [87]. In small-breed dogs, C3 is the most often reported disc to be affected [79, 87, 90–92] compared to C6–C7 in large-breed dogs [87]. On reviewing case reports of all dogs, regardless of size, C5–C6 [94] and C6–C7 predominate [90].

Thoracolumbar disc disease represents the majority of all case presentations for IVDD [78, 79, 88]. These patients guard their back and therefore may appear to be stiff in gait or even when just standing. They also may present with paraparesis or paraplegia, knuckling, and loss of deep pain [63]. When the thoracolumbar region of the spine is affected by IVDD, T12–T13 and T13–L1 are most often implicated in chondrodystrophic breeds [67, 79, 82, 95–102]. By contrast, T13–L1 and L1–L2 predominate followed by L2–L3 in large-breed dogs [85, 86].

Knuckling is an important clinical sign to note because it may indicate the development of IVDD. It may also spur the clinician to assess the patient for the presence or absence of deep pain, which if present indicates progression of IVDD in such a way that surgical management would be advised.

At the same time, it is important that the clinician does not have tunnel vision and recognizes that non-neurologic conditions can also cause knuckling, specifically [103]:

- osteoarthritis;
- hip dysplasia;
- cranial cruciate ligament rupture.

In these orthopedic-based conditions, there is knuckling, but without true proprioceptive deficits.

Ideally, each paw should be tested at least twice for proprioceptive deficits to be certain that the results are repeatable. The clinician should note whether the patient corrects or fails to correct each paw placement, and the clinician should be cognizant of the relative time it takes to right each foot. If one or more feet are sluggish compared with the others, the astute clinician should make a note of this in the medical record as it may assist with lesion localization.

Assessment of this reflex is technically easy and should be well tolerated by the veterinary patient in that it does not induce pain or discomfort. For cat-sized dogs that are intolerant of this test because they do not like having their feet touched, tactile and visual placement tests or hopping may be more fruitful [1, 2].

Recall from Section 8.4 that the tactile placement test is performed with the cat-sized patient held by the clinician, facing forwards, in front of a horizontal surface. The clinician covers the dog's eyes so that it cannot see what is directly in front of it. With the dog's visual field obstructed, the clinician then moves the dog toward the horizontal surface so that the dorsal aspects of its distal forelimbs come into contact with the table's edge. As soon as the dog contacts the table edge, it should respond by placing its paws on the table. Both forelimbs can be tested simultaneously, although occasionally a normal patient will not respond on the side that is being held. In this case, the patient should be re-tested holding the opposite side. Note that the test is primarily used to test the forelimbs – it is appreciably less reliable when used to assess the hind limbs [1, 14, 15, 104]. A patient that has proprioceptive deficits in the forelimbs is unlikely to replace its paws [1].

Recall from Section 8.4 that the visual placement test is identical with the tactile placement test with one exception: the patient's visual field is unobstructed. As the cat-sized dog is advanced toward the horizontal surface, it typically flexes its forelimbs in advance of contacting the table's edge, then extends both forelimbs to bear weight on the table's surface [1, 13, 15].

If the dog remains uncooperative, proprioception can be assessed by placing a sheet of paper under one foot of the standing dog. The clinician then slowly slides the paper away from being directly under the dog's body. A dog with normal proprioception will pull its foot back to a normal standing posture whereas a dog with an abnormal response will fall over in the direction in which the paper is moving [1].

Whereas both the tactile and visual placement tests are primarily associated with the forelimbs, the hopping test can be used to evaluate reliably both forelimb and hind limb function. The patient is lifted off the ground and supported with the exception of the limb being tested. That limb is then brought into contact with the floor, bearing the patient's weight as the limb is moved laterally. Because this sideways motion displaces the center of gravity of the patient, the patient "falls" toward the newly established center of gravity, causing a "hopping" motion in the normal patient [1, 13–15, 104]. Each limb should be tested and contralateral sides should be compared to detect subtle weakness and asymmetry.

Note that the patient's size represents the primary limitation. The author would be unable to hop a Great Dane!

Hemi-hopping, otherwise referred to as hemi-walking, is a variation of the hopping test that tests ipsilateral limbs concurrently. To test the patient's left forelimb and left hind limb, its right forelimb and right hind limb are lifted off the ground as it is pushed to the left. By contrast, to test the patient's right forelimb and right hind limb, its left forelimb and left hind limb are lifted off the ground as it is pushed to the right [13–15, 46, 104].

Wheel-barrowing is yet another variation of hopping that tests forelimbs or hind limbs concurrently [1, 13–15]:

- To test both forelimbs, the patient is supported under the abdomen. Without the hind limbs coming into contact with the ground, the patient is encouraged to move forward. In a normal patient, the forelimbs will alternate movements.

- To test both hind limbs, the patient is supported under each axillary region with its thoracic end raised so that the forelimbs do not come into contact with the ground. With the patient standing, in effect, upright on both hind limbs, it is encouraged to move backwards.

Abnormal patients will either stumble because they lose their foot placement or they will knuckle [13].

16.5 Assessing for Other Abnormal Movements

Involuntary movements tend to be of less clinical significance in veterinary patients than in human patients; however, these can be self-reported by the client or documented clinically. These so-called dyskinesias often have blurred definitions in the veterinary literature and may be difficult to describe because of perceived overlap between them [1, 14]. The three most commonly identified dyskinesias in veterinary medicine are

1) tremors;
2) tics;
3) myoclonus.

Tremors are rhythmic trembling of one or more body parts that involve antagonistic muscle groups. They may be focal or generalized. They may be triggered by metabolic disturbances such as hypocalcemia or they may be clinical signs of toxicosis as from mycotoxins or metaldehyde. Pharmacologic toxicosis is also possible such as through overdoses of phenylpropanolamine [14, 105].

Idiopathic head tremor syndrome (IHTS) has anecdotally been reported in the veterinary medical literature in a number of breeds, especially Doberman Pinschers, English Bulldogs, Boxers, and Labrador Retrievers [106–108]. The etiology of IHTS is poorly understood, and it is often misinterpreted as a seizure disorder [106, 107]. It is believed to be heritable in Doberman Pinschers, but the genetic link in other breeds has not yet been established [106, 109]. Stress is thought to precipitate and/or aggravate IHTS in nearly 50% of case presentations involving Doberman Pinschers [107]. In most cases, tremors are short-lived [106] and may be interrupted 66.7% of the time through client interaction with the patient in the form of verbal communication, tactile stimulation, or offering the patient a toy or treat [107]. Affected dogs tend to retain their alertness throughout episodes of IHTS, and although IHTS may be visibly distressing to a client, it is not painful and should not detract from quality of life [106]. In fact, many patients with IHTS experience spontaneous resolution of signs such that IHTS may only impact a patient for a fraction of its life for reasons that are beyond current understanding [106].

When tremors are associated with goal-oriented movement, as when a dog lowers its head into its food bowl, they are further categorized as intention tremors. Intention tremors in the dog may be due to:

- congenital cerebellar malformation such as cerebellar vermian hypoplasia or cerebellar agenesis [110, 111];
- infectious disease such as parvovirus [112];
- neurodegenerative disease such as cerebellar cortical abiotrophy [113, 114];
- metabolic storage disorders such as mucopolysaccharidosis [115] and gangliosidosis [116].

Intention tremors may also be idiopathic [117].

In contrast to a tremor, a tic is a contraction of one or more muscle groups. When they occur in veterinary patients, tics often involve the facial muscles.

Myoclonus is an exaggerated or violent tic, with an extremely intense, albeit brief, muscle contraction that results in a very pronounced jerking of the affected body part. Myoclonus may be seen in dogs that:

- are recovering from encephalitis secondary to canine distemper virus [14, 118, 119];
- are being induced and/or are recovering from anesthetic cocktails [120, 121];
- are experiencing an adverse reaction to an administered drug such as intrathecal administration of morphine [122, 123].

16.6 Evaluating the Spinal Reflexes

Recall from Section 8.6 that a reflex is an automatic, spontaneous response to a stimulus that is hard-wired into the body. The patient does not have to think about it for it to occur [2, 124].

At its most basic, a spinal reflex occurs when a peripheral receptor receives a stimulus. The receptor transmits the message to a sensory neuron that synapses with interneurons within an integration center – in this case, the spinal cord. The outcome is a "reply" sent via interneurons to a part of the body that can do something in response to the initial stimulus. The resultant action is effected by the motor neuron [124].

Spinal reflexes are considered to be normal only when all components of this "communication" are functional. There must be an intact pathway. If there is not, it is up to the clinician to determine which part of the pathway is "broken." When there is a "break" in the pathway, the quality of one or more reflexes may be impacted and observed on neurologic examination [13].

Abnormal reflexes may be described as [1, 14, 15]:

- exaggerated;
- weak;
- absent.

Recognizing the quality of the reflex compared with what is expected in a normal patient may help to assist with the localization of a neurologic lesion.

Note that reflexes may be impacted by patient stress or excitement. For example, exaggerated reflexes are common in hyperexcitable patients. If a reflex is exaggerated, yet the patient displays no deficits in postural reactions or gait, then the patient is likely to be normal [125].

Reflexes may also be impacted by age. For example, the patellar reflex is often diminished in senior dogs that are otherwise neurologically sound [126].

Another way to facilitate lesion localization is to break the spinal cord into various segments [2, 15]:

- C1–C5;
- C6–T2;
- T3–L3;
- L4–L6;
- L7–S3.

The segments are grouped in such a way that each cluster has a characteristic mix of neurologic signs [2, 14, 15]:

- C1–C5 lesions cause so-called upper motor neuron (UMN) signs in all four limbs. UMN signs are characterized by loss of muscle inhibition. This causes an increase in muscle tone and exaggerated reflexes.
- C6–T2 lesions cause mixed signs. The thoracic limbs demonstrate lower motor neuron (LMN) signs, characterized by decreased muscle tone and decreased to absent reflexes. In contrast, the pelvic limbs demonstrate UMN signs.
- T3–L3 lesions cause zero abnormalities in the thoracic limbs; however, they cause UMN signs in the pelvic limbs.
- L4–L6 lesions cause zero abnormalities in the thoracic limbs; however, they cause LMN signs in the pelvic limbs.
- L7–S3 lesions also cause LMN signs to the tail and perineum.

Different nerves are associated with each spinal segment cluster. Spinal reflexes can be used to test different spinal cord segments to assess the integrity of their associated nerves [2, 14, 15].

Note that not all reflexes are equally reliable. Some are much more difficult to elicit than others. Others rely on user ability and experience to improve the accuracy and reproducibility of the clinician's assessment. The two most reliable spinal reflexes that can be performed in the dog are [2]:

1) the patellar reflex;
2) the withdrawal or flexor reflex.

Both are present in the neonatal puppy; however, they may be difficult to appreciate [16].

There is not one right way to perform these reflexes. Depending upon where and by whom the clinician was trained, patient positioning may vary. It becomes less important that the dog is positioned in dorsal recumbency, as suggested by Garosi [2] and de Lahunta and Glass [104], or in lateral recumbency, as suggested by Thomas and Dewey [15]. Of greater significance is the repeatability of the results obtained when eliciting each reflex. Repeatability is more likely when both the clinician and patient are comfortable, and when the clinician has had extensive practice with eliciting each reflex in order to make an accurate determination as to its quality.

For both the patellar and the withdrawal reflexes, the author prefers that the dog be placed in lateral recumbency. The patellar reflex evaluates whether or not the femoral nerve and the associated L4–L6 segments of the spinal cord are intact. With the patient restrained in lateral recumbency, the clinician uses one hand to support the limb that is "up" by seating this hand under the medial thigh. The stifle of the "up" limb is positioned so that it is partially flexed. The clinician then uses his other hand to swing the plexor firmly and smoothly to make contact with the patellar ligament. The stifle should respond by automatically extending [2, 14, 15, 104].

If the patellar reflex is weak or absent, then a lesion is likely to be present within the femoral nerve itself or within the L4–L6 spinal segments. However, severe stifle disease can also result in the same weak or absent patellar reflex, reminding the clinician of the importance of evaluating the patient as a whole rather than taking into consideration only the results of the neurologic examination, which are not intended to stand alone. Accurate lesion localization requires the clinician to integrate all diagnostic findings to create a clinical picture that best fits a given patient [2].

If the patellar reflex is exaggerated and there are no concurrent abnormalities in gait and postural reactions, the patient is likely to be overexcited or tense, without true neurologic disease. However, an exaggerated patellar reflex in combination with other gait and postural deficits is likely suggestive of an UMN lesion cranial to L4 [2]. The patellar reflex may also appear to be exaggerated if the flexor muscles of the stifle, those that typically counteract stifle extension that is elicited in the reflex arc, have decreased tone as from a lesion within the sciatic nerve or spinal cord segments caudal to L6 [2].

The withdrawal reflex assesses the integrity of different nerves and different spinal segments depending upon whether it is performed on a thoracic or a hind limb. When performed in the thoracic limb, the withdrawal evaluates the C6–T2 spinal cord segments as well as the musculocutaneous, axillary, median, ulnar, and radial nerves. When performed in the hind limb, the withdrawal reflex evaluates the L7–S1 segments and the sciatic nerve. [2, 14, 15, 104].

With the patient restrained in lateral recumbency, the clinician pinches interdigital skin or a nail bed on each limb, one limb at a time, with the limb being tested held in extension. When the thoracic limb is tested, the patient should automatically respond by flexing the shoulder, elbow, and carpus to pull the limb away from the clinician. When the pelvic limb is tested, the patient should automatically respond by flexing the hip, stifle, and hock to pull the limb away from the clinician. The contralateral limb should be unaffected, meaning that if the right hind limb is evaluated for the withdrawal reflex, the left hind limb should not respond. If the contralateral limb extends when the opposite limb is being tested for the withdrawal reflex, an abnormal crossed-extensor reflex is present and requires further investigation [2, 14, 15, 104]. The only exception is in a newborn puppy up to 17 days of age, during which time a crossed extensor reflex can be considered normal [16, 127].

A third spinal reflex that should be performed in the neurologic examination of every patient, feline or canine, is the perineal or anal reflex. Recall that this assesses anal tone. To determine if there is appropriate tone, the clinician touches the anal rim with a gloved forefinger. An anus with normal tone will "wink" as the anal sphincters close. Decreased or absent tone is suggestive of a lesion in the S1–S3 segments or dysfunctional anal innervation from branches of the pudendal nerve [15]. In addition, the perineal reflex also results in flexion of the tail. Failure of the patient to tail-tuck suggests that there may be a lesion within the caudal spinal cord segments [15]. In a neonatal puppy up to 3 weeks of age, stimulation of the perineal region also triggers elimination [16].

A fourth spinal reflex that may be performed is the panniculus or cutaneous trunci reflex. The clinician uses a hemostat to gently pinch the skin lateral to the spine, beginning in the lumbosacral region and moving cranially, one vertebra at a time. Both the patient's left and right lateral sides should be tested. When performed in the normal patient, the panniculus reflex results in contraction of the cutaneous trunci muscles. This contraction will be evident as a twitch over the thoracolumbar region due to the integrity of the lateral thoracic nerve and C8–T1 spinal segments [14, 15]. If contraction of the cutaneous trunci muscles is not evident at a discrete cutoff point, then a lesion is likely to be present anywhere from one to four segments cranially [15].

Additional spinal reflexes may be tested in the dog, but are beyond the scope of this text given that their reliability and reproducibility are highly user dependent. In the thoracic limb, these include [2, 14, 15, 104]:

- the extensor carpi radialis or triceps reflex, which assesses the integrity of the radial nerve in the thoracic limb and C7–T1 spinal cord segments;
- the biceps reflex, which evaluates the spinal cord segments C6–C8 and also the musculocutaneous nerve.

In the pelvic limb, the author does not routinely test for the gastrocnemius reflex. This evaluates the sciatic nerve and primarily L7–S1 segments; however, this reflex is difficult to elicit in a normal patient, let alone one with neurologic dysfunction [15].

16.7 Assessing the Cranial Nerves

After evaluating the gait and postural reactions, the clinician typically assesses the cranial nerves [104]. Recall from Section 8.7 that there are 12 pairs of cranial nerves and that they are numbered in order from where they arise within the brain, from cranial to caudal [15]:

- CN I: the olfactory nerve.
- CN II: the optic nerve.
- CN III: the oculomotor nerve.
- CN IV: the trochlear nerve.
- CN V: the trigeminal nerve.
- CN VI: the abducent nerve.
- CN VII: the facial nerve.
- CN VIII: the vestibulocochlear nerve.
- CN IX: The glossopharyngeal nerve.
- CN X: the vagus nerve.
- CN XI: the accessory nerve.
- CN XII: the hypoglossal nerve.

Recall also from Section 8.7 that not all of the cranial nerve pairs are routinely tested during a routine physical examination.

16.7.1 Reviewing the Ocular Reflexes Associated with the Cranial Nerves

CN II is one of several components in the visual pathway that conveys the special sense of vision to a patient. For a patient to be visual, the dog must have a functional eye, retina, CN II, optic tract, and occipital cortex. To assess a patient's vision, the clinician may observe whether or not the patient visually tracks an object such as a cotton ball that is dropped from a height, as from a hand to the ground. This rudimentary test is effective at differentiating visual from avisual patients if the patient is alert, aware, and observant. However, it cannot establish the fineness of the patient's vision, the clarity and crispness of the patient's sight [13, 15].

Another rudimentary test of the patient's vision is to create an obstacle course or maze within the examination room or treatment area. The maze need not be extravagant – it may consist of a series of cardboard boxes or open cage doors. The purpose of the maze is to test an ambulatory patient's ability to navigate through the obstacles by observing them and changing course accordingly [13].

Pupil size is dependent upon a balance between sympathetic and parasympathetic pathways. The former is in many ways tied to the attitude and emotional status of the patient: stress as triggered by "fight or flight" tends to dilate both pupils due to abundant sympathetic stimulation. By contrast, parasympathetic pathways facilitate pupillary response to the amount of ambient light: strong light tends to induce pupillary constriction or miosis whereas low ambient lighting causes pupillary dilation or mydriasis. CN III has a parasympathetic component that is responsible for facilitating miosis [2].

Pupil size should be bilaterally symmetrical. When pupils are asymmetric, the patient is said to have anisocoria (Figure 16.5a). There are innumerable causes of anisocoria in the dog. However, broad categories of possible differentials include the following:

- central nervous system neoplasia such as meningioma or choroid plexus carcinoma [128, 129];
- cerebrovascular incident [130];
- parasitic disease such as tick paralysis [131];

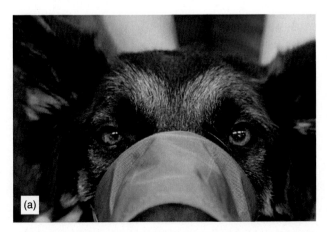
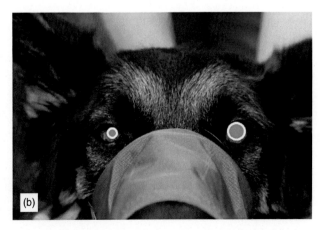

Figure 16.5 (a) This patient is demonstrating anisocoria. The right pupil is smaller than the left. (b) The same patient with the pupils drawn in to highlight the degree of asymmetry. Source (a), (b): Courtesy of Elizabeth Robbins, DVM.

- infectious disease such as rickettsial ehrlichiosis [132];
- eye contact with toxic plant *Datura stramonium* [133];
- drug toxicity such as bromism, an overdose of potassium bromide [134];
- parasympathetic denervation of the iris sphincter muscle [135, 136].

To elicit a pupillary light reflex (PLR), CN II and CN III must be functional. Recall from Section 3.2.8 that there are two variations of PLRs: direct and consensual. To perform a direct PLR, a bright light is shone into the eye that is being evaluated. If CN II and CN III are intact, then CN III will modulate entry of the light into the eye by constricting the pupil. A normal pupil should constrict in response to the light. In addition, the pupil of the contralateral eye should also constrict. This is referred to as the consensual PLR [1, 13, 15, 104].

PLRs are age-dependent. They are absent at birth, but they develop in puppies as early as 5–14 days of age [16].

PLRs can also be altered by anesthetic agents or combinations thereof. For example, injectable anesthetic agents, in particular a triple cocktail of atropine, xylazine, and ketamine, depress PLRs [137, 138].

PLRs are most often used in lesion localization for patients that present for apparent blindness. However, recall from Section 3.2.8 that positive PLRs do not guarantee that the patient is visual. Normal PLRs will be present in a patient that is cortically blind. This explains why multiple tests are required in order for lesion localization to be accurate [139, 140].

If the patient is visual yet lacks one or both PLRs and/or exhibits pupil asymmetry, then there is a lesion either in CN III or in the sympathetic innervation of the eye [13]. Horner's syndrome is an example of the latter and is characterized by miosis of the affected eye [141]. In addition, there is concurrent enophthalmos, ptosis (drooping of the upper eyelid), and a pronounced nictitating membrane [141].

When Horner's syndrome occurs in the dog, it is often idiopathic, particularly in the Golden Retriever [142–146]. When a cause for Horner's syndrome is identified, it may include the following [145, 146]:

- trauma to the head and neck;
- trauma to the brachial plexus;
- trauma to the inner ear, most often sustained during aggressive ear flushing;
- chronic otitis media;
- chronic otitis interna;
- intracranial neoplasia;
- intrathoracic neoplasia.

In addition to the PLR, the menace response tests the integrity of CN II in addition to CN VII. To perform the menace response, the clinician makes a threatening gesture toward each eye. A patient with a positive menace response must first see the threat and then blink as a protective function. It is important that the clinician takes care not to touch the eyelids themselves in the process or to create excessive air currents, because although the outcome may be the same (the patient blinks), it will be due to touch as a stimulus rather than vision [139, 140].

Puppies develop a menace response in both eyes during the first 4 weeks of life [16], although it may take until 2–3 months of age for it to become consistent [13].

One additional ocular reflex should be reviewed at this time. Recall the palpebral reflex, as discussed in Section 3.2.8. The palpebral reflex tests CN V and CN VII. The clinician touches the medial canthus of each eyelid. A neurologically normal dog with this reflex intact will blink due to tactile stimulation. In order to do so, the dog must first sense the clinician's contact via CN V and then blink via CN VII. [139, 140]

Puppies develop the palpebral reflex within the first 3 days of life [16].

16.7.2 Reviewing the Cranial Nerves Associated with Ocular Movement

Coordinated movement of the eyes is facilitated by CN III, IV, and VI [13, 15, 104], which innervate the extraocular muscles. Strabismus results when there is dysfunction in one or more of the extraocular muscles. The resulting misalignment between the eyes prevents them from directing their gaze at the same point in space at the same time. As a result, binocular vision and depth perception may be compromised [147–150].

In veterinary medicine, strabismus typically stems from underlying neuropathy. The direction of the strabismus confers which cranial nerve is impacted:

- Ventrolateral strabismus involves CN III.
- Rotatory strabismus involves CN IV.
- Medial strabismus involves CN VI.

Strabismus can occur in one or both eyes. Unlike cats, in which strabismus is common and may be breed-related, particularly in Siamese cats [139, 151–153], dogs tend not to have strabismus unless there is an underlying medical condition. For example, canine strabismus may result from retrobulbar masses or abscesses [154, 155]. Rarely are there congenital defects such as osteoma cutis: the presence of bone within the eyelid distorts the eye's ability to conform to the globe and ultimately results in strabismus [156].

16.7.3 Reviewing the Cranial Nerves Associated with Tactile Sensation

The role of CN V in the sensory portion of the palpebral reflex via its ophthalmic branch has already been reviewed. In this reflex, CN V is responsible for sensing tactile stimulation at the level of the medial canthus.

The ophthalmic branch of CN V can also be assessed when the clinician touches a saline-moistened cotton-tipped applicator to the cornea. This so-called corneal reflex requires the ophthalmic branch of CN V to recognize tactile stimulation, which then alerts CN VI to retract the globe [15].

CN V is also responsible for detecting tactile sensation in other regions of the face. For instance, facial sensation can be assessed by taking the tips of a hemostat or cotton-tipped applicator and touching the nasal septum. A patient with an intact maxillary branch of CN V will pull away from the stimulus. A patient that does not attempt to escape the stimulus likely has a lesion in the maxillary branch of CN V [15].

The maxillary branch of CN V can also be assessed when the upper lip adjacent to the maxillary canine tooth is pinched. The author makes use of this technique much less commonly in the dog because in her opinion it is more aversive than the aforementioned technique and is more likely to result in fractious behavior on the part of the patient [15]. For similar reasons, the author does not tend to test the mandibular branch of CN V: the lower lip adjacent to the mandibular canine tooth is pinched and the patient is expected to withdraw its head [15].

16.7.4   Reviewing the Cranial Nerves Associated with Muscle Movement Other than Ocular

CN V, VII, and XI innervate select muscle groups within the body. When these muscles exhibit changes in form or function, their associated cranial nerves may be implicated [15]:

- The muscles of mastication are innervated by CN V. Dysfunction within CN V may lead to atrophy of the temporalis or masseter muscles or a weak or "dropped" jaw.
- The positions of the eyelids and lip folds are innervated by CN VII. If ptosis is present or if lip folds are droopy, dysfunction of CN VII may be considered.
- The trapezius muscle, which straddles the dorsal shoulder and upper back, is innervated by CN XI. Dysfunction of this nerve will lead to atrophy of this muscle. However, this atrophy may be so subtle that it is rarely, if ever, appreciated in the affected patient.

16.7.5   Reviewing the Cranial Nerves Associated with Digestion

CN IX, X, and XII assist with digestion. When these digestive functions are observed to be dysfunctional by either the client or the clinician on physical examination, their associated cranial nerves may be implicated [15]:

- CN IX and X help to coordinate the swallowing reflex. Patients with deficits in one or both of these nerves

may have a client-reported history of dysphagia or regurgitation. In the dog, a finger is often advanced into the caudal pharyngeal region to elicit a gag in order to confirm that both nerves are functional.
- The tongue is innervated by CN XII. A patient with a deficit in this nerve may have difficulty lapping up water or prehending food. The patient may also have "tongue droop," meaning that the tongue involuntarily hangs out of the mouth. The author may grab the tongue of a canine patient with gauze to assess tongue strength. If the tongue is weak, there may be dysfunction within CN XII.

16.7.6   Reviewing the Cranial Nerves Associated with Maintaining Posture

The vestibular portion of CN VIII helps the body to maintain itself in equilibrium. The patient is able to sense changes in head position without losing balance. The patient is also able to keep images focused on the retina when the head is turning by moving the eyes in the opposite direction to the head due to coordination between the eyes and the vestibular apparatus [15].

A patient with a dysfunctional vestibular portion of CN VIII may exhibit a head tilt, abnormal (rather than physiologic) nystagmus, or ataxia with a broad-based stance.

16.8   Assessing Nociception

Recall from Section 8.8 that nociception refers to the patient's perception of pain as an aversive experience that can result from either an actual or an anticipated stimulus [157–160]. Perception of pain is unique to the individual [160]. Pain perception may be influenced by the patient's age, health status, and past experiences [158]. Pain may be acute or chronic; it may also be additive [160]. Furthermore, pain is not just the immediate sensation, but also the after-effects: how pain alters the patient's emotional status becomes equally important [159–161].

Veterinary patients present a challenge to clinicians because they cannot articulate in words recognizable in the human language what it is that they are experiencing. Human patients can identify and convey the timeline of pain (onset, duration, progression), the intensity of the pain, and the pain's characteristics (stabbing, burning, throbbing, tingling, etc.). Veterinary patients rely upon owners and the veterinary team to pick up on behavioral or other observational cues that may be suggestive that pain exists [159, 160].

The burden is therefore on the clinician to anticipate, recognize, intervene, manage, and reevaluate pain not just during surgical procedures or hospital stays, but at each and every visit [160, 161]. This has been referred to in the medical literature as the PLATTER approach [161]:

- **PL**an;
- **A**nticipate;
- **T**rea**T**;
- **E**valuate;
- **R**eturn.

This acronym serves as an important reminder that to manage pain effectively, the clinician must invest in a patient-tailored plan that is revised as needed rather than falling back upon the old-school, cookie-cutter approach to pharmacologic therapy. Drugs may still represent one appropriate arm of therapy. However, effective pain management may also need to take into consideration proper nursing care, gentle handling, behavioral therapy, exercise, nutrition and weight management, range of motion exercises and other physiotherapy, therapeutic laser, and other complementary modalities [158].

Pain used to be considered an afterthought, but is now considered to be as important to every patient as obtaining the temperature, pulse, and respiratory rate. Some practices have automatically inserted it into the medical record as the fourth vital sign [160, 161].

Review Section 8.8 to recall some of the more frequently employed pain scales in veterinary medicine, including the Melbourne Pain Scale [162, 163] and the composite scale that was created by Colorado State University Veterinary Teaching Hospital [164, 165]. These assess canine posture, activity, mental status, vocalization, and response to palpation to create an understanding of the potential for pain in any given patient.

When considering pain recognition in dogs and cats, pupil size, heart rate, and respiratory rate are inconsistent. Behavior is still considered to be the superior indicator [160, 166].

Understanding the patient's "normal" behavior is critical to the identification of new behaviors, particularly those that are consistently out of character. For example, a dog that is consistently people-friendly within the clinic environment should be flagged as a potential concern if that same dog suddenly disengages, hides itself from observers, and/or resorts to defensive aggression [160].

Additional behavior changes that may reflect underlying pain in dogs include changes in activity, changes in appetite, the guarding of surgical wounds, and changes in elimination habits [160].

Posture can be a significant behavioral cue. A canine patient that is curled up, sleeping, in a normal position is less likely to be in pain than a dog that is hunched up under itself, particularly if the tucked up-dog is attempting to disappear from sight. This dog may be experiencing psychologic pain as from stress or true physical pain, particularly if it is observed to be hunched in the

postoperative period. Additional postural cues that may be indicative of pain in a dog is a head held low, or a patient that is constantly shifting weight from one limb to another [160].

Facial expressions can be telling when it comes to recognizing pain or the potential for pain in the clinic setting. Dogs that exhibit a furrowed brow, tense facial muscles, flattened ears, and drawn-back lips may be in pain and/or anxious [159].

The utility of composite scales is that they are technically easy to use and encourage the veterinary team to rely heavily on observation – not just once, but at repeated intervals – emphasizing again the importance of continuity of care. Few scales have been assessed for validity and reliability. At this point, it likely matters less which scale is used in a clinical setting and more that pain is being considered in each and every veterinary patient, not just those undergoing surgery [160].

Composite scales also paint a more complete picture of patient well-being by evaluating multiple criteria rather than just one. The clinician is more likely to identify areas where the patient deviates from its norm because more aspects of the patient are observed and recorded.

For example, let us consider three separate patients with three different locations of physical pain that can be induced by various maneuvers in the physical examination:

- A dog with structural brain disease demonstrates a pain response when the clinician applies firm and constant pressure on the skull just above the zygomatic arch.
- A dog with neck pain resists movement of the neck in the direction that elicits pain.
- A dog with a lumbosacral lesion reacts painfully when firm, downward pressure is applied to the sacrum.

Despite the fact that pain is present in all three dogs, the pain response between them is likely to vary. Not all dogs may react in the same way, and not all dogs may experience the the same intensity of pain. If all three dogs in the scenario outlined were painful, yet only one criterion was observed, one or more dogs may be wrongly labeled as non-painful.

By using composite scales to observe more variables, the definition of what constitutes pain is broadened. This allows the astute clinician to recognize that pain is expressed in multiple forms that may include, but are not limited to:

- The patient attempting to escape.
- The patient's attention being drawn to the area that was touched. A patient that was looking away from the clinician may suddenly turn its head in the clinician's direction.

- The patient vocalizing (growling, crying, whimpering, whining).
- The patient attempting to physically harm the clinician.

Moreover, the repeated use of composite scales in the same patient over time helps to improve the veterinary team's understanding of how each patient responds to external and internal stimuli, and how medical intervention in response to the perceived pain has impacted the extent of the painful response that the patient is displaying.

In addition to making use of composite scales, it is important that clinicians test the intactness of pain pathways, from a neurologic perspective, to assess whether aversive stimuli are making it through the spinal cord as signals to the brain, where they are consciously perceived. A failure to perceive pain is informative and may help the clinician to localize the lesion by identifying where the signal is successfully received in the patient versus where it is not.

When clinicians test the integrity of pain pathways, they are interested in two different types of pain [1, 15]:

1) superficial pain;
2) deep pain.

Recall that superficial pain originates in the skin. To test a patient's perception of superficial pain, the clinician uses a hemostat to grasp a skin fold at the site of interest. The clinician waits for the patient to settle, then gradually increases the "squeeze" of the hemostat to pinch the skin. Pinching ceases as soon as the patient provides an appropriate response [1, 15]:

- The patient may twitch the skin.
- The patient may react vocally.
- The patient may try to bite.
- The patient may try to escape.

All of these responses are indicative that the noxious event was felt.

In contrast to superficial pain, deep pain arises deep to the skin and its pathways are less likely to be damaged than those at the body's surface. Accordingly, deep pain is only tested when the patient fails to respond to the clinician's attempts to elicit a superficial pain test [1, 15].

To assess a patient's ability to perceive deep pain, the clinician begins by pinching the toes or the tail with his fingers. If this elicits no response, the clinician graduates from using fingertips to a hemostat. As with the superficial pain test, the clinician gradually increases the "squeeze" of the hemostat to pinch with incrementally greater force to elicit a response. A limb withdrawal is not enough; this merely tells the clinician that the reflex is intact. The clinician is looking for the patient to react by turning its head in the direction of the stimulus, vocalizing, or attempting to bite [1, 15].

The absence of deep pain, as from severe spinal cord compression or other lesions, is suggestive of severe damage at the level of the spinal cord and carries a guarded prognosis for recovery.

References

1 van Nes, J.J., Meij, B.P., and van Ham, L. (2009) Nervous system, in *Medical History and Physical Examination in Companion Animals* (eds. A. Rijnberk and F.J. van Sluijs), Saunders Elsevier, St. Louis, pp. 160–174.
2 Garosi, L. (2009) Neurological examination of the cat. How to get started. *Journal of Feline Medicine and Surgery*, **11** (5), 340–348.
3 Chrisman, C.L. (2006) The neurologic examination. *Clinician's Brief*, January, 11–16.
4 Sammut, V. (2005) *Skills Laboratory, Part 1: Performing a Neurologic Examination*, http://veterinarymedicine.dvm360.com/skills-laboratory-part-1-performing-neurologic-examination (accessed 16 January 2016).
5 Plessas, I.N., Rusbridge, C., Driver, C.J. *et al.* (2012) Long-term outcome of Cavalier King Charles spaniel dogs with clinical signs associated with Chiari-like malformation and syringomyelia. *Veterinary Record*, **171**(20), 501.
6 Rusbridge, C., Carruthers, H., Dube, M.P. *et al.* (2007) Syringomyelia in cavalier King Charles spaniels: the relationship between syrinx dimensions and pain. *Journal of Small Animal Practice*, **48** (8), 432–436.

7 Rusbridge, C., MacSweeny, J.E., Davies, J.V. *et al.* (2000) Syringohydromyelia in Cavalier King Charles spaniels. *Journal of the American Animal Hospital Association*, **36** (1), 34–41.
8 Rusbridge, C. (1997) Persistent scratching in Cavalier King Charles spaniels. *Veterinary Record*, **141** (7), 179.
9 Wrzosek, M., Plonek, M., Nicpon, J. *et al.* (2015) Retrospective multicenter evaluation of the "fly-catching syndrome" in 24 dogs: EEG, BAER, MRI, CSF findings and response to antiepileptic and antidepressant treatment. *Epilepsy & Behavior*, **53**, 184–189.
10 Cash, W.C., and Blauch, B.S. (1979) Jaw snapping syndrome in eight dogs. *Journal of the American Veterinary Medical Association*, **175** (7), 709–710.
11 Manteca, X. (1994) Fly snapping syndrome in dogs. *Veterinary Quarterly*, **16** (Suppl.), 49.
12 Overall, K.L. and Dunham, A.E. (2002) Clinical features and outcome in dogs and cats with obsessive–compulsive disorder: 126 cases (1989–2000). *Journal of the American Veterinary Medical Association*, **221** (10), 1445–1452.
13 Averill, D.R., Jr. (1981) The neurologic examination. *Veterinary Clinics of North America: Small Animal Practice*, **11** (3), 511–521.

14 Thomas, W.B. (2000) Initial assessment of patients with neurologic dysfunction. *Veterinary Clinics of North America: Small Animal Practice*, **30** (1), 1–24, v.

15 Thomas, W.B. and Dewey, C.W. (2008) Performing the neurologic examination, in *A Practical Guide to Canine and Feline Neurology*, 2nd edn. (ed. C.W. Dewey), Wiley-Blackwell, Ames, IA, pp. 53–74.

16 Lavely, J.A. (2006) Pediatric neurology of the dog and cat. *Veterinary Clinics of North America: Small Animal Practice*, **36** (3), 475–501, v.

17 Fox, M.W. (1963) Conditioned reflexes and the innnate behaviour of the neonate dog. *Journal of Small Animal Practice*, **4**, 85–99.

18 Kustritz, M.V.R. (2011) History and physical examination of the neonate, in *Small Animal Pediatrics: The First 12 Months of Life* (eds. M.E. Peterson and M.A. Kutzler), Saunders Elsevier, St. Louis, pp. 20–27.

19 Hoskins, J.D. and Partington, B.P. (2001) Physical examination and diagnostic imaging procedures, in *Veterinary Pediatrics: Dogs and Cats from Birth to Six Months*, 3rd edn. (ed. J.D. Hoskins), Saunders Elsevier, Philadelphia, pp. 6–7.

20 Breazile, J.E. (1978) Neurologic and behavioral development in the puppy. *Veterinary Clinics of North America: Small Animal Practice*, **8**, 109–112.

21 Mason, L.K., Harvey, C.E., and Orsher, R.J. (1988) Total ear canal ablation combined with lateral bulla osteotomy for end-stage otitis in dogs. Results in thirty dogs. *Veterinary Surgery*, **17** (5), 263–268.

22 Little, C.J.L., Lane, J.G., Gibbs, C., and Pearson, G.R. (1991) Inflammatory middle-ear disease of the dog – the clinical and pathological features of cholesteatoma, a complication of otitis-media. *Veterinary Record*, **128** (14), 319–322.

23 Thomsen, B., Garosi, L., Skerritt, G. *et al.* (2016) Neurological signs in 23 dogs with suspected rostral cerebellar ischaemic stroke. *Acta Veterinaria Scandinavica*, **58** (1), 40.

24 Joseph, R.J., Greenlee, P.G., Carrillo, J.M., and Kay, W.J. (1988) Canine cerebrovascular disease – clinical and pathological findings in 17 cases. *Journal of the American Animal Hospital Association*, **24** (5), 569–576.

25 Wessmann, A., Chandler, K., and Garosi, L. (2009) Ischaemic and haemorrhagic stroke in the dog. *Veterinary Journal*, **180** (3), 290–303.

26 Schunk, K.L. (1988) Disorders of the vestibular system. *Veterinary Clinics of North America: Small Animal Practice*, **18** (3), 641–665.

27 Rossmeisl, J.H., Jr. (2010) Vestibular disease in dogs and cats. *Veterinary Clinics of North America: Small Animal Practice*, **40** (1), 81–100.

28 Kornegay, J.N. (1991) Ataxia, head tilt, nystagmus. Vestibular diseases. *Problems in Veterinary Medicine*, **3** (3), 417–425.

29 Troxel, M.T., Drobatz, K.J., and Vite, C.H. (2005) Signs of neurologic dysfunction in dogs with central versus peripheral vestibular disease. *Journal of the American Veterinary Medical Association*, **227** (4), 570–574.

30 Garosi, L.S., Lowrie, M.L., and Swinbourne N.F. (2012) Neurological manifestations of ear disease in dogs and cats. *Veterinary Clinics of North America: Small Animal Practice*, **42** (6), 1143–1160.

31 Cerda-Gonzalez, S. and Dewey, C.W. (2010) Congenital diseases of the craniocervical junction in the dog. *Veterinary Clinics of North America: Small Animal Practice*, **40** (1), 121–141.

32 Pritchard, J.C., Jacob, M.E., Ward, T.J. *et al.* (2016) *Listeria monocytogenes* septicemia in an immunocompromised dog. *Veterinary Clinical Pathology*, **45** (2), 254–259.

33 Goodman, R.A., Hawkins, E.C., Olby, N.J. *et al.* (2003) Molecular identification of *Ehrlichia ewingii* infection in dogs: 15 cases (1997–2001). *Journal of the American Veterinary Medical Association*, **222** (8), 1102–1107.

34 Irwin, P.J. and Parry, B.W. (1999) Streptococcal meningoencephalitis in a dog. *Journal of the American Animal Hospital Association*, **35** (5), 417–422.

35 Simpson, K.W., Khan, K.N.M., Podell, M. *et al.* (1993) Systemic mycosis caused by *Acremonium* sp in a dog. *Journal of the American Veterinary Medical Association*, **203** (9), 1296–1299.

36 Peterson, K., Vanadurongvan, K., Burrish, H. *et al.* (1996) Animal rabies – South Dakota, 1995 (Reprinted from *MMWR*, 1996, **45**, 164–166). *JAMA*, **275** (13), 982.

37 Monroe, W.E. (1989) Clinical signs associated with pseudorabies in dogs. *Journal of the American Veterinary Medical Association*, **195** (5), 599–602.

38 O'Neill, E.J., Merrett, D., and Jones, B. (2005) Granulomatous meningoencephalomyelitis in dogs: a review. *Irish Veterinary Journal*, **58** (2), 86–92.

39 Alley, M.R., Jones, B.R., and Johnstone, A.C. (1983) Granulomatous meningoencephalomyelitis of dogs in New Zealand. *New Zealand Veterinary Journal*, **31** (7), 117–119.

40 McKeown, H.M. (2002) Hypothyroidism in a boxer dog. *Canadian Veterinary Journal/Revue Vétérinaire Canadienne*, **43** (7), 553–555.

41 Boothe, H.W., Hobson, H.P., and McDonald, D.E. (1996) Treatment of traumatic separation of the auricular and annular cartilages without ablation: results in five dogs. *Veterinary Surgery*, **25** (5), 376–379.

42 Cizinauskas, S., Lang, J., Maier, R. *et al.* (2001) Paradoxical vestibular disease with trigeminal nerve-sheath tumor in a dog. *Schweizer Archiv für Tierheilkunde*, **143** (8), 419–425.

43 Pumarola, M., Anor, S., Borras, D., and Ferrer, I. (1996) Malignant epithelioid schwannoma affecting the trigeminal nerve of a dog. *Veterinary Pathology*, **33** (4), 434–436.

44 Bagley, R.S., Gavin, P.R., Moore, M.P. *et al.* (1999) Clinical signs associated with brain tumors in dogs: 97 cases (1992–1997). *Journal of the American Veterinary Medical Association*, **215** (6), 818–819.

45 Zaki, F.A. and Nafe, L.A. (1980) Choroid-plexus tumors in the dog. *Journal of the American Veterinary Medical Association*, **176** (4), 328–330.

46 Parent, J.M. (2006) The cat with a head tilt, vestibular ataxia, or nystagmus, in *Problem-Based Feline Medicine* (ed. J. Rand), Saunders Elsevier, Philadelphia, pp. 835–851.

47 Chrisman, C.L. (2006) The neurologic examination. *Clinician's Brief*, January, 11–16.

48 Ingram, E.A., Kale, D.C., and Balfour, R.J. (2013) Hemilaminectomy for thoracolumbar Hansen Type I intervertebral disk disease in ambulatory dogs with or without neurologic deficits: 39 cases (2008–2010). *Veterinary Surgery*, **42** (8), 924–931.

49 Ruddle, T.L., Allen, D.A., Schertel, M.D. *et al.* (2006) Outcome and prognostic factors in nonambulatory Hansen Type I intervertebral disc extrusions: 308 cases. *Veterinary and Comparative Orthopaedics and Traumatology*, **19**(1), 29–34.

50 Bley, T., Lang, J., Jaggy, A. *et al.* (2007) Lumbar spinal 'juxtaarticular' cyst in a Gordon setter. *Journal of Veterinary Medicine. A: Physiology, Pathology, Clinical Medicine*, **54** (9), 494–498.

51 Rohdin, C., Nyman, H.T., Wohlsein, P., and Jaderlund, K.H. (2014) Cervical spinal intradural arachnoid cysts in related, young pugs. *Journal of Small Animal Practice*, **55** (4), 229–234.

52 Webb, A.A. (1999) Intradural spinal arachnoid cyst in a dog. *Canadian Veterinary Journal/Revue Vétérinaire Canadienne*, **40** (8), 588–589.

53 Schueler, R.O., Roush, J.K., and Oyster, R.A. (1993) Spinal ganglioneuroma in a dog. *Journal of the American Veterinary Medical Association*, **203** (4), 539–541.

54 Galan, A., Gamito, A., Carletti, B.E. *et al.* (2014) Uncommon acute neurologic presentation of canine distemper in 4 adult dogs. *Canadian Veterinary Journal/Revue Vétérinaire Canadienne*, **55** (4), 373–378.

55 Raw, M.E., Pearson, G.R., Brown, P.J., and Baumgartner, W. (1992) Canine distemper infection associated with acute nervous signs in dogs. *Veterinary Record*, **130** (14), 291–293.

56 Lane, L.V., Meinkoth, J.H., Brunker, J. *et al.* (2012) Disseminated prototothecosis diagnosed by evaluation of CSF in a dog. *Veterinary Clinical Pathology*, **41** (1), 147–152.

57 Goncalves, R., Carrera, I., Garosi, L. *et al.* (2011) Clinical and topographic magnetic resonance imaging characteristics of suspected thalamic infarcts in 16 dogs. *Veterinary Journal*, **188** (1), 39–43.

58 Cook, J.R. (1998) Fibrocartilaginous embolism. *Veterinary Clinics of North America: Small Animal Practice*, **18** (3), 581–592.

59 Kortz, G.D., Meier, W.A., Higgins, R.J. *et al.* (1997) Neuronal vacuolation and spinocerebellar degeneration in young Rottweiler dogs. *Veterinary Pathology*, **34** (4), 296–302.

60 Cooper, C., Gutierrez-Quintana, R., Penderis, J., and Goncalves, R. (2015) Osseous associated cervical spondylomyelopathy at the C2–C3 articular facet joint in 11 dogs. *Veterinary Record*, **177** (20), 522.

61 Pintus, D., Cancedda, M.G., Macciocu, S. *et al.* (2016) Pathological findings in a Dachshund-cross dog with neuroaxonal dystrophy. *Acta Veterinaria Scandinavica*, **58** (1), 37.

62 Ruddle, T.L., Allen, D.A., Shertel, E.R. *et al.* (2006) Outcome and prognostic factors in non-ambulatory Hansen Type I intervertebral disc extrusions: 300 cases. *Veterinary and Comparative Orthopaedics and Traumatology*, **19** (1), 29–34.

63 Brisson, B.A. (2010) Intervertebral disc disease in dogs. *Veterinary Clinics of North America: Small Animal Practice*, **40** (5), 829.

64 King, A.S. and Smith, R.N. (1955) A comparison of the anatomy of the intervertebral disc in dog and man: with reference to herniation of the nucleus pulposus. *British Veterinary Journal*, **3**, 135–149.

65 Evans, H.E. (ed.) (1993) *Miller's Anatomy of the Dog*, 3rd edn., Saunders Elsevier, Philadelphia.

66 Modic, M.T., Masaryk, T.J., Ross, J.S., and Carter, J.R. (1988) Imaging of degenerative disk disease. *Radiology*, **168** (1), 177–186.

67 Hansen, H.J. (1952) A pathologic–anatomical study on disc degeneration in dog, with special reference to the so-called enchondrosis intervertebralis. *Acta Orthopaedica Scandinavica Supplementum*, **11**, 1–117.

68 Ghosh, P., Taylor, T.K., and Braund, K.G. (1977) The variation of the glycosaminoglycans of the canine intervertebral disc with ageing. I. Chondrodystrophoid breed. *Gerontology*, **23** (2), 87–98.

69 Hansen, H.J. (1959) Comparative views of the pathology of disk degeneration in animals. *Laboratory Investigation*, **8**, 1242–1265.

70 Ghosh, P., Taylor, T.K., and Braund, K.G. (1976) A comparative chemical and histological study of the chondrodystrophoid and nonchondrodystrophoid canine intervertebral disc. *Veterinary Pathology*, **13**, 414–427.

71 Ghosh, P., Taylor, T.K., Braund, K.G., and Larsen, L.H. (1976) The collagenous and non-collagenous protein of the canine intervertebral disc and their variation with age, spinal level and breed. *Gerontology*, **22** (3), 124–134.

72 Ghosh, P., Taylor, T.K., and Braund, K.G. (1977) Variation of the glycosaminoglycans of the intervertebral disc with ageing. II. Non-chondrodystrophoid breed. *Gerontology*, **23** (2), 99–109.

73 Dallman, M.J., Moon, M.L., and Giovannittijensen, A. (1991) Comparison of the width of the intervertebral-disk space and radiographic changes before and after intervertebral-disk fenestration in dogs. *American Journal of Veterinary Research*, **52** (1), 140–145.

74 Jensen, V.F. (2001) Asymptomatic radiographic disappearance of calcified intervertebral disc material in the Dachshund. *Veterinary Radiology & Ultrasound*, **42** (2), 141–148.

75 Jensen, V.F. and Arnbjerg, J. (2001) Development of intervertebral disk calcification in the Dachshund: a prospective longitudinal radiographic study. *Journal of the American Animal Hospital Association*, **37** (3), 274–282.

76 Jensen, V.F., Beck, S., Christensen, K.A., and Arnbjerg, J. (2008) Quantification of the association between intervertebral disk calcification and disk herniation in Dachshunds. *Journal of the American Veterinary Medical Association*, **233** (7), 1090–1095.

77 Stigen, O. (1991) Calcification of intervertebral discs in the Dachshund. A radiographic study of 327 young dogs. *Acta Veterinaria Scandinavica*, **32**, 197–203.

78 Goggin, J.E., Li, A.S., and Franti, C.E. (1970) Canine intervertebral disk disease: characterization by age, sex, breed, and anatomic site of involvement. *American Journal of Veterinary Research*, **31** (9), 1687–1692.

79 Gage, E.D. (1975) Incidence of clinical disc disease in the dog. *Journal of the American Animal Hospital Association*, **11**, 135–138.

80 Ball, M.U., Mcguire, J.A., Swaim, S.F., and Hoerlein, B.F. (1982) Patterns of occurrence of disk disease among registered Dachshunds. *Journal of the American Veterinary Medical Association*, **180** (5), 519–522.

81 Priester, W.A. (1976) Canine intervertebral disc disease – occurrence by age, breed, and sex among 8,117 cases. *Theriogenology*, **6**, 293–303.

82 Brown, N.O., Helphrey, M.L., and Prata, R.G. (1977) Thoracolumbar disk disease in the dog: a retrospective analysis of 187 cases. *Journal of the American Animal Hospital Association*, **13**, 665–672.

83 Besalti, O., Pekcan, Z., Sirin, Y.S., and Erbas, G. (2006) Magnetic resonance imaging findings in dogs with thoracolumbar intervertebral disk disease: 69 cases (1997–2005). *Journal of the American Veterinary Medical Association*, **228** (6), 902–908.

84 Levine, J.M., Levine, G.J., Kerwin, S.C. *et al.* (2006) Association between various physical factors and acute thoracolumbar intervertebral disk extrusion or protrusion in Dachshunds. *Journal of the American Veterinary Medical Association*, **229** (3), 370–375.

85 Cudia, S.P. and Duval, J.M. (1997) Thoracolumbar intervertebral disk disease in large, nonchondrodystrophic dogs: a retrospective study. *Journal of the American Animal Hospital Association*, **33** (5), 456–460.

86 Macias, C., McKee, W.M., May, C., and Innes, J.F. (2002) Thoracolumbar disc disease in large dogs: a study of 99 cases. *Journal of Small Animal Practice*, **43** (10), 439–446.

87 Cherrone, K.L., Dewey, C.W., Coates, J.R., and Bergman, R.L. (2004) A retrospective comparison of cervical intervertebral disk disease in nonchondrodystrophic large dogs versus small dogs. *Journal of the American Animal Hospital Association*, **40** (4), 316–320.

88 Hansen, H.J. (1951) A pathologic–anatomical interpretation of disc degeneration in dogs. *Acta Orthopaedica Scandinavica Supplementum*, **20**, 280–293.

89 Denny, H.R. (1978) The surgical management of cervical disc protrusions in the dog: a review of 40 cases. *Journal of Small Animal Practice*, **19**, 251–257.

90 Ryan, T.M., Platt, S.R., Llabres-Diaz, F.J. *et al.* (2008) Detection of spinal cord compression in dogs with cervical intervertebral disc disease by magnetic resonance imaging. *Veterinary Record*, **163** (1), 11–15.

91 Seim, H.B. and Prata, R.G. (1982) Ventral decompression for the treatment of cervical disk disease in the dog – a review of 54 cases. *Journal of the American Animal Hospital Association*, **18** (2), 233–240.

92 Morgan, P.W., Parent, J., and Holmberg, D.L. (1993) Cervical pain secondary to intervertebral disc disease in dogs – radiographic findings and surgical implications. *Progress in Veterinary Neurology*, **4** (3), 76–80.

93 Gill, P.J., Lippincott, C.L., and Anderson, S.M. (1996) Dorsal laminectomy in the treatment of cervical intervertebral disk disease in small dogs: a retrospective study of 30 cases. *Journal of the American Animal Hospital Association*, **32** (1), 77–80.

94 Hillman, R.B., Kengeri, S.S., and Waters, D.J. (2009) Reevaluation of predictive factors for complete recovery in dogs with nonambulatory tetraparesis secondary to cervical disk herniation. *Journal of the American Animal Hospital Association*, **45** (4), 155–163.

95 Hoerlein, B.F. (1953) Intervertebral disc protrusions in the dog. Incidence and pathological lesions. *American Journal of Veterinary Research*, **14**, 260–269.

96 Knecht, C.D. (1972) Results of surgical treatment for thoracolumbar disc protrusion. *Journal of Small Animal Practice*, **13**, 449–453.

97 Levine, J.M., Fosgate, A.V., and Rushing, C.R. (2009) Magnetic resonance imaging in dogs with neurological impairment due to acute thoracic and lumbar intervertebral disc herniation. *Journal of Veterinary Internal Medicine*, **23**, 1220–1226.

98 Brisson, B.A., Moffatt, S.L., Swayne, S.L., and Parent, J.M. (2004) Recurrence of thoracolumbar intervertebral disk extrusion in chondrodystrophic dogs after surgical decompression with or without prophylactic fenestration: 265 cases (1995–1999). *Journal of the American Veterinary Medical Association*, **224** (11), 1808–1814.

99 Tanaka, H., Nakayama, M., and Takase, K. (2004) Usefulness of myelography with multiple views in diagnosis of circumferential location of disc material in dogs with thoracolumber intervertebral disc herniation. *Journal of Veterinary Medical Science*, **66** (7), 827–833.

100 McKee, W.M. (1992) A comparison of hemilaminectomy (with concomitant disc fenestration) and dorsal laminectomy for the treatment of thoracolumbar disc protrusion in dogs. *Veterinary Record*, **130** (14), 296–300.

101 Gambardella, P.C. (1980) Dorsal decompressive laminectomy for treatment of thoracolumbar disc disease in dogs: a retrospective study of 98 cases. *Veterinary Surgery*, **9**, 24–26.

102 Scott, H.W. (1997) Hemilaminectomy for the treatment of thoracolumbar disc disease in the dog: a

follow-up study of 40 cases. *Journal of Small Animal Practice*, **38** (11), 488–494.

103 Parent, J. (2010) Clinical approach and lesion localization in patients with spinal diseases. *Veterinary Clinics of North America: Small Animal Practice*, **40** (5), 733.

104 de Lahunta, A. and Glass, E. (2009) The neurologic examination, in *Veterinary Neuroanatomy and Clinical Neurology*, 4th edn. (eds. A. de Lahunta, E. Glass, and M. Kent), Saunders Elsevier, St. Louis, pp. 487–501.

105 Peterson, K.L., Lee, J.A., and Hovda, L.R. (2011) Phenylpropanolamine toxicosis in dogs: 170 cases (2004–2009). *Journal of the American Veterinary Medical Association*, **239** (11), 1463–1469.

106 Shell, L.G., Berezowski, J., Rishniw, M. *et al.* (2015) Clinical and breed characteristics of idiopathic head tremor syndrome in 291 dogs: a retrospective study. *Veterinary Medicine International*, **2015**, 165463.

107 Wolf, M., Bruehschwein, A., Sauter-Louis, C. *et al.* (2011) An inherited episodic head tremor syndrome in Doberman pinscher dogs. *Movement Disorders*, **26** (13), 2381–2386.

108 Guevar, J., De Decker, S., Van Ham, L.M. *et al.* (2014) Idiopathic head tremor in English bulldogs. *Movement Disorders*, **29** (2), 191–194.

109 de Lahunta, A., Glass, E.N., and Kent, M. (2006) Classifying involuntary muscle contractions. *Compendium: Continuing Education for the Practicing Veterinarian*, **28** (7), 516.

110 Lim, J.H., Kim, D.Y., Yoon, J.H. *et al.* (2008) Cerebellar vermian hypoplasia in a Cocker Spaniel. *Journal of Veterinary Science*, **9** (2), 215–217.

111 Harari, J., Miller, D., Padgett, G.A., and Grace, J. (1983) Cerebellar agenesis in two canine littermates. *Journal of the American Veterinary Medical Association*, **182** (6), 622–623.

112 Schatzberg, S.J., Haley, N.J., Barr, S.C. *et al.* (2003) Polymerase chain reaction (PCR) amplification of parvoviral DNA from the brains of dogs and cats with cerebellar hypoplasia. *Journal of Veterinary Internal Medicine*, **17** (4), 538–544.

113 Nibe, K., Kita, C., Morozumi, M. *et al.* (2007) Clinicopathological features of canine neuroaxonal dystrophy and cerebellar cortical abiotrophy in Papillon and Papillon-related dogs. *Journal of Veterinary Medical Science*, **69** (10), 1047–1052.

114 Olby, N., Blot, S., Thibaud, J.L. *et al.* (2004) Cerebellar cortical degeneration in adult American Staffordshire Terriers. *Journal of Veterinary Internal Medicine*, **18** (2), 201–208.

115 Jolly, R.D., Ehrlich, P.C., Franklin, R.J. *et al.* (2001) Histological diagnosis of mucopolysaccharidosis IIIA in a wire-haired Dachshund. *Veterinary Record*, **148** (18), 564–567.

116 Yamato, O., Ochiai, K., Masuoka, Y. *et al.* (2000) GM1 gangliosidosis in Shiba dogs. *Veterinary Record*, **146** (17), 493–496.

117 Cheeseman, M.T., Kelly, D.F., and Horsfall, K.L. (1995) Multisystemic inflammatory disease in a Borzoi dog. *Journal of Small Animal Practice*, **36** (1), 22–24.

118 Schubert, T., Clemmons, R., Miles, S., and Draper, W. (2013) The use of botulinum toxin for the treatment of generalized myoclonus in a dog. *Journal of the American Animal Hospital Association*, **49** (2), 122–127.

119 Koutinas, A.F., Polizopoulou, Z.S., Baumgaertner, W. *et al.* (2002) Relation of clinical signs to pathological changes in 19 cases of canine distemper encephalomyelitis. *Journal of Comparative Pathology*, **126** (1), 47–56.

120 Ferreira, J.P., Dzikit, T.B., Zeiler, G.E. *et al.* (2015) Anaesthetic induction and recovery characteristics of a diazepam–ketamine combination compared with propofol in dogs. *Journal of the South African Veterinary Association*, **86** (1), 1258.

121 Cattai, A., Rabozzi, R., Natale, V., and Franci, P. (2015) The incidence of spontaneous movements (myoclonus) in dogs undergoing total intravenous anaesthesia with propofol. *Veterinary Anaesthesia and Analgesia*, **42** (1), 93–98.

122 Iff, I., Valeskini, K., and Mosing, M. (2012) Severe pruritus and myoclonus following intrathecal morphine administration in a dog. *Canadian Veterinary Journal/Revue Vétérinaire Canadienne*, **53** (9), 983–986.

123 da Cunha, A.F., Carter, J.E., Grafinger, M. *et al.* (2007) Intrathecal morphine overdose in a dog. *Journal of the American Veterinary Medical Association*, **230** (11), 1665–1668.

124 Jennings, D.P. and Bailey, J.G. (2004) Spinal control of posture and movement, in *Dukes' Physiology of Domestic Animals*, 12th edn. (ed. W.O. Reece), Comstock, Ithaca, NY, pp. 892–903.

125 Fingeroth, J.M. and Thomas, W.B. (eds.) (2015) *Advances in Intervertebral Disc Disease in Dogs and Cats*, Wiley-Blackwell, Ames, IA.

126 Levine, J.M., Hillman, R.B., Erb, H.N., and de Lahunta, A. (2002) The influence of age on patellar reflex response in the dog. *Journal of Veterinary Internal Medicine*, **16** (3), 244–246.

127 Hoskins, J.D. (1990) Clinical evaluation of the kitten – from birth to 8 weeks of age. *Compendium: Continuing Education for the Practicing Veterinarian*, **12** (9), 1215.

128 Pastorello, A., Constantino-Casas, F., and Archer, J. (2010) Choroid plexus carcinoma cells in the cerebrospinal fluid of a Staffordshire Bull Terrier. *Veterinary Clinical Pathology*, **39** (4), 505–510.

129 Webb, A.A., Cullen, C.L., Rose, P. *et al.* (2005) Intracranial meningioma causing internal ophthalmoparesis in a dog. *Veterinary Ophthalmology*, **8** (6), 421–425.

130 Garosi, L., McConnell, J.F., Platt, S.R. *et al.* (2006) Clinical and topographic magnetic resonance characteristics of suspected brain infarction in 40 dogs. *Journal of Veterinary Internal Medicine*, **20** (2), 311–321.

131 Holland, C.T. (2008) Asymmetrical focal neurological deficits in dogs and cats with naturally occurring tick paralysis (*Ixodes holocyclus*): 27 cases (1999–2006). *Australian Veterinary Journal*, **86** (10), 377–384.

132 Goodman, R.A., Hawkins, E.C., Olby, N.J. *et al.* (2003) Molecular identification of *Ehrlichia ewingii* infection in dogs: 15 cases (1997–2001). *Journal of the American Veterinary Medical Association*, **222** (8), 1102–1107.

133 Hansen, P. and Clerc, B. (2002) Anisocoria in the dog provoked by a toxic contact with an ornamental plant: *Datura stramonium*. *Veterinary Ophthalmology*, **5** (4), 277–279.

134 Yohn, S.E., Morrison, W.B., and Sharp, P.E. (1992) Bromide toxicosis (bromism) in a dog treated with potassium bromide for refractory seizures. *Journal of the American Veterinary Medical Association*, **201** (3), 468–470.

135 Gerding, P.A., Brightman, A.H., and Brogdon, J.D. (1986) Pupillotonia in a dog. *Journal of the American Veterinary Medical Association*, **189** (11), 1477.

136 Sarchahi, A.A. (2007) Pupillotonia in a Spitz dog: a case report. *Iranian Journal of Veterinary Research*, **8** (4), 370–373.

137 Kim, J., Heo, J., Ji, D., and Kim, M.S. (2015) Quantitative assessment of pupillary light reflex in normal and anesthetized dogs: a preliminary study. *Journal of Veterinary Medical Science*, **77** (4), 475–478.

138 Whiting, R.E.H., Yao, G., Narfstrom, K. *et al.* (2013) Quantitative assessment of the canine pupillary light reflex. *Investigative Ophthalmology and Visual Science*, **54** (8), 5432–5440.

139 Rijnberk, A. and van Sluijs, F.S. (eds.) (2009) *Medical History and Physical Examination in Companion Animals*, Saunders Elsevier, St. Louis.

140 de Lahunta, A., Glass, E., and Kent, M. (eds.) (2009) *Veterinary Neuroanatomy and Clinical Neurology*, 4th edn., Saunders Elsevier, St. Louis.

141 Bagley, R.S. (2006) The cat with anisocoria or abnormally dilated or constricted pupils, in *Problem-Based Feline Medicine* (ed. J. Rand), Saunders Elsevier, Philadelphia, pp. 870–889.

142 Simpson, K.M., Williams, D.L., and Cherubini, G.B. (2015) Neuropharmacological lesion localization in idiopathic Horner's syndrome in Golden Retrievers and dogs of other breeds. *Veterinary Ophthalmology*, **18** (1), 1–5.

143 Boydell, P. (1995) Idiopathic Horner's syndrome in the Golden Retriever. *Journal of Small Animal Practice*, **36** (9), 382–384.

144 van Hagen, M.A., Kwakernaak, C.M., Boeve, M.H., and Stades, F.C. (1999) Horner's syndrome in the dog: a retrospective study. *Tijdschrift voor Diergeneeskunde*, **124** (20), 600–602 (in Dutch).

145 Morgan, R.V. and Zanotti, S.W. (1989) Horner's syndrome in dogs and cats: 49 cases (1980–1986). *Journal of the American Veterinary Medical Association*, **194** (8), 1096–1099.

146 Kern, T.J., Aromando, M.C., and Erb, H.N. (1989) Horner's syndrome in dogs and cats: 100 cases (1975–1985). *Journal of the American Veterinary Medical Association*, **195** (3), 369–373.

147 Maggs, D.J., Miller, P.E., and Ofri, R. (2013) *Slatter's Fundamentals of Veterinary Ophthalmology*, 5th edn., Saunders Elsevier, St. Louis.

148 Gunton, K.B., Wasserman, B.N., and DeBenedictis, C. (2015) Strabismus. *Primary Care*, **42** (3), 393–407.

149 Campos, E.C. (2008) Why do the eyes cross? A review and discussion of the nature and origin of essential infantile esotropia, microstrabismus, accommodative esotropia, and acute comitant esotropia. *Journal of AAPOS*, **12** (4), 326–331.

150 Ketring, K.L. and Glaze, M.B. (2012) *Atlas of Feline Ophthalmology*, 2nd edn., Wiley-Blackwell, Ames, IA.

151 Rengstorff, R.H. (1976) Strabismus measurements in the Siamese cat. *American Journal of Optometry and Physiological Optics*, **53** (10), 643–646.

152 Blake, R. and Crawford, M.L. (1974) Development of strabismus in Siamese cats. *Brain Research*, **77** (3), 492–496.

153 Hyde, J.E. (1962) Cross-eyedness: a study in Siamese cats. *American Journal of Ophthalmology*, **53**, 70–75.

154 Betbeze, C. (2015) Management of orbital diseases. *Topics in Companion Animal Medicine*, **30** (3), 107–117.

155 van der Woerdt, A. (2008) Orbital inflammatory disease and pseudotumor in dogs and cats. *Veterinary Clinics of North America: Small Animal Practice*, **38** (2), 389–401, vii–viii.

156 Hindley, K.E., Billson, F.M., Piripi, S. *et al.* (2016) Primary isolated osteoma cutis causing eyelid deformation and strabismus in a dog. *Veterinary Ophthalmology*, **19** (5), 439–443.

157 de Lahunta, A. and Glass, E. (2009) General sensory systems: general proprioception and general somatic afferent, in *Veterinary Neuroanatomy and Clinical Neurology*, 4th edn. (eds. A. de Lahunta, E. Glass, and M. Kent), Saunders Elsevier, St. Louis, pp. 221–242.

158 Epstein, M., Rodan, I., Griffenhagen, G. *et al.* (2015) 2015 AAHA/AAFP Pain Management Guidelines for Dogs and Cats. *Journal of the American Animal Hospital Association*, **51** (2), 67–84.

159 Balakrishnan, A. and Benasutti, E. (2012) Pain assessment in dogs and cats. *Today's Veterinary Practice*, March/April, 68–74.

160 Mathews, K., Kronen, P.W., Lascelles, D. *et al.* (2014) Guidelines for recognition, assessment and treatment of pain: WSAVA Global Pain Council members and co-authors of this document. *Journal of Small Animal Practice*, **55** (6), E10–E68.

161 AAHA/AAFP Pain Management Guidelines Task Force Members, Hellyer, P., Rodan, I. *et al.* (2007) AAHA/AAFP Pain Management Guidelines for Dogs and Cats. *Journal of Feline Medicine and Surgery*, **9** (6), 466–480.

162 Hansen, B.D. (2003) Assessment of pain in dogs: veterinary clinical studies. *ILAR Journal*, **44** (3), 197–205.

163 Firth, A.M. and Haldane, S.L. (1999) Development of a scale to evaluate postoperative pain in dogs. *Journal of the American Veterinary Medical Association*, **214** (5), 651–659.

164 Hellyer, P.W., Uhrig, S.R., and Robinson, S.G. (2006) *Feline Pain*, http://csu-cvmbs.colostate.edu/Documents/anesthesia-pain-management-pain-score-feline.pdf (accessed 30 May 2016).

165 Hellyer, P.W., Uhrig, S.R., and Robinson, S.G. (2006) *Canine Pain*, http://csu-cvmbs.colostate.edu/Documents/anesthesia-pain-management-pain-score-canine.pdf (accessed 30 May 2016).

166 Brondani, J.T., Luna, S.P., and Padovani, C.R. (2011) Refinement and initial validation of a multidimensional composite scale for use in assessing acute postoperative pain in cats. *American Journal of Veterinary Research*, **72** (2), 174–183.

Index

Performing the Small Animal Physical Examination, First Edition. Ryane E. Englar.
© 2017 John Wiley & Sons, Inc. Published 2017 by John Wiley & Sons, Inc.